PHARMACOGENETICS AND INDIVIDUALIZED THERAPY

PHARMACOGENETICS AND INDIVIDUALIZED THERAPY

Edited by

Anke-Hilse Maitland-van der Zee
Utrecht University
Utrecht, The Netherlands

Ann K. Daly
Newcastle University,
Newcastle upon Tyne, UK

WILEY
A JOHN WILEY & SONS, INC., PUBLICATION

Published by John Wiley & Sons, Inc., Hoboken, New Jersey
Published simultaneously in Canada

Library of Congress Cataloging-in-Publication Data:

Pharmacogenetics and individualized therapy / edited by Anke-Hilse Mailand-van der Zee, Ann K. Daly.
p. ; cm.
Includes bibliographical references and index.
ISBN 978-0-470-43354-6 (cloth)
1. Pharmacogenetics. I. Maitland-van der Zee, Anke-Hilse. II. Daly, Ann K.
[DNLM: 1. Pharmacogenetics–methods. 2. Drug Therapy–methods. 3. Individualized Medicine–methods. QV 38]
RM301.3.G45P396 2011
615′.19–dc23 2011015209

10 9 8 7 6 5 4 3 2 1

CONTENTS

PREFACE

Pharmacogenetics and individualized therapy is a rapidly evolving field that is likely to have important consequences for clinical practice in the coming decades. This book is aimed at a general audience including advanced undergraduate and graduate students in medicine, pharmacy, pharmacology, and other related disciplines as well as researchers based in either academia or the pharmaceutical industry. Some familiarity with basic pharmacology and genetics is assumed.

This book is organized in five parts. Part I describes the basic principles of pharmacogenetics including factors relevant to drug disposition (phase I and phase II metabolizing enzymes, and drug transporters) and the role of pharmacodynamics (drug targets).

Part II includes discussions of state-of-the art pharmacogenetics in many important therapeutic areas [cardiovascular, psychiatry, cancer, asthma/chronic obstructive pulmonary disease (COPD), adverse drug reactions, transplantation, inflammatory bowel disease, pain medication].

Part III describes ethical and related issues in implementing pharmacogenetics into clinical practice.

In Part IV important developments in the techology supporting pharmacogenetics research are discussed. More recent developments in genotyping techniques provide opportunities for genotyping over 1 million single-nucleotide polymorphisms in many patients at affordable prices. Further developments in analysis techniques provide investigators with the opportunity to consider gene–environment and epistatic interactions as well as the possibility of whole-genome sequencing.

Part V discusses the impact of pharmacogenetics in the pharmaceutical industry and also the role that pharmacogenetics currently plays in the registration process.

It has been a privilege to interact with the distinguished expert authors who have provided chapters for this book, and we would like to express our sincere gratitude to them for their excellent contributions. We also wish to thank Lisa Gilhuijs-Pederson, PhD for assistance in editing this book.

Ann K. Daly, PhD

Anke-Hilse Maitland-van der Zee, PharmD PhD

CONTRIBUTORS

Katherine J. Aitchison, Institute of Psychiatry, King's College London, London, UK

Martin Armstrong, Clinical Development and Medical Affairs, Shire AG, Geneva, Switzerland

Maria Arranz, Institute of Psychiatry, King's College London, London, UK

Anthonius de Boer, Faculty of Science, Utrecht Institute for Pharmaceutical Sciences (UIPS), Division of Pharmacoepidemiology and Pharmacotherapy, Utrecht University, Utrecht, The Netherlands

Daniel K. Burns, Deane Drug Discovery Institute, Duke University, Durham, North Carolina, USA

Angel Carracedo, Galician Foundation of Genomic Medicine (SERGAS), University of Santiago de Compostela, Santiago de Compostela, Spain

Ingolf Cascorbi, Institute of Experimental and Clinical Pharmacology, University Hospital Schleswig–Holstein, Kiel, Germany

Martina Cornel, Department of Human Genetics/EMGO Institute for Health Care and Research, VU University Medical Center, Amsterdam, The Netherlands and Center for Society and Genomics, Radboud University, Nijmegen, The Netherlands

Sarah Curran, Institute of Psychiatry, King's College London, London, UK

Ann K. Daly, Institute of Cellular Medicine, Newcastle University Medical School, Newcastle upon Tyne, UK

Vita Dolžan, Institute of Biochemistry, Faculty of Medicine, University of Ljubljana, Ljubljana, Slovenia

Markus Grube, Department of Pharmacology, Ernst Moritz Arndt-University of Greifswald, Greifswald, Germany

Shiew-Mei Huang, Office of Clinical Pharmacology, Center for Drug Evaluation and Research, Food and Drug Administration, Silver Spring, Maryland, USA

Susanne Karner, Dr. Margarete Fischer-Bosch Institute of Clinical Pharmacology, Stuttgart, Germany

Myong-Jin Kim, Office of Clinical Pharmacology, Center for Drug Evaluation and Research, Food and Drug Administration, Silver Spring, Maryland, USA

Olaf H. Klungel, Faculty of Science, Utrecht Institute of Pharmaceutical Sciences (UIPS), Division of Pharmacoepidemiology and Pharmacotherapy, Utrecht University, Utrecht, The Netherlands

Gerard H. Koppelman, Pediatric Pulmonology and Pediatric Allergology, Beatrix Childrens Hospital, University Medical Center Groningen, Groningen, The Netherlands

Ellen S. Koster, Faculty of Science, Utrecht Institute of Pharmaceutical Sciences (UIPS), Division of Pharmacoepidemiology and Pharmacotherapy, Utrecht University, Utrecht, The Netherlands

Heyo K. Kroemer, Department of Pharmacology, Ernst Moritz Arndt-University of Greifswald, Greifswald, Germany

Lawrence J. Lesko, Office of Clinical Pharmacology, Center for Drug Evaluation and Research, Food and Drug Administration, Silver Spring, Maryland, USA

Jörn Lötsch, Pharmazentrum Frankfurt and Department of Clinical Pharmacology, Johann Wolfgang Goethe-University Hospital, Frankfurt, Germany

Anke-Hilse Maitland-van der Zee, Faculty of Science, Utrecht Institute of Pharmaceutical Sciences (UIPS), Division of Pharmacoepidemiology and Pharmacotherapy, Utrecht University, Utrecht, The Netherlands

Sharon Marsh, Faculty of Pharmacy and Pharmaceutical Sciences, University of Alberta, Edmonton, Alberta, Canada

Henriette E. Meyer zu Schwabedissen, Department of Pharmacology, Ernst Moritz Arndt-University of Greifswald, Greifswald, Germany

Alison A. Motsinger-Reif, Bioinformatics Research Center, Department of Statistics, North Carolina State University, Raleigh, North Carolina, USA

Ruth I. Ohlsen, Institute of Psychiatry, King's College London, London, UK

Bas J. M. Peters, Faculty of Science, Utrecht Institute for Pharmaceutical Sciences (UIPS), Division of Pharmacoepidemiology and Pharmacotherapy, Utrecht University, Utrecht, The Netherlands

Toine Pieters, Faculty of Science, Utrecht Institute for Pharmaceutical Sciences (UIPS), Division of Pharmacoepidemiology and Pharmacotherapy, Utrecht University, Utrecht, The Netherlands; and Department of Medical Humanities, VU University Medical Center, Amsterdam, The Netherlands

Munir Pirmohamed, Institute of Translational Medicine, University of Liverpool, Liverpool, UK

Jan A. M. Raaijmakers, Faculty of Science, Utrecht Institute of Pharmaceutical Sciences (UIPS), Division of Pharmacoepidemiology and Pharmacotherapy, Utrecht University, Utrecht, The Netherlands

Elke Schaeffeler, Dr. Margarete Fischer-Bosch Institute of Clinical Pharmacology, Stuttgart, Germany

Tom Schalekamp, Faculty of Science, Utrecht Institute for Pharmaceutical Sciences (UIPS), Division of Pharmacoepidemiology and Pharmacotherapy, Utrecht University, Utrecht, The Netherlands

Matthias Schwab, Dr. Margarete Fischer-Bosch Institute of Clinical Pharmacology, Stuttgart, Germany and Institute of Experimental and Clinical Pharmacology and Toxicology, University Hospital, Tübingen, Germany

Beatriz Sobrino, Galician Foundation of Genomic Medicine (SERGAS), University of Santiago de Compostela, Santiago de Compostela, Spain

Scott S. Sundseth, Cabernet Pharmaceuticals, Durham, North Carolina, USA

Alexander Teml, Dr. Margarete Fischer-Bosch Institute of Clinical Pharmacology, Stuttgart, Germany

Evangelia M. Tsapakis, Institute of Psychiatry, King's College London, London, UK

Susanne Vijverberg, Faculty of Science, Utrecht Institute for Pharmaceutical Sciences (UIPS), Division of Pharmacoepidemiology and Pharmacotherapy, Utrecht University, Utrecht, The Netherlands

Nora S. Vyas, Institute of Psychiatry, King's College London, London, UK

Issam Zineh, Office of Clinical Pharmacology, Center for Drug Evaluation and Research, Food and Drug Administration, Silver Spring, Maryland, USA

CHAPTER 1

Pharmacogenetics: A Historical Perspective

ANN K. DALY

Newcastle University, Newcastle upon Tyne, UK

1.1 INTRODUCTION

It has been known for thousands of years that some individuals show toxic responses following consumption of fava beans, especially in countries bordering the Mediterranean. This is probably the earliest pharmacogenetic observation, although the biological basis for this has been established only quite recently (see Section 1.2). The foundation for much of modern pharmacogenetics came from experiments on chemical metabolism during the 19th century. These studies included the establishment that benzoic acid undergoes conjugation with glycine *in vivo* in both humans and animals, that benzene is oxidized to phenol in both dogs and humans and that some compounds can undergo conjugation with acetate (for a review, see Ref. 1).

1.2 EARLY PHARMACOGENETICS STUDIES (FROM 1900 TO 1970)

The development of genetics and Mendelian inheritance together with observations by Archibald Garrod on the possibility of variation in chemical metabolism in the early 20th century has been well reviewed elsewhere see [2]. Probably the first direct pharmacogenetic study was reported in 1932 when Synder's study on the ability to taste phenylthiocarbamide within families showed that this trait was genetically determined [3]. The gene responsible for this variation and common genetic polymorphisms have only recently been identified (for a perspective, see Ref. 4).

Pharmacogenetics and Individualized Therapy, First Edition.
Edited by Anke-Hilse Maitland-van der Zee and Ann K. Daly.

Although not a prescribed drug, phenylthiocarbamide shows homology to drugs such as propylthiouracil.

The initial drug-specific pharmacogenetics observations appeared in the literature during the 1950s. These were concerned with three widely used drugs at that time, that are all still used today: isoniazid, primaquine, and succinylcholine. The earliest observation concerned primaquine, which was found by Alf Alving to be associated with acute hemolysis in a small number of individuals [5]. Subsequent work by Alving and colleagues found that this toxicity was due to absence of the enzyme glucose-6-phosphate dehydrogenase in red blood cells of affected individuals [6]. The molecular genetic basis of this deficiency was later established by Ernest Beutler and colleagues in 1988 [7].

Isoniazid was first used against tuberculosis in the early 1950s, although it had been developed originally a number of years previously as an antidepressant. As reviewed recently, its use in tuberculosis patients represented an important advance in treatment of this disease [8]. Variation between individuals in urinary excretion profiles was described by Hettie Hughes [9], who soon afterwards also found an association between the metabolic profile and the incidence of a common adverse reaction, peripheral neuritis, with those showing slow conversion of the parent drug to acetylisoniazid more susceptible [10]. Further studies by several different workers, particularly Mitchell and Bell [11], Harris [12], and David Price Evans [13], led to the conclusion that isoniazid acetylation was subject to a genetic polymorphism and that some individuals ($\sim$10% of East Asians but 50% of Europeans) were slow acetylators. Slow acetylation was shown to be a recessive trait. As summarized in Section 1.4, the biochemical and genetic basis of slow acetylation is now well understood.

Also during the 1950s, a rare adverse response to the muscle relaxant succinylcholine was found to be due to an inherited deficiency in the enzyme cholinesterase [14]. Succinylcholine is used as a muscle relaxant during surgery, and those with the deficiency show prolonged paralysis (succinylcholine apnea). This observation was then further developed by Werner Kalow, who showed that the deficiency is inherited as an autosomal recessive trait and devised a biochemical test to screen for the deficiency, as he described in a description of his early work [15]. The gene encoding this enzyme, which is now usually referred to as *butyrylcholinesterase*, has been well studied, and a number of different mutations responsible for the deficiency have been identified. However, the original biochemical test is still the preferred method for identifying those affected by succinylcholine apnea due to the rarity of both the problem and the number of different mutations.

While these initial studies showing the clear role for genetics in determining adverse responses to primaquine, isoniazid, and succinylcholine were in progress, the general importance of the area was increasingly recognized. Arno Motulsky published a key review on the relationship between biochemical genetics and drug reactions that highlighted the adverse reactions to primaquine and succinylcholine in 1957 [16]. The term *pharmacogenetics* was first used in 1959 by Friedrich Vogel in an article on human genetics written in German [17] and was soon adopted by others working in the field.

1.3 PHARMACOGENETICS OF DRUG OXIDATION

As described in Section 1.1, studies in the 19th century had demonstrated oxidation of benzene to phenol in vivo [1]. Pioneering studies on drug metabolism, especially those in the laboratories of the Millers and of Brodie and Gillette during the 1950s, showed that many drugs undergo oxidative metabolism in the presence of NADPH and molecular oxygen in liver microsomes [18,19]. In 1962, Omura and Sato described cytochrome P450 from a rat liver microsome preparation as a hemoprotein that showed a peak at 450 nm in the presence of carbon monoxide and dithionite [20]. Shortly afterwards Ron Estabrook, David Cooper, and Otto Rosenthal showed that cytochrome P450 had steroid hydroxylase activity [21], and further studies confirmed its role in the metabolism of drugs such as codeine, aminopyrene, and acetanilide [22]. At this time, it was still assumed that cytochrome P450 was a single enzyme, but evidence for multiple forms emerged in the late 1960s [23,24] with purification of a range of rat and rabbit enzymes achieved during the 1970s [25,26].

Independent metabolism studies on two newly developed drugs sparteine and debrisoquine in Germany by Michel Eichelbaum and in the United Kingdom by Robert Smith in the mid 1970s resulted in findings indicating that some individuals were unable to oxidize these drugs, although the majority of individuals showed normal metabolism [27,28]. These studies estimated that 10% of Europeans showed absence of activity, and the term *poor metabolizer* was first used. At this time, the enzymes responsible for this absence of activity were not known, but further studies confirmed that the deficiency in metabolism of both drugs cosegregated [29] and that the trait was inherited recessively [30]. It became clear that a number of different drugs, including tricyclic antidepressants, were also metabolized by this enzyme [31]. Studies on human liver microsomes confirmed that the enzyme responsible was a cytochrome P450 [32,33], and this enzyme was then purified to homogeneity [34]. The availability of antibodies to the purified protein facilitated the cloning of the relevant cDNA by Frank Gonzalez and colleagues, who initially termed the gene CYPIID1 [35]. On the basis of emerging data for cytochrome P450 genes in humans and other animal species, it was decided subsequently that the gene encoding the debrisoquine/sparteine hydroxylase should be termed CYP2D6. Studies on human genomic DNA led to the identification of several polymorphisms in CYP2D6 associated with the poor metabolizer phenotype, including the most common splice site variant, a large deletion, and a small deletion [36–40]. A major additional contribution to the field was made in 1993 by Johansson, Ingelman-Sundberg, and colleagues, who described the phenomenon of ultrarapid metabolizers with one or more additional copies of CYP2D6 present [41]. These ultrarapid metabolizers had been previously identified on the basis of poor response to tricyclic antidepressants, and this was one of the first accounts of copy number variation in the human genome. Agreement regarding the current nomenclature for variant alleles in CYP2D6 and other cytochromes P450 was reached in 1996 [42].

In an approach similar to that used in the discovery of the CYP2D6 polymorphism, Kupfer and Preisig found that some individuals showed absence of metabolism of the anticonvulsant *S*-mephenytoin [43]. It was demonstrated that *S*-mephenytoin metabolism did not cosegregate with that of debrisoquine and sparteine, as this polymorphism was due to a separate gene defect. Identification of the gene responsible for *S*-mephenytoin hydroxylase proved difficult initially, probably because the relevant enzyme was expressed at a low level in the liver. The gene, now termed CYP2C19, was cloned by Goldstein and Meyer and colleagues in 1994, and the two most common polymorphisms associated with absence of *S*-mephenytoin hydroxylase activity were identified [44,45].

A number of other cytochrome P450 genes are now known to be subject to functionally significant polymorphisms. In the case of one of these, CYP2C9, which metabolizes a range of drugs, including warfarin, tolbutamide, and nonsteroidal antiinflammatory drugs, some evidence for the existence of a polymorphism appeared in 1979 when a trimodal distribution in the metabolism of tolbutamide was reported [46]. Subsequently, it was shown that tolbutamide metabolism was distinct from debrisoquine metabolism [47]. The enzyme involved was purified and cloned and later named CYP2C9 [48,49]. Analysis of CYP2C9 cDNA sequences provided evidence for the presence of coding region polymorphisms resulting in amino acid substitutions, and expression studies suggested these were functionally significant [48,50,51]. Genotyping of patients undergoing warfarin treatment confirmed the functional importance of the two most common coding region CYP2C9 polymorphisms [52–54].

Using a similar approach involving comparison of cloned cDNA sequences, evidence for a nonsynonymous polymorphism in CYP2A6 was obtained [55]. Following expression studies and population screening, it was demonstrated that this polymorphism was associated with a rare absence of CYP2A6 activity, but additional polymorphisms (including a large deletion) in CYP2A6 that also lead to loss of activity have been reported [56].

Biochemical studies on human liver demonstrated that some individuals express an additional cytochrome P450 with homology but not identity to the major drug metabolizing P450 CYP3A4 [57–59]. Expression of this isoform, now termed CYP3A5, is also determined by a common genetic polymorphism affecting splicing that was first identified by Erin Schutz and colleagues in 2001 [60].

From the early studies in the 1970s, it is now clear that at least four CYPs, namely, CYP2D6, CYP2C19, CYP2A6, and CYP3A5, are subject to polymorphisms leading to absence of enzyme activity in significant numbers of individuals and that CYP2C9 activity is very low (although not completely absent) in some individuals. There are also a large number of polymorphisms leading to smaller changes in cytochrome P450 activities (see Chapter 3 for more details). Current knowledge of phenotype–genotype relationships within the cytochrome P450 family is now more comprehensive than for the majority of human genes, although a better understanding of some aspects such as regulation of gene expression is still needed.

1.4 PHARMACOGENETICS OF DRUG CONJUGATION

As discussed in Section 1.2, a polymorphism affecting conjugation of drugs such as isoniazid with acetyl CoA had been known to exist since the 1950s. Other conjugation polymorphisms were subsequently described from phenotyping studies. In particular, Richard Weinshilboum identified several polymorphisms affecting methylation of xenobiotics and endogenous compounds by measurement of enzymatic activities in blood cells. He described the most pharmacologically important of these polymorphisms, in thiopurine methyltransferase (TPMT), in 1980 [61]. Approximately 1 in every 300 Europeans lacks this enzyme with lower activity observed in heterozygotes. Other conjugation polymorphisms identified by phenotypic approaches included a deficiency in the glutathione *S*-transferase M1 (GSTM1), which affects 50% of Europeans and was originally detected by measurement of *trans*-stilbene oxide conjugation in lymphocytes [62]. The classic paper by Motulsky on genetic variability in metabolism [16] mentioned the mild hyperbilirubinemia described previously by Gilbert in 1901 and usually referred to as *Gilbert's syndrome* [63]. This was later shown to relate to impaired activity in glucuronidation by a form of the enzyme UDP-glucuronosyltransferase, and there were suggestions that glucuronidation of prescribed drugs might also be affected in this syndrome [64].

With the development of molecular cloning techniques, the basis of the various conjugation polymorphisms known previously became clear during the late 1980s and early 1990s, and evidence also emerged for additional functionally significant polymorphisms by sequence comparisons. The molecular basis of the GSTM1 deficiency was established quite early in 1988, probably because it is due to a large gene deletion that was readily detectable by a number of different approaches [65]. Cloning of the NAT2 cDNA, encoding the enzyme responsible for isoniazid metabolism, was achieved in 1991 by Blum and Meyer with two common variant alleles with several base substitutions in their coding regions found to be associated with absence of activity [66]. Other inactive variants were identified elsewhere [67,68], and, as in the case of the cytochrome P450 alleles, a standardized nomenclature system was developed [69]. In the case of TPMT, gene cloning and identification of two common alleles associated with absence of activity was achieved in 1996 [70,71]. The most common variant allele giving rise to Gilbert's syndrome was identified in the same year and found to be a TA insertion in the promoter region of the UGT1A1 gene, which encodes the major UDP-glucuronosyltransferase responsible for bilirubin conjugation [72].

Genotyping for the TPMT polymorphisms in patients being prescribed 6-mercaptopurine or azathioprine and the UGT1A1 variant associated with Gilbert's disease in patients receiving irinotecan are now recommended but not mandated by the US Food and Drug Administration (FDA). Knowledge of genotype can enable either dose adjustment or an alternative drug to be prescribed.

1.5 PHARMACOGENETIC STUDIES ON RECEPTORS AND TRANSPORTERS

Progress on pharmacogenetics of drug receptors and other targets has been slower mainly because phenotypic evidence for the existence of functionally significant polymorphisms was generally not available. However, as discussed in

Chapter 5, data from the human genome sequencing project have provided new insights into this area. Studies on polymorphisms in both the adrenergic receptor and dopamine receptor genes appeared in the early 1990s with Stephen Liggett leading in the area of adrenergic receptors [73]. As discussed in Chapter 6, polymorphisms in the various adrenergic receptors have been demonstated to be of considerable relevance to drug response, especially for the $\beta 2$-receptor, but the overall pharmacological importance of polymorphisms in dopamine receptors is still less well established.

Among other drug targets, vitamin K epoxide reductase, the target for coumarin anticoagulants, which is also discussed in detail in Chapter 6, is another example of a gene with well-established pharmacogenetics. In particular, limited phenotypic data from the 1970s suggested that the target for warfarin was subject to interindividual variation in some individuals with resistance to the drug occurring in some families [74]. The gene encoding vitamin K epoxide reductase in humans was finally identified only in 2004 [75,76], but this advance quickly led to identification of isolated mutations associated with warfarin resistance and also to common genetic polymorphisms affecting response to anticoagulants [77–79].

1.6 PHARMACOGENOMICS, GENOMEWIDE STUDIES, AND PERSONALIZED MEDICINE

As reviewed by Meyer [2], the term *pharmacogenomics* first appeared in the literature in 1997. One of the first articles using this term [80] described its relevance to personalized medicine. Pharmacogenomics is often described as the whole-*genome* application of *pharmacogenetics*. There is clearly a large overlap between the two disciplines, but pharmacogenomics is broader and may involve the development of new drugs to target specific genes as well as more effective use of existing medicines. Prior to the 1990s, pharmacogenetic studies were concerned with the effects of single genes, but in the era of pharmacogenomics, the combined effects of a number of genes on a particular phenotype is typically investigated.

Probably the best example of an area in which there has been some implementation of pharmacogenomics is in cancer chemotherapy. Although pharmacogenetic polymorphisms such as TPMT (see Section 1.4) are important in determining the metabolism of selected drugs used in chemotherapy and their possible toxicity, it was realised that tumor genotype and phenotype in addition to host genotype will be predictors of response. The licensing of trastuzumab (Herceptin) as a targeted therapy for breast tumors in 1998 is the earliest example of a drug used as a personalized medicine on the basis of tumor phenotype (for review, see Ref. 81). A test to determine estrogen receptor status is needed before the drug is prescribed as only tumors that are estrogen receptor–positive respond. Other similar drugs followed, most notably imatinib (Glivec) in 2001. Imatinib is a tyrosine kinase inhibitor effective only in tumors with a particular chromosomal translocation [81]. In a separate development, it is now possible to classify tumors by signature for expression of a number of different genes and to use this signature to predict the most appropriate cancer chemotherapy regimen. As discussed by Bonnefoi and colleagues [82], clinical trials are now in progress in breast cancer patients to confirm previous retrospective trials showing that determining mRNA expression levels for a set of either 21 or 70 genes in tumor tissue was of value in predicting whether patients with early-stage breast cancer should undergo chemotherapy or be treated only by hormone therapy.

Another area of pharmacogenomics that is currently developing is the use of genomewide association studies to identify genotypes associated with either drug response or drug toxicity. Such studies have been widely reported for complex polygenic diseases with some interesting novel genes affecting disease susceptibility already identified [83]. A number of genomewide association studies on drug response or adverse reactions have appeared since 2007 [84–86], but these have generally pointed to only one or two genes having a major effect rather than the larger number of genes each with a small effect typically seen in the complex polygenic disease studies. Further similar studies, especially on serious adverse drug reactions, are already in progress.

1.7 CONCLUSION

During 1957–1997, pharmacogenetics evolved to pharmacogenomics. There has been considerable further progress in the subsequent 12 years. Our understanding of single gene effects, especially in relation to drug metabolism, is now comprehensive, but our understanding of effects by multiple genes is still limited. In addition, we still need to translate the range of well-validated and clinically relevant pharmacogenetic discoveries that have been made over the years into more widespread use in patient care. Despite the predictions that we are entering an era of personalized medicine [80], except for the few examples discussed in Sections 1.5 and 1.6 in relation to cancer treatment, this has not yet occurred to any great extent.

REFERENCES

1. Conti A, Bickel MH. History of drug-metabolism—discoveries of major pathways in 19th-century. *Drug Metab. Rev.* 1977;**6**:1–50.
2. Meyer UA. Pharmacogenetics—five decades of therapeutic lessons from genetic diversity. *Nat. Rev. Genet.* 2004;**5**:669–676.
3. Snyder LH. Studies in human inheritance IX. The inheritance of taste deficiency in man. *Ohio J. Sci.* 1932;**32**:436–468.
4. Wooding S. Phenylthiocarbamide: A 75-year adventure in genetics and natural selection. *Genetics* 2006;**172**:2015–2023.
5. Clayman CB, Arnold J, Hockwald RS, Yount EH Jr, Edgcomb JH, Alving AS. Toxicity of primaquine in Caucasians. *J. Am. Med. Assoc. (JAMA)* 1952;**149**:1563–1568.
6. Alving AS, Carson PE, Flanagan CL, Ickes CE. Enzymatic deficiency in primaquine-sensitive erythrocytes. *Science* 1956;**124**:484–485.

7. Hirono A, Beutler E. Molecular cloning and nucleotide sequence of cDNA for human glucose-6-phosphate dehydrogenase variant A(−). *Proc. Natl. Acad. Sci. USA* 1988;**85**:3951–3954.
8. Rieder HL. Fourth-generation fluoroquinolones in tuberculosis. *Lancet* 2009;**373**:1148–1149.
9. Hughes HB. On the metabolic fate of isoniazid. *J. Pharmacol. Exp. Ther.* 1953;**109**:444–452.
10. Hughes HB, Biehl JP, Jones AP, Schmidt LH. Metabolism of isoniazid in man as related to the occurrence of peripheral neuritis. *Am. Rev. Tuberc.* 1954;**70**:266–273.
11. Mitchell RS, Bell JC. Clinical implications of isoniazid, PAS and streptomycin blood levels in pulmonary tuberculosis. *Trans. Am. Clin. Climatol. Assoc.* 1957;**69**:98–102; *discussion*. 103–105.
12. Harris HW, Knight RA, Selin MJ. Comparison of isoniazid concentrations in the blood of people of Japanese and European descent; therapeutic and genetic implications. *Am. Rev. Tuberc.* 1958;**78**:944–948.
13. Evans DAP, Manley KA, McKusick VA. Genetic control of isoniazid metabolism in man. *Br. Med. J.* 1960;**2**:485–491.
14. Lehmann H, Ryan E. The familial incidence of low pseudocholinesterase level. *Lancet* 1956;**271**:124.
15. Kalow W. The Pennsylvania State University College of Medicine 1990 Bernard B. Brodie Lecture. Pharmacogenetics: Past and future. *Life Sci.* 1990;**47**:1385–1397.
16. Motulsky AG. Drug reactions enzymes, and biochemical genetics. *J. Am. Med. Assoc.* 1957;**165**:835–837.
17. Vogel F. Moderne probleme der humangenetik. *Ergebnisse der Innere Medizinische und Kinderheilkunde* 1959;**12**:52–62.
18. Conney AH, Miller EC, Miller JA. Substrate-induced synthesis and other properties of benzpyrene hydroxylase in rat liver. *J. Biol. Chem.* 1957;**228**:753–766.
19. Brodie BB, Gillette JR, La Du BN. Enzymatic metabolism of drugs and other foreign compounds. *Annu. Rev. Biochem.* 1958;**27**:427–454.
20. Omura T, Sato R. A new cytochrome in liver microsomes. *J. Biol. Chem.* 1962; **237**:1375–1376.
21. Cooper DY, Estabrook RW, Rosenthal O. The stoichiometry of C21 hydroxylation of steroids by adrenocortical microsomes. *J. Biol. Chem.* 1963;**238**:1320–1323.
22. Cooper DY, Levin S, Narasimhulu S, Rosenthal O. Photochemical action spectrum of the terminal oxidase of mixed function oxidase systems. *Science* 1965; **147**:400–402.
23. Sladek NE, Mannering GJ. Induction of drug metabolism. I. Differences in the mechanisms by which polycyclic hydrocarbons and phenobarbital produce their inductive effects on microsomal N-demethylating systems. *Mol. Pharmacol.* 1969;**5**:174–185.
24. Alvares AP, Schilling G, Levin W, Kuntzman R. Studies on the induction of CO-binding pigments in liver microsomes by phenobarbital and 3-methylcholanthrene. *Biochem. Biophys. Res. Commun.* 1967;**29**:521–526.
25. Cheng KC, Schenkman JB. Purification and characterization of two constitutive forms of rat liver microsomal cytochrome P-450. *J. Biol. Chem.* 1982;**257**:2378–2385.

26. Wiebel FJ, Selkirk JK, Gelboin HV, Haugen DA, van der Hoeven TA, Coon MJ. Position-specific oxygenation of benzo(a)pyrene by different forms of purified cytochrome P-450 from rabbit liver. *Proc. Natl. Acad. Sci. USA* 1975;**72**:3917–3920.
27. Eichelbaum M, Spannbrucker N, Steincke B, Dengler HJ. Defective N-oxidation of sparteine in man: A new pharmacogenetic defect. *Eur. J. Clin. Pharmacol.* 1979;**17**:153–155.
28. Mahgoub A, Idle JR, Dring LG, Lancaster R, Smith RL. Polymorphic hydroxylation of debrisoquine in man. *Lancet* 1977;**ii**:584–586.
29. Bertilsson L, Dengler HJ, Eichelbaum M, Schulz HU. Pharmacogenetic covariation of defective N-oxidation of sparteine and 4-hydroxylation of debrisoquine. *Eur. J. Clin. Pharmacol.* 1980;**17**:153–155.
30. Evans DAP, Mahgoun A, Sloan TP, Idle JR, Smith RL. A family and population study of the genetic polymorphism of debrisoquine oxidation in a white British population. *J. Med. Genet.* 1980;**17**:102–105.
31. Bertilsson L, Eichelbaum M, Mellstrom B, Sawe J, Schultz NV, Sjoqvist F. Nortryptyline and antipyrine clearance in relation to debrisoquine hydroxylation in man. *Life Sci.* 1980;**27**:1673–1677.
32. Kahn GC, Boobis AR, Murray S, Brodie MJ, Davies DS. Assay and characterisation of debrisoquine 4-hydroxylase activity of microsomal fractions of human liver. *Br. J. Clin. Pharmacol.* 1982;**13**:637–645.
33. Meier PJ, Mueller HK, Dick B, Meyer UA. Hepatic monooxygenase activities in subjects with a genetic defect in drug oxidation. *Gastroenterology* 1983;**85**:682–692.
34. Distelrath LM, Reilly PEB, Martin MV, Davis GG, Wilkinson GR, Guengerich FP. Purification and characterisation of the human liver cytochromes P450 involved in debrisoquine 4-hydroxylation and phenacetin O-deethylation, two prototypes for genetic polymorphism in oxidative drug metabolism. *J. Biol. Chem.* 1985;**260**:9057–9067.
35. Gonzalez FJ, Vilbois F, Hardwick JP, McBride OW, Nebert DW, Gelboin HV, et al. Human debrisoquine 4-hydroxylase (P450IID1): cDNA and deduced amino acid sequence and assignment of the *CYP2D* locus to chromosome 22. *Genomics* 1988;**2**:174–179.
36. Heim M, Meyer UA. Genotyping of poor metabolisers by allele-specific PCR amplification. *Lancet* 1990;**2**:529–532.
37. Gough AC, Miles JS, Spurr NK, Moss JE, Gaedigk A, Eichelbaum M, et al. Identification of the primary gene defect at the cytochrome P450 *CYP2D* locus. *Nature* 1990;**347**:773–776.
38. Hanioka N, Kimura S, Meyer UA, Gonzalez FJ. The human *CYP2D* locus associated with a common genetic defect in drug oxidation: a G_{1934} to A base change in intron 3 of a mutant *CYP2D6* allele results in an aberrant 3′ splice recognition site. *Am. J. Hum. Genet.* 1990;**47**:994–1001.
39. Kagimoto M, Heim M, Kagimoto K, Zeugin T, Meyer UA. Multiple mutations of the human cytochrome P450IID6 gene (CYP2D6) in poor metabolisers of debrisoquine. *J. Biol. Chem.* 1990;**265**:17209–17214.
40. Gaedigk A, Blum M, Gaedigk R, Eichelbaum M, Meyer UA. Deletion of the entire cytochrome P450 gene as a cause of impaired drug metabolism in poor metabolizers of the debrisoquine/sparteine polymorphism. *Am. J. Hum. Genet.* 1991;**48**:943–950.
41. Johansson I, Lundqvist E, Bertilsson L, Dahl M-L, Sjoqvist F, Ingelman-Sundberg M. Inherited amplification of an active gene in the cytochrome P450 *CYP2D* locus as a cause

of ultrarapid metabolism of debrisoquine. *Proc. Natl. Acad. Sci. USA* 1993;**90**:11825–11829.

42. Daly AK, Brockmoller J, Broly F, Eichelbaum M, Evans WE, Gonzalez FJ, et al. Nomenclature for human CYP2D6 alleles. *Pharmacogenetics* 1996;**6**:193–211.
43. Kupfer A, Preisig R. Pharmacogenetics of mephenytoin: A new drug hydroxylation polymorphism in man. *Eur. J. Clin. Pharmacol.* 1984;**26**:753–759.
44. de Morais SMF, Wilkinson GR, Blaisdell J, Meyer UA, Nakamura K, Goldstein JA. Identification of a new genetic defect responsible for the polymorphism of *(S)*-mephenytoin metabolism in Japanese. *Mol. Pharmacol.* 1994;**46**:594–598.
45. de Morais SMF, Wilkinson GR, Blaisdell J, Nakamura K, Meyer UA, Goldstein JA. The major genetic defect responsible for the polymorphism of *S*-mephenytoin metabolism in humans. *J. Biol. Chem.* 1994;**269**:15419–15422.
46. Scott J, Poffenbarger PL. Pharmacogenetics of tolbutamide metabolism in humans. *Diabetes* 1978;**28**:41–51.
47. Miners JO, Smith KJ, Robson RA, McManus ME, Veronese ME, Birkett DJ. Tolbutamide hydroxylation by human liver microsomes. Kinetic characterisation and relationship to other cytochrome P-450 dependent xenobiotic oxidations. *Biochem. Pharmacol.* 1988;**37**:1137–1144.
48. Kimura S, Pastewka J, Gelboin HV, Gonzalez FJ. cDNA and amino acid sequences of two members of the human P450IIC gene subfamily. *Nucleic Acids Res.* 1987;**15**:10053–10054.
49. Meehan RR, Gosden JR, Rout D, Hastie ND, Friedberg T, Adesnik M, et al. Human cytochrome P450 PB-1: A multigene family involved in mephenytoin and steroid oxidations that maps to chromosome 10. *Am. J. Hum. Genet.* 1988;**42**:26–37.
50. Rettie AE, Wienkers LC, Gonzalez FJ, Trager WF, Korzekwa KR. Impaired (*S*)-warfarin metabolism catalysed by the R144C allelic variant of CYP2C9. *Pharmacogenetics* 1994;**4**:39–42.
51. Sullivan-Close TH, Ghanayem BI, Bell DA, Zhang Z-Y, Kaminsky LS, Shenfield GM, et al. The role of the *CYP2C9*-Leu359 allelic variant in the tolbutamide polymorphism. *Pharmacogenetics* 1996;**6**:341–349.
52. Furuya H, FernandezSalguero P, Gregory W, Taber H, Steward A, Gonzalez FJ, et al. Genetic polymorphism of CYP2C9 and its effect on warfarin maintenance dose requirement in patients undergoing anticoagulation therapy. *Pharmacogenetics* 1995;**5**:389–392.
53. Steward DJ, Haining RL, Henne KR, Davis G, Rushmore TH, Trager WF, et al. Genetic association between sensitivity to warfarin and expression of CYP2C9*3. *Pharmacogenetics* 1997;**7**:361–367.
54. Aithal GP, Day CP, Kesteven PJL, Daly AK. Association of polymorphisms in the cytochrome P450 CYP2C9 with warfarin dose requirement and risk of bleeding complications. *Lancet* 1999;**353**:717–719.
55. Fernandez-Salguero P, Hoffman SMG, Cholerton S, Mohrenweiser H, Raunio H, Pelkonen O, et al. A genetic polymorphism in coumarin 7-hydroxylation: Sequence of the human *CYP2A* genes and identification of variant *CYP2A6* alleles. *Am. J. Hum. Genet.* 1995;**57**:651–660.
56. Oscarson M, McLellan RA, Gullsten H, Yue QY, Lang MA, Bernal ML, et al. Characterisation and PCR-based detection of a CYP2A6 gene deletion found at a high frequency in a Chinese population. *FEBS Lett* 1999;**448**:105–110.

57. Aoyama T, Yamano S, Waxman DJ, Lapenson DP, Meyer UA, Fischer V, et al. Cytochrome P450 hPCN3, a novel cytochrome P450 IIA gene product that is differentially expressed in adult human liver. *J. Biol. Chem.* 1989;**264**:10388–10395.
58. Schuetz JD, Molowa DT, Guzelian PS. Characterization of a cDNA encoding a new member of the glucocorticoid-responsive cytochromes P450 in human liver. *Arch. Biochem. Biophys.* 1989;**274**:355–365.
59. Wrighton SA, Ring BJ, Watkins PB, VandenBranden M. Identification of a polymorphically expressed member of the human cytochrome P-450III family. *Mol. Pharmacol.* 1989;**36**:97–105.
60. Kuehl P, Zhang J, Lin Y, Lamba J, Assem M, Schuetz J, et al. Sequence diversity in CYP3A promoters and characterization of the genetic basis of polymorphic CYP3A5 expression. *Nat. Genet.* 2001;**27**:383–391.
61. Weinshilboum R, Sladek SL. Mercaptopurine pharmacogenetics: Monogenic inheritance of erythrocyte thiopurine methyltransferase activity. *Am. J. Hum. Genet.* 1980;**32**:651–662.
62. Seidegard J, Pero RW. The hereditary transmission of high glutathione transferase-activity towards trans-stilbene oxide in human mononuclear leukocytes. *Hum. Genet.* 1985;**69**:66–68.
63. Gilbert C, Lereboullet P. La cholemie simple familiale. *Semaine Med.* 1901;**21**:241–243.
64. Macklon AF, Savage RL, Rawlins MD. Gilbert syndrome and drug metabolism. *Clin. Pharmacokin.* 1979;**4**:223–232.
65. Seidegard J, Vorachek WR, Pero RW, Pearson WR. Hereditary differences in the expression of the human glutathione *S*-transferase active on *trans*-stilbene oxide are due to a gene deletion. *Proc. Natl. Acad. Sci. USA* 1988;**85**:7293–7297.
66. Blum M, Demierre A, Grant DM, Heim M, Meyer UA. Molecular mechanism of slow acetylation of drugs and carcinogens in humans. *Proc. Natl. Acad. Sci. USA* 1991;**88**:5237–5241.
67. Vatsis KP, Martell KJ, Weber WW. Diverse point mutations in the human gene for polymorphic *N*-acetyltransferase. *Proc. Natl. Acad. Sci. USA* 1991;**88**:6333–6337.
68. Hickman D, Sim E. *N*-acetyltransferase polymorphism. Comparison of phenotype and genotype in humans. *Biochem. Pharmacol.* 1991;**42**:1007–1014.
69. Vatsis KP, Weber WW, Bell DA, Dupret J-M, Evans DAP, Grant DM, et al. Nomenclature for *N*-acetyltransferases. *Pharmacogenetics* 1995;**5**:1–17.
70. Szumlanski C, Otterness D, Her C, Lee D, Brandriff B, Kelsell D, et al. Thiopurine methyltransferase pharmacogenetics: Human gene cloning and characterization of a common polymorphism. *DNA Cell Biol.* 1996;**15**:17–30.
71. Tai H-L, Krynetski EY, Yates CR, Loennechen T, Fessing MY, Krynetskaia NF, et al. Thiopurine *S*-methyltransferase deficiency: two nucleotide transitions define the most prevalent mutant allele associated with loss of catalytic activity in Caucasians. *Am. J. Hum. Genet.* 1996;**58**:694–702.
72. Monaghan G, Ryan M, Seddon R, Hume R, Burchell B. Genetic variation in bilirubin UDP-glucuronosyltransferase gene promoter and Gilbert's syndrome. *Lancet* 1996;**347**:578–581.
73. Green SA, Cole G, Jacinto M, Innis M, Liggett SB. A polymorphism of the human beta 2-adrenergic receptor within the fourth transmembrane domain alters ligand binding and functional properties of the receptor. *J. Biol. Chem.* 1993;**268**:23116–23121.

74. O'Reilly RA. The second reported kindred with hereditary resistance to oral anticoagulant drugs. *New Engl. J. Med.* 1970;**282**:1448–1451.
75. Rost S, Fregin A, Ivaskevicius V, Conzelmann E, Hortnagel K, Pelz HJ, et al. Mutations in VKORC1 cause warfarin resistance and multiple coagulation factor deficiency type 2. *Nature* 2004;**427**:537–541.
76. Li T, Chang CY, Jin DY, Lin PJ, Khvorova A, Stafford DW. Identification of the gene for vitamin K epoxide reductase. *Nature* 2004;**427**:541–544.
77. D'Andrea G, D'Ambrosio RL, Di Perna P, Chetta M, Santacroce R, Brancaccio V, et al. A polymorphism in VKORC1 gene is associated with an inter-individual variability in the dose-anticoagulant effect of warfarin. *Blood* 2005;**105**:645–649.
78. Rieder MJ, Reiner AP, Gage BF, Nickerson DA, Eby CS, McLeod HL, et al. Effect of VKORC1 haplotypes on transcriptional regulation and warfarin dose. *N. Engl. J. Med.* 2005;**352**:2285–2293.
79. Sconce EA, Khan TI, Wynne HA, Avery P, Monkhouse L, King BP, et al. The impact of CYP2C9 and VKORC1 genetic polymorphism and patient characteristics upon warfarin dose requirements: Proposal for a new dosing regimen. *Blood* 2005;**106**:2329–2333.
80. Marshall A. Laying the foundations for personalized medicines. *Nat. Biotechnol.* 1997;**15**:954–957.
81. Ross JS, Schenkein DP, Pietrusko R, Rolfe M, Linette GP, Stec J, et al. Targeted therapies for cancer 2004. *Am. J. Clin. Pathol.* 2004;**122**:598–609.
82. Bonnefoi H, Underhill C, Iggo R, Cameron D, Predictive signatures for chemotherapy sensitivity in breast cancer: Are they ready for use in the clinic? *Eur. J. Cancer* 2009;**45**:1733–1743.
83. Burton PR, Clayton DG, Cardon LR, Craddock N, Deloukas P, Duncanson A, et al., Genome-wide association study of 14,000 cases of seven common diseases and 3, *000 shared controls. Nature* 2007;**447**:661–678.
84. Cooper GM, Johnson JA, Langaee TY, Feng H, Stanaway IB, Schwarz UI, et al. A genome-wide scan for common genetic variants with a large influence on warfarin maintenance dose. *Blood* 2008;**112**:1022–1027.
85. Link E, Parish S, Armitage J, Bowman L, Heath S, Matsuda F, et al. SLCO1B1 variants and statin-induced myopathy—a genomewide study. *N. Engl. J. Med.* 2008;**359**:789–799.
86. Daly AK, Donaldson PT, Bhatnagar P, Shen Y, Pe'er I, Floratos A, et al. HLA-B*5701 genotype is a major determinant of drug-induced liver injury due to flucloxacillin. *Nat. Genet.* 2009;**41**:816–819.

PART I

PHARMACOGENETICS: RELATIONSHIP TO PHARMACOKINETICS AND PHARMACODYNAMICS

CHAPTER 2

Pharmacogenetics in Drug Metabolism: Role of Phase I Enzymes

VITA DOLŽAN

Faculty of Medicine, University of Ljubljana, Ljubljana, Slovenia

2.1 INTRODUCTION

Phase I drug metabolizing enzymes (DMEs) catalyze the first step in metabolism of xenobiotics such as drugs and carcinogens. Most of these enzymes, especially cytochromes P450 (P450s or CYPs), metabolically activate xenobiotics to reactive electrophilic forms that are then conjugated to endogenous compounds by phase II DMEs: UDP-glucuronosyltransferases (UGTs), *N*-acetyltransferases (NATs), glutathione-*S*-transferases (GSTs), or others (reviewed in Chapter 3). All these metabolic processes transform the xenobiotic to a more water-soluble form that can be transported from the cells (as reviewed in Chapter 4) to be eliminated from the body.

Although nearly 80% of phase I biotransformation reactions are catalyzed by P450s, also other, non-P450 enzymes play an important role in metabolism of xenobiotics, especially in metabolic activation of some clinically important drugs. These non-P450 enzymes belong to various classes; of particular importance are dehydrogenases, oxidases, esterases, epoxide hydrolases, and others. Of these non-P450 enzymes, dehydrogenases are not reviewed in this chapter. The role of dihydropyrimidine dehydrogenase (DPD) in cancer treatment is reviewed in Chapter 8, while alcohol and aldehyde dehydrogenases (ADH and ALDH, respectively) play a major role in alcohol toxicity and are mainly of toxicological importance.

Most phase I enzymes exhibit variability in their expression level and activity, and in about 40% of these enzymes a large extent of this variability is due to genetic polymorphism [1,2]. As these genetic polymorphisms alter enzyme activity, they may lead to interindividual differences in the metabolism of drugs and could therefore influence drug plasma levels and drug response. By using enzyme-specific

Pharmacogenetics and Individualized Therapy, First Edition.
Edited by Anke-Hilse Maitland-van der Zee and Ann K. Daly.

probe drugs individuals can be grouped into four phenotype groups according to their metabolic rate: poor metabolizers (PMs) lacking functional enzyme due to homozygosity for two defective alleles, intermediate metabolizers (IMs) heterozygous for one defective allele or carrying two alleles with reduced activity, and extensive metabolizers (EMs) with two normal alleles and ultrarapid metabolizers (UMs) carrying gene duplication or multiple gene copies. The rate of metabolism for a certain drug can differ 1000-fold between the PMs and UMs. Such patients may require dose adjustments as a standard population based dosing may result in a higher risk for adverse effects due to high plasma levels in PMs or in unresponsiveness to treatment in UMs [3,4].

A meta-analysis performed in the United States revealed that serious ADRs occur in 6.7% of all hospitalized patients, while 0.3% of all hospitalized patients develop fatal adverse drug reactions (ADRs) [5]. It has been shown that among the drugs that are cited in the ADR reports 56% are metabolized by polymorphic phase I enzymes and that 86% of these enzymes are actually P450s. On the contrary, only 20% of drugs that are substrates for enzymes not known to be polymorphic were cited in the ADR reports [6].

2.2 CYTOCHROMES P450

Cytochromes P450 (P450s or CYPs) are a large and ubiquitous superfamily of heme–thiolate proteins. Their name originates from their particular spectral properties, namely, when reduced with carbon monoxide (CO) these proteins have an absorbance peak at approximately 450 nm. These enzymes catalyze several types of oxidation, but also reduction reactions of a great number of endogenous and exogenous substrates. In humans the majority of the P450 enzymes are expressed in the liver, while some are expressed in other tissues such as gastrointestinal tract, central nervous system, lung, trachea, nasal and olfactory mucosa, skin, and adrenal gland [7–9]. Expression of some P450 enzymes, such as CYP1B1 and CYP2W, has also been detected in tumour tissue [10,11].

The human genome encodes 59 P450 proteins that are categorized into 18 families and 43 subfamilies on the basis of their sequence similarities [12]. The nomenclature of CYPs is well established. The abbreviation CYP indicates cytochrome P450, while the first Arabic number designates the family that includes sequences that are more than 40% identical at the aminoacid level. The letter that follows indicates the subfamily characterized by sequence identity higher than 55%, and the next Arabic number indicates the individual enzyme (CYP2C9). In certain families several subfamilies have been identified, such as in CYP2 (12 subfamilies with 16 active genes and 14 pseudogenes) and CYP4 (5 subfamilies with 12 active genes and 8 pseudogenes), whereas in others only a single active gene product has been reported (CYP17, CYP19, CYP21). Genes are written in italics and the separate alleles are designated by a star and the number that follows (*CYP2C9*2*). The corresponding gene products (mRNA, cDNA and proteins) are written non-italicized and in all–capital letters [13–15]. Cytochrome P450 (CYP) Allele Nomenclature Committee website publishes peer-reviewed information on human CYP alleles regarding their nucleotide changes, their functional consequences, and links to publications where the allele has been identified and characterized, making it a website particularly interesting for researchers in the field of pharmacogenetics [15–17].

Cytochromes P450 are monooxygenases, and one of the most typical reactions that they catalyze is hydroxylation, where one atom of molecular oxygen is incorporated into a substrate and the other is reduced to water using NADPH as the source of the electrons. However, P450s catalyse more than 40 different types of reactions, predominantly oxidations, such as aliphatic and aromatic hydroxylations, dealkylations, demethylations, epoxidations, oxidative group transfers, and the oxidative cleavage of C–N, C–O, C–C, or C–S bonds, but occasionally they can also catalyze reduction reactions [18,19].

Cytochromes P450 are involved in the metabolism of structurally very diverse substrates, either of endogenous origin or foreign to the body (xenobiotics). Enzymes from families CYP1–CYP3 primarily metabolize xenobiotics and have broad substrate specificities. More than 2000 substrates for these enzymes have been identified so far, including the majority of clinically used drugs, chemical carcinogens and other organic compounds [20]. In particular, three families: CYP1, CYP2, and CYP3 account for a total of 75–80% of the phase I metabolism of xenobiotics as whole and for 65–70% of the clearance of clinically used drugs [21]. Among them, CYP3A, CYP2D6, CYP2C9, and CYP2C19 account for the majority of P450-mediated drug metabolism, while CYP1A2, CYP2B6, CYP2C8, and CYP2E1 play an important role in metabolism of a smaller number of clinically important drugs [2]. Members of family CYP4 participate in the metabolism of both exogenous and endogenous substrates, while families CYP5 to CYP51 play a vital role in the metabolism of endogenous, physiologically important substrates such as sterols and bile acids, fatty acids, eicosanoids, and fat-soluble vitamins. Although these enzymes are not involved in drug metabolism, they are becoming increasingly important as potential targets for drug treatment in conditions such as cancer, hypercholesterolemia, vascular and neurological diseases, and steroid hormone disorders.

The biotransformation reactions catalyzed by drug metabolizing P450s result mostly in inactivation of a drug as they attenuate its biologic activity and accelerate its clearance from the body. However, these P450s also participate in bioactivation of some prodrugs to their clinically active form. In some of the biotransformation reactions catalyzed by P450s more reactive electrophilic metabolites are produced that may play a role in drug toxicity (acetaminophen is a classical example), but it is not yet elucidated how many of the ADRs can be attributed to this process [22,23].

2.2.1 CYP2D6

CYP2D6 is one of the most studied P450s. CYP2D6 accounts for less than 5% of total P450s in liver [24,25]; however, it is involved in the oxidation of 20–25% of all drugs in clinical use. Another important site of CYP2D6 expression is brain, where it plays an important role in metabolism of psychotropic drugs as well as endogenous substrates [26,27].

The interindividual variability in the capacity to hydroxylate an antihypertensive drug debrisoquine was reported in the late 1970s [28,29]. At the same time, a similar report was published regarding an antiarrythmic drug sparteine [30], and it was shown that the deficiency in this metabolism was inherited as an autosomal recessive trait. Later it was demonstrated that both drugs are metabolized by the same enzyme, debrisoquine–sparteine hydroxylase [31]. Since then many substrates and reactions were reported for CYP2D6. When the human *CYP2D6* gene was finally cloned in the late 1980s [32,33] it was shown that most of the individuals with deficient capacity to metabolize these drugs carry inactivating mutations in this gene [34–36].

2.2.1.1 CYP2D6 Polymorphism

CYP2D6 is a part of a cluster of three genes arranged in tandem with two pseudogenes, *CYP2D8P* and *CYP2D7P*, on chromosome 22q13.1 [37]. It is a highly polymorphic gene with 120 alleles variants characterized to date. Several nucleotide changes may be present on one allele, or a specific change may be shared among several alleles [16]. *CYP2D6* genotypes usually exhibit large interethnic differences and genetic variability of CYP2D6 is high also among individuals of the same population [38].

In Caucasians, the most frequent deficiency (null) allele is *CYP2D6*4*, carrying a G > A point mutation in the splice site of intron 3/exon 4 causing a splicing defect and resulting in an altered reading frame that introduces a premature stop codon. As the frequency of this allele is 20–25% in Caucasians, it represents 70–90% of all deficient phenotypes. Nevertheless, this allele is rare in other populations with a frequency of around 6–7% in Africans and African-Americans [39,40] and around 1% or less in Orientals [41–43].

The second most common deficiency allele is *CYP2D6*5*, characterized by deletion of the entire *CYP2D6* gene [36] that occurs with a frequency of 3–6% in most of the populations. Most of the other nonfunctional alleles have low frequencies in different populations. They are due mostly to SNPs or small insertions or deletions that alter splicing and/or the reading frame, leading to premature stop codons, while fewer mutations result in a full-length nonfunctional proteins. Deletions resulting in hybrid *CYP2D6/2D7* genes were also reported (*CYP2D6*13*) [44].

Several alleles causing decreased, but not absent enzyme activity have also been described. In Orientals the high frequencies of *CYP2D6*10* allele (around 50%) explained the lower capacity to hydroxylate debrisoquine compared to the Caucasians. *CYP2D6*10* allele is characterised by a SNP causing Pro30Ser amino acid substitution that leads to an unstable enzyme with decreased catalytic activity. This allele is rare in Caucasians and has a frequency of about 2% [45]. A similar shift in the metabolic ratio for debrisoquine hydroxylation was found in Africans from Zimbabwe and was ascribed to the high frequency of *CYP2D6*17* allele that carries nonsynonymous mutations [46]. This allele occurs with different frequencies in African populations: 34% in Zimbabwe [47], 28% in Ghana [40], 17% in Tanzania [48], and 9% in Ethiopia [49], however, it is almost absent in Europen Caucasians [40]. More recently *CYP2D6*41* allele was identified in Caucasian individuals with reduced metabolic capacity [50], and it was shown that the molecular deficit is caused by a SNP 2988G>A located in intron 6 that leads to alternative splicing and substantially increases the ratio between the splice variant lacking the entire exon 6 and has a premature stop codon at position 291 and the normal transcript [51].

Following the observation of extremely rapid metabolism of nortriptyline in some individuals [4], alleles carrying multiple copies of functional *CYP2D6* genes were identified [52,53], and individuals carrying up to 13 functional *CYP2D6* copies on one allele have been found [49,52]. These *CYP2D6*N×2* alleles represent approximately 3% of *CYP2D6* alleles in Caucasians and 4.5% in African–Americans [54]. The frequency of CYP2D6 gene duplications increase with a gradient from north to south of Europe and are 1–2% in Sweden [55], 3.6% in Germany [45], 7–10% in Spain [56,57], and 10% in Sicily [58]. Haplotypes with multiple gene copies were more frequent among Ethiopians (29%) [49] and in Saudi Arabia (20%) [59]. However, the finding that only 10–30% of Caucasian and UMs actually carry *CYP2D6* gene duplications led to a search of other possible genetic causes for enhanced metabolism [60]. A *CYP2D6*53* allele leading to increased activity was identified and characterized in a Japanese population [61].

2.2.1.2 CYP2D6 Genotyping

Rapidly developing genotyping techniques permit the identification of molecular defects causing genetic variability in metabolic capacity for CYP2D6 substrates. Genotyping is however complicated by the presence of two highly homologous pseudogenes within the same locus and by the diversity of mutations; a considerable part of variability is due not only to SNPs but also to insertions or deletions and copy number variations such as gene deletions or duplications.

CYP2D6 gene duplications and gene deletions were initially determined by Southern blotting that was later replaced by long-distance PCR (XL-PCR) [53]. The long amplicon of the *CYP2D6* gene region was then used as a template for subsequent allele-specific PCR reactions for and restriction analysis to detect the most frequent variant alleles [45]. Several gene copy number assays based on quantitative PCR were developed [62,63] and are now commercially available for research use.

The number of polymorphisms that have to be genotyped for an accurate phenotype prediction is still debated. Several laboratories demonstrated that in Caucasians genotyping for a limited number of *CYP2D6* alleles predicts PMs with close to 100% accuracy [45,56,64,65]. It was estimated that on the basis of the allele frequency data, as little as one to two extra-long PCR (XL-PCR) reactions followed by a maximum of six nested amplifications allow accurate prediction of an individual's genotype, while as few as four nested amplifications suffice to identify 97.9% of PMs [66]. However, testing for only a few alleles may lead to false classification of PMs as EMs and in one study testing for 24 *CYP2D6* alleles was recommended in African-Americans [54].

Since the first allele-specific PCR test to identify the two most common defective *CYP2D6* alleles [67], a number of approaches was developed for *CYP2D6* genotyping [68]. Traditional approaches were based on PCR amplification coupled to various post-PCR detection methods such as allele specific PCR [67], and restriction fragment length polymorphism (PCR-RFLP) [45] for the analysis of known mutations or single-stranded conformation polymorphism (SSCP) analysis for the detection of both known and unknown mutations [69]. All these methods require considerable optimization and are laborious, especially if testing a large number of alleles. More recently, real-time PCR methods (TaqMan) have greatly simplified SNP genotyping as the use of universal reaction conditions allowed simultaneous analysis of different SNPs [70]. Also the introduction of microarrays simplified genetic testing for many variants in parallel [71]. The first microarray-based pharmacogenetic test, the Roche AmpliChip CYP 450 test [72], was approved for clinical use in Europe in September 2004 and by the FDA in January 2005 [73]. Using over 15,000 oligonucleotide probes, this chip enables testing for 20 *CYP2D6* alleles and 7 *CYP2D6* duplications along with 3 *CYP2C19* alleles and facilitates pharmacogenetics testing in the clinical environment [74]. Its use has advanced most in psychiatry [75], and the potentials of *CYP2D6* genotyping in oncology [76] have been also recognized by the FDA [77].

2.2.1.3 CYP2D6 Genotype–Phenotype Correlations

An estimation of individual's metabolic capacity for CYP2D6 substrates can be obtained by phenotyping and several probe drugs are available [78]. Alternatively, phenotype can be deduced from genotype data. As CYP2D6 is not inducible, genetic polymorphism is the major determinant of its activity and the genotype correlates well with the metabolic capacity for various drugs [71]. Correlations between the phenotype and genotype have been extensively studied, providing a rather well-understood molecular basis for the variation in CYP2D6 activity [79].

Many different approaches were used to predict the metabolic capacity (phenotype) from genotype [80]. Traditionally genotypes were categorized into PMs, IMs, EMs, and UMs according to the number of active alleles. Individuals carrying two nonfunctional alleles lack any CYP2D6 enzyme activity and are phenotypically PMs. The prevalence of PMs is approximately 7% in Caucasians and 1–3% in other populations. Subjects with one nonfunctional allele and one allele that codes for an enzyme with decreased activity were defined as intermediate metabolizers (IMs). Several pharmacokinetic studies suggested that the metabolic capacity in IMs is severely reduced and may be comparable to that of PMs, especially long-term treatment [81]. Among Caucasians more than 50% of all IMs carry *CYP2D6*41/*0* genotype, while **9* and **10* alleles account for no more than 20% of all IMs. Subjects with at least one functional allele have normal metabolic capacity and are classified as EMs. Ultrarapid metabolizers have three or more copies of the active *CYP2D6* allele and display extremely high enzyme activity.

It was shown that genotyping correctly identifies PMs, but it is difficult to quantitatively predict catalytic activity among IMs and EMs [64]. In addition, there are inconsistencies in the assignment of IM phenotype, as some clinical studies classified genotypes such as *CYP2D6*2/*10* or *CYP2D6*10/*10* as IMs and not EMs [82]. Ethnicity also plays a role, as it was shown that among subjects carrying *CYP2D6*2* allele, CYP2D6 activity was considerably slower in African-Americans compared to Caucasians [83]. IM phenotype is of clinical importance in East Asian population because of the high frequency of *CYP2D6**10* allele [42]. The prediction of phenotype is also difficult in carriers of *CYP2D6**17* allele, frequent in Africans and African-Americans [54,84], as it was shown to be substrate-dependent [83].

One problem of phenotype prediction based on the genotyping data is that it is based on the assumption that a given allele has comparable activity toward all CYP2D6 substrates [83] and does not account for the observations that the metabolic capacity of a particular variant allele may be substrate dependant [82,85,86]. Enzyme activity was also shown to be influenced by nongenetic factors such as dietary habits [87]. The prediction is further complicated by the large number of possible genotypes that have to be interpreted in a way that will allow application to clinical settings. The CYP2D6 activity score model was proposed for the translation of genotype information into a qualitative and comprehensive measure of phenotype [88]. In this model values were assigned to particular alleles: score 0 was assigned to nonfunctional *CYP2D6* alleles **3*, **4*, **4×N*, **5*, **6*, **7*, **16*, **36*, **40*, **42*, and **56B*, score 0.5 was assigned to alleles with decreased function **9*, **10*, **17*, **29*, **41*, **45*, and **46*, score 1 was assigned to functional alleles **1*, **2*, **35*, **43*, **45*, and **46*; and score 2 was assigned to duplicated alleles **1×N*, **2×N*, and **35×N*. Besides simplifying the genotype information, this model predicts the probability for a subject with a certain score to present with a certain phenotype [88].

2.2.1.4 Clinical Implications of CYP2D6 Variability

CYP2D6 is involved in the metabolism of 20–25% of all drugs in clinical use, including many antidepressants, antipsychotics, antiepileptics, antiarythmics, and opioids.

The clinical relevance has been most consistently shown for PMs that may suffer from ADRs at the usual doses of drugs with narrow therapeutic window or do not respond to prodrugs that require metabolic activation by CYP2D6. On the other hand, at usual doses UMs may lack the therapeutic effect of drugs or may exhibit toxicity of prodrugs that require metabolic activation by CYP2D6. The clinical relevance of the IM and EM phenotype is not so clear.

Nearly half of the drugs that are metabolized by CYP2D6 are used in psychiatry, and these drugs are typically associated with a delayed therapeutic response, narrow therapeutic window, and a multitude of ADRs. A number of studies investigated the influence of CYP2D6 genetic variability on antipsychotic and antidepressant pharmacokinetics, occurrence of ADRs, and treatment efficacy. Although the data show that *CYP2D6* polymorphism significantly influences haloperidol and risperidone pharmacokinetics [58,89–93], the data on influence on treatment outcome and ADRs occurrence are less conclusive, largely because studies have been small and retrospective. The same applies to the studies on antidepressants [4,94,95]. Nevertheless, the association between the CYP2D6 PM phenotype and antipsychotics or antidepressants induced ADRs was confirmed by systematic reviews [82,96]. In UMs a trend toward lower therapeutic efficacy was reported [4]. A large case–control study established that CYP2D6 PMs suffered 2.5–6-fold higher risk of risperidone ADRs and were more often discontinued from risperidone because of ADRs [97]. CYP2D6 PM and UM phenotypes also appeared to be associated with higher treatment costs due to longer hospitalization [98].

On the basis of the therapeutic drug monitoring and genotyping data, dosing adjustments for antipsychotics and antidepressants were recommended for patients who are CYP2D6 PMs [82]. Fewer attempts have been made toward the implementation of pharmacogenetic testing for guided drug selection, despite the observations that the first antipsychotic prescribed for a patient by a psychiatrist may not be the best choice for that individual [99] and that the risk of switching to another antidepressant is higher in PMs than EMs [100].

CYP2D6 also plays a crucial role in the metabolism of tamoxifen, which is an estrogen receptor modulator widely used for the endocrine treatment of all stages of hormone-receptor-positive breast cancer. Although many CYPs are involved in the metabolism of tamoxifen, CYP2D6 is crucial for the biotransformation of tamoxifen to endoxifen, the key metabolite with around 100 times greater affinity for the estrogen receptor than the parent compound. Women with nonfunctional *CYP2D6* alleles would thus achieve lower plasma concentrations of endoxifen [101]. Similarly, tamoxifen response was influenced by the concomitant treatment with selective serotonin reuptake inhibitors (SSRIs) that inhibit CYP2D6 [102]. Pharmacogenetics of tamoxifen treatment is discussed in more detail in Chapter 8.

As codeine, oxycodone, hydrocodone and tramadol are prodrugs activated by CYP2D6, PMs may lack the analgesic effects from codeine-like drugs, while in UMs higher plasma concentrations of morphine and its glucuronides were measured after codeine administration [103] and toxic responses were reported [104,105]. Infant death was reported in a breastfeeding mother that was UM for CYP2D6 and was treated with codeine [106].

Regarding cardiovascular drugs, PMs were reported to have a 4–5-fold increase in the risk for ADRs on treatment with metoprolol, a ß-adrenoreceptor antagonist [107].

2.2.1.5 CYP2D6 in Endogenous Metabolism

CYP2D6 is also expressed in brain, where it plays an important role in the metabolism not only of drugs but also of endogenous substrates, such as neuroactive steroids and neurotransmitters [26,108], suggesting a link between CYP2D6 and personality traits in healthy individuals as well as psychiatric and neurologic disorders [109–111].

2.2.2 CYP2C Subfamily

The *CYP2C* gene subfamily includes four genes that cluster on chromosomal location 10q24 [112] in the following order from centromere to telomere: *CYP2C18–CYP2C19–CYP2C9–CYP2C8* [113].

The crystal structures of CYP2C8 and CYP2C9 are available for both unliganded forms and complexes with respective substrates [114–116]. *CYP2C18* does not seem to translate to functional protein [117], while the other genes are expressed predominantly in the liver and constitute 30–40% of the hepatic microsomal

P450s and participate in the metabolism of about 20% of clinically prescribed drugs [24]. They are also expressed in extrahepatic tissues, where they are implicated in the endogenous metabolism of arachidonic acid and some steroids. CYP2C9 and CYP2C19 polymorphism is of great clinical significance as they are involved in metabolism of many drugs with narrow therapeutic window. Lately, more information is emerging also on the pharmacogenetic importance of CYP2C8.

2.2.3 CYP2C8

CYP2C8 constitutes about 7% of total liver P450s [24] and is involved in the metabolism of approximately 5% of clinically used drugs, especially antidiabetics, antimalarials, and taxanes [118].

2.2.3.1 CYP2C8 Polymorphism

Up to now 16 alleles have been described for *CYP2C8* gene [16]. Variants of wild-type *CYP2C8**1A* allele due to SNPs in 5′-regulatory region have been reported, but they did not influence respective protein levels [119]. *CYP2C8**2* codes for a Ile269Phe substitution and was found mostly in Africans and African-Americans with an allele frequency of around 16–18% [118,120]. *CYP2C8**3* coding for Arg139Lys and Lys399Arg has an allele frequency of 13% in Caucasians and 2% in African-Americans and is in strong linkage disequilibrium with *CYP2C9**2* [121]. *CYP2C8**4* codes for a protein with Ile264Met substitution and has a frequency of 8% in Caucasians, but is not found in other races. The frequency of polymorphic *CYP2C8* alleles appears to be very low in Asians [122].

2.2.3.2 Clinical Implications of CYP2C8 Polymorphism

CYP2C8 plays a major role in disposition of therapeutic drugs such as the anticancer drug paclitaxel [123], the antidiabetes drugs repaglinide, rosiglitazone, and troglitazone [124]; the antiarrhythmic drug amiodarone [125]; and the HMG-CoA reductase inhibitor cerivastatin [126,127]. Many substrates are shared with CYP3A4, but usually different metabolic products are generated [123].

The CYP2C8 gene codes for the principal enzyme involved in the elimination and detoxification of paclitaxel. The protein products of *CYP2C8**2* and *CYP2C8**3* allele exhibited only 15% and 50%, respectively, of the activity toward paclitaxel hydroxylation *in vitro* as compared to wild-type protein [118,119]. Nevertheless, the impact of this variability on paclitaxel treatment is not so clear. In breast cancer patients no major association was found between *ABCB1*, *ABCG2*, *CYP1B1*, CYP3A4, *CYP3A5*, and *CYP2C8* genotypes and paclitaxel clearance [128]. Also relatively large clinical studies failed to show any significant association of *CYP2C8* polymorphism and paclitaxel treatment response and survival in advanced head and neck cancer, advanced non-small-cell lung cancer or ovarian cancer [129,130]. Although a study of 38 ovarian cancer patients reported lower clearance of paclitaxel in patients heterozygous for *CYP2C8**3* when stratified according to the *ABCB1 G2677T/A* genotype and the exposure to paclitaxel correlated to the degree of neurotoxicity [131], a larger study revealed no significant associations between

CYP2C8 genotype and either outcome or toxicity of combined carboplatin and taxane regimens after cytoreductive surgery of advanced ovarian cancer [132].

CYP2C8 genotype was also shown to influence the pharmacokinetics of glucose-lowering meglitinides, but the clinical importance of altered metabolism remains to be determined [133]. Most of the studies were performed on small numbers of healthy volunteers, while large-scale studies on diabetic patients on long-term treatment are lacking [134,135]. There are also no data as to whether *CYP2C8* genotype modifies the risk of micro- and macrovascular complications in patients with diabetes mellitus. Surprisingly, *CYP2C8*3* carriers had higher repaglinide clearance and lower plasma concentrations compared to wild-type carriers, but no statistically significant differences in the blood glucose response to repaglinide were observed between the genotypes [136,137]. Similarly, *CYP2C8*3* carriers had significantly lower rosiglitazone area under the plasma concentration–time curve (AUC) and significantly higher rosiglitazone oral clearance as compared with *CYP2C8* wild-type homozygotes [138]. Although *CYP2C8* genotype significantly predicted rosiglitazone disposition, it did not influence its glucose-lowering effect [139].

Decreased metabolism of (*R*)-ibuprofen was observed in carriers of *CYP2C8*3* [140]. The *CYP2C8*4* allele, along with variant UGT2B7 and ABCC2, also led to increased risk of diclofenac hepatotoxicity, possibly due to formation or accumulation of reactive diclofenac metabolites [141].

As CYP2C8 is the predominant P450 involved in the disposition of many antimalarials such as amodiaquine, chloroquine, and dapsone, the relatively high occurrence of *CYP2C8*2* allele in Africans may have implications for fighting malaria in this region [142]. Impaired activation of antimalarial amodiaquine to the active metabolite *N*-desethylaminodiaquine has been observed in *CYP2C8*2*, leading to increased risk of severe ADRs [143]. In another study *CYP2C8*2* displayed defective metabolism of amodiaquine, while *CYP2C8*3* showed markedly decreased activity. No evidence was reported for influence of *CYP2C8* genotype on amodiaquine efficacy or toxicity, but this remains to be investigated in larger samples [144]. Besides genetic variability drug interactions may also influence the efficacy and toxicity of antimalarials. Coadministration of antiretroviral drugs such as efavirenz, saquinavir, lopinavir, and tipranavir that are potent CYP2C8 inhibitors at clinically relevant concentrations may be of particular importance [144].

2.2.3.3 CYP2C8 Genotyping

No diagnostic kits are available, but reliable methods that are suitable for both research and routine laboratory use were developed for genotyping *CYP2C8*2*, **3*, and **4* alleles either by classical PCR-RFLP, simple multiplex PCR [145] or by faster and more cost-effective real-time PCR methods [146,147].

2.2.3.4 CYP2C8 in Endogenous Metabolism

CYP2C8, besides other CYP2C enzymes, participates in the metabolism of retinoids and arachidonic acid [148,149]. Arachidonic acid is metabolized to biologically active epoxides [150] that affect many physiologic processes, including water reabsorption and sodium transport in the kidney, inflammation, vascular smooth muscle tone, and platelet aggregation [151,152]. Increased secretion of arachidonic acid metabolites was observed in carriers of high-activity *CYP2C8* alleles compared to the low-activity genotypes [153]. Nevertheless, few of the studies confirmed a major role of CYP2C genetic variability in the risk for hypertension [120] or cardiovascular diseases [154,155].

2.2.4 CYP2C9

Of the CYP2C family, CYP2C9 is the major enzyme found in the human liver, constituting 18–30% of total hepatic P450 [156,157]. CYP2C9 is not expressed in fetal liver, but its levels rise rapidly in the first 3 months after birth [158]. CYP2C9 is distinguished from other human CYP2C enzymes by a preference for substrates bearing a negative charge at physiological pH, although it also metabolizes neutral or positively charged substrates [159]. It participates in disposition of about 10–20% of commonly prescribed drugs, many of which have narrow therapeutic indices [20], so subjects with slow metabolism may be at increased risk of ADRs when prescribed drugs extensively metabolized by CYP2C9.

2.2.4.1 CYP2C9 Polymorphism

CYP2C9 is polymorphic, and 34 alleles and 7 variants with major interethnic differences in frequency distribution were reported [16]. The *CYP2C9*2* allele carries a point mutation in exon 3 causing Arg144Cys substitution [160], while the *CYP2C9*3* allele carries a point mutation in exon 7 causing Ile359Leu substitution [161,162]. It was demonstrated both *in vitro* and *in vivo* that these two allelic variants of *CYP2C9* gene influenced the metabolic activity of the enzyme. The CYP2C9.2 and CYP2C9.3 proteins expressed *in vitro* demonstrate approximately 12% and 5%, respectively, of the wild-type enzyme activity [160,162], however, the reduction in activity was highly dependent on the substrate [163]. Mean clearances in homozygous carriers of the *CYP2C9*3* allele were below 25% that of the wild type for *S*-warfarin, tolbutamide, glipizide, celecoxib, and fluvastatin. In the more frequent heterozygous carriers the clearances were within 40–75% [164].

Alleles *CYP2C9*2* and *CYP2C9*3* are the two most common alleles in Caucasian populations with allelic frequencies of 8–14% and 4–16%, respectively. Their frequencies in African populations were 4% and 2%, respectively [164]. *CYP2C9*2* allele was not detected, while *CYP2C9*3* allele was found only in heterozygous form in 3.5% of the Asian populations. Many new alleles with decreased catalytic activity were discovered by sequencing of individuals from different racial groups, but their frequencies in various populations may be too low to be of clinical significance. *CYP2C9*4* has been identified only in Japanese patients, while *CYP2C9*5*, coding for Asp360Glu and *CYP2C9*6*, characterized by deletion of adenine at nucleotide 818 that results in a frameshift causing a null allele were found only among African-Americans with a frequency of 1.7% and 0.6%, respectively [165–167].

2.2.4.2 Clinical Implications of CYP2C9 Polymorphism

CYP2C9 polymorphism has clinical implications for several commonly prescribed drugs such as oral anticoagulants, hypoglycemic agents, angiotensin-2 antagonists, HMG-CoA-reductase inhibitors (statins), many nonsteroidal antiinflammatory drugs (NSAIDs), and antiepileptics and other drugs [168,169].

The most important and widely replicated clinical implication of *CYP2C9* polymorphism is related to oral anticoagulant treatment (for further information, see Chapter 6). Warfarin is the most widely prescribed oral anticoagulant for reducing thromboembolic events; however, in Europe, acenocoumarol and phenprocoumon are also used. They act by interfering with the recycling of vitamin K in the liver, which leads to reduced activation of several clotting factors. Oral anticoagulant treatment can be difficult to manage because of the narrow therapeutic index of these drugs and wide interindividual variability in the dose required to achieve the desired therapeutic effect. Despite careful monitoring of prothrombin time expressed as international normalized ratio (INR), bleeding events are likely to occur and the risk of serious bleeding ranges from 1.3 to 4.2 per 100 patient years of exposure [170].

Warfarin is available as a racemate, and CYP2C9 is the major enzyme responsible for 7-hydroxylation of *S*-warfarin, while CYP1A2, CYP2C19, and CYP3A4 are responsible for oxidative metabolism of less potent (*R*)-enantiomer [171]. Several clinical studies have demonstrated that *CYP2C9* polymorphisms significantly influence warfarin pharmacokinetics by reducing (*S*)-warfarin metabolic clearance, consequently lowering maintenance dose requirements. The effects of CYP2C9 polymorphisms on the pharmacokinetics and anticoagulant response is most pronounced in warfarin and least in phenprocoumon [172]. A systematic review and a meta-analysis of 39 studies comprising 7907 patients showed that, compared to the *CYP2C9*1/*1* genotype, dose requirement was lower for 19.6% in *CYP2C9*1/*2*, 33.7% in CYP2C9*1/*3, 36.0% in *CYP2C9*2/*2*, 56.7% in *CYP2C9*2/*3*, and 78.1% in *CYP2C9*3/*3* genotype carriers [173]. However, pharmacogenetic models could explain only 37% of interpatient variability in warfarin dose requirement when accounting for *CYP2C9* genotype and nongenetic factors [174].

To explain the variability observed within the different *CYP2C9* genotype groups, polymorphisms in genes encoding components of the coagulation cascade were investigated [175,176]. VKORC1, the enzyme inhibited by warfarin, is discussed in detail in Chapter 5. All studies on warfarin dose requirement agree that around 12–18% of variability is predicted by *CYP2C9* genotype but about 30% by *VKORC1* genotype. Altogether approximately 50–60% of variability in warfarin dose requirement can be predicted by both pharmacogenetic and nongenetic factors [176–178].

CYP2C9 also plays a major role in clearance of approximately half of the nonsteroidal anti-inflammatory drugs (NSAIDs), including diclofenac, oxicams, ibuprofen, flurbiprofen, and indomethacin. In ibuprofen disposition, CYP2C8 may also play a role, while CYP3A also participates in elimination of celecoxib, valdecoxib, and meloxicam. CYP2C9 was found to play only a minor role in pharmacokinetics of sulindac, naproxen, ketoprofen, diclofenac, rofecoxib, and etoricoxib. Although it is generally accepted that cardiovascular and gastointestinal adverse effects of NSAIDs are related to their mechanism of action, subjects with polymorphic alleles may have increased exposure and indeed, a greater risk of adverse effects was observed in some, but not all studies [179]. For drugs that are metabolized mainly by CYP2C9, the association of variant *CYP2C9* alleles and the risk of acute gastrointestinal bleeding showed a gene–dose effect. Besides *CYP2C9*2* and **3* alleles also *CYP2C8*3* showed increased risk of developing acute gastrointestinal bleeding during the use of NSAID that are CYP2C8 or CYP2C9 substrates [180,181]. Although more data and larger studies are needed to confirm the association between *CYP2C9* genotype and adverse effects of NSAIDs [182], it was proposed that *CYP2C9* polymorphisms might be considered in treatment strategies because of the widespread use of NSAIDs, especially in aging populations [183]. There was also great concern that *CYP2C8* or *CYP2C9* polymorphisms may modify the protective effect of regular NSAID use on the risk of colorectal carcinoma, but no such interaction was found [184].

CYP2C9 is also the main enzyme in the disposition of sulfonylurea drugs (tolbutamide, glibenclamide, glimepiride, glipizide) and nateglinide while rosiglitazone is also metabolized by CYP2C8. Although the majority of the studies was performed on small numbers of healthy volunteers, many indicated that the *CYP2C9*3* allele was associated with decreased clearance of sulfonylureas [134]. Compared to carriers of the *CYP2C9*1/*1* wild-type genotype, oral clearance of sulfonylurea was 50–80% of normal in *CYP2C9*1/*3* genotype and 20% in subjects with *CYP2C9*3/*3* genotype, but the resulting differences in drug effects were much less pronounced [164]. Only scarce data exist on the clinical implications of this genetic variability on adverse drug effects or clinical outcomes in patients ingesting oral antidiabetics; however, carriers of polymorphic *CYP2C9* alleles were reported to experience higher incidences of hypoglicaemia on treatment with sulfonylurea drugs [133]. Among sulfonylureas, the tolbutamide dose requirement was most affected by *CYP2C9*3* genotype [185]. Considering pharmacokinetic data, dose adjustments based on *CYP2C9* genotypes were proposed to help reduce the incidence of ADRs [135].

2.2.4.3 CYP2C9 in Endogenous Metabolism

Besides its role in drug metabolism CYP2C9 contributes to the metabolism of fatty acids, prostanoids, and steroid hormones, but our understanding of the role of CYP2C9 in endogenous metabolism is limited. As CYP2C9 participates in the oxidation of arachidonic acid to several physiologically active metabolites, it may play an important role in the regulation of vascular renal, pulmonary, and cardiac function and vascular homeostasis and inflammatory response, but more clinical studies are needed [186,187].

2.2.5 CYP2C19

CYP2C19 is expressed predominantly in liver, where it accounts for around 3% of total hepatic CYPs and is involved in metabolism of about 5% of all drugs. It is also expressed in fetal liver at relatively constant levels throughout gestation, but postnatal increases in CYP2C19 are observed within the first year of life [158]. It is particularly important for metabolism of several antidepressants, proton pump inhibitors, and antiepileptics.

CYP2C19 was first described as *S*-mephenytoin hydroxylase. Approximately 10-fold difference in oral clearance was described between EMs and PMs of *S*-mephenytoin, and about 3% of Caucasians throughout the world are PMs of *S*-mephenytoin [188–190]. Large interethnic differences exist in the distribution of EM and PM genotypes. Among Africans 4–7% are PMs [169]. The frequency of PMs is much higher in Orientals and ranges from 12% to 22% [3,189,191], however, in the Vanuatu islands in Melanesia the frequency of PMs is 70% [192].

2.2.5.1 CYP2C19 Polymorphism

The interindividual variability in CYP2C19 activity is determined mainly by the genetic polymorphisms of this enzyme. Seven variant alleles (*CYP2C19*2–*8*) that code for a non-functional enzyme have been described to date (as of 2011) [16]. *CYP2C19*2* allele (first reported as m1) is characterized by 681G > A substitution in exon 5 that creates an aberrant splice site and produces a premature stop codon leading to a truncated inactive protein product that lacks the heme-binding region [193]. This allele accounts for 93% of the defective alleles in Caucasians and 75% in Orientals [193,194]. *CYP2C19*3* allele (first reported as m2) is extremely rare in Caucasians; however, it accounts for approximately 25% of all inactive alleles in Orientals. It is characterized by 636G > A substitution in exon 4 that also creates a premature stop codon [195]. Additional nonfunctional, however rare alleles have been described in individuals with decreased ability to metabolize the probe drugs (*CYP2C19*4–*8*) [196–200], while most of the other rare alleles (*CYP2C19*9–*15*) were discovered by direct sequencing and still need to be characterized regarding their function [201].

A novel variant allele, *CYP2C19*17* has been reported. This allele is characterized by two SNPs in the promoter region, –3402C > T and -806C > T, the later is associated with increased transcriptional activity that leads to ultrarapid metabolism of some CYP2C19 substrates [202]. This allele is particularly frequent in Caucasian populations—a frequency of 18% was reported in Swedes and Ethiopians [202], 19.61% in Greeks [203] and 25,1% in healthy German women [204], but it is rare in Oriental populations with a frequency of 1,2–4% in Chinese [194,202] and 1.3% in Japanese [205], indicating that *CYP2C19*17* plays a minor role in Oriental populations.

2.2.5.2 Clinical Implications of CYP2C19 Polymorphism

There is considerable evidence for the clinical significance of *CYP2C19* polymorphism. Among other drugs, CYP2C19 is particularly important for the metabolism of proton pump inhibitor (PPI) omeprazole and related compounds. Altered CYP2C19 activity does not seem to increase the risk for ADRs of PPIs, although 5-fold higher exposure to the drug was observed in PMs compared to EMs of CYP2C19. Several studies reported higher levels of systemic drug exposure and a better pharmacodynamic response (more effective acid suppression) as well as a more favorable therapeutic response (improved duodenal and gastric ulcer healing) in CYP2C19

PMs during treatment with omeprazole and lansoprazole [206,207]. Several studies showed that the efficacy of omeprazole- and lansoprazole-based triple therapies for eradication of *Helicobacter pylori* (*H. pylori*) infection is significantly higher in homozygous or heterozygous carriers of *CYP2C19* deficiency alleles, while the eradication rates of rabeprazole therapy were not dependent on *CYP2C19* genotype [208]. Also in Chinese and Japanese patients treated for gastroesophageal reflux disease (GERD) with rabeprazole, the healing of erosive lesions did not depend on *CYP2C19* genotype [209,210]. Similarly, in GERD patients treated with esomeprazole that is predominantly metabolized by CYP3A4 rather than CYP2C19, the healing rate was not dependent on *CYP2C19* genotype [211].

As *CYP2C19**17* allele was associated with 2-fold decrease in omeprazole disposition due to ultrarapid metabolism in healthy volunteers, homozygous carriers of this allele were reported to be at risk of subtherapeutic drug exposure and therapeutic failure [202,212], however, this allele did not influence the efficacy of *H. pylori* eradication with pantoprazole [213]. This result is in accordance with the observations of previous studies where the presence of *CYP2C19**2* allele had a more pronounced effect on the metabolism of other CYP2C19 substrates, such as escitalopram and omeprazole than did the presence of *CYP2C19**17* allele [214,215].

CYP2C19 also plays an important role in elimination of several antidepressants. In general, CYP2C19 PMs are reported to achieve higher plasma levels of antidepressants than are EMs. Although no simple relationship exists between dosage, plasma levels, and clinical outcome of antidepressants, PMs are more likely to suffer from adverse effects and withdrawal from the treatment. Only a few studies investigated the influence of *CYP2C19**17* allele on the disposition and efficacy of antidepressants. Homozygous carriers of *CYP2C19**17* allele had significantly lower mean serum concentrations of escitalopram than EMs [215], however plasma levels of sertraline were not influenced by *CYP2C19**17* allele [216]. Among 14 different antidepressants, *CYP2C19* genotype based dose adjustments were published for amitryptyline, citalopram, clorimipramine, imipramine, moclobemide, and trimipramine [217]. Overall, regardless of the substrate *CYP2C19,* defective alleles seem to have a greater influence on drug disposition than *CYP2C19**17* allele [216].

Diazepam is partially demethylated by CYP2C19, and the high frequency of mutated alleles in Orientals is probably the reason why such populations have a slower metabolism and are treated with lower doses of diazepam than Caucasians [3].

CYP2C19 also plays an important role in the conversion of clopidrogrel into an active thiol metabolite that inhibits platelet aggregation and is an important part of the treatment for patients with ischemic heart disease. Although several CYP enzymes may be involved in the metabolic activation of clopidogrel, thus far the clinical relevance was reported only for carriers of defective *CYP2C19* alleles [218,219]. Plasma levels of the active metabolite of clopidogrel were one-third lower in healthy carriers of at least one nonfunctional *CYP2C19* allele compared to noncarriers, while among patients with acute coronary syndromes *CYP2C19* polymorphism significantly increased the risk of death from cardiovascular causes [220] and the risk of stent thrombosis [221]. Also among young survivors of acute myocardial infarction, the risk of recurrent arterial thrombotic events was greatly increased in carriers of at least one copy of *CYP2C19*2* allele [222]. Similarly, among patients with acute myocardial infarction, those carrying two nonfunctional *CYP2C19* alleles had a higher rate of subsequent cardiovascular events than did the noncarriers. This effect was particularly marked among the patients undergoing percutaneous coronary intervention [223].

Given the important role of CYP2C19 in the bioactivation of clopidogrel, drugs that inhibit CYP2C19 may also reduce the antiplatelet effect of clopidogrel. Increasing evidence suggests that some proton pump inhibitors inhibit CYP2C19 [224,225] and thus potentially lead to an increased risk of adverse cardiac outcomes and deaths [226]. In fact, among patients receiving acetylsalicylic acid and clopidogrel following acute myocardial infarction, concomitant therapy with proton pump inhibitors other than pantoprazole was associated with a loss of beneficial effects of clopidogrel and increased risk of reinfarction [227]. Despite these findings, it remains to be investigated whether genotyping for *CYP2C19* would help to stratify the risk for adverse events in patients with acute coronary syndrome as many other factors also influence the pharmacodynamic response to clopidogrel [228].

Although genetic variability is the main determinant of the interindividual variability in CYP2C19 activity, other factors such as age, use of interacting drugs, and chronic disease were also shown to contribute to this variability [229–231]. Mild liver disease significantly decreased the capacity to hydroxylate mephenytoin, while metabolic capacity of cytochromes CYP1A2, CYP2D6, and CYP2E1 was compromised only in patients with moderate to severe liver disease [231]. In human hepatocytes inflammatory cytokines downregulate CYP2C19 mRNA expression [232]. Also in patients with congestive heart failure, an inverse relationship between TNF-α and IL6 (interleukin 6) plasma concentrations and the activity of CYP2C19 was reported [233]. Decreased activity of CYP2C19 was also observed in patients with advanced cancer, resulting in a conversion of phenotype to PM in 25–37% of the patients with normal genotype [234,235]. Therefore any attempts to individualize the treatment using genotyping approach would significantly underestimate the number of phenotypical PMs among advanced cancer patients [235]. As CYP2C19 is involved in a disposition of a number of chemotherapeutic agents, cyclophosphamide included [236], decreased activity of this enzyme may influence the efficacy and toxicity of these agents, particularly in Oriental populations.

2.2.5.3 CYP2C19 in Endogenous Metabolism

Similar to other members of CYP2C family, CYP2C19 also metabolizes arachidonic acid to epoxyeicosanoid acids, which are involved in vascular tone and inflammation. Increased circulating levels of inflammatory markers were found in women from the Stanislas cohort homozygous for the defective allele *CYP2C19*2,* and it was suggested that *CYP2C19* may be considered a new candidate gene for cardiovascular risk via inflammation [237]. So far these associations were studied mostly in cardiovascular diseases, but not in other inflammatory processes, such as rheumatoid arthritis. However, a study on leflunomide treated rheumatoid arthritis patients reported that frequencies of polymorphic *CYP2C9* and *CYP2C19* alleles in patients were not significantly higher than in general healthy population [238].

Another clinically important role of CYP2C19 in endogenous metabolism has emerged as CYP2C19 and CYP3A4 were reported to contribute to extraadrenal 21-hydroxylation of progesterone but not 17-hydroxy progesterone. It was proposed that these enzymes may ameliorate mineralocorticoid deficiency, but not glucocorticoid deficiency, in patients with congenital adrenal hyperplasia (CAH) due to 21-hydroxylase (*CYP21A2*) gene mutations. Indeed, one of five patients with a CAH phenotype milder than that predicted by *CYP21A2* genotype was homozygous for *CYP2C19**17* allele [239].

2.2.6 CYP3A Subfamily

The CYP3A subfamily represents the most abundantly expressed CYPs in human liver, as well as in the gut, where they are involved in the metabolism of 50% of all drugs currently on the market [240]. The human CYP3A locus carries four genes and two pseudogenes, probably arising through gene duplication. Only *CYP3A4*, *CYP3A5*, *CYP3A7*, and *CYP3A43* encode active enzymes relevant for drug metabolism.

The CYP3A subfamily accounts for more than 50% of all CYP-dependent drug metabolism, including HMG-CoA reductase inhibitors such as simvastatin and atorvastatin, the immunosuppressants cyclosporine A and tacrolimus, macrolide antibiotics such as erythromycin, antihistamines, and anticancer agents [240].

CYP3A enzymes have similar substrate specificities [241], and most of the drugs that are metabolized by CYP3A enzymes are also substrates of *p*-glycoprotein. Huge interindividual variability in CYP3A expression levels and activity exists. The variability in clearance of CYP3A substrates was greater than 10-fold *in vivo* and around 30-fold *in vitro* [242]. Genetic factors were estimated to account for 70–90% of this variability; however, environmental or endogenous factors may lead to even greater level of variability due to induction or inhibition of the enzyme [243]. Inducers such as rifampicin, anticonvulsants such as carbamazepine or phenytoin, glucocorticoids, and hyperforin in St. John's wort significantly decrease plasma levels of coadministered CYP3A4 substrates, due to increased clearance, and may lead to therapeutic failure. A classical example is decreased effectiveness of oral contraceptives in patients on rifampicin [244]. On the other hand, a number of drugs such as the antifungal ketoconazole, HIV protease inhibitors, some macrolide antibiotics, and antidepressants belonging to selective serotonin reuptake inhibitors and even food constituents such as grapefruit juice inhibit CYP3A4, and when coadministered, significantly increase the plasma levels of CYP3A substrates, resulting in drug toxicity [245]. Because many drugs that are metabolized by CYP3A4 are coadministered, these drug interactions frequently lead to ADRs and seem to be clinically more relevant than genetic polymorphism [246].

2.2.7 CYP3A4

CYP3A4 is the most abundantly expressed CYP in human liver and small intestine, where it accounts for 30–40% of total CYP content. Intestinal CYP3A4 plays a major role in the first-pass metabolism of orally administered drugs. CYP3A4 is also expressed in other parts of gastrointestinal tract, kidney, and pancreas.

2.2.7.1 CYP3A4 Polymorphism

Following observations of the large extent of variability in CYP3A activity as being due to genetic factors [243], a large number of sequencing and phenotype–genotype correlation studies were performed, but they failed to identify a common functional polymorphism, and no correlation was found between the genotype and the phenotype [247]. Most *CYP3A4* alleles occur at low allele frequency (<1–2%) or are prevalent only in specific populations [248]. *In vitro* some alleles lead to absent (**20*), decreased (**8, *11, *13, *17*), or increased activity (**18*), but only limited genotype–phenotype association was observed [249]. The only allele that appears to influence the CYP3A4 expression is the promoter variant *CYP3A4*1B*, characterized by –392A > G polymorphism that is present with 35–67% allele frequency in African-Americans and 2–10% frequency in Caucasians but is absent in Asians. *CYP3A4*18* allele that codes for Leu293Pro substitution was not found in Caucasians, but occurs with an allele frequency of 10% in Chinese. This population specific frequency distribution may result in increased disposition of CYP3A4 substrates in Africans and Asians [250].

2.2.7.2 Clinical Implications of CYP3A4 Polymorphism

In general, it was suggested that genetic variability of CYP3A4 may be of limited importance as a pharmacogenetic marker due to a low frequency of *CYP3A4* polymorphic alleles in Caucasians and a limited genotype–phenotype relationship [249].

CYP3A4 polymorphism seems to play a role in treatment with antiretroviral agents. *CYP3A4*1B* decreased absorption of indinavir, which may be problematic because plasma levels correlate with decrease in viral load [251]. Besides *CYP2B6*, also *CYP2A6* and *CYP3A4* influenced efavirenz pharmacokinetics in HIV patients [252].

CYP3A4 also plays an important role in metabolism of more than 33% of anticancer agents such as docetaxel, irinotecan, etoposide, tamoxifen, and cyclosporine, so cancer treatment may be influenced by *CYP3A4* variability. CYP3A4 was implicated in increased risk of cancer-treatment-related complications, especially secondary malignant neoplasms [253]. Enhanced docetaxel clearance was demonstrated in patients carrying the *CYP3A4*1B* allele, suggesting that these patients may be undertreated and have poorer therapeutic outcome [254]. Cancer treatment with CYP3A4 substrates was also shown to be compromised by drug interactions. In cancer patients treated with docetaxel in combination with the potent CYP3A4 inhibitor ketoconazole, a 49% decrease in docetaxel clearance was found [255]. On the contrary, formation of the cytotoxic irinotecan metabolites was significantly decreased on induction of CYP3A4 [256,257].

2.2.7.3 CYP3A4 in Endogenous Metabolism

CYP3A4 is involved in metabolism of endogenous substrates such as steroid hormones, and bile acids and xenobiotics such as food constituents and environmental pollutants and its polymorphism were frequently studied in relation to cancer risk [258]. Increased metabolism of estrogens and testosterone was observed in *CYP3A4*18* allele *in vitro*, and the presence of this allele was associated with low bone mineral density [259].

2.2.8 CYP3A5

CYP3A5 is the major CYP expressed in kidney, but has also been detected in other extrahepatic tissues [260]. CYP3A5 is expressed in fetal and adult liver in about 25% of Caucasians and more than 50% of African-Americans [261], but the level is usually less than that of CYP3A4. However, because of genetic polymorphism, CYP3A5 may account for more than 50% of CYP3A content in liver in some individuals [262].

2.2.8.1 CYP3A5 Polymorphism

Of 11 polymorphic alleles and 15 variants reported to date [16], *CYP3A5*3* and *CYP3A5*6* alleles result in severely decreased or absent CYP3A5 expression in the liver due to alternative splicing that leads to protein truncation [247,263]. As 80% of Caucasians and 30% of Africans are homozygous for *CYP3A5*3* allele, they do not express CYP3A4 in liver. *CYP3A5*6* allele is found in 15% of African-Americans, but is very rare in Caucasians.

2.2.8.2 Clinical Implications of CYP3A5 Polymorphism

As nonfunctional *CYP3A5* alleles occur with high frequency, they may be of clinical importance for drug treatment; however, it is difficult to predict the impact of *CYP3A5* polymorphism on total CYP3A activity in the liver, due to a large substrate overlap with CYP3A4. In addition, it is difficult to determine the contribution of a particular allele to increased CYP3A activity due to linkage between *CYP3A4*1B* and *CYP3A5*1*.

CYP3A5 polymorphism may be of importance for treatment with immunosuppressive drugs as they have a narrow therapeutic index and exhibit large interpatient variability regarding both pharmacokinetics and pharmacodynamics. In general, the influence of *CYP3A5*1* and *CYP3A5*3* on tacrolimus pharmacokinetics is well established, while data on cyclosporine A and sirolimus disposition are not conclusive [264]. Carriers of *CYP3A5*1* allele associated with hepatic expression of CYP3A5 had significantly lower tacrolimus exposure and more nephrotoxicity within 5 years of kidney transplantation, but it was not possible to determine whether this toxicity is due to increased production of toxic metabolites due to genetic variability in CYP3A5 expression or due to increased exposure to corticosteroids, known inducers of CYP3A enzymes [265]. On the contrary, patients with *CYP3A5*3* showed higher dose-adjusted blood concentrations of tacrolimus [266]. It was shown that an adult renal transplant recipient with a *CYP3A5*1/*3* genotype requires a 1.5 times higher starting dose of tacrolimus compared to *CYP3A5*3* homozygous patients to reach the predefined target exposure and adequate immunosuppression early after transplantation [267].

2.2.9 CYP3A7

CYP3A7 is the major CYP detected in the embryonic, fetal, and newborn liver, although it was detected also in some adult livers, but at much lower levels than CYP3A4. Only a few substrates have been studied for CYP3A7-dependent metabolism, and hydroxylation of dehydroepiandrosterone sulfate (DHEA-S) was suggested to be its most physiologically important role during fetal life [268]. After birth CYP3A7 appears to be silenced, and CYP3A4 expression increases rapidly, reaching 50% of adult levels between 6 and 12 months of age [260,269].

2.2.9.1 CYP3A7 Polymorphism

*CYP3A7*1C* allele was reported to cause persistent CYP3A7 activity during adult life and resulted in nearly 50% reduction in DHEA-S levels in healthy elderly individuals [270]. *CYP3A7*2* allele is characterized by a SNP in exon 11 that leads to Thr409Arg substitution and occurs with an allele frequency of 8% in Caucasians, 17% in Saudi Arabians, 28% in Chinese and 62% in Tanzanians. This allele encoded a functional enzyme with a higher detoxification capacity than *CYP3A7*1* allele, but its impact on fetal drug clearance and endogenous metabolism is not clear. Fetal livers that expressed CYP3A7.2 also expressed CYP3A5 protein, and linkage disequilibrium was found between the *CYP3A7*2* and *CYP3A5*1*. Linkage disequilibrium was also observed between *CYP3A7*1* and *CYP3A5*3*, resulting in CYP3A7.1 but no CYP3A5 expression and lower detoxification capacity [271].

2.2.10 CYP3A43

CYP3A43 shares over 70% amino acid sequence homology with other CYP3A enzymes, but as it represents only 0.1–0.2% of total CYP3A content in adult human liver, it is unlikely to play an important role in drug metabolism. Besides liver, it was found also in testis, kidney, pancreas, and prostate [272,273].

2.2.10.1 CYP3A43 Polymorphism

Of 5 variants reported in CYP3A43, *CYP3A43*2* leads to a frameshift mutation causing a premature stop codon, while *CYP3A43*3* causes amino acid substitution (P340A). The functional role of these mutations remains to be elucidated [274].

2.2.11 CYP1A2

CYP1A2 is expressed mainly in the liver, where it may account for 10–15% of the total CYP content. Large interindividual differences were observed in the metabolic capacity for caffeine, a test substrate for CYP1A2. Although this variability is due mainly to genetic factors as shown by twin studies [275], environmental factors also influence the activity. Smoking is a potent inducer of *CYP1A2* gene, and patients who are smokers would be expected to have a higher rate of CYP1A2-mediated drug disposition.

2.2.11.1 CYP1A2 Polymorphism

In total, 16 different alleles in *CYP1A2* have been reported, with an additional 21 different variants described for *CYP1A2*1* allele [16], but there are no common functional polymorphisms. In smokers, *CYP1A2*1C* (-3860G>A) caused significantly reduced rate of caffeine 3-demethylation [276], while *CYP1A2*1F* (−163C>A) resulted in higher inducibility by smoking [277] or omeprazole [278]. The *CYP1A2*1K* allele (–739, –729T, and –163A) resulted in lower constitutive CYP1A2 activity [279].

2.2.11.2 Clinical Implications of CYP1A2 Polymorphism

CYP1A2 is involved in the metabolism of atypical antipsychotics such as clozapine and olanzepine. As the prevalence of smokers is higher among psychiatric patients than in the general population (around 80% compared to 25%) [280], CYP1A2 was suggested to play an important role in metabolism of atypical antipsychotics, especially in subjects on long-term treatment. Many studies investigated the association of *CYP1A2* polymorphisms with development of tardive dyskinesia, as this is a frequent and potentially irreversible extrapyramidal side effect of long-term antipsychotic treatment, but the results were not concordant. No association was observed in German [281] or Chinese [282] schizophrenia patients, while an association of *CYP1A2*1C* with higher risk for developing tardive dyskinesia was observed among north Indian patients who were smokers and treated only with typical antipsychotics [283].

2.2.12 CYP2A6

CYP2A6 is expressed at medium to low levels in liver, where it accounts for 0.2–13% of total CYP content [24]. It was also detected in lung, trachea, and nasal and oesophageal mucosa. CYP2A6 exhibits large interindividual and interethnic variability in levels of expression and activity, due largely to genetic polymorphisms.

2.2.12.1 CYP2A6 Polymorphism

CYP2A6 is highly polymorphic. It has 78 alleles and variants and many additional SNPs where the haplotype has not yet been determined; however, the frequency of nonfunctional and deficiency alleles is low in Caucasians [284]. *CYP2A6*1B* displays several variants and occurs with an allele frequency of 37.5% in the Japanese population. *CYP2A6*1B1* variant carries gene conversion in the 3′-flanking region and was associated with increased metabolic capacity [276]. The most important defective allele is *CYP2A6*4*, carrying a gene deletion that occurs with a frequency of 7–22% in Asians but only 0.5–1% in Caucasians [285]. Large interindividual variations in the rate of nicotine metabolism were reported within groups of individuals having the same *CYP2A6* genotype possibly due to CYP2B6 also contributing to metabolism [286].

2.2.12.2 Clinical Implications of CYP2A6 Polymorphism

CYP2A6 is the major enzyme involved in oxidation of nicotine to cotinine. As nicotine is primarily responsible for the addictive properties of cigarettes, it is generally accepted that individuals with reduced nicotine metabolism due to low CYP2A6 activity smoke less [287]. A 2009 multicenter study found a rare variant resulting in decreased activity associated with reduced risk of the upper aerodigestive tract cancer [288]. As frequency of defective alleles is higher in Asians compared to Caucasians, they also have lower smoking related cancer risk [289,290]. This may be due to decreased metabolism of procarcinogens from tobacco smoke to carcinogenic tobacco-specific nitrosamines [291]. The effect of nicotine metabolism on risk of cigarette smoking associated health problems such as other cancers and cardiovascular and pulmonary disorders remains to be determined [292–294].

CYP2A6 is also involved in metabolism of clinically important drugs such as coumarin, halothane, valproic acid, and disulfiram. Along with CYP1A2 and CYP2C8, it activates prodrug tegafur to active anticancer drug 5′-fluorouracil [295,296]. As patients with defective *CYP2A6* alleles exhibit significantly decreased plasma levels of 5′-fluorouracil, genotyping for *CYP2A6*4* allele was proposed to increase the efficacy of treatment with tegafur in Japanese patients [297].

2.2.13 CYP2B6

CYP2B6 has long been considered to have a minor role in drug metabolism; however, the list of clinically relevant substrates of this enzyme is growing. CYP2B6 is expressed mainly in liver, where it constitutes about 3–5% of the total microsomal P450 pool [298–301], but it was also detected at lower levels in extrahepatic tissues, including intestine, kidney, lung, skin, and the brain [9,299,302]. CYP2B6 expression levels in human livers vary 20–250-fold between individuals, while CYP2B6 activity in liver microsomes varies more than 100-fold [303–305]. Transcriptional regulation is considered to be one of the major contributors to this variability. CYP2B6 is highly inducible by phenobarbital-type compounds as well as many other typical inducers of CYP3A4 in a dose-dependent manner [306–308]. Constitutive androstane receptor (CAR), pregnane X receptor (PXR), glucocorticoid receptor (GR), and vitamin D receptor were shown to mediate transcriptional activation in response to xenobiotic exposure [309].

2.2.13.1 CYP2B6 Polymorphism

Besides the differences in gene regulation, genetic polymorphisms largely contribute to interindividual variability in CYP2B6 activity. CYP2B6 is highly polymorphic, and currently 29 alleles and a number of variants have been described [16]. Several SNPs cause amino acid substitutions and are found at frequencies up to 30% in Caucasian populations [301], but are less frequent in Japanese [310]. Most of these SNPs were associated with moderately decreased expression and activity [301]; however, some novel nonsynonymous SNPs actually result in phenotypic null alleles [311]. Several SNPs associated with polymorphic *CYP2B6* expression were also identified in the promoter region and in the introns [312].

*CYP2B6*4* characterized by amino acid substitution Lys262Arg was associated with increased clearance of the probe drug bupropion [313]. One of the most frequently studied alleles is *CYP2B6*6* characterized by two SNPs 516G>T in exon 4 and 785A>G in exon 5, that lead to amino acid substitutions Gln172His and Lys262Arg. It was shown that 516G>T leads to aberrant splicing, reduced levels of CYP2B6 mRNA that lacks exons 4–6 and to decreased CYP2B6 expression [314,315]. The activity of this allele seems to be substrate-dependent, as it was higher for cyclophosphamide [316] and lower for efavirenz [317,318].

Besides genetic polymorphisms, CYP2B6 activity also varies according to sex and ethnicity. CYP2B6 activity was 3.6- and 5.0-fold higher in Hispanic females than in Caucasian or African-American females [312].

2.2.13.2 Clinical Implications of CYP2B6 Polymorphism

Whereas CYP2B6 participates in the disposition of a few precarcinogens and some important therapeutic drugs such as artemisinin, ketamine, propofol, bupropion, and the HIV1 reverse transcriptase inhibitors nevirapine and efavirenz, it is involved in the metabolic activation of the cytotoxic prodrugs cyclophosphamide, ifosfamide, thiotepa, and procarbazine. Although CYP2B6 contributes only 20% to ifosfamide activation (compared to 40% of the prodrug activated by CYP3A4), it contributes more than 80% to cyclophosphamide activation (compared to the 4% share of CYP3A4) [319,320]. Regarding the important role of CYP2B6 in the metabolism of many clinically important drugs, polymorphisms of this enzyme are likely to affect their pharmacokinetics. In addition, substrates such as cyclophosphamide, ifosfamide, anti-HIV drug efavirenz, and antimalarial artemisinin can affect their clearance or toxicity as they accelerate their own metabolism due to induction of CYP2B6 [308,321], while the anticancer agent thiotepa inhibits CYP2B6 [322].

Many studies showed that *CYP2B6*6* carriers have reduced capacity to metabolize the probe drug bupropion [323] and efavirenz (EFV) [317,318]. This allele is particularly common in Africans (frequency close to 50%) [324] and more common in African-Americans (20–30%) than in European Americans (3%) and is associated with significantly greater efavirenz plasma exposure and central nervous system (CNS) side effects during HIV therapy [325]. The *CYP2B6*6* allele occurred at a high frequency of 49% in HIV patients from Zimbabwe and was associated with high EFV concentrations. Predictions showed that a 35% dose reduction would maintain drug exposure within the therapeutic range in homozygous *CYP2B6*6* patients [326] and indeed successful HIV1 suppression and reduced EFV-associated CNS symptoms were achieved with reduced dose in a clinical trial [327]. There is increasing evidence that *CYP2B6* genotyping may be useful to complement an individualization strategy based on plasma drug determinations to increase the safety and tolerability of EFV [328].

Regarding the activation of cyclophosphamide, homozygotes for *CYP2B6*6* showed significantly higher clearance and shorter half-life of the drug than did heterozygotes and homozygotes for *CYP2B6*1* [316]. The potency of cyclophosphamide activation was also affected by polymorphisms in the promoter region and introns in the *CYP2B6* and was related to leukocytopenia in Japanese patients with malignant lymphoma or breast cancer [329].

Stimulants such as ecstasy [330] and nicotine [331] are partly metabolized by CYP2B6, and *CYP2B6*6* allele was associated with faster nicotine and cotinine clearance, especially among individuals exhibiting decreased activity *CYP2A6* genotypes [286]. CYP2B6 is also the primary enzyme involved in the metabolism of the antidepressant and antismoking drug bupropion; therefore this drug is preferred for both *in vitro* and *in vivo* phenotyping [332,333]. Carriers of *CYP2B6*6* allele treated with bupropion had higher abstinence rates than did placebo-treated smokers at the end of treatment as well as at the 6-month follow-up [334].

2.2.14 CYP2E1

CYP2E1 metabolizes a small number of clinically important drugs such as halogenated anesthetics (enflurane, halothane, isoflurane, methoxyflurane, sevoflurane), acetaminophen (paracetamol), and theophylline [240]. CYP2E1 is of greater toxicological than clinical importance because of its role in the metabolism and toxicity of alcohol and solvents. Besides alcohol dehydrogenase, CYP2E1 is the second major enzyme involved in ethanol oxidation to acetaldehyde, a highly reactive and toxic metabolite. Reactive species are generated in this process and may contribute to liver injury and other alcohol-induced diseases [335]. CYP2E1 also activates many low-molecular-weight xenobiotics (nitrosamines, styrene, aniline, benzene, and many other solvents, especially halogenated hydrocarbons) to hepatotoxic or carcinogenic products [336].

In addition to human liver, CYP2E1 is expressed in other tissues, including brain [337]. Regulation of CYP2E1 expression and activity is complex and involves transcriptional activation, mRNA stabilization, increased mRNA translation efficiency, and decreased protein degradation [338]. CYP2E1 is induced by ethanol. This induction is accompanied with the proliferation of the endoplasmic reticulum that results in enhanced activity of other P450s and in tolerance to other drugs due to increased metabolism. CYP2E1 is also induced by isoniazid. In livers of patients with chronic hepatitis C viral infection, mRNAs encoding CYP2E1 were downregulated, due at least in part to the elevated production of proinflammatory cytokines [339]. Moderate to severe liver disease also decreased CYP2E1 enzyme activity [231].

Interindividual variability was observed in the expression of hepatic CYP2E1 in humans [337]. Subjects also differed with respect to CYP2E1 inducibility by ethanol [340]. Genetic diversity of CYP2E1 may be increased by alternative splicing. Alternatively spliced mRNA transcripts were detected in cancer cell lines and were predicted to lead to truncated non-functional proteins [341].

2.2.14.1 CYP2E1 Polymorphism

The *CYP2E1* gene is not very polymorphic as only 13 variants were described to date [16]. Especially the coding region seems very conserved. Among the three alleles that code for an amino acid substitution—*CYP2E1*2* (Arg76His), *CYP2E1*3* (Val389Ile), and *CYP2E1*4* (Val179Ile)—reduced protein levels and catalytic activity were observed only in *CYP2E1*2* [342–344].

Several polymorphisms have been identified in the 5′-flanking region, including a repeat polymorphism consisting of either six (*CYP2E1*1C*) or eight (*CYP2E1*1D*) sequence repeats. Although this repeat polymorphism had no effect on constitutive expression [345], increased activity was observed after alcohol exposure and in obese subjects with eight repeats [346]. Other polymorphisms identified so far do not appear to be of functional importance [343].

2.2.14.2 Clinical Implications of CYP2E1 Polymorphism

Although the *CYP2E1*2* polymorphism has been widely studied in toxicogenetics, especially in regard to its role in alcohol metabolism, oxidative stress, and susceptibility to alcohol-related diseases and cancer, the results of most of these studies are not conclusive and are not reviewed here.

Regarding drug treatment, CYP2E1 may play an important role in the metabolism of anesthetics [347] and acetaminophen (paracetamol) toxicity [348]. As *CYP2E1* genotype influenced acetaminophen metabolism [349], genetic variability may increase the risk of developing liver failure on acetaminophen overdose.

CYP2E1 participates in metabolism of the antituberculosis drug isoniazid (besides NAT2), and many studies investigated the association between *CYP2E1* polymorphism and isoniazid-induced hepatotoxicity, but with conflicting results. Two studies demonstrated higher risk for hepatotoxicity in patients homozygous for wild-type allele [350,351]; but no association between polymorphic alleles and isoniazid-induced hepatotoxicity has been observed in more recent studies [352–354].

Theophylline is partly metabolized by CYP2E1 (besides CYP2A1), and hydroxylation of theophylline was reported to be affected by *CYP2E1* promoter polymorphism in asthma patients [355].

2.2.14.3 CYP2E1 in Endogenous Metabolism

It has been proposed that CYP2E1 enables ketone utilization [356,357], so it may have an important physiological role in starvation, obesity, and diabetes. CYP2E1 was upregulated in diabetic patients, and the clearance of several CYP2E1 substrates was higher in obese than nonobese individuals [358].

2.3 NON-P450 PHASE I ENZYMES

2.3.1 Flavin-Containing Monoxygenases

Flavin-containing monoxygenases (FMOs) constitute a family of microsomal flavoproteins containing a single flavin adenine dinucleotide (FAD). They catalyze monoxygenation of many nitrogen-, sulfur-, and other nucleophile-containing xenobiotics, including drugs [359].

Flavin-containing monoxygenases represent the second most important monoxygenase system, besides P450s, involved in xenobiotic metabolism. There are many similarities as well as differences between both classes of enzymes. Both have similar intracellular and tissue localization and catalyze monoxygenation reactions, but the catalytic cycle of both monoxygenases is different and FMOs do not require a reductase to transfer electrons from NADPH. Despite overlapping substrate specificities, different metabolites are usually produced. In addition, biotransformation reactions catalyzed by FMOs mostly decrease the pharmacological activity and/or toxicity of the compound. In contrast to P450s, FMOs are not inducible by xenobiotics, so the risk for ADRs due to drug–drug interactions may be low for drugs metabolized by FMOs, and the contribution of FMOs in drug metabolism may be advantageous [360].

Although it was proposed that FMOs may play an important role in drug metabolism, their role is not as widely documented as that of P450s and clinical studies are lacking. It was shown that FMOs metabolize endogenous substrates such as biogenic amines and trimethylamine, lipoic acid, and sulfhydryls, such as cysteamine and methionine, but the physiological role of FMOs is not elucidated [359].

The nomenclature for human FMOs is similar to that for P450s and is based on nucleotide sequence similarities. Genes with more than 82% sequence similarity are grouped within a family, and the italicized abbreviation *FMO* is used to designate a gene or an allele [361].

Six *FMO* gene families, each with a single member, have been identified in humans, along with five pseudogenes. The similarity in exon/intron organization of *FMO* genes suggests that the FMO family members may have arisen from gene duplication events [362].

The functional diversity of FMOs is determined by their developmental- and tissue-specific expression pattern [363]. There is also considerable interindividual and interethnic variability in the levels of FMOs. Most of this variability is presumed to be due to genetic variability, as these enzymes are not readily induced by xenobiotics. SNPs contributing to genetic variability in human FMOs as missense, nonsense, deletion, and truncation mutants that can affect FMO function have been reported [364–366]. The major alleles of *FMO2* and *FMO6* encode nonfunctional proteins due to a nonsense mutation and splice-site abnormalities, respectively [367,368]. Splice variants were also detected in other FMOs [369].

2.3.2 FMO1

Human FMO1 represents the major FMO in fetal liver, where its activity is approximately 32% of CYP3A7's, but it is not detectable in adult liver [370,371]. In adults, FMO1 represents the most prevalent FMO in kidney. It is also expressed at points of xenobiotic entry in the body such as intestinal mucosa, esophagus, and nasal mucosa [372]. FMO1 was reported to participate (besides several P450s) in the metabolism of disulfiram, an aldehyde dehydrogenase inhibitor used to support the treatment of alcohol dependence [373]. FMO1 may also play a role in extrahepatic metabolism of pesticides [374].

2.3.2.1 FMO1 Poymorphisms and Their Clinical Implications

Several SNPs were reported in *FMO1*. Many of them are synonymous or do not affect catalytic activity, but some SNPs leading to missense or nonsense mutations were described as well [375]. Because FMO1 is the major form in fetal human liver, these variants may be important in pediatric drug disposition. They may also contribute to altered metabolism in fetus on maternal exposure to xenobiotics such as pesticides [374].

2.3.3 FMO2

2.3.3.1 FMO2 Poymorphisms and Their Clinical Implications

Although FMO2 represents the dominant FMO expressed in adult lung [376], most Caucasians and Asians are homozygous for *FMO2*2A* allele, which codes for Gln472Stop truncation mutation, so they do not express a functional protein [367]. However, around 26% of African-Americans, 7% of Puerto Ricans, and 2% of Mexicans carry one normal *FMO2*1* allele and express a functional full-length protein [377,378]. These individuals may be at higher risk for pulmonary toxicity of chemicals containing thioureas [379], but on the other hand they may be protected against toxicity of some thioether organophosphate insecticides metabolized by FMO2 to sulfoxides that are less toxic than oxon metabolites produced by P450s [380].

FMO2 also catalyzes bioactivation of second-generation antituberculosis drugs such as ethionamide and thiacetazone. It was proposed that carriers of *FMO2*1* allele might suffer from decreased antimicrobial effect or even toxicity of these drugs. FMO2 variability may be clinically important in regions such as sub-Saharan Africa, where tuberculosis presents a major health problem and the frequency of *FMO2*1* allele carriers is high [381].

2.3.4 FMO3

Human FMO3 is responsible for the majority of FMO-mediated hepatic metabolism as it is the major FMO present in adult human liver, with levels approaching 0.5% of the total microsomal and 60% of the CYP3A protein levels [382]. FMO3 levels in lung, kidney, fetal liver, and small intestine are much lower [383]. In brain, FMO3 levels are less than 1% of levels in adult liver [384].

2.3.4.1 FMO3 Poymorphisms and Their Clinical Implications

Human microsomal FMO3 levels have been reported to differ by 2–20-fold, presumably due to genetic variability [371,382]. Large interethnic differences exist in the distribution of *FMO3* polymorphisms [385]. In total, 283 *FMO3* SNPs have been listed so far in the GeneCards database; 25 of them lead to amino acid substitution, and five are nonsense and/or frameshift mutations [386]. *FMO3* promoter haplotype variants that result either in increase or in decrease of transcriptional activity were also reported [387].

A phenotype–genotype correlation was observed and in particular missense and nonsense *FMO3* mutations (e.g., Pro153Leu, Met66Ile, Glu305Stop) were shown to cause severe deficiency in metabolism of trimethylamine (TMA), derived from dietary precursors such as choline, to the odorless TMA *N*-oxide [364]. Homozygous individuals may excrete as much as 90% of dietary TMA unmetabolized in their urine, sweat, and breath, and they suffer from the characteristic fish-like odor, thus trimethylaminuria is also called "fish-like odor syndrome" [388,389]. Between 0.1% and 1% of Caucasians suffer from this disease, however, a larger prevalence is observed in some parts of the world, especially in the tropics [388,389]. Many individuals with trimethylaminuria manifest additional metabolic and psychosocial symptomatology that might be due to a disturbance of endogenous metabolism of biogenic amines. Adverse reactions from tyramine, other amines, and sulfur-containing drugs were observed in several patients with this condition [388]. It has been suggested that tricyclic antidepressants may potentiate the symptoms in patients suffering from mild or severe trimethylaminuria, but no clinical evidence has been published.

It was proposed that FMO3 is the most important FMO in drug metabolism, but clinical studies assesing the impact of *FMO3* polymorphisms on drug metabolism are scarce. FMO3 catalyzes tamoxifen *N*-oxygenation, which represents a detoxication pathway, in contrast to P450-mediated tamoxifen activation [390]. As it was suggested that the benefits of tamoxifen treatment may depend on the rate of metabolic activation versus detoxication, *FMO3* polymorphisms may influence breast cancer therapy and chemoprevention [391].

Variability of *FMO3* may also influence the benefits of chemoprevention with the nonsteroidal antiinflammatory drug (NSAID) sulindac. Among patients with familial adenomatous polyposis, carriers of SNPs that decrease FMO3 activity were shown to benefit more from the chemopreventive efect of sulindac sulfide [392,393].

Caffeine oxidation in healthy subjects and metabolism of clozapine in schizophrenia patients were not influenced by common *FMO3* SNPs [394]. More recently, *FMO3* polymorphisms have been associated with the symptomatology of schizophrenia and adverse effects of olanzepine treatment, but associations with different SNPs were observed in different ethnic groups [395].

2.3.5 FMO4, FMO5, and FMO6

Both FMO4 and FMO5 are expressed in adult liver and to a lesser extent in kidney, fetal liver, small intestine, lung, and also brain. All three FMOs exhibit genetic polymorphism [375]. Although FMO5 represents $\geq$50% of the total FMO transcripts in adult human liver, the role of FMO5 in drug or chemical metabolism remains to be established [382,383]. It is, however, believed that FMO4 and FMO5 do not contribute significantly to drug metabolism in humans as they display very restricted substrate specificity [383,396]. On the basis of sequence analysis of *FMO6* 70% amino acid sequence identity with human FMO3 was predicted, but alternative splicing creates shorter transcripts that do not encode a functional enzyme [368].

2.3.6 Quinone Oxidoreductases

Quinone oxidoreductases are cytosolic flavoproteins that catalyze metabolic reduction of a variety of quinone compounds, including bioreductive chemotherapeutic drugs, such as mitomycin C and anthracyclines, and may thus play a role in cancer chemotherapy [397]. Two quinone oxidoreductases with similar substrate specificities were identified, however, they differ in their requirement for the electron donating cofactors. NAD(P)H:quinone oxidoreductase 1 (NQO1) can use either NADH or NADPH [397], while NRH:quinone oxidoreductase 2 (NQO2) requires dihydronicotinamide riboside (NRH) as the electron donor [398]. As both enzymes catalyze the two-electron reduction of quinones to hydroquinones, which can be removed by conjugation, NQOs may protect from the formation of more reactive semiquinones and reactive-oxygen species (ROS) produced by the one-electron reduction catalyzed by P450s [399]. Of both enzymes, NQO1 is better characterized than NQO2.

2.3.7 NQO1

NQO1 is expressed in all types of tissues, but inter- and intraindividual variability in enzyme activity has been observed [400]. *NQO1* gene is expressed at higher levels in several tumor tissue types, including liver and colon, as compared to normal tissues of similar origin, thus it may serve as the target of bioreductive chemotherapeutic drugs [401–403]. *NQO1* gene expression is induced as a part of the oxidative stress-triggered defense mechanism that includes the coordinated induction of >24 other genes. Also, prooxidant drugs, such as anthracyclines, induce NQO1 activity [404].

In general, NQO1 provides protection against toxicity of quinones, free-radical damage, oxidative stress, and neoplasia, but on the other hand it activates cytotoxic antitumor quinones such as mitomycin C, leading to the production of ROS and DNA alkylation [405].

2.3.7.1 NQO1 Polymorphism

In general, *NQO1* is not highly polymorphic and only two functional SNPs have been identified so far. The *NQO1*2* allele carries a 609C>T SNP in exon 6 that codes for Pro187Ser substitution. Ubiquitination and rapid degradation of the variant protein lead to deficiency in NQO1 enzyme activity [406]. Significant interethnic differences in *NQO1*2* allele frequencies were observed. Approximately 5% of Caucasians and African-Americans and around 20% of Asians may be homozygous and completely lack NQO1 activity, while a further 20–25% of Caucasians or Africans and 34–52% of Asians may be heterozygous for this allele and have low to intermediate NQO1 activity [407,408]. The *NQO1*3* allele carries 465C>T SNP in exon 4 and codes for Arg139Trp substitution, associated with reduced enzyme activity [409]. The frequency of this allele in Caucasians and Asians is around 5% and 4%, respectively [408].

2.3.7.2 Clinical Implications of NQO1 Polymorphism

As NQO1 plays an important role in the metabolism of bioreductive chemotherapeutic drugs and elevated NQO1 activity was observed in certain tumors, it has been proposed that *NQO1* genotyping might help in the selection of patients who would benefit most from a specific anticancer regimen. In agreement with these suggestions, reduced tumor NQO1 activity and decreased survival were observed in carriers of *NQO1*2* compared to noncarriers treated for disseminated peritoneal cancer with intraperitoneal mitomycin C perfusion [410]. However, in women with metastatic breast cancer *NQO1* polymorphism was not associated with the efficacy or toxicity of the sequentially administered low-dose mitomycin C and irinotecan [411].

No association was found between the *NQO1*2* polymorphism and the risk of anthracycline-related congestive heart failure [412,413]; however, in independent studies this polymorphism increased the risk of secondary malignant neoplasms after treatment for childhood acute lymphoblastic leukemia [414,415].

Studies of the role of *NQO1* polymorphism in the risk for tardive dyskinesia during long-term antipsychotic treatment are still inconclusive: the initial study showed an association that was not confirmed in the meta-analysis of five later studies [416].

Although NQO1 participates in the reduction of vitamin K to vitamin K hydroquinone [417], no association was observed between *NQO1* polymorphism and warfarin dose requirement [418,419].

2.3.7.3 NQO1 in Endogenous Metabolism

Besides its role in the cellular defense against electrophilic and oxidative stress, NQO1 has multiple physiological functions [420] that might be influenced by its genetic variability. It is involved in the reduction of CoQ [421], in the maintenance of intracellular levels of bioactive vitamin E, and in the reduction of vitamin K [417]. NQO1 may also be involved in scavenging superoxide within the cell and may influence p53-dependent stress responses by p53 stabilization [422].

2.3.8 NQO2

NQO2 is the second member of quinone oxidoreductase family of proteins. Similar to NQO1, NQO2 is also expressed in all types of tissues [423], and variability in NQO2 activity has been observed in tumor tissues. NQO2 was downregulated in tumor hepatic tissue [403], but its expression was detected in superficial bladder tumors and in intraperitoneal metastases in ovarian cancer [424].

Despite 54% homology with human NQO1 [425], NQO2 has little endogenous enzyme activity. The addition of its electron donor NRH potentiates its activity, so it may be considered a potential therapeutic target in tumors expressing NQO2 [398,424]. More recently, NQO2 was shown to play a role in mediating the antiproliferative effects of resveratrol, a grape-derived polyphenol under intensive study for its potential in cancer prevention [426]. The off-target binding of Abl kinase inhibitor imatinib to the active site of NQO2 has been documented, but potential implications of this binding for the treatment of chronic myelogenous leukemia patients are not known [427].

2.3.8.1 NQO2 Polymorphisms and Their Clinical Implications

Human *NQO2* gene is highly polymorphic, but most of the polymorphisms are located in the promoter region or do not lead to amino acid substitutions [428]. The 29-bp (basepair) insertion/deletion polymorphism in the promoter region resulted in a differential expression of NQO2. Higher NQO2 expression and increased susceptibility to Parkinson's disease was observed in carriers of the allele without the 29-bp insertion [429,430]. This promoter polymorphism is highly linked with the 14055T>C SNP in exon 3, resulting in Phe47Leu substitution and lower NQO2 enzyme activity relative to wild-type allele. It was proposed that tumors homozygous for this polymorphism may be unresponsive to some bioreductive anticancer agents [424]. NQO2 polymorphisms were also associated with clozapine-induced agranulocytosis in schizophrenia patients [431].

2.3.8.2 NQO2 in Endogenous Metabolism

Information on the physiological role of NQO2 is scarce. NQO2 binds melatonin (MT3 receptor), but its function in central control of circadian rhythm is not known [432]. Deficiency of NQO2 may influence TNF signalling [433] as well as p53-dependent stress responses [434,435].

2.3.9 Esterases

Esterases are hydrolysis enzymes that split an ester into an acid and an alcohol. A wide range of esterases exist that differ in their substrate specificity, protein structure, and biological function [436]. Most pharmacogenetic information is available on carboxylesterases, butyrylcholinesterases, and paraoxonases, so only these enzymes will be reviewed.

2.3.10 Carboxylesterases (CES)

Carboxylesterases (CES) constitute a multigene family that may have evolved from a common ancestral gene. According to the sequence alignment of the encoding genes, they were classified into five major groups displaying 80% sequence identity within a group (ranging from CES1 to CES5) and several subgroups. The majority of CESs that have been identified belong to the CES1 or CES2 family [437]. CES3 shares about 40% sequence identity with CES1 and CES2 [438].

Carboxylesterases are localized in the endoplasmic reticulum of many tissues. CES1 and CES2 expression is the highest in liver, where they play an important role in systemic clearance of esters. CES1, but not CES2, is expressed in monocytes/macrophages. CES1 also plays an important role in renal clearance, while CES2 plays a role in the clearance of orally administered drugs through the small intestine and colon. CES3 expression is highest in liver, followed by colon and small intestine [439]. A large interindividual variability in CES expression was observed in both normal and tumor tissue. Approximately 6% of total CES2 transcripts in colon tissue were found to be alternatively spliced to inactive CES2Δ [458–473] variant that lacked irinotecan hydrolase activity [440].

Carboxylesterases efficiently hydrolyze a variety of xenobiotics and endogenous substrates with ester, thioester, or amide bonds to more soluble acid, alcohol, and amine products and are involved in drug metabolism and xenobiotic detoxication [439]. CES1 and CES2 differ in their substrate specificity. CES1 acts on structurally distinct compounds, but prefers substrates with a small alcohol group and large acyl group. In contrast, CES2 mainly hydrolyzes substrates with a large alcohol group and small acyl group [441]. This finding is in agreement with reports that several angiotensin-converting enzyme (ACE) inhibitors that are ethyl esters with large acyl groups are hydrolyzed by CES1, while the local anesthetic procaine and the anticholinergic drug oxybutynin with large alcohol substitutes are substrates for CES2 [442]. CES1 and CES2 are both involved in hydrolysis of heroin, but the methyl ester of cocaine is hydrolyzed by CES1, and benzoyl esters of cocaine are hydrolyzed by CES2 and butyrylcholinesterase [443].

Carboxylesterases play an important role in metabolic activation of prodrugs that are ester derivatives of therapeutic agents [441]. Although CES1, CES2, and CES3 all metabolize irinotecan (CPT11) and its oxidative metabolites to the active metabolite SN38, a potent topoisomerase I inhibitor, CES2 showed the highest catalytic activity and CES3, the lowest [438].

2.3.10.1 CES1 Polymorphisms and Their Clinical Implications

Significant interindividual variability was observed in the disposition of some of the CES1 substrates, and polymorphisms were identified in *CES1* gene that can lead to clinically significant alteration in pharmacokinetics and drug responses to CES1 substrates. In the *CES1* promoter region, –816A > C substitution resulted in increased transcriptional activity and enhanced antihypertensive response to imidapril, a prodrug for ACE inhibitor [444]. The polymorphic allele was later shown to be closely linked to the haplotype with two putative Sp1 binding sites and higher trancription activity as compared to the major haplotype withouth any Sp1 binding sites [445].

More recently, two functional polymorphisms were identified in the CES1 coding region. The 428G > A transition in exon 4 codes for Gly143Glu substitution and leads to severely reduced CES1 hydrolytic activity. The frequency of the polymorphic 143Glu allele was reported to be 3.7%, 4.3%, 2.0%, and 0% in white, black, Hispanic, and Asian populations, respectively. A rare 1-bp deletion (780delT) in exon 6 results in a frameshift (Asp260fs) and premature truncation of the protein that has completely lost hydrolytic activity [446]. Both CES1 variants were recently shown to be deficient regarding activation of the antihypertensive prodrug trandolapril [447]. Both variants also result in impaired activation of the antiviral prodrug oseltamivir, widely used in the treatment and prophylaxis of influenza A and B as well as avian influenza [448].

2.3.10.2 CES1 in Endogenous Metabolism

As CES1 has been implicated in hydrolysis of stored cholesterol esters in macrophage foam cells and in release of free cholesterol for high-density lipoprotein-mediated cholesterol efflux [449], it might play a role in cholesterol homeostasis and athersoclerosis [450].

2.3.11 Butyrylcholinesterase

Two types of cholinesterases exist, which differ in their tissue distribution, substrate specificity, and sensitivity to various inhibitors. Acetylcholinesterase (AChE) is present mainly in muscles and nervous tissue and has a very specialized function in neural transmission. Butyrylcholinesterase (BChE) is produced in liver and is present in plasma and all the tissues and participates in drug metabolism. BChE hydrolyses the neuromuscular blocking agents, such as succinylcholine and mivacurium, used during general anaesthesia. In the 1960s, it was first recognized that the abnormal response to the muscle relaxant drug succinylcholine administered to surgery patients to facilitate tracheal intubation is due to an inherited alteration in serum butyrylcholinesterase [451] (for more detailed discussion, see Chapter 1).

2.3.11.1 BCHE Polymorphisms and Their Clinical Implications

Until now more than 60 different variants have been reported to code for enzymes with absent or significantly decreased activity. People with *BCHE* variants experience an extensively prolonged apnea in response to muscle relaxants [452,453].

2.3.11.2 BChE in Endogenous Metabolism

The physiological role of BChE is not clear; however, the recently developed BCHE knockout mouse model might help to unravel some of its roles in metabolism and disease [454]. In elderly nondemented individuals the presence of reduced-activity butyrylcholinesterase variants correlated with preserved attentional performance and reduced rate of cognitive decline, so it was proposed that besides acetylcholinesterase, butyrylcholinesterase also plays a role in attention span and memory [455]. It has been proposed that butyrylcholinesterase genotyping may contribute to pharmacogenetics-based treatment of dementia, as dementia patients with normal butyrylcholinesterase showed the highest improvement in attention span during cholinesterase inhibitor therapy [456]. Similarly, female patients with normal BChE benefited more from rivastigmine treatment for Alzheimer's disease [455], while patients with BChE deficiency are expected to be intolerant of standard doses of anti-Alzheimer's drugs, such as donepezil [457].

2.3.12 Paraoxonases

Paraoxonases (PONs) belong to arylesterases and share no sequence similarity with carboxyesterases or cholinesterases. Three esterases with over 80% of deduced aminoacid sequence similarity belong to this family: PON1, PON2, and PON3 [458]. PON1 and PON3 are expressed in liver and excreted in blood, where they associate with high-density lipoprotein (HDL) particles [459]. PON2 is not present in blood, but is expressed widely in a number of tissues, including liver, lungs, brain, and heart [460].

Besides displaying paraoxonase activity, which is important for metabolism of organophosphates (paraoxon and diazoxon), warfare agents (soman and sarin), and aromatic esters (phenylacetate), PON1 also has arylesterase activity and hydrolyzes a large number of aromatic and aliphatic lactones, such as statin lactones (simvastatin and lovastatin) and the diuretic spironolactone [461]. PON1 may thus play an important role in the disposition of dietary lactones. PON2 and PON3 lack paraoxonase activity, but they share the lactonase activity of PON1 [462]. PON1 is the most widely investigated and best understood enzyme of the paraoxonase family.

2.3.12.1 PON1 Polymorphisms and Their Clinical Implications

Expression levels and activity of PON1 are largely determined by common polymorphisms in the PON1 gene. Among polymorphisms identified in the promoter region of the human *PON1* gene, the –107C > T SNP influenced PON1 expression and serum levels [463].

Two SNPs that result in amino acid substitution were reported in *PON1*. The first codes for Leu55Met substitution; however, its influence of PON1 protein levels is due largely to linkage with –107C > T SNP in the promoter region [464]. The Gln192Arg substitution had no effect of PON1 esterase activity, while its influence on paraoxonase activity was substrate-specific [465].

PON1 may be an important effect modifier of the success of the statin treatment. A reciprocal interaction was observed between statins and PON1; statins were found to influence PON1 activity, concentration, and gene expression, while *PON1* genotypes significantly predicted changes of HDL cholesterol during statin treatment in a number of populations [466].

Two noncoding SNPs (rs854548 and rs854555) in *PON1* were associated with the response to anti-TNF treatment in a recent genomewide association study in rheumatoid arthritis patients prospectively followed after beginning anti-TNF therapy with adalimumab, etanercept, or infliximab, but the mechanism of this interaction remains to be clarified [467].

2.3.12.2 PON1 in Endogenous Metabolism

As PON1 is believed to attenuate the oxidation of LDL, it may thus participate in cardiovascular protection, but epidemiological studies reported conflicting results [466,468]. *PON1* polymorphisms may also influence the risk of diabetic complications [469].

2.3.13 Epoxide Hydrolases (EHs)

Epoxide hydrolases (EHs) are a special class of hydrolases that transform endogenous and exogenous epoxides to usually less reactive and less mutagenic diols. These reactions are particulary important for detoxification of the chemically reactive epoxides that arise from the oxidative metabolism of endogenous compounds and xenobiotics, including P450 reactions [470]. Five epoxide hydrolases that differ in molecular weight, subcellular localization, and substrate specificity have been identified: microsomal EH (EPHX1), soluble EH (EPHX2), a soluble hepoxilin A (3) hydrolase, leukotriene A(4) hydrolase, and microsomal cholesterol 5,6-oxide hydrolase [471]. The last three enzymes have very limited and unique substrate specificities and do not participate in drug metabolism.

2.3.14 Microsomal Epoxide Hydrolase (EPHX1)

Microsomal epoxide hydrolase (EPHX1 or mEH) metabolizes a broad array of epoxide substrates, including epoxide metabolites of certain antiepileptic medications, such as phenytoin and carbamazepine, and many environmental epoxides, such as those derived from polycyclic aromatic hydrocarbons (PAHs) [472]. Their association with cancer risk and xenobiotic toxicity has been extensively investigated in epidemiological studies, but these studies are not reviewed here.

EPHX1 has a broad tissue distribution and substrate specificity [473]. The highest concentrations are found in liver, gonads, kidneys, lungs, and bronchial epithelial cells [474]. EPHX1 is inducible, and an increase in its enzyme activity was observed in tuberculosis patients treated with rifampicin, ethambutol, and isoniazid [475].

2.3.14.1 EPHX1 Polymorphisms and Their Clinical Implications

EPHX1 is highly polymorphic. Although more than 100 SNPs have been identified in the *EPHX1* gene region, only a few are characterized and show effects on hydrolase activity *in vitro*. The 337T > C SNP in exon 3 results in Tyr113His substitution and decreased enzyme activity, while 416A > G in exon 4 leads to His139Arg substitution and increased enzyme activity [476]

Clinical studies investigating the implications of *EPHX1* polymorphism in drug treatment are scarce. Both functional SNPs influenced the maintenance dose of carbamazepine in patients treated for epilepsy [477], but were not associated with risk of adverse reactions to anticonvulsants [478,479].

Initial observations that homozygotes for *EPHX1* 139Arg polymorphism require higher warfarin doses than do noncarriers [480] were not replicated, and *EPHX1* polymorphism was not associated with warfarin dose requirement in larger studies [418].

Variability in *EPHX1* may also have implications for lung cancer treatment as it influenced EPHX1 expression levels and survival in non-small-cell lung cancer (NSCLC) patients treated with adriamycin-containing chemotherapy regimens [481].

2.3.14.2 EPHX1 in Endogenous Metabolism

Identification of two SNPs resulting in decreased mRNA and protein levels (–4238T>A in the promoter region and 2557C>G in intron 1) in a patient with extremely elevated serum bile salt levels in the absence of observable hepatocellular injury, suggested that microsomal epoxide hydrolase participates in the sodium-dependent uptake of bile acids into hepatocytes [482].

2.3.15 Cytosolic Epoxide Hydrolase (EPHX2)

Cytosolic (soluble) epoxide hydrolase (EPHX2, also cEH or sEH) differs from the microsomal form regarding its substrate specificity, molecular weight, and immunologic reactivity. The role of EPHX2 in the metabolism of endogenous substrates has been more widely studied than its role in drug metabolism. Microsomal P450-mediated oxidation of polyunsaturated fatty acids results in formation of epoxides that are excellent substrates for EPHX2 [483].

2.3.15.1 EPHX2 Polymorphisms and Their Clinical Implications

Greater than 500-fold interindividual variability in EPHX2 activity was observed in human lymphocytes and liver microsomes, and a large extent of this variability could be explained by genetic variability in coding and regulatory regions of the gene [475,484]. Many common polymorphisms were observed in *EPHX2* that result in amino acid substitution and alter enzyme activites [485–487].

As EPHX2 participates in disposition of endogenous epoxide intermediates and may thus play a role in vascular tone homeostasis, inflammation, response to ischemia, and other physiological processes, the association of *EPHX2* polymorphism and susceptibility for neurological, cardiovascular and lung diseases, and inflammation has been widely investigated in epidemiological studies [488–491].

REFERENCES

1. Nebert DW, Ingelman-Sundberg M, Daly AK. Genetic epidemiology of environmental toxicity and cancer susceptibility: Human allelic polymorphisms in drug-metabolizing enzyme genes, their functional importance, and nomenclature issues. *Drug Metab. Rev.* 1999;**31**:467–487.
2. Ingelman-Sundberg M. Genetic susceptibility to adverse effects of drugs and environmental toxicants. The role of the CYP family of enzymes. *Mutat. Res.* 2001;**482**: 11–19.
3. Bertilsson L. Geographical/interracial differences in polymorphic drug oxidation. Current state of knowledge of cytochromes P450 (CYP) 2D6 and 2C19. *Clin. Pharmacokinet.* 1995;**29**:192–209.
4. Bertilsson L, Aberg-Wistedt A, Gustafsson LL, Nordin C. Extremely rapid hydroxylation of debrisoquine: A case report with implication for treatment with nortriptyline and other tricyclic antidepressants. *Ther. Drug Monit.* 1985;**7**:478–480.
5. Lazarou J, Pomeranz BH, Corey PN. *Incidence of adverse drug reactions in hospitalized patients: A meta-analysis of prospective studies. JAMA* 1998;**279**:1200–1205.
6. Phillips KA, Veenstra DL, Oren E, Lee JK, Sadee W. Potential role of pharmacogenomics in reducing adverse drug reactions: A systematic review. *JAMA* 2001;**286**: 2270–2279.
7. Ding X, Kaminsky LS. Human extrahepatic cytochromes P450: function in xenobiotic metabolism and tissue-selective chemical toxicity in the respiratory and gastrointestinal tracts. *Annu. Rev. Pharmacol. Toxicol.* 2003;**43**:149–173.
8. Meyer RP, Gehlhaus M, Knoth R, Volk B. Expression and function of cytochrome p450 in brain drug metabolism. *Curr. Drug Metab.* 2007;**8**:297–306.
9. Yengi LG, Xiang Q, Pan J, et al. Quantitation of cytochrome P450 mRNA levels in human skin. *Anal. Biochem.* 2003;**316**:103–110.
10. Murray GI, Taylor MC, McFadyen MC, et al. Tumor-specific expression of cytochrome P450 CYP1B1. *Cancer Res.* 1997;**57**:3026–3031.
11. Karlgren M, Gomez A, Stark K, et al. Tumor-specific expression of the novel cytochrome P450 enzyme, CYP2W1. *Biochem. Biophys. Res. Commun.* 2006;**341**:451–458.
12. `http://drnelson.utmem.edu/human.P450.table.html` (accessed 11/09).
13. Nelson DR, Koymans L, Kamataki T, et al. P450 superfamily: Update on new sequences, gene mapping, accession numbers and nomenclature. *Pharmacogenetics* 1996;**6**:1–42.
14. Oscarson M, Ingelman-Sundberg M. CYPalleles: A web page for nomenclature of human cytochrome P450 alleles. *Drug Metab. Pharmacokinet.* 2002;**17**:491–495.

15. Sim SC, Ingelman-Sundberg M. The human cytochrome P450 Allele Nomenclature Committee Web site: Submission criteria, procedures, and objectives. *Meth. Mol. Biol.* 2006;**320**:183–191.
16. `http://www.cypalleles.ki.se/` (accessed 11/09).
17. Ingelman-Sundberg M, Oscarson M, Daly AK, Garte S, Nebert DW. Human cytochrome P-450 (CYP) genes: A web page for the nomenclature of alleles. *Cancer Epidemiol. Biomark. Prev.* 2001;**10**:1307–1308.
18. Guengerich FP. Common and uncommon cytochrome P450 reactions related to metabolism and chemical toxicity. *Chem. Res. Toxicol.* 2001;**14**:611–650.
19. Meunier B, de Visser SP, Shaik S. Mechanism of oxidation reactions catalyzed by cytochrome p450 enzymes. *Chem. Rev.* 2004;**104**:3947–3980.
20. Rendic S. Summary of information on human CYP enzymes: Human P450 metabolism data. *Drug Metab. Rev.* 2002;**34**:83–448.
21. Evans WE, Relling MV. Pharmacogenomics: Translating functional genomics into rational therapeutics. *Science* 1999;**286**:487–491.
22. Liebler DC, Guengerich FP. Elucidating mechanisms of drug-induced toxicity. *Nat. Rev. Drug Discov.* 2005;**4**:410–420.
23. Guengerich FP. Cytochrome P450s and other enzymes in drug metabolism and toxicity. *Am. Assoc. Pharm. Sci. J.* 2006;**8**:E101–E111.
24. Shimada T, Yamazaki H, Mimura M, Inui Y, Guengerich FP. Interindividual variations in human liver cytochrome P-450 enzymes involved in the oxidation of drugs, carcinogens and toxic chemicals: Studies with liver microsomes of 30 Japanese and 30 Caucasians. *J. Pharmacol. Exp. Ther.* 1994;**270**:414–423.
25. Zanger UM, Fischer J, Raimundo S, et al., Comprehensive analysis of the genetic factors determining expression and function of hepatic CYP2D6. *Pharmacogenetics* 2001;**11**:573–585.
26. Gervasini G, Carrillo JA, Benitez J. Potential role of cerebral cytochrome P450 in clinical pharmacokinetics: Modulation by endogenous compounds. *Clin. Pharmacokinet.* 2004;**43**:693–706.
27. Dutheil F, Dauchy S, Diry M, et al. , Xenobiotic-metabolizing enzymes and transporters in the normal human brain: Regional and cellular mapping as a basis for putative roles in cerebral function, *Drug Metab. Dispos.* 2009;**37**:1528–1538.
28. Mahgoub A, Idle JR, Dring LG, Lancaster R, Smith RL. Polymorphic hydroxylation of debrisoquine in man. *Lancet* 1977;**2**:584–586.
29. Tucker GT, Silas JH, Iyun AO, Lennard MS, Smith AJ. Polymorphic hydroxylation of debrisoquine. *Lancet* 1977;**2**:718.
30. Eichelbaum M, Spannbrucker N, Steincke B, Dengler HJ. Defective N-oxidation of sparteine in man: A new pharmacogenetic defect. *Eur. J. Clin. Pharmacol.* 1979;**16**:183–187.
31. Eichelbaum M, Bertilsson L, Sawe J, Zekorn C. Polymorphic oxidation of sparteine and debrisoquine: related pharmacogenetic entities. *Clin. Pharmacol. Ther.* 1982;**31**:184–186.
32. Gonzalez FJ, Vilbois F, Hardwick JP, et al. Human debrisoquine 4-hydroxylase (P450IID1): cDNA and deduced amino acid sequence and assignment of the CYP2D locus to chromosome 22. *Genomics* 1988;**2**:174–179.
33. Kimura S, Umeno M, Skoda RC, Meyer UA, Gonzalez FJ. The human debrisoquine 4-hydroxylase (CYP2D) locus: Sequence and identification of the polymorphic CYP2D6 gene, a related gene, and a pseudogene, *Am. J. Hum. Genet.* 1989;**45**:889–904.

34. Broly F, Gaedigk A, Heim M, Eichelbaum M, Morike K, Meyer UA. Debrisoquine/sparteine hydroxylation genotype and phenotype: Analysis of common mutations and alleles of CYP2D6 in a European population, *DNA Cell Biol.* 1991;**10**:545–558.
35. Kagimoto M, Heim M, Kagimoto K, Zeugin T, Meyer UA. Multiple mutations of the human cytochrome P450IID6 gene (CYP2D6) in poor metabolizers of debrisoquine. Study of the functional significance of individual mutations by expression of chimeric genes. *J. Biol. Chem.* 1990;**265**:17209–17214.
36. Gaedigk A, Blum M, Gaedigk R, Eichelbaum M, Meyer UA. Deletion of the entire cytochrome P450 CYP2D6 gene as a cause of impaired drug metabolism in poor metabolizers of the debrisoquine/sparteine polymorphism. *Am. J. Hum. Genet.* 1991;**48**:943–950.
37. Heim MH, Meyer UA. Evolution of a highly polymorphic human cytochrome P450 gene cluster: CYP2D6. *Genomics* 1992;**14**:49–58.
38. Bradford LD. CYP2D6 allele frequency in European Caucasians, Asians, Africans and their descendants. *Pharmacogenomics* 2002;**3**:229–243.
39. Leathart JB, London SJ, Steward A, Adams JD, Idle JR, Daly AK. CYP2D6 phenotype-genotype relationships in African-Americans and Caucasians in Los Angeles. *Pharmacogenetics* 1998;**8**:529–541.
40. Griese EU, Asante-Poku S, Ofori-Adjei D, Mikus G, Eichelbaum M. Analysis of the CYP2D6 gene mutations and their consequences for enzyme function in a West African population. *Pharmacogenetics* 1999;**9**:715–723.
41. Wang SL, Huang JD, Lai MD, Liu BH, Lai ML. Molecular basis of genetic variation in debrisoquin hydroxylation in Chinese subjects: Polymorphism in RFLP and DNA sequence of CYP2D6. *Clin. Pharmacol. Ther.* 1993;**53**:410–418.
42. Johansson I, Oscarson M, Yue QY, Bertilsson L, Sjoqvist F, Ingelman-Sundberg M. Genetic analysis of the Chinese cytochrome P4502D locus: Characterization of variant CYP2D6 genes present in subjects with diminished capacity for debrisoquine hydroxylation. *Mol. Pharmacol.* 1994;**46**:452–459.
43. Dahl ML, Yue QY, Roh HK, et al. Genetic analysis of the CYP2D locus in relation to debrisoquine hydroxylation capacity in Korean, Japanese and Chinese subjects. *Pharmacogenetics* 1995;**5**:159–164.
44. Daly AK, Fairbrother KS, Andreassen OA, London SJ, Idle JR, Steen VM. Characterization and PCR-based detection of two different hybrid CYP2D7P/CYP2D6 alleles associated with the poor metabolizer phenotype. *Pharmacogenetics* 1996;**6**: 319–328.
45. Sachse C, Brockmoller J, Bauer S, Roots I. Cytochrome P450 2D6 variants in a Caucasian population: Allele frequencies and phenotypic consequences. *Am. J. Hum. Genet.* 1997;**60**:284–295.
46. Oscarson M, Hidestrand M, Johansson I, Ingelman-Sundberg M. A combination of mutations in the CYP2D6*17 (CYP2D6Z) allele causes alterations in enzyme function. *Mol. Pharmacol.* 1997;**52**:1034–1040.
47. Masimirembwa C, Persson I, Bertilsson L, Hasler J, Ingelman-Sundberg M. A novel mutant variant of the CYP2D6 gene (CYP2D6*17) common in a black African population: Association with diminished debrisoquine hydroxylase activity. *Br. J. Clin. Pharmacol.* 1996;**42**:713–719.
48. Wennerholm A, Johansson I, Massele AY, et al., Decreased capacity for debrisoquine metabolism among black Tanzanians: Analyses of the CYP2D6 genotype and phenotype. *Pharmacogenetics* 1999;**9**:707–714.

49. Aklillu E, Persson I, Bertilsson L, Johansson I, Rodrigues F, Ingelman-Sundberg M. Frequent distribution of ultrarapid metabolizers of debrisoquine in an ethiopian population carrying duplicated and multiduplicated functional CYP2D6 alleles. *J. Pharmacol. Exp. Ther.* 1996;**278**:441–446.

50. Raimundo S, Toscano C, Klein K, et al. A novel intronic mutation, 2988G > A, with high predictivity for impaired function of cytochrome P450 2D6 in white subjects, *Clin. Pharmacol. Ther.* 2004;**76**:128–138.

51. Toscano C, Klein K, Blievernicht J, et al. Impaired expression of CYP2D6 in intermediate metabolizers carrying the *41 allele caused by the intronic SNP 2988G > A: Evidence for modulation of splicing events. *Pharmacogenet. Genomics* 2006; **16**:755–766.

52. Johansson I, Lundqvist E, Bertilsson L, Dahl ML, Sjoqvist F, Ingelman-Sundberg M. Inherited amplification of an active gene in the cytochrome P450 CYP2D locus as a cause of ultrarapid metabolism of debrisoquine. *Proc. Natl. Acad. Sci. USA* 1993;**90**: 11825–11829.

53. Lundqvist E, Johansson I, Ingelman-Sundberg M. Genetic mechanisms for duplication and multiduplication of the human CYP2D6 gene and methods for detection of duplicated CYP2D6 genes. *Gene* 1999;**226**:327–338.

54. Cai WM, Nikoloff DM, Pan RM, et al. CYP2D6 genetic variation in healthy adults and psychiatric African-American subjects: Implications for clinical practice and genetic testing. *Pharmacogenomics J.* 2006;**6**:343–350.

55. Dahl ML, Johansson I, Bertilsson L, Ingelman-Sundberg M, Sjoqvist F. Ultrarapid hydroxylation of debrisoquine in a Swedish population. Analysis of the molecular genetic basis. *J. Pharmacol. Exp. Ther.* 1995;**274**:516–520.

56. Agundez JA, Ledesma MC, Ladero JM, Benitez J. Prevalence of CYP2D6 gene duplication and its repercussion on the oxidative phenotype in a white population. *Clin. Pharmacol. Ther.* 1995;**57**:265–269.

57. Bernal ML, Sinues B, Johansson I, et al. Ten percent of North Spanish individuals carry duplicated or triplicated CYP2D6 genes associated with ultrarapid metabolism of debrisoquine. *Pharmacogenetics* 1999;**9**:657–660.

58. Scordo MG, Spina E, Facciola G, Avenoso A, Johansson I, Dahl ML. Cytochrome P450 2D6 genotype and steady state plasma levels of risperidone and 9-hydroxyrisperidone. *Psychopharmacology* (Berlin) 1999;**147**:300–305.

59. McLellan RA, Oscarson M, Seidegard J, Evans DA, Ingelman-Sundberg M. Frequent occurrence of CYP2D6 gene duplication in Saudi Arabians. *Pharmacogenetics* 1997;**7**:187–191.

60. Lovlie R, Daly AK, Matre GE, Molven A, Steen VM. Polymorphisms in CYP2D6 duplication-negative individuals with the ultrarapid metabolizer phenotype: a role for the CYP2D6*35 allele in ultrarapid metabolism? *Pharmacogenetics* 2001;**11**:45–55.

61. Sakuyama K, Sasaki T, Ujiie S, et al. Functional characterization of 17 CYP2D6 allelic variants (CYP2D6. 2 10, 14A-B, 18, 27, 36, 39, 47–51, 53–55, and 57). *Drug Metab. Dispos.* 2008;**36**:2460–2467.

62. Schaeffeler E, Schwab M, Eichelbaum M, Zanger UM. CYP2D6 genotyping strategy based on gene copy number determination by TaqMan real-time PCR. *Hum. Mutat.* 2003;**22**:476–485.

63. Bodin L, Beaune PH, Loriot MA. Determination of cytochrome P450 2D6 (CYP2D6) gene copy number by real-time quantitative PCR. *J. Biomed. Biotechnol.* 2005;**2005**:248–253.

64. Griese EU, Zanger UM, Brudermanns U, et al. Assessment of the predictive power of genotypes for the in-vivo catalytic function of CYP2D6 in a German population. *Pharmacogenetics* 1998;**8**:15–26.

65. Marez D, Legrand M, Sabbagh N, et al. Polymorphism of the cytochrome P450 CYP2D6 gene in a European population: Characterization of 48 mutations and 53 alleles, their frequencies and evolution. *Pharmacogenetics* 1997;**7**:193–202.

66. Gaedigk A, Gotschall RR, Forbes NS, Simon SD, Kearns GL, Leeder JS. Optimization of cytochrome P4502D6 (CYP2D6) phenotype assignment using a genotyping algorithm based on allele frequency data. *Pharmacogenetics* 1999;**9**:669–682.

67. Heim M, Meyer UA. Genotyping of poor metabolisers of debrisoquine by allele-specific PCR amplification. *Lancet* 1990;**336**, 529–532.

68. Daly AK. Development of analytical technology in pharmacogenetic research. *Naunyn. Schmiedebergs. Arch. Pharmacol.* 2004;**369**:133–140.

69. Broly F, Marez D, Sabbagh N, et al. An efficient strategy for detection of known and new mutations of the CYP2D6 gene using single strand conformation polymorphism analysis. *Pharmacogenetics* 1995;**5**:373–384.

70. Molden E, Johansen PW, Boe GH, et al. Pharmacokinetics of diltiazem and its metabolites in relation to CYP2D6 genotype. *Clin. Pharmacol. Ther.* 2002;**72**:333–342.

71. Chou WH, Yan FX, Robbins-Weilert DK, et al. Comparison of two CYP2D6 genotyping methods and assessment of genotype-phenotype relationships. *Clin. Chem.* 2003;**49**:542–551.

72. `http://www.roche.com/home/products/prod_diag_amplichip.htm` (accessed 11/09).

73. `http://www.fda.gov/MedicalDevices/ProductsandMedicalProcedures/DeviceApprovalsandClearances/Recently-ApprovedDevices/ucm078879.htm` (accessed 11/09).

74. de Leon J, Susce MT, Johnson M, et al. DNA microarray technology in the clinical environment: The AmpliChip CYP450 test for CYP2D6 and CYP2C19 genotyping. *CNS Spectrums* 2009;**14**:19–34.

75. de Leon J, Arranz MJ, Ruano G. Pharmacogenetic testing in psychiatry: A review of features and clinical realities, *Clin. Lab. Med.* 2008;**28**:599–617.

76. Beverage JN, Sissung TM, Sion AM, Danesi R, Figg WD. CYP2D6 polymorphisms and the impact on tamoxifen therapy. *J. Pharm. Sci.* 2007;**96**:2224–2231.

77. `http://www.fda.gov/ohrms/dockets/ac/06/briefing/2006-4248B1-01-FDA-Tamoxifen%20Background%20Summary%20Final.pdf` (accessed 11/09).

78. Frank D, Jaehde U, Fuhr U. Evaluation of probe drugs and pharmacokinetic metrics for CYP2D6 phenotyping. *Eur. J. Clin. Pharmacol.* 2007;**63**:321–333.

79. Ingelman-Sundberg M. Genetic polymorphisms of cytochrome P450 2D6 (CYP2D6): Clinical consequences, evolutionary aspects and functional diversity. *Pharmacogenomics J.* 2005;**5**:6–13.

80. Kirchheiner J. CYP2D6 phenotype prediction from genotype: Which system is the best? *Clin. Pharmacol. Ther.* 2008;**83**, 225–227.

81. Rau T, Heide R, Bergmann K, et al. Effect of the CYP2D6 genotype on metoprolol metabolism persists during long-term treatment. *Pharmacogenetics* 2002; **12**:465–472.

82. Kirchheiner J, Nickchen K, Bauer M, et al. Pharmacogenetics of antidepressants and antipsychotics: The contribution of allelic variations to the phenotype of drug response. *Mol. Psychiatry.* 2004;**9**:442–473.

83. Gaedigk A, Bradford LD, Marcucci KA, Leeder JS. Unique CYP2D6 activity distribution and genotype-phenotype discordance in black Americans. *Clin. Pharmacol. Ther.* 2002;**72**:76–89.

84. Wennerholm A, Dandara C, Sayi J, et al. The African-specific CYP2D617 allele encodes an enzyme with changed substrate specificity. *Clin. Pharmacol. Ther.* 2002;**71**:77–88.

85. Bogni A, Monshouwer M, Moscone A, et al. Substrate specific metabolism by polymorphic cytochrome P450 2D6 alleles. *Toxicol. In Vitro* 2005;**19**:621–629.

86. Shen H, He MM, Liu H, et al. Comparative metabolic capabilities and inhibitory profiles of CYP2D6.1, CYP2D6.10, and CYP2D6.17. *Drug Metab. Dispos.* 2007;**35**:1292–1300.

87. Aklillu E, Herrlin K, Gustafsson LL, Bertilsson L, Ingelman-Sundberg M. Evidence for environmental influence on CYP2D6-catalysed debrisoquine hydroxylation as demonstrated by phenotyping and genotyping of Ethiopians living in Ethiopia or in Sweden. *Pharmacogenetics* 2002;**12**:375–383.

88. Gaedigk A, Simon SD, Pearce RE, Bradford LD, Kennedy MJ, Leeder JS. The CYP2D6 activity score: Translating genotype information into a qualitative measure of phenotype. *Clin. Pharmacol. Ther.* 2008;**83**:234–242.

89. Bertilsson L, Dahl ML, Dalen P, Al-Shurbaji A. Molecular genetics of CYP2D6: Clinical relevance with focus on psychotropic drugs. *Br. J. Clin. Pharmacol.* 2002; **53**:111–122.

90. Nyberg S, Dahl ML, Halldin C. A PET study of D2 and 5-HT2 receptor occupancy induced by risperidone in poor metabolizers of debrisoquin and risperidone. *Psychopharmacology (Berlin)* 1995;**119**:345–348.

91. Suzuki A, Otani K, Mihara K, et al. Effects of the CYP2D6 genotype on the steady-state plasma concentrations of haloperidol and reduced haloperidol in Japanese schizophrenic patients. *Pharmacogenetics* 1997;**7**:415–418.

92. Mihara K, Suzuki A, Kondo T, et al. Effects of the CYP2D6*10 allele on the steady-state plasma concentrations of haloperidol and reduced haloperidol in Japanese patients with schizophrenia. *Clin. Pharmacol. Ther.* 1999;**65**:291–294.

93. Brockmoller J, Kirchheiner J, Schmider J, et al. The impact of the CYP2D6 polymorphism on haloperidol pharmacokinetics and on the outcome of haloperidol treatment. *Clin. Pharmacol. Ther.* 2002;**72**:438–452.

94. Meyer JW, Woggon B, Kupfer A. Importance of oxidative polymorphism on clinical efficacy and side-effects of imipramine—a retrospective study. *Pharmacopsychiatry* 1988;**21**:365–366.

95. Steimer W, Zopf K, von Amelunxen S, et al. Amitriptyline or not, that is the question: Pharmacogenetic testing of CYP2D6 and CYP2C19 identifies patients with low or high risk for side effects in amitriptyline therapy. *Clin. Chem.* 2005;**51**:376–385.

96. de Leon J, Armstrong SC, Cozza KL. Clinical guidelines for psychiatrists for the use of pharmacogenetic testing for CYP450 2D6 and CYP450 2C19. *Psychosomatics* 2006;**47**:75–85.

97. de Leon J, Susce MT, Pan RM, Fairchild M, Koch WH, Wedlund PJ. The CYP2D6 poor metabolizer phenotype may be associated with risperidone adverse drug reactions and discontinuation. *J. Clin. Psychiatry.* 2005;**66**:15–27.

98. Chou WH, Yan FX, de Leon J, et al. Extension of a pilot study: impact from the cytochrome P450 2D6 polymorphism on outcome and costs associated with severe mental illness. *J. Clin. Psychopharmacol.* 2000;**20**:246–251.
99. Lieberman JA, Stroup TS, McEvoy JP, et al. Effectiveness of antipsychotic drugs in patients with chronic schizophrenia. *New Engl. J. Med.* 2005;**353**:1209–1223.
100. Bijl MJ, Visser LE, Hofman A, et al. Influence of the CYP2D6*4 polymorphism on dose, switching and discontinuation of antidepressants. *Br. J. Clin. Pharmacol.* 2008; **65**:558–564.
101. Lim HS, Ju Lee H, Seok Lee K, Sook Lee E, Jang IJ, Ro J. Clinical implications of CYP2D6 genotypes predictive of tamoxifen pharmacokinetics in metastatic breast cancer. *J. Clin. Oncol.* 2007;**25**:3837–3845.
102. Jin Y, Desta Z, Stearns V, et al. CYP2D6 genotype, antidepressant use, and tamoxifen metabolism during adjuvant breast cancer treatment. *J. Natl. Cancer Inst.* 2005; **97**:30–39.
103. Kirchheiner J, Schmidt H, Tzvetkov M, et al. Pharmacokinetics of codeine and its metabolite morphine in ultra-rapid metabolizers due to CYP2D6 duplication. *Pharmacogenomics J.* 2007;**7**:257–265.
104. Dalen P, Frengell C, Dahl ML, Sjoqvist F. Quick onset of severe abdominal pain after codeine in an ultrarapid metabolizer of debrisoquine. *Ther. Drug Monit.* 1997;**19**: 543–544.
105. Halling J, Weihe P, Brosen K. CYP2D6 polymorphism in relation to tramadol metabolism: A study of faroese patients. *Ther. Drug Monit.* 2008;**30**:271–275.
106. Koren G, Cairns J, Chitayat D, Gaedigk A, Leeder SJ. Pharmacogenetics of morphine poisoning in a breastfed neonate of a codeine-prescribed mother. *Lancet* 2006;**368**:704.
107. Wuttke H, Rau T, Heide R, et al. Increased frequency of cytochrome P450 2D6 poor metabolizers among patients with metoprolol-associated adverse effects. *Clin. Pharmacol. Ther.* 2002;**72**:429–437.
108. Siegle I, Fritz P, Eckhardt K, Zanger UM, Eichelbaum M. Cellular localization and regional distribution of CYP2D6 mRNA and protein expression in human brain. *Pharmacogenetics* 2001;**11**:237–245.
109. Kirchheiner J, Lang U, Stamm T, Sander T, Gallinat J. Association of CYP2D6 genotypes and personality traits in healthy individuals. *J. Clin. Psychopharmacol.* 2006;**26**:440–442.
110. Gonzalez I, Penas-Lledo EM, Perez B, Dorado P, Alvarez M, A LL. Relation between CYP2D6 phenotype and genotype and personality in healthy volunteers. *Pharmacogenomics* 2008;**9**:833–840.
111. Dorado P, Penas-Lledo EM, Llerena A. CYP2D6 polymorphism: implications for antipsychotic drug response, schizophrenia and personality traits. *Pharmacogenomics* 2007;**8**:1597–1608.
112. Gray IC, Nobile C, Muresu R, Ford S, Spurr NK. A 2.4-megabase physical map spanning the CYP2C gene cluster on chromosome 10q24. *Genomics* 1995;**28**:328–332.
113. de Morais SM, Schweikl H, Blaisdell J, Goldstein JA. Gene structure and upstream regulatory regions of human CYP2C9 and CYP2C18. *Biochem. Biophys. Res. Commun.* 1993;**194**:194–201.
114. Schoch GA, Yano JK, Sansen S, Dansette PM, Stout CD, Johnson EF. Determinants of cytochrome P450 2C8 substrate binding: Structures of complexes with montelukast, troglitazone, felodipine, and 9-cis-retinoic acid. *J. Biol. Chem.* 2008;**283**:17227–17237.

115. Schoch GA, Yano JK, Wester MR, Griffin KJ, Stout CD, Johnson EF. Structure of human microsomal cytochrome P450 2C8. Evidence for a peripheral fatty acid binding site. *J. Biol. Chem.* 2004;**279**:9497–9503.

116. Williams PA, Cosme J, Ward A, Angove HC, Matak Vinkovic D, Jhoti H. Crystal structure of human cytochrome P450 2C9 with bound warfarin. *Nature* 2003;**424**:464–468.

117. Furuya H, Meyer UA, Gelboin HV, Gonzalez FJ. Polymerase chain reaction-directed identification, cloning, and quantification of human CYP2C18 mRNA. *Mol. Pharmacol.* 1991;**40**:375–382.

118. Dai D, Zeldin DC, Blaisdell JA, et al. Polymorphisms in human CYP2C8 decrease metabolism of the anticancer drug paclitaxel and arachidonic acid. *Pharmacogenetics* 2001;**11**:597–607.

119. Bahadur N, Leathart JB, Mutch E, et al. CYP2C8 polymorphisms in Caucasians and their relationship with paclitaxel 6alpha-hydroxylase activity in human liver microsomes. *Biochem. Pharmacol.* 2002;**64**:1579–1589.

120. Dreisbach AW, Japa S, Sigel A, et al. The Prevalence of CYP2C8, 2C9, 2J2, and soluble epoxide hydrolase polymorphisms in African Americans with hypertension. *Am. J. Hypertens.* 2005;**18**:1276–1281.

121. Yasar U, Lundgren S, Eliasson E, et al. Linkage between the CYP2C8 and CYP2C9 genetic polymorphisms. *Biochem. Biophys. Res. Commun.* 2002;**299**:25–28.

122. Nakajima M, Fujiki Y, Noda K, et al. Genetic polymorphisms of CYP2C8 in Japanese population. *Drug Metab. Dispos.* 2003;**31**:687–690.

123. Rahman A, Korzekwa KR, Grogan J, Gonzalez FJ, Harris JW. Selective biotransformation of taxol to 6 alpha-hydroxytaxol by human cytochrome P450 2C8. *Cancer Res.* 1994;**54**:5543–5546.

124. Yamazaki H, Shibata A, Suzuki M, et al. Oxidation of troglitazone to a quinone-type metabolite catalyzed by cytochrome P-450 2C8 and P-450 3A4 in human liver microsomes. *Drug Metab. Dispos.* 1999;**27**:1260–1266.

125. Ohyama K, Nakajima M, Nakamura S, Shimada N, Yamazaki H, Yokoi T. A significant role of human cytochrome P450 2C8 in amiodarone N-deethylation: An approach to predict the contribution with relative activity factor. *Drug Metab. Dispos.* 2000;**28**:1303–1310.

126. Muck W. Clinical pharmacokinetics of cerivastatin. *Clin. Pharmacokinet.* 2000;**39**:99–116.

127. Totah RA, Rettie AE. Cytochrome P450 2C8: substrates, inhibitors, pharmacogenetics, and clinical relevance. *Clin. Pharmacol. Ther.* 2005;**77**:341–352.

128. Henningsson A, Marsh S, Loos WJ, et al. Association of CYP2C8, CYP3A4, CYP3A5, and ABCB1 polymorphisms with the pharmacokinetics of paclitaxel. *Clin. Cancer Res.* 2005;**11**:8097–8104.

129. Grau JJ, Caballero M, Campayo M, et al. Gene single nucleotide polymorphism accumulation improves survival in advanced head and neck cancer patients treated with weekly paclitaxel. *Laryngoscope* 2009;**119**:1484–1490.

130. Gandara DR, Kawaguchi T, Crowley J, et al. Japanese-US common-arm analysis of paclitaxel plus carboplatin in advanced non-small-cell lung cancer: A model for assessing population-related pharmacogenomics. *J. Clin. Oncol.* 2009;**27**:3540–3546.

131. Green H, Soderkvist P, Rosenberg P, et al. Pharmacogenetic studies of Paclitaxel in the treatment of ovarian cancer. *Basic Clin. Pharmacol. Toxicol.* 2009;**104**:130–137.

132. Marsh S, Paul J, King CR, Gifford G, McLeod HL, Brown R. Pharmacogenetic assessment of toxicity and outcome after platinum plus taxane chemotherapy in ovarian cancer: The Scottish Randomised Trial in Ovarian Cancer. *J. Clin. Oncol.* 2007; **25**:4528–4535.
133. Holstein A, Beil W. Oral antidiabetic drug metabolism: pharmacogenomics and drug interactions. *Expert Opin. Drug Metab. Toxicol.* 2009;**5**:225–241.
134. Bozkurt O, de Boer A, Grobbee DE, Heerdink ER, Burger H, Klungel OH. Pharmacogenetics of glucose-lowering drug treatment: A systematic review. *Mol. Diagn. Ther.* 2007;**11**:291–302.
135. Kirchheiner J, Roots I, Goldammer M, Rosenkranz B, Brockmoller J. Effect of genetic polymorphisms in cytochrome p450 (CYP) 2C9 and CYP2C8 on the pharmacokinetics of oral antidiabetic drugs: Clinical relevance. *Clin. Pharmacokinet.* 2005;**44**:1209–1225.
136. Niemi M, Leathart JB, Neuvonen M, Backman JT, Daly AK, Neuvonen PJ. Polymorphism in CYP2C8 is associated with reduced plasma concentrations of repaglinide. *Clin. Pharmacol. Ther.* 2003;**74**:380–387.
137. Niemi M, Backman JT, Kajosaari LI, et al. Polymorphic organic anion transporting polypeptide 1B1 is a major determinant of repaglinide pharmacokinetics. *Clin. Pharmacol. Ther.* 2005;**77**:468–478.
138. Aquilante CL, Bushman LR, Knutsen SD, Burt LE, Rome LC, Kosmiski LA. Influence of SLCO1B1 and CYP2C8 gene polymorphisms on rosiglitazone pharmacokinetics in healthy volunteers. *Hum. Genomics* 2008;**3**:7–16.
139. Kirchheiner J, Thomas S, Bauer S, et al. Pharmacokinetics and pharmacodynamics of rosiglitazone in relation to CYP2C8 genotype. *Clin. Pharmacol. Ther.* 2006;**80**:657–667.
140. Martinez C, Garcia-Martin E, Blanco G, Gamito FJ, Ladero JM, Agundez JA. The effect of the cytochrome P450 CYP2C8 polymorphism on the disposition of (R)-ibuprofen enantiomer in healthy subjects. *Br. J. Clin. Pharmacol.* 2005;**59**:62–69.
141. Daly AK, Aithal GP, Leathart JB, Swainsbury RA, Dang TS, Day CP. Genetic susceptibility to diclofenac-induced hepatotoxicity: Contribution of UGT2B7, CYP2C8, and ABCC2 genotypes. *Gastroenterology* 2007;**132**:272–281.
142. Gil JP, Gil Berglund E. CYP2C8 and antimalaria drug efficacy. *Pharmacogenomics* 2007;**8**:187–198.
143. Rower S, Bienzle U, Weise A, et al. Short communication: high prevalence of the cytochrome P450 2C8*2 mutation in Northern Ghana. *Trop. Med. Int. Health* 2005;**10**:1271–1273.
144. Parikh S, Ouedraogo JB, Goldstein JA, Rosenthal PJ, Kroetz DL. Amodiaquine metabolism is impaired by common polymorphisms in CYP2C8: Implications for malaria treatment in Africa. *Clin. Pharmacol. Ther.* 2007;**82**:197–203.
145. Muthiah YD, Lee WL, Teh LK, Ong CE, Salleh MZ, Ismail R. A simple multiplex PCR method for the concurrent detection of three CYP2C8 variants. *Clin. Chim. Acta* 2004; **349**:191–198.
146. Weise A, Grundler S, Zaumsegel D, et al. Development and evaluation of a rapid and reliable method for cytochrome P450 2C8 genotyping. *Clin. Lab.* 2004;**50**:141–148.
147. Weise A, Lambertz U, Thome N, et al. A fast and reliable single-run method for genotyping of the human cytochrome P450 2C8 gene for different ethnic groups. *Clin. Lab.* 2006;**52**:599–603.

148. Zeldin DC, Moomaw CR, Jesse N, et al. Biochemical characterization of the human liver cytochrome P450 arachidonic acid epoxygenase pathway. *Arch. Biochem. Biophys.* 1996;**330**:87–96.

149. Nadin L, Murray M. Participation of CYP2C8 in retinoic acid 4-hydroxylation in human hepatic microsomes. *Biochem. Pharmacol.* 1999;**58**:1201–1208.

150. Rifkind AB, Lee C, Chang TK, Waxman DJ. Arachidonic acid metabolism by human cytochrome P450s 2C8, 2C9, 2E1, and 1A2: Regioselective oxygenation and evidence for a role for CYP2C enzymes in arachidonic acid epoxygenation in human liver microsomes. *Arch. Biochem. Biophys.* 1995;**320**:380–389.

151. Node K, Huo Y, Ruan X, et al. Anti-inflammatory properties of cytochrome P450 epoxygenase-derived eicosanoids. *Science* 1999;**285**:1276–1279.

152. Hoagland KM, Maier KG, Moreno C, Yu M, Roman RJ. Cytochrome P450 metabolites of arachidonic acid: Novel regulators of renal function. *Nephrol. Dial. Transplant.* 2001;**16**:2283–2285.

153. Kirchheiner J, Meineke I, Fuhr U, Rodriguez-Antona C, Lebedeva E, Brockmoller J. Impact of genetic polymorphisms in CYP2C8 and rosiglitazone intake on the urinary excretion of dihydroxyeicosatrienoic acids. *Pharmacogenomics* 2008;**9**:277–288.

154. Yasar U, Bennet AM, Eliasson E, et al. Allelic variants of cytochromes P450 2C modify the risk for acute myocardial infarction. *Pharmacogenetics* 2003;**13**:715–720.

155. Lee CR, North KE, Bray MS, Couper DJ, Heiss G, Zeldin DC. CYP2J2 and CYP2C8 polymorphisms and coronary heart disease risk: The atherosclerosis risk in communities (ARIC) study. *Pharmacogenet. Genomics* 2007;**17**:349–358.

156. Lasker JM, Wester MR, Aramsombatdee E, Raucy JL. Characterization of CYP2C19 and CYP2C9 from human liver: Respective roles in microsomal tolbutamide, S-mephenytoin, and omeprazole hydroxylations. *Arch. Biochem. Biophys.* 1998;**353**:16–28.

157. Rodrigues AD, Lin JH. Screening of drug candidates for their drug–drug interaction potential. *Curr. Opin. Chem. Biol.* 2001;**5**:396–401.

158. Hines RN. Ontogeny of human hepatic cytochromes P450. *J. Biochem. Mol. Toxicol.* 2007;**21**:169–175.

159. Mancy A, Broto P, Dijols S, Dansette PM, Mansuy D. The substrate binding site of human liver cytochrome P450 2C9: An approach using designed tienilic acid derivatives and molecular modeling. *Biochemistry* 1995;**34**:10365–10375.

160. Rettie AE, Korzekwa KR, Kunze KL, et al. Hydroxylation of warfarin by human cDNA-expressed cytochrome P-450: A role for P-4502C9 in the etiology of (S)-warfarin-drug interactions. *Chem. Res. Toxicol.* 1992;**5**:54–59.

161. Sullivan-Klose TH, Ghanayem BI, Bell DA, et al. The role of the CYP2C9-Leu359 allelic variant in the tolbutamide polymorphism. *Pharmacogenetics* 1996;**6**:341–349.

162. Haining RL, Hunter AP, Veronese ME, Trager WF, Rettie AE. Allelic variants of human cytochrome P450 2C9: Baculovirus-mediated expression, purification, structural characterization, substrate stereoselectivity, and prochiral selectivity of the wild-type and I359L mutant forms. *Arch. Biochem. Biophys.* 1996;**333**:447–458.

163. Lee CR, Goldstein JA, Pieper JA. Cytochrome P450 2C9 polymorphisms: A comprehensive review of the in-vitro and human data. *Pharmacogenetics* 2002;**12**:251–263.

164. Kirchheiner J, Brockmoller J. Clinical consequences of cytochrome P450 2C9 polymorphisms. *Clin. Pharmacol. Ther.* 2005;**77**:1–16.

165. Yasar U, Aklillu E, Canaparo R, et al. Analysis of CYP2C9*5 in Caucasian, Oriental and black-African populations. *Eur. J. Clin. Pharmacol.* 2002;**58**:555–558.

166. Allabi AC, Gala JL, Desager JP, Heusterspreute M, Horsmans Y. Genetic polymorphisms of CYP2C9 and CYP2C19 in the Beninese and Belgian populations. *Br. J. Clin. Pharmacol.* 2003;**56**:653–657.

167. Kidd RS, Curry TB, Gallagher S, Edeki T, Blaisdell J, Goldstein JA. Identification of a null allele of CYP2C9 in an African-American exhibiting toxicity to phenytoin. *Pharmacogenetics* 2001;**11**:803–808.

168. Miners JO, Birkett DJ. Cytochrome P4502C9: An enzyme of major importance in human drug metabolism. *Br. J. Clin. Pharmacol.* 1998;**45**:525–538.

169. Goldstein JA. Clinical relevance of genetic polymorphisms in the human CYP2C subfamily. *Br. J. Clin. Pharmacol.* 2001;**52**:349–355.

170. Aithal GP, Day CP, Kesteven PJ, Daly AK. Association of polymorphisms in the cytochrome P450 CYP2C9 with warfarin dose requirement and risk of bleeding complications. *Lancet* 1999;**353**:717–719.

171. Kaminsky LS, Zhang ZY. Human P450 metabolism of warfarin. *Pharmacol. Ther.* 1997;**73**:67–74.

172. Beinema M, Brouwers JR, Schalekamp T, Wilffert B. Pharmacogenetic differences between warfarin, acenocoumarol and phenprocoumon. *Thromb. Haemost.* 2008;**100**: 1052–1057.

173. Lindh JD, Holm L, Andersson ML, Rane A. Influence of CYP2C9 genotype on warfarin dose requirements—a systematic review and meta-analysis. *Eur. J. Clin. Pharmacol.* 2009;**65**:365–375.

174. Herman D, Locatelli I, Grabnar I, et al. Influence of CYP2C9 polymorphisms, demographic factors and concomitant drug therapy on warfarin metabolism and maintenance dose. *Pharmacogenomics J.* 2005;**5**:193–202.

175. Shikata E, Ieiri I, Ishiguro S, et al. Association of pharmacokinetic (CYP2C9) and pharmacodynamic (factors II, VII, IX, and X; proteins S and C; and gamma-glutamyl carboxylase) gene variants with warfarin sensitivity. *Blood* 2004;**103**:2630–2635.

176. Herman D, Peternel P, Stegnar M, Breskvar K, Dolzan V. The influence of sequence variations in factor VII, gamma-glutamyl carboxylase and vitamin K epoxide reductase complex genes on warfarin dose requirement. *Thromb. Haemost.* 2006;**95**: 782–787.

177. Schwarz UI, Ritchie MD, Bradford Y, et al. Genetic determinants of response to warfarin during initial anticoagulation. *New Engl. J. Med.* 2008;**358**:999–1008.

178. Wadelius M, Chen LY, Lindh JD, et al. The largest prospective warfarin-treated cohort supports genetic forecasting. *Blood* 2009;**113**:784–792.

179. Pilotto A, Seripa D, Franceschi M, et al. Genetic susceptibility to nonsteroidal anti-inflammatory drug-related gastroduodenal bleeding: Role of cytochrome P450 2C9 polymorphisms. *Gastroenterology* 2007;**133**:465–471.

180. Blanco G, Martinez C, Ladero JM, et al. Interaction of CYP2C8 and CYP2C9 genotypes modifies the risk for nonsteroidal anti-inflammatory drugs-related acute gastrointestinal bleeding. *Pharmacogenet. Genomics* 2008;**18**:37–43.

181. Agundez JA, Garcia-Martin E, Martinez C. Genetically based impairment in CYP2C8- and CYP2C9-dependent NSAID metabolism as a risk factor for gastrointestinal bleeding: Is a combination of pharmacogenomics and metabolomics required to improve personalized medicine? *Expert Opin. Drug Metab. Toxicol.* 2009;**5**:607–620.

182. Cross JT, Poole EM, Ulrich CM. A review of gene-drug interactions for nonsteroidal anti-inflammatory drug use in preventing colorectal neoplasia. *Pharmacogenomics J.* 2008;**8**, 237–247.

183. Ali ZK, Kim RJ, Ysla FM. CYP2C9 polymorphisms: considerations in NSAID therapy. *Curr. Opin. Drug Discov. Devel.* 2009;**12**:108–114.

184. McGreavey LE, Turner F, Smith G, et al. No evidence that polymorphisms in CYP2C8, CYP2C9, UGT1A6, PPARdelta and PPARgamma act as modifiers of the protective effect of regular NSAID use on the risk of colorectal carcinoma. *Pharmacogenet. Genomics* 2005;**15**:713–721.

185. Becker ML, Visser LE, Trienekens PH, Hofman A, van Schaik RH, Stricker BH. Cytochrome P450 2C9 *2 and *3 polymorphisms and the dose and effect of sulfonylurea in type II diabetes mellitus. *Clin. Pharmacol. Ther.* 2008;**83**:288–292.

186. Makita K, Falck JR, Capdevila JH. Cytochrome P450, the arachidonic acid cascade, and hypertension: new vistas for an old enzyme system. *FASEB J.* 1996;**10**:1456–1463.

187. Roman RJ. P-450 metabolites of arachidonic acid in the control of cardiovascular function. *Physiol. Rev.* 2002;**82**:131–185.

188. Alvan G, Bechtel P, Iselius L, Gundert-Remy U. Hydroxylation polymorphisms of debrisoquine and mephenytoin in European populations. *Eur. J. Clin. Pharmacol.* 1990;**39**:533–537.

189. Bertilsson L, Lou YQ, Du YL, et al. Pronounced differences between native Chinese and Swedish populations in the polymorphic hydroxylations of debrisoquin and S-mephenytoin. *Clin. Pharmacol. Ther.* 1992;**51**:388–397.

190. Xie HG, Stein CM, Kim RB, Wilkinson GR, Flockhart DA, Wood AJ. Allelic, genotypic and phenotypic distributions of S-mephenytoin 4′-hydroxylase (CYP2C19) in healthy Caucasian populations of European descent throughout the world. *Pharmacogenetics* 1999;**9**:539–549.

191. Nakamura K, Goto F, Ray WA, et al. Interethnic differences in genetic polymorphism of debrisoquin and mephenytoin hydroxylation between Japanese and Caucasian populations. *Clin. Pharmacol. Ther.* 1985;**38**:402–408.

192. Kaneko A, Kaneko O, Taleo G, Bjorkman A, Kobayakawa T. High frequencies of CYP2C19 mutations and poor metabolism of proguanil in Vanuatu. *Lancet* 1997;**349**: 921–922.

193. de Morais SM, Wilkinson GR, Blaisdell J, Nakamura K, Meyer UA, Goldstein JA. The major genetic defect responsible for the polymorphism of S-mephenytoin metabolism in humans. *J. Biol. Chem.* 1994;**269**:15419–15422.

194. Chen L, Qin S, Xie J, et al. Genetic polymorphism analysis of CYP2C19 in Chinese Han populations from different geographic areas of mainland China. *Pharmacogenomics* 2008;**9**:691–702.

195. de Morais SM, Wilkinson GR, Blaisdell J, Meyer UA, Nakamura K, Goldstein JA. Identification of a new genetic defect responsible for the polymorphism of (S)-mephenytoin metabolism in Japanese. *Mol. Pharmacol.* 1994;**46**:594–598.

196. Ferguson RJ, De Morais SM, Benhamou S, et al. A new genetic defect in human CYP2C19: Mutation of the initiation codon is responsible for poor metabolism of S-mephenytoin. *J. Pharmacol. Exp. Ther.* 1998;**284**:356–361.

197. Xiao ZS, Goldstein JA, Xie HG, et al. Differences in the incidence of the CYP2C19 polymorphism affecting the S-mephenytoin phenotype in Chinese Han and Bai

populations and identification of a new rare CYP2C19 mutant allele. *J. Pharmacol. Exp. Ther.* 1997;**281**:604–609.

198. Ibeanu GC, Blaisdell J, Ghanayem BI, et al. An additional defective allele, CYP2C19*5, contributes to the S-mephenytoin poor metabolizer phenotype in Caucasians. *Pharmacogenetics* 1998;**8**:129–135.
199. Ibeanu GC, Goldstein JA, Meyer U, et al. Identification of new human CYP2C19 alleles (CYP2C19*6 and CYP2C19*2B) in a Caucasian poor metabolizer of mephenytoin. *J. Pharmacol. Exp. Ther.* 1998;**286**:1490–1495.
200. Ibeanu GC, Blaisdell J, Ferguson RJ, et al. A novel transversion in the intron 5 donor splice junction of CYP2C19 and a sequence polymorphism in exon 3 contribute to the poor metabolizer phenotype for the anticonvulsant drug S-mephenytoin. *J. Pharmacol. Exp. Ther.* 1999;**290**:635–640.
201. Blaisdell J, Mohrenweiser H, Jackson J, et al. Identification and functional characterization of new potentially defective alleles of human CYP2C19. *Pharmacogenetics* 2002;**12**:703–711.
202. Sim SC, Risinger C, Dahl ML, et al. A common novel CYP2C19 gene variant causes ultrarapid drug metabolism relevant for the drug response to proton pump inhibitors and antidepressants. *Clin. Pharmacol. Ther.* 2006: **79**:103–113.
203. Ragia G, Arvanitidis KI, Tavridou A, Manolopoulos VG. Need for reassessment of reported CYP2C19 allele frequencies in various populations in view of CYP2C19*17 discovery: The case of Greece. *Pharmacogenomics* 2009;**10**:43–49.
204. Justenhoven C, Hamann U, Pierl CB, et al. CYP2C19*17 is associated with decreased breast cancer risk. *Breast Cancer Res. Treat.* 2009;**115**:391–396.
205. Sugimoto K, Uno T, Yamazaki H, Tateishi T. Limited frequency of the CYP2C19*17 allele and its minor role in a Japanese population. *Br. J. Clin. Pharmacol.* 2008;**65**:437–439.
206. Klotz U. Clinical impact of CYP2C19 polymorphism on the action of proton pump inhibitors: A review of a special problem. *Int. J. Clin. Pharmacol. Ther.* 2006; **44**:297–302.
207. Klotz U. Impact of CYP2C19 polymorphisms on the clinical action of proton pump inhibitors (PPIs). *Eur. J. Clin. Pharmacol.* 2009;**65**:1–2.
208. Zhao F, Wang J, Yang Y, et al. Effect of CYP2C19 genetic polymorphisms on the efficacy of proton pump inhibitor-based triple therapy for Helicobacter pylori eradication: A meta-analysis. *Helicobacter* 2008;**13**:532–541.
209. Lee YC, Lin JT, Wang HP, Chiu HM, Wu MS. Influence of cytochrome P450 2C19 genetic polymorphism and dosage of rabeprazole on accuracy of proton-pump inhibitor testing in Chinese patients with gastroesophageal reflux disease. *J. Gastroenterol. Hepatol.* 2007;**22**:1286–1292.
210. Yamano HO, Matsushita HO, Yanagiwara S. Plasma concentration of rabeprazole after 8-week administration in gastroesophageal reflux disease patients and intragastric pH elevation. *J. Gastroenterol. Hepatol.* 2008;**23**:534–540.
211. Lou HY, Chang CC, Sheu MT, Chen YC, Ho HO. Optimal dose regimens of esomeprazole for gastric acid suppression with minimal influence of the CYP2C19 polymorphism. *Eur. J. Clin. Pharmacol.* 2009;**65**:55–64.
212. Baldwin RM, Ohlsson S, Pedersen RS, et al. Increased omeprazole metabolism in carriers of the CYP2C19*17 allele; a pharmacokinetic study in healthy volunteers. *Br. J. Clin. Pharmacol.* 2008;**65**:767–774.

213. Kurzawski M, Gawronska-Szklarz B, Wrzesniewska J, Siuda A, Starzynska T, Drozdzik M. Effect of CYP2C19*17 gene variant on Helicobacter pylori eradication in peptic ulcer patients. *Eur. J. Clin. Pharmacol.* 2006;**62**:877–880.

214. Ohlsson Rosenborg S, Mwinyi J, Andersson M, et al. Kinetics of omeprazole and escitalopram in relation to the CYP2C19*17 allele in healthy subjects. *Eur. J. Clin. Pharmacol.* 2008;**64**:1175–1179.

215. Rudberg I, Mohebi B, Hermann M, Refsum H, Molden E. Impact of the ultrarapid CYP2C19*17 allele on serum concentration of escitalopram in psychiatric patients. *Clin. Pharmacol. Ther.* 2008;**83**:322–327.

216. Rudberg I, Hermann M, Refsum H, Molden E. Serum concentrations of sertraline and N-desmethyl sertraline in relation to CYP2C19 genotype in psychiatric patients. *Eur. J. Clin. Pharmacol.* 2008;**64**:1181–1188.

217. Kirchheiner J, Brosen K, Dahl ML, et al. CYP2D6 and CYP2C19 genotype-based dose recommendations for antidepressants: a first step towards subpopulation-specific dosages. *Acta Psychiatr. Scand.* 2001;**104**:173–192.

218. Hulot JS, Bura A, Villard E, et al. Cytochrome P450 2C19 loss-of-function polymorphism is a major determinant of clopidogrel responsiveness in healthy subjects. *Blood* 2006;**108**:2244–2247.

219. Frere C, Cuisset T, Morange PE, et al. Effect of cytochrome p450 polymorphisms on platelet reactivity after treatment with clopidogrel in acute coronary syndrome. *Am. J. Cardiol.* 2008;**101**:1088–1093.

220. Mega JL, Close SL, Wiviott SD, et al. Cytochrome p-450 polymorphisms and response to clopidogrel. *New Engl. J. Med.* 2009;**360**:354–362.

221. Sibbing D, Stegherr J, Latz W, et al. Cytochrome P450 2C19 loss-of-function polymorphism and stent thrombosis following percutaneous coronary intervention. *Eur. Heart J.* 2009;**30**:916–922.

222. Collet JP, Hulot JS, Pena A, et al. Cytochrome P450 2C19 polymorphism in young patients treated with clopidogrel after myocardial infarction: A cohort study. *Lancet* 2009;**373**:309–317.

223. Simon T, Verstuyft C, Mary-Krause M, et al. Genetic determinants of response to clopidogrel and cardiovascular events. *New Engl. J. Med.* 2009;**360**:363–375.

224. Li XQ, Andersson TB, Ahlstrom M, Weidolf L. Comparison of inhibitory effects of the proton pump-inhibiting drugs omeprazole, esomeprazole, lansoprazole, pantoprazole, and rabeprazole on human cytochrome P450 activities. *Drug Metab. Dispos.* 2004;**32**: 821–827.

225. Siller-Matula JM, Spiel AO, Lang IM, Kreiner G, Christ G, Jilma B. Effects of pantoprazole and esomeprazole on platelet inhibition by clopidogrel. *Am. Heart. J.* 2009;**157**:148.e1–148.e5.

226. Small DS, Farid NA, Payne CD, et al. Effects of the proton pump inhibitor lansoprazole on the pharmacokinetics and pharmacodynamics of prasugrel and clopidogrel. *J. Clin. Pharmacol.* 2008;**48**:475–484.

227. Juurlink DN, Gomes T, Ko DT, et al. A population-based study of the drug interaction between proton pump inhibitors and clopidogrel. *Canad. Med. Assoc. J.* 2009;**180**: 713–718.

228. Storey RF. Clopidogrel in acute coronary syndrome: To genotype or not? *Lancet* 2009;**373**:276–278.

229. Bebia Z, Buch SC, Wilson JW, et al. Bioequivalence revisited: Influence of age and sex on CYP enzymes. *Clin. Pharmacol. Ther.* 2004;**76**:618–627.

230. Parkinson A, Mudra DR, Johnson C, Dwyer A, Carroll KM. The effects of gender, age, ethnicity, and liver cirrhosis on cytochrome P450 enzyme activity in human liver microsomes and inducibility in cultured human hepatocytes. *Toxicol. Appl. Pharmacol.* 2004;**199**:193–209.

231. Frye RF, Zgheib NK, Matzke GR, et al. Liver disease selectively modulates cytochrome P450–mediated metabolism. *Clin. Pharmacol. Ther.* 2006;**80**:235–245.

232. Aitken AE, Morgan ET. Gene-specific effects of inflammatory cytokines on cytochrome P450 2C, 2B6 and 3A4 mRNA levels in human hepatocytes. *Drug Metab. Dispos.* 2007;**35**:1687–1693.

233. Frye RF, Schneider VM, Frye CS, Feldman AM. Plasma levels of TNF-alpha and IL-6 are inversely related to cytochrome P450-dependent drug metabolism in patients with congestive heart failure. *J. Card. Fail.* 2002;**8**:315–319.

234. Williams ML, Bhargava P, Cherrouk I, Marshall JL, Flockhart DA, Wainer IW. A discordance of the cytochrome P450 2C19 genotype and phenotype in patients with advanced cancer. *Br. J. Clin. Pharmacol.* 2000;**49**:485–488.

235. Helsby NA, Lo WY, Sharples K, et al. CYP2C19 pharmacogenetics in advanced cancer: Compromised function independent of genotype. *Br. J. Cancer* 2008;**99**:1251–1255.

236. Timm R, Kaiser R, Lotsch J, et al. Association of cyclophosphamide pharmacokinetics to polymorphic cytochrome P450 2C19. *Pharmacogenomics J.* 2005;**5**:365–373.

237. Bertrand-Thiebault C, Berrahmoune H, Thompson A, et al. Genetic Polymorphism of CYP2C19 gene in the Stanislas cohort. A link with inflammation. *Ann. Hum. Genet.* 2008;**72**:178–183.

238. Bohanec Grabar P, Rozman B, Tomsic M, Suput D, Logar D, Dolzan V. Genetic polymorphism of CYP1A2 and the toxicity of leflunomide treatment in rheumatoid arthritis patients. *Eur. J. Clin. Pharmacol.* 2008;**64**:871–876.

239. Gomes LG, Huang N, Agrawal V, Mendonca BB, Bachega TA, Miller WL. Extraadrenal 21-hydroxylation by CYP2C19 and CYP3A4: Effect on 21-hydroxylase deficiency. *J. Clin. Endocrinol. Metab.* 2009;**94**:89–95.

240. `http://medicine.iupui.edu/flockhart/` (accessed 11/09).

241. Williams JA, Ring BJ, Cantrell VE, et al. Comparative metabolic capabilities of CYP3A4, CYP3A5, and CYP3A7. *Drug Metab. Dispos.* 2002;**30**:883–891.

242. Westlind A, Lofberg L, Tindberg N, Andersson TB, Ingelman-Sundberg M. Interindividual differences in hepatic expression of CYP3A4: Relationship to genetic polymorphism in the 5′-upstream regulatory region. *Biochem. Biophys. Res. Commun.* 1999;**259**:201–205.

243. Ozdemir V, Kalowa W, Tang BK, et al. Evaluation of the genetic component of variability in CYP3A4 activity: a repeated drug administration method. *Pharmacogenetics* 2000;**10**:373–388.

244. Brockmoller J, Roots I. Assessment of liver metabolic function. Clinical implications. *Clin. Pharmacokinet.* 1994;**27**:216–248.

245. Veronese ML, Gillen LP, Burke JP, et al. Exposure-dependent inhibition of intestinal and hepatic CYP3A4 in vivo by grapefruit juice. *J. Clin. Pharmacol.* 2003;**43**:831–839.

246. Ohno Y, Hisaka A, Ueno M, Suzuki H. General framework for the prediction of oral drug interactions caused by CYP3A4 induction from in vivo information. *Clin. Pharmacokinet.* 2008;**47**:669–680.

247. Kuehl P, Zhang J, Lin Y, et al. Sequence diversity in CYP3A promoters and characterization of the genetic basis of polymorphic CYP3A5 expression. *Nat. Genet.* 2001;**27**:383–391.

248. Floyd MD, Gervasini G, Masica AL, et al. Genotype-phenotype associations for common CYP3A4 and CYP3A5 variants in the basal and induced metabolism of midazolam in European- and African-American men and women. *Pharmacogenetics* 2003;**13**: 595–606.

249. He P, Court MH, Greenblatt DJ, Von Moltke LL. Genotype-phenotype associations of cytochrome P450 3A4 and 3A5 polymorphism with midazolam clearance in vivo. *Clin. Pharmacol. Ther.* 2005;**77**:373–387.

250. Lamba JK, Lin YS, Thummel K, et al. Common allelic variants of cytochrome P4503A4 and their prevalence in different populations. *Pharmacogenetics* 2002;**12**:121–132.

251. Bertrand J, Treluyer JM, Panhard X, et al. Influence of pharmacogenetics on indinavir disposition and short-term response in HIV patients initiating HAART. *Eur. J. Clin. Pharmacol.* 2009;**65**:667–678.

252. Arab-Alameddine M, Di Iulio J, Buclin T, et al. Pharmacogenetics-based population pharmacokinetic analysis of efavirenz in HIV-1-infected individuals. *Clin. Pharmacol. Ther.* 2009;**85**:485–494.

253. Kelly KM, Perentesis JP. Polymorphisms of drug metabolizing enzymes and markers of genotoxicity to identify patients with Hodgkin's lymphoma at risk of treatment-related complications. *Ann. Oncol.* 2002;**13**(Suppl. 1):34–39.

254. Tran A, Jullien V, Alexandre J, et al. Pharmacokinetics and toxicity of docetaxel: role of CYP3A, MDR1, and GST polymorphisms. *Clin. Pharmacol. Ther.* 2006;**79**:570–580.

255. Engels FK, Ten Tije AJ, Baker SD, et al. Effect of cytochrome P450 3A4 inhibition on the pharmacokinetics of docetaxel. *Clin. Pharmacol. Ther.* 2004;**75**:448–454.

256. Friedman HS, Petros WP, Friedman AH, et al. Irinotecan therapy in adults with recurrent or progressive malignant glioma. *J. Clin. Oncol.* 1999;**17**:1516–1525.

257. Mathijssen RH, Verweij J, de Bruijn P, Loos WJ, Sparreboom A. Effects of St. John's wort on irinotecan metabolism. *J. Natl. Cancer Inst.* 2002;**94**:1247–1249.

258. Keshava C, McCanlies EC, Weston A. CYP3A4 polymorphisms—potential risk factors for breast and prostate cancer: A HuGE review. *Am. J. Epidemiol.* 2004;**160**:825–841.

259. Kang YS, Park SY, Yim CH, et al. The CYP3A4*18 genotype in the cytochrome P450 3A4 gene, a rapid metabolizer of sex steroids, is associated with low bone mineral density. *Clin. Pharmacol. Ther.* 2009;**85**:312–318.

260. de Wildt SN, Kearns GL, Leeder JS, van den Anker JN. Cytochrome P450 3A: Ontogeny and drug disposition. *Clin. Pharmacokinet.* 1999;**37**:485–505.

261. Wandel C, Witte JS, Hall JM, Stein CM, Wood AJ, Wilkinson GR. CYP3A activity in African American and European American men: Population differences and functional effect of the CYP3A4*1B5′-promoter region polymorphism. *Clin. Pharmacol. Ther.* 2000;**68**:82–91.

262. Wrighton SA, Ring BJ, Watkins PB, VandenBranden M. Identification of a polymorphically expressed member of the human cytochrome P-450III family. *Mol. Pharmacol.* 1989;**36**:97–105.

263. Lee SJ, Usmani KA, Chanas B, et al. Genetic findings and functional studies of human CYP3A5 single nucleotide polymorphisms in different ethnic groups. *Pharmacogenetics* 2003;**13**:461–472.

264. Wang J. CYP3A polymorphisms and immunosuppressive drugs in solid-organ transplantation. *Expert. Rev. Mol. Diagn.* 2009;**9**:383–390.

265. Kuypers DR. Kidney transplantation: Current issues and future prospects. *Acta. Clin. Belg.* 2007;**62**:208–217.

266. Jun KR, Lee W, Jang MS, et al. Tacrolimus concentrations in relation to CYP3A and ABCB1 polymorphisms among solid organ transplant recipients in Korea. *Transplantation* 2009;**87**:1225–1231.

267. Press RR, Ploeger BA, den Hartigh J, et al. Explaining variability in tacrolimus pharmacokinetics to optimize early exposure in adult kidney transplant recipients. *Ther. Drug Monit.* 2009;**31**:187–197.

268. Kitada M, Kato T, Ohmori S, et al. Immunochemical characterization and toxicological significance of P-450HFLb purified from human fetal livers. *Biochim. Biophys. Acta.* 1992;**1117**:301–305.

269. Stevens JC, Hines RN, Gu C, et al. Developmental expression of the major human hepatic CYP3A enzymes. *J. Pharmacol. Exp. Ther.* 2003;**307**:573–582.

270. Smit P, van Schaik RH, van der Werf M, et al. A common polymorphism in the CYP3A7 gene is associated with a nearly 50% reduction in serum dehydroepiandrosterone sulfate levels. *J. Clin. Endocrinol. Metab.* 2005;**90**:5313–5316.

271. Rodriguez-Antona C, Jande M, Rane A, Ingelman-Sundberg M. Identification and phenotype characterization of two CYP3A haplotypes causing different enzymatic capacity in fetal livers. *Clin. Pharmacol. Ther.* 2005;**77**:259–270.

272. Westlind A, Malmebo S, Johansson I, et al. Cloning and tissue distribution of a novel human cytochrome p450 of the CYP3A subfamily, CYP3A43. *Biochem. Biophys. Res. Commun.* 2001;**281**:1349–1355.

273. Domanski TL, Finta C, Halpert JR, Zaphiropoulos PG. cDNA cloning and initial characterization of CYP3A43, a novel human cytochrome P450. *Mol. Pharmacol.* 2001;**59**:386–392.

274. Cauffiez C, Lo-Guidice JM, Chevalier D, et al. First report of a genetic polymorphism of the cytochrome P450 3A43 (CYP3A43) gene: Identification of a loss-of-function variant. *Hum. Mutat.* 2004;**23**:101.

275. Rasmussen BB, Brix TH, Kyvik KO, Brosen K. The interindividual differences in the 3-demthylation of caffeine alias CYP1A2 is determined by both genetic and environmental factors. *Pharmacogenetics* 2002;**12**:473–478.

276. Nakajima M, Yokoi T, Mizutani M, Kinoshita M, Funayama M, Kamataki T. Genetic polymorphism in the 5′-flanking region of human CYP1A2 gene: effect on the CYP1A2 inducibility in humans. *J. Biochem.* 1999;**125**:803–808.

277. Sachse C, Brockmoller J, Bauer S, Roots I. Functional significance of a C−>A polymorphism in intron 1 of the cytochrome P450 CYP1A2 gene tested with caffeine. *Br. J. Clin. Pharmacol.* 1999;**47**:445–449.

278. Han XM, Ouyang DS, Chen XP, et al. Inducibility of CYP1A2 by omeprazole in vivo related to the genetic polymorphism of CYP1A2. *Br. J. Clin. Pharmacol.* 2002; **54**:540–543.

279. Aklillu E, Carrillo JA, Makonnen E, et al. Genetic polymorphism of CYP1A2 in Ethiopians affecting induction and expression: Characterization of novel haplotypes with single-nucleotide polymorphisms in intron 1. *Mol. Pharmacol.* 2003;**64**:659–669.

280. Smith SS, Fiore MC. The epidemiology of tobacco use, dependence, and cessation in the United States. *Primary Care* 1999;**26**:433–461.

281. Schulze TG, Schumacher J, Muller DJ, et al. Lack of association between a functional polymorphism of the cytochrome P450 1A2 (CYP1A2) gene and tardive dyskinesia in schizophrenia. *Am. J. Med. Genet.* 2001;**105**:498–501.

282. Chong SA, Tan EC, Tan CH, Mythily. Smoking and tardive dyskinesia: lack of involvement of the CYP1A2 gene. *J. Psychiatry. Neurosci.* 2003;**28**:185–189.

283. Tiwari AK, Deshpande SN, Rao AR, et al. Genetic susceptibility to tardive dyskinesia in chronic schizophrenia subjects: I. Association of CYP1A2 gene polymorphism. *Pharmacogenomics J.* 2005;**5**:60–69.

284. Oscarson M. Genetic polymorphisms in the cytochrome P450 2A6 (CYP2A6) gene: Implications for interindividual differences in nicotine metabolism. *Drug Metab. Dispos.* 2001;**29**:91–95.

285. Oscarson M, McLellan RA, Gullsten H, et al. Characterisation and PCR-based detection of a CYP2A6 gene deletion found at a high frequency in a Chinese population. *FEBS Lett.* 1999;**448**:105–110.

286. Ring HZ, Valdes AM, Nishita DM, et al. Gene-gene interactions between CYP2B6 and CYP2A6 in nicotine metabolism. *Pharmacogenet. Genomics* 2007;**17**: 1007–1015.

287. Audrain-McGovern J, Al Koudsi N, Rodriguez D, Wileyto EP, Shields PG, Tyndale RF. The role of CYP2A6 in the emergence of nicotine dependence in adolescents. *Pediatrics* 2007;**119**:e264–e274.

288. Canova C, Hashibe M, Simonato L, et al. Genetic associations of 115 polymorphisms with cancers of the upper aerodigestive tract across 10 European countries: The ARCAGE project. *Cancer Res.* 2009;**69**:2956–2965.

289. Ariyoshi N, Miyamoto M, Umetsu Y, et al. Genetic polymorphism of CYP2A6 gene and tobacco-induced lung cancer risk in male smokers. *Cancer Epidemiol. Biomarkers Prev.* 2002;**11**:890–894.

290. Derby KS, Cuthrell K, Caberto C, et al. Nicotine metabolism in three ethnic/racial groups with different risks of lung cancer. *Cancer Epidemiol. Biomarkers Prev.* 2008;**17**: 3526–3535.

291. Upadhyaya P, Hecht SS. Identification of adducts formed in the reactions of 5′-acetoxy-N′-nitrosonornicotine with deoxyadenosine, thymidine, and DNA. *Chem. Res. Toxicol.* 2008;**21**:2164–2171.

292. MacLeod SL, Chowdhury P. The genetics of nicotine dependence: Relationship to pancreatic cancer. *World J. Gastroenterol.* 2006;**12**:7433–7439.

293. Landi S, Gemignani F, Moreno V, et al. A comprehensive analysis of phase I and phase II metabolism gene polymorphisms and risk of colorectal cancer. *Pharmacogenet. Genomics* 2005;**15**:535–546.

294. Minematsu N, Nakamura H, Iwata M, et al. Association of CYP2A6 deletion polymorphism with smoking habit and development of pulmonary emphysema. *Thorax* 2003;**58**:623–628.

295. Komatsu T, Yamazaki H, Shimada N, Nakajima M, Yokoi T. Roles of cytochromes P450 1A2, 2A6, and 2C8 in 5-fluorouracil formation from tegafur, an anticancer prodrug, in human liver microsomes. *Drug Metab. Dispos.* 2000;**28**:1457–1463.

296. Kajita J, Fuse E, Kuwabara T, Kobayashi H. The contribution of cytochrome P450 to the metabolism of tegafur in human liver. *Drug Metab. Pharmacokinet.* 2003; **18**:303–309.
297. Kaida Y, Inui N, Suda T, Nakamura H, Watanabe H, Chida K. The CYP2A6*4 allele is determinant of S-1 pharmacokinetics in Japanese patients with non-small-cell lung cancer. *Clin. Pharmacol. Ther.* 2008;**83**:589–594.
298. Code EL, Crespi CL, Penman BW, Gonzalez FJ, Chang TK, Waxman DJ. Human cytochrome P4502B6: Interindividual hepatic expression, substrate specificity, and role in procarcinogen activation. *Drug Metab. Dispos.* 1997;**25**:985–993.
299. Gervot L, Rochat B, Gautier JC, et al. Human CYP2B6: Expression, inducibility and catalytic activities. *Pharmacogenetics* 1999;**9**:295–306.
300. Hanna IH, Reed JR, Guengerich FP, Hollenberg PF. Expression of human cytochrome P450 2B6 in Escherichia coli: Characterization of catalytic activity and expression levels in human liver. *Arch. Biochem. Biophys.* 2000;**376**:206–216.
301. Lang T, Klein K, Fischer J, et al. Extensive genetic polymorphism in the human CYP2B6 gene with impact on expression and function in human liver. *Pharmacogenetics* 2001;**11**:399–415.
302. Miksys S, Lerman C, Shields PG, Mash DC, Tyndale RF. Smoking, alcoholism and genetic polymorphisms alter CYP2B6 levels in human brain. *Neuropharmacology* 2003;**45**:122–132.
303. Ekins S, Vandenbranden M, Ring BJ, et al. Further characterization of the expression in liver and catalytic activity of CYP2B6. *J. Pharmacol. Exp. Ther.* 1998;**286**:1253–1259.
304. Wang H, Faucette S, Sueyoshi T, et al. A novel distal enhancer module regulated by pregnane X receptor/constitutive androstane receptor is essential for the maximal induction of CYP2B6 gene expression. *J. Biol. Chem.* 2003;**278**:14146–14152.
305. Goodwin B, Moore LB, Stoltz CM, McKee DD, Kliewer SA. Regulation of the human CYP2B6 gene by the nuclear pregnane X receptor. *Mol. Pharmacol.* 2001;**60**:427–431.
306. Faucette SR, Sueyoshi T, Smith CM, Negishi M, Lecluyse EL, Wang H. Differential regulation of hepatic CYP2B6 and CYP3A4 genes by constitutive androstane receptor but not pregnane X receptor. *J. Pharmacol. Exp. Ther.* 2006;**317**:1200–1209.
307. Faucette SR, Wang H, Hamilton GA, et al. Regulation of CYP2B6 in primary human hepatocytes by prototypical inducers. *Drug Metab. Dispos.* 2004;**32**:348–358.
308. Wang H, Faucette S, Moore R, Sueyoshi T, Negishi M, LeCluyse E. Human constitutive androstane receptor mediates induction of CYP2B6 gene expression by phenytoin. *J. Biol. Chem.* 2004;**279**:29295–29301.
309. Wang H, Tompkins LM. CYP2B6: New insights into a historically overlooked cytochrome P450 isozyme. *Curr. Drug Metab.* 2008;**9**:598–610.
310. Hiratsuka M, Takekuma Y, Endo N, et al. Allele and genotype frequencies of CYP2B6 and CYP3A5 in the Japanese population. *Eur. J. Clin. Pharmacol.* 2002;**58**: 417–421.
311. Lang T, Klein K, Richter T, et al. Multiple novel nonsynonymous CYP2B6 gene polymorphisms in Caucasians: Demonstration of phenotypic null alleles. *J. Pharmacol. Exp. Ther.* 2004;**311**:34–43.
312. Lamba V, Lamba J, Yasuda K, et al. Hepatic CYP2B6 expression: Gender and ethnic differences and relationship to CYP2B6 genotype and CAR (constitutive androstane receptor) expression. *J. Pharmacol. Exp. Ther.* 2003;**307**:906–922.

313. Kirchheiner J, Klein C, Meineke I, et al. Bupropion and 4-OH-bupropion pharmacokinetics in relation to genetic polymorphisms in CYP2B6. *Pharmacogenetics* 2003;**13**:619–626.

314. Hofmann MH, Blievernicht JK, Klein K, et al. Aberrant splicing caused by single nucleotide polymorphism c.516G > T [Q172H], a marker of CYP2B6*6, is responsible for decreased expression and activity of CYP2B6 in liver. *J. Pharmacol. Exp. Ther.* 2008;**325**:284–292.

315. Desta Z, Saussele T, Ward B, et al. Impact of CYP2B6 polymorphism on hepatic efavirenz metabolism in vitro. *Pharmacogenomics* 2007;**8**:547–558.

316. Xie HJ, Yasar U, Lundgren S, et al. Role of polymorphic human CYP2B6 in cyclophosphamide bioactivation. *Pharmacogenomics J.* 2003;**3**:53–61.

317. Tsuchiya K, Gatanaga H, Tachikawa N, et al. Homozygous CYP2B6*6 (Q172H and K262R) correlates with high plasma efavirenz concentrations in HIV-1 patients treated with standard efavirenz-containing regimens. *Biochem. Biophys. Res. Commun.* 2004;**319**:1322–1326.

318. Wang J, Sonnerborg A, Rane A, et al. Identification of a novel specific CYP2B6 allele in Africans causing impaired metabolism of the HIV drug efavirenz. *Pharmacogenet. Genomics* 2006;**16**:191–198.

319. Huang Z, Roy P, Waxman DJ. Role of human liver microsomal CYP3A4 and CYP2B6 in catalyzing N-dechloroethylation of cyclophosphamide and ifosfamide. *Biochem. Pharmacol.* 2000;**59**:961–972.

320. Roy P, Yu LJ, Crespi CL, Waxman DJ. Development of a substrate-activity based approach to identify the major human liver P-450 catalysts of cyclophosphamide and ifosfamide activation based on cDNA-expressed activities and liver microsomal P-450 profiles. *Drug Metab. Dispos.* 1999;**27**:655–666.

321. Faucette SR, Zhang TC, Moore R, et al. Relative activation of human pregnane X receptor versus constitutive androstane receptor defines distinct classes of CYP2B6 and CYP3A4 inducers. *J. Pharmacol. Exp. Ther.* 2007;**320**:72–80.

322. Rae JM, Soukhova NV, Flockhart DA, Desta Z. Triethylenethiophosphoramide is a specific inhibitor of cytochrome P450 2B6: Implications for cyclophosphamide metabolism. *Drug Metab. Dispos.* 2002;**30**:525–530.

323. Hesse LM, He P, Krishnaswamy S, et al. Pharmacogenetic determinants of interindividual variability in bupropion hydroxylation by cytochrome P450 2B6 in human liver microsomes. *Pharmacogenetics* 2004;**14**:225–238.

324. Klein K, Lang T, Saussele T, et al. Genetic variability of CYP2B6 in populations of African and Asian origin: Allele frequencies, novel functional variants, and possible implications for anti-HIV therapy with efavirenz. *Pharmacogenet. Genomics* 2005;**15**:861–873.

325. Haas DW, Ribaudo HJ, Kim RB, et al. Pharmacogenetics of efavirenz and central nervous system side effects: An Adult AIDS clinical trials group study. *AIDS* 2004;**18**: 2391–2400.

326. Nyakutira C, Roshammar D, Chigutsa E, et al. High prevalence of the CYP2B6 516G-> T(*6) variant and effect on the population pharmacokinetics of efavirenz in HIV/AIDS outpatients in Zimbabwe. *Eur. J. Clin. Pharmacol.* 2008;**64**:357–365.

327. Gatanaga H, Hayashida T, Tsuchiya K, et al. Successful efavirenz dose reduction in HIV type 1-infected individuals with cytochrome P450 2B6 *6 and *26. *Clin. Infect. Dis.* 2007;**45**:1230–1237.

328. Rotger M, Colombo S, Furrer H, et al. Influence of CYP2B6 polymorphism on plasma and intracellular concentrations and toxicity of efavirenz and nevirapine in HIV-infected patients. *Pharmacogenet. Genomics* 2005;**15**:1–5.

329. Nakajima M, Komagata S, Fujiki Y, et al. Genetic polymorphisms of CYP2B6 affect the pharmacokinetics/pharmacodynamics of cyclophosphamide in Japanese cancer patients. *Pharmacogenet. Genomics* 2007;**17**:431–445.

330. Kreth K, Kovar K, Schwab M, Zanger UM. Identification of the human cytochromes P450 involved in the oxidative metabolism of "Ecstasy"-related designer drugs. *Biochem. Pharmaçol.* 2000;**59**:1563–1571.

331. Yamazaki H, Inoue K, Hashimoto M, Shimada T. Roles of CYP2A6 and CYP2B6 in nicotine C-oxidation by human liver microsomes. *Arch. Toxicol.* 1999; **73**:65–70.

332. Faucette SR, Hawke RL, Lecluyse EL, et al. Validation of bupropion hydroxylation as a selective marker of human cytochrome P450 2B6 catalytic activity. *Drug Metab. Dispos.* 2000;**28**:1222–1230.

333. Hesse LM, Venkatakrishnan K, Court MH, et al. CYP2B6 mediates the in vitro hydroxylation of bupropion: Potential drug interactions with other antidepressants. *Drug Metab. Dispos.* 2000;**28**:1176–1183.

334. Lee AM, Jepson C, Hoffmann E, et al. CYP2B6 genotype alters abstinence rates in a bupropion smoking cessation trial. *Biol. Psychiatry* 2007;**62**:635–641.

335. Cederbaum AI, Lu Y, Wu D. Role of oxidative stress in alcohol-induced liver injury. *Arch. Toxicol.* 2009;**83**:519–548.

336. Guengerich FP, Kim DH, Iwasaki M. Role of human cytochrome P-450 IIE1 in the oxidation of many low molecular weight cancer suspects. *Chem. Res. Toxicol.* 1991;**4**:168–179.

337. Powell H, Kitteringham NR, Pirmohamed M, Smith DA, Park BK. Expression of cytochrome P4502E1 in human liver: Assessment by mRNA, genotype and phenotype. *Pharmacogenetics* 1998;**8**:411–421.

338. Koop DR, Tierney DJ. Multiple mechanisms in the regulation of ethanol-inducible cytochrome P450IIE1. *Bioessays* 1990;**12**:429–435.

339. Nakai K, Tanaka H, Hanada K, et al. Decreased expression of cytochromes P450 1A2, 2E1, and 3A4 and drug transporters Na + -taurocholate-cotransporting polypeptide, organic cation transporter 1, and organic anion-transporting peptide-C correlates with the progression of liver fibrosis in chronic hepatitis C patients. *Drug Metab. Dispos.* 2008;**36**:1786–1793.

340. Lucas D, Menez C, Girre C, et al. Cytochrome P450 2E1 genotype and chlorzoxazone metabolism in healthy and alcoholic Caucasian subjects. *Pharmacogenetics* 1995;**5**: 298–304.

341. Bauer M, Herbarth O, Aust G, Graebsch C. Molecular cloning and expression of novel alternatively spliced cytochrome P450 2E1 mRNAs in humans. *Mol. Cell. Biochem.* 2005;**280**:201–207.

342. Hu Y, Oscarson M, Johansson I, et al. Genetic polymorphism of human CYP2E1: Characterization of two variant alleles. *Mol. Pharmacol.* 1997;**51**:370–376.

343. Fairbrother KS, Grove J, de Waziers I, et al. Detection and characterization of novel polymorphisms in the CYP2E1 gene. *Pharmacogenetics* 1998;**8**:543–552.

344. Hanioka N, Tanaka-Kagawa T, Miyata Y, et al. Functional characterization of three human cytochrome p450 2E1 variants with amino acid substitutions. *Xenobiotica* 2003;**33**:575–586.

345. Hu Y, Hakkola J, Oscarson M, Ingelman-Sundberg M. Structural and functional characterization of the 5′-flanking region of the rat and human cytochrome P450 2E1 genes: Identification of a polymorphic repeat in the human gene. *Biochem. Biophys. Res. Commun.* 1999;**263**:286–293.

346. McCarver DG, Byun R, Hines RN, Hichme M, Wegenek W. A genetic polymorphism in the regulatory sequences of human CYP2E1: Association with increased chlorzoxazone hydroxylation in the presence of obesity and ethanol intake. *Toxicol. Appl. Pharmacol.* 1998;**152**:276–281.

347. Restrepo JG, Garcia-Martin E, Martinez C, Agundez JA. Polymorphic drug metabolism in anaesthesia. *Curr. Drug Metab.* 2009;**10**:236–246.

348. Lee SS, Buters JT, Pineau T, Fernandez-Salguero P, Gonzalez FJ. Role of CYP2E1 in the hepatotoxicity of acetaminophen. *J. Biol. Chem.* 1996;**271**:12063–12067.

349. Ueshima Y, Tsutsumi M, Takase S, Matsuda Y, Kawahara H. Acetaminophen metabolism in patients with different cytochrome P-4502E1 genotypes. *Alcohol Clin. Exp. Res.* 1996;**20**:25A–28A.

350. Huang YS, Chern HD, Su WJ, et al. Cytochrome P450 2E1 genotype and the susceptibility to antituberculosis drug-induced hepatitis. *Hepatology* 2003;**37**:924–930.

351. Vuilleumier N, Rossier MF, Chiappe A, et al. CYP2E1 genotype and isoniazid-induced hepatotoxicity in patients treated for latent tuberculosis. *Eur. J. Clin. Pharmacol.* 2006;**62**:423–429.

352. Cho HJ, Koh WJ, Ryu YJ, et al. Genetic polymorphisms of NAT2 and CYP2E1 associated with antituberculosis drug-induced hepatotoxicity in Korean patients with pulmonary tuberculosis. *Tuberculosis (Edinb)* 2007;**87**:551–556.

353. Fukino K, Sasaki Y, Hirai S, et al. Effects of N-acetyltransferase 2 (NAT2), CYP2E1 and glutathione-S-transferase (GST) genotypes on the serum concentrations of isoniazid and metabolites in tuberculosis patients. *J. Toxicol. Sci.* 2008;**33**:187–195.

354. Yamada S, Tang M, Richardson K, et al. Genetic variations of NAT2 and CYP2E1 and isoniazid hepatotoxicity in a diverse population. *Pharmacogenomics* 2009;**10**: 1433–1445.

355. Yoon Y, Park HD, Park KU, Kim JQ, Chang YS, Song J. Associations between CYP2E1 promoter polymorphisms and plasma 1,3-dimethyluric acid/theophylline ratios. *Eur. J. Clin. Pharmacol.* 2006;**62**:627–631.

356. Johansson I, Eliasson E, Norsten C, Ingelman-Sundberg M. Hydroxylation of acetone by ethanol- and acetone-inducible cytochrome P-450 in liver microsomes and reconstituted membranes. *FEBS Lett.* 1986;**196**:59–64.

357. Bondoc FY, Bao Z, Hu WY, et al. Acetone catabolism by cytochrome P450 2E1: Studies with CYP2E1-null mice. *Biochem. Pharmacol.* 1999;**58**:461–463.

358. Kotlyar M, Carson SW. Effects of obesity on the cytochrome P450 enzyme system. *Int. J. Clin. Pharmacol. Ther.* 1999;**37**:8–19.

359. Krueger SK, Williams DE. Mammalian flavin-containing monooxygenases: Structure/ function, genetic polymorphisms and role in drug metabolism. *Pharmacol. Ther.* 2005; **106**:357–387.

360. Cashman JR., Some distinctions between flavin-containing and cytochrome P450 monooxygenases. *Biochem. Biophys. Res. Commun.* 2005;**338**:599–604.

361. Lawton MP, Cashman JR, Cresteil T, et al. A nomenclature for the mammalian flavin-containing monooxygenase gene family based on amino acid sequence identities. *Arch. Biochem. Biophys.* 1994;**308**:254–257.

362. Hernandez D, Janmohamed A, Chandan P, Phillips IR, Shephard EA. Organization and evolution of the flavin-containing monooxygenase genes of human and mouse: Identification of novel gene and pseudogene clusters. *Pharmacogenetics* 2004;**14**: 117–130.

363. Hines RN. Developmental and tissue-specific expression of human flavin-containing monooxygenases 1 and 3. *Expert. Opin. Drug Metab. Toxicol.* 2006;**2**:41–49.

364. Hernandez D, Addou S, Lee D, Orengo C, Shephard EA, Phillips IR. Trimethylaminuria and a human FMO3 mutation database. *Hum. Mutat.* 2003;**22**:209–213.

365. Cashman JR., Human flavin-containing monooxygenase (form 3): Polymorphisms and variations in chemical metabolism. *Pharmacogenomics* 2002;**3**:325–339.

366. Zhou J, Shephard EA. Mutation, polymorphism and perspectives for the future of human flavin-containing monooxygenase 3. *Mutat. Res.* 2006;**612**:165–171.

367. Dolphin CT, Beckett DJ, Janmohamed A, et al. The flavin-containing monooxygenase 2 gene (FMO2) of humans, but not of other primates, encodes a truncated, nonfunctional protein. *J. Biol. Chem.* 1998;**273**:30599–30607.

368. Hines RN, Hopp KA, Franco J, Saeian K, Begun FP. Alternative processing of the human FMO6 gene renders transcripts incapable of encoding a functional flavin-containing monooxygenase. *Mol. Pharmacol.* 2002;**62**:320–325.

369. Lattard V, Zhang J, Cashman JR., Alternative processing events in human FMO genes. *Mol. Pharmacol.* 2004;**65**:1517–1525.

370. Yeung CK, Lang DH, Thummel KE, Rettie AE. Immunoquantitation of FMO1 in human liver, kidney, and intestine. *Drug Metab. Dispos.* 2000;**28**:1107–1111.

371. Koukouritaki SB, Simpson P, Yeung CK, Rettie AE, Hines RN. Human hepatic flavin-containing monooxygenases 1 (FMO1) and 3 (FMO3) developmental expression. *Pediatr. Res.* 2002;**51**:236–243.

372. Hines RN, Cashman JR, Philpot RM, Williams DE, Ziegler DM. The mammalian flavin-containing monooxygenases: Molecular characterization and regulation of expression. *Toxicol. Appl. Pharmacol.* 1994;**125**:1–6.

373. Pike MG, Mays DC, Macomber DW, Lipsky JJ. Metabolism of a disulfiram metabolite, S-methyl N,N-diethyldithiocarbamate, by flavin monooxygenase in human renal microsomes. *Drug Metab. Dispos.* 2001;**29**:127–132.

374. Furnes B, Schlenk D. Extrahepatic metabolism of carbamate and organophosphate thioether compounds by the flavin-containing monooxygenase and cytochrome P450 systems. *Drug Metab. Dispos.* 2005;**33**:214–218.

375. Furnes B, Feng J, Sommer SS, Schlenk D. Identification of novel variants of the flavin-containing monooxygenase gene family in African Americans. *Drug Metab. Dispos.* 2003;**31**:187–193.

376. Zhang J, Cashman JR., Quantitative analysis of FMO gene mRNA levels in human tissues. *Drug Metab. Dispos.* 2006;**34**:19–26.

377. Whetstine JR, Yueh MF, McCarver DG, et al. Ethnic differences in human flavin-containing monooxygenase 2 (FMO2) polymorphisms: Detection of expressed protein in African-Americans. *Toxicol. Appl. Pharmacol.* 2000;**168**:216–224.

378. Krueger SK, Siddens LK, Martin SR, et al. Differences in FMO2*1 allelic frequency between Hispanics of Puerto Rican and Mexican descent. *Drug Metab. Dispos.* 2004;**32**:1337–1340.

379. Henderson MC, Krueger SK, Stevens JF, Williams DE. Human flavin-containing monooxygenase form 2 S-oxygenation: Sulfenic acid formation from thioureas and oxidation of glutathione. *Chem. Res. Toxicol.* 2004;**17**:633–640.

380. Henderson MC, Krueger SK, Siddens LK, Stevens JF, Williams DE. S-oxygenation of the thioether organophosphate insecticides phorate and disulfoton by human lung flavin-containing monooxygenase 2. *Biochem. Pharmacol.* 2004;**68**:959–967.

381. Francois AA, Nishida CR, de Montellano PR, Phillips IR, Shephard EA. Human flavin-containing monooxygenase 2.1 catalyzes oxygenation of the antitubercular drugs thiacetazone and ethionamide. *Drug Metab. Dispos.* 2009;**37**:178–186.

382. Overby LH, Carver GC, Philpot RM. Quantitation and kinetic properties of hepatic microsomal and recombinant flavin-containing monooxygenases 3 and 5 from humans. *Chem. Biol. Interact.* 1997;**106**:29–45.

383. Dolphin CT, Cullingford TE, Shephard EA, Smith RL, Phillips IR. Differential developmental and tissue-specific regulation of expression of the genes encoding three members of the flavin-containing monooxygenase family of man, FMO1, FMO3 and FM04. *Eur. J. Biochem.* 1996;**235**:683–689.

384. Cashman JR, Zhang J. Interindividual differences of human flavin-containing monooxygenase 3: Genetic polymorphisms and functional variation. *Drug Metab. Dispos.* 2002;**30**:1043–1052.

385. Phillips IR, Shephard EA. Flavin-containing monooxygenases: Mutations, disease and drug response. *Trends. Pharmacol. Sci.* 2008;**29**:294–301.

386. `http://www.genecards.org/` (accessed 11/09).

387. Koukouritaki SB, Poch MT, Cabacungan ET, McCarver DG, Hines RN. Discovery of novel flavin-containing monooxygenase 3 (FMO3) single nucleotide polymorphisms and functional analysis of upstream haplotype variants. *Mol. Pharmacol.* 2005;**68**: 383–392.

388. Treacy EP, Akerman BR, Chow LM, et al. Mutations of the flavin-containing monooxygenase gene (FMO3) cause trimethylaminuria, a defect in detoxication. *Hum. Mol. Genet.* 1998;**7**:839–845.

389. Mitchell SC, Smith RL. Trimethylamine and odorous sweat. *J. Inherit. Metab. Dis.* 2003;**26**:415–416.

390. Parte P, Kupfer D. Oxidation of tamoxifen by human flavin-containing monooxygenase (FMO) 1 and FMO3 to tamoxifen-N-oxide and its novel reduction back to tamoxifen by human cytochromes P450 and hemoglobin. *Drug Metab. Dispos.* 2005;**33**:1446–1452.

391. Krueger SK, Vandyke JE, Williams DE, Hines RN. The role of flavin-containing monooxygenase (FMO) in the metabolism of tamoxifen and other tertiary amines. *Drug Metab. Rev.* 2006;**38**:139–147.

392. Hisamuddin IM, Wehbi MA, Chao A, et al. Genetic polymorphisms of human flavin monooxygenase 3 in sulindac-mediated primary chemoprevention of familial adenomatous polyposis. *Clin. Cancer Res.* 2004;**10**:8357–8362.

393. Hisamuddin IM, Wehbi MA, Schmotzer B, et al. Genetic polymorphisms of flavin monooxygenase 3 in sulindac-induced regression of colorectal adenomas in familial adenomatous polyposis. *Cancer Epidemiol. Biomarkers. Prev.* 2005;**14**:2366–2369.

394. Sachse C, Ruschen S, Dettling M, et al. Flavin monooxygenase 3 (FMO3) polymorphism in a white population: Allele frequencies, mutation linkage, and functional effects on clozapine and caffeine metabolism. *Clin. Pharmacol. Ther.* 1999;**66**: 431–438.

395. Cashman JR, Zhang J, Nelson MR, Braun A. Analysis of flavin-containing monooxygenase 3 genotype data in populations administered the anti-schizophrenia agent olanzapine. *Drug Metab. Lett.* 2008;**2**:100–114.

396. Overby LH, Buckpitt AR, Lawton MP, Atta-Asafo-Adjei E, Schulze J, Philpot RM. Characterization of flavin-containing monooxygenase 5 (FMO5) cloned from human and guinea pig: Evidence that the unique catalytic properties of FMO5 are not confined to the rabbit ortholog. *Arch. Biochem. Biophys.* 1995;**317**:275–284.

397. Ross D, Siegel D. NAD(P)H:quinone oxidoreductase 1 (NQO1, DT-diaphorase), functions and pharmacogenetics. *Methods Enzymol.* 2004;**382**:115–144.

398. Wu K, Knox R, Sun XZ, et al. Catalytic properties of NAD(P)H:quinone oxidoreductase-2 (NQO2), a dihydronicotinamide riboside dependent oxidoreductase. *Arch. Biochem. Biophys.* 1997;**347**:221–228.

399. Joseph P, Jaiswal AK. NAD(P)H:quinone oxidoreductase1 (DT diaphorase) specifically prevents the formation of benzo[a]pyrene quinone-DNA adducts generated by cytochrome P4501A1 and P450 reductase. *Proc. Natl. Acad. Sci. USA* 1994;**91**: 8413–8417.

400. Siegel D, Ross D. Immunodetection of NAD(P)H:quinone oxidoreductase 1 (NQO1) in human tissues. *Free Radical Biol. Med.* 2000;**29**:246–253.

401. Cresteil T, Jaiswal AK. High levels of expression of the NAD(P)H:quinone oxidoreductase (NQO1) gene in tumor cells compared to normal cells of the same origin. *Biochem. Pharmacol.* 1991;**42**:1021–1027.

402. Belinsky M, Jaiswal AK. NAD(P)H:quinone oxidoreductase1 (DT-diaphorase) expression in normal and tumor tissues. *Cancer Metast. Rev.* 1993;**12**:103–117.

403. Strassburg A, Strassburg CP, Manns MP, Tukey RH. Differential gene expression of NAD(P)H:quinone oxidoreductase and NRH:quinone oxidoreductase in human hepatocellular and biliary tissue. *Mol. Pharmacol.* 2002;**61**:320–325.

404. Jaiswal AK. Nrf2 signaling in coordinated activation of antioxidant gene expression. *Free Radical Biol. Med.* 2004;**36**:1199–1207.

405. Begleiter A, Leith MK, Curphey TJ, Doherty GP. Induction of DT-diaphorase in cancer chemoprevention and chemotherapy. *Oncol. Res.* 1997;**9**:371–382.

406. Siegel D, Anwar A, Winski SL, Kepa JK, Zolman KL, Ross D. Rapid polyubiquitination and proteasomal degradation of a mutant form of NAD(P)H:quinone oxidoreductase 1. *Mol. Pharmacol.* 2001;**59**:263–268.

407. Kelsey KT, Ross D, Traver RD, et al. Ethnic variation in the prevalence of a common NAD(P)H quinone oxidoreductase polymorphism and its implications for anti-cancer chemotherapy. *Br. J. Cancer* 1997;**76**:852–854.

408. Gaedigk A, Tyndale RF, Jurima-Romet M, Sellers EM, Grant DM, Leeder JS. NAD(P)H: quinone oxidoreductase: Polymorphisms and allele frequencies in Caucasian, Chinese and Canadian Native Indian and Inuit populations. *Pharmacogenetics* 1998;**8**:305–313.

409. Pan SS, Forrest GL, Akman SA, Hu LT. NAD(P)H:quinone oxidoreductase expression and mitomycin C resistance developed by human colon cancer HCT 116 cells. *Cancer Res.* 1995;**55**:330–335.

410. Fleming RA, Drees J, Loggie BW, et al. Clinical significance of a NAD(P)H: Quinone oxidoreductase 1 polymorphism in patients with disseminated peritoneal cancer receiving intraperitoneal hyperthermic chemotherapy with mitomycin C. *Pharmacogenetics* 2002;**12**:31–37.

411. Mrozek E, Kolesar J, Young D, Allen J, Villalona-Calero M, Shapiro CL. Phase II study of sequentially administered low-dose mitomycin-C (MMC) and irinotecan (CPT-11) in women with metastatic breast cancer (MBC). *Ann. Oncol.* 2008;**19**:1417–1422.

412. Wojnowski L, Kulle B, Schirmer M, et al. NAD(P)H oxidase and multidrug resistance protein genetic polymorphisms are associated with doxorubicin-induced cardiotoxicity. *Circulation.* 2005;**112**:3754–3762.

413. Blanco JG, Leisenring WM, Gonzalez-Covarrubias VM, et al. Genetic polymorphisms in the carbonyl reductase 3 gene CBR3 and the NAD(P)H:quinone oxidoreductase 1 gene NQO1 in patients who developed anthracycline-related congestive heart failure after childhood cancer. *Cancer* 2008;**112**:2789–2795.

414. Blanco JG, Edick MJ, Hancock ML, et al. Genetic polymorphisms in CYP3A5, CYP3A4 and NQO1 in children who developed therapy-related myeloid malignancies. *Pharmacogenetics.* 2002;**12**:605–611.

415. Stanulla M, Dynybil C, Bartels DB, et al. The NQO1 C609T polymorphism is associated with risk of secondary malignant neoplasms after treatment for childhood acute lymphoblastic leukemia: A matched-pair analysis from the ALL-BFM study group. *Haematologica* 2007;**92**:1581–1582.

416. Zai CC, Tiwari AK, Basile V, et al. Oxidative stress in tardive dyskinesia: Genetic association study and meta-analysis of NADPH quinine oxidoreductase 1 (NQO1) and Superoxide dismutase 2 (SOD2, MnSOD) genes. *Prog. Neuropsychopharmacol. Biol. Psychiatry* 2010;**34**:50–56.

417. Gong X, Gutala R, Jaiswal AK. Quinone oxidoreductases and vitamin K metabolism. *Vitam. Horm.* 2008;**78**:85–101.

418. Wadelius M, Chen LY, Eriksson N, et al. Association of warfarin dose with genes involved in its action and metabolism. *Hum. Genet.* 2007;**121**:23–34.

419. Momary KM, Shapiro NL, Viana MA, Nutescu EA, Helgason CM, Cavallari LH. Factors influencing warfarin dose requirements in African-Americans. *Pharmacogenomics* 2007;**8**:1535–1544.

420. Ross D. Quinone reductases multitasking in the metabolic world. *Drug Metab. Rev.* 2004;**36**:639–654.

421. Beyer RE, Segura-Aguilar J, Di Bernardo S, et al. The role of DT-diaphorase in the maintenance of the reduced antioxidant form of coenzyme Q in membrane systems. *Proc. Natl. Acad. Sci. USA* 1996;**93**:2528–2532.

422. Asher G, Lotem J, Cohen B, Sachs L, Shaul Y. Regulation of p53 stability and p53-dependent apoptosis by NADH quinone oxidoreductase 1. *Proc. Natl. Acad. Sci. USA* 2001;**98**:1188–1193.

423. Jaiswal AK. Human NAD(P)H:quinone oxidoreductase2. Gene structure, activity, and tissue-specific expression. *J. Biol. Chem.* 1994;**269**:14502–14508.

424. Jamieson D, Wilson K, Pridgeon S, et al. NAD(P)H:quinone oxidoreductase 1 and nrh: quinone oxidoreductase 2 activity and expression in bladder and ovarian cancer and lower NRH:quinone oxidoreductase 2 activity associated with an NQO2 exon 3 single-nucleotide polymorphism. *Clin. Cancer Res.* 2007;**13**:1584–1590.

425. Jaiswal AK, McBride OW, Adesnik M, Nebert DW. Human dioxin-inducible cytosolic NAD(P)H:menadione oxidoreductase. cDNA sequence and localization of gene to chromosome 16. *J. Biol. Chem.* 1988;**263**:13572–13578.

426. Hsieh TC. Antiproliferative effects of resveratrol and the mediating role of resveratrol targeting protein NQO2 in androgen receptor-positive, hormone-non-responsive CWR22Rv1 cells. *Anticancer Res.* 2009;**29**:3011–3017.

427. Winger JA, Hantschel O, Superti-Furga G, Kuriyan J. The structure of the leukemia drug imatinib bound to human quinone reductase 2 (NQO2). *BMC Struct. Biol.* 2009;**9**:7.

428. Iida A, Sekine A, Saito S, et al. Catalog of 320 single nucleotide polymorphisms (SNPs) in 20 quinone oxidoreductase and sulfotransferase genes. *J. Hum. Genet.* 2001;**46**: 225–240.

429. Harada S, Fujii C, Hayashi A, Ohkoshi N. An association between idiopathic Parkinson's disease and polymorphisms of phase II detoxification enzymes: Glutathione S-transferase M1 and quinone oxidoreductase 1 and 2. *Biochem. Biophys. Res. Commun.* 2001;**288**:887–892.

430. Wang W, Le WD, Pan T, Stringer JL, Jaiswal AK. Association of NRH:quinone oxidoreductase 2 gene promoter polymorphism with higher gene expression and increased susceptibility to Parkinson's disease. *J. Gerontol. A Biol. Sci. Med. Sci.* 2008;**63**:127–134.

431. Ostrousky O, Meged S, Loewenthal R, et al. NQO2 gene is associated with clozapine-induced agranulocytosis. *Tissue Antigens* 2003;**62**:483–491.

432. Nosjean O, Ferro M, Coge F, et al. Identification of the melatonin-binding site MT3 as the quinone reductase 2. *J. Biol. Chem.* 2000;**275**:31311–31317.

433. Ahn KS, Gong X, Sethi G, Chaturvedi MM, Jaiswal AK, Aggarwal BB. Deficiency of NRH:quinone oxidoreductase 2 differentially regulates TNF signaling in keratinocytes: Up-regulation of apoptosis correlates with down-regulation of cell survival kinases. *Cancer Res.* 2007;**67**:10004–10011.

434. Gong X, Kole L, Iskander K, Jaiswal AK. NRH:quinone oxidoreductase 2 and NAD(P)H: quinone oxidoreductase 1 protect tumor suppressor p53 against 20s proteasomal degradation leading to stabilization and activation of p53. *Cancer Res.* 2007;**67**: 5380–5388.

435. Yu KD, Di GH, Yuan WT, et al. Functional polymorphisms, altered gene expression and genetic association link NRH:quinone oxidoreductase 2 to breast cancer with wild-type p53. *Hum. Mol. Genet.* 2009;**18**:2502–2517.

436. Coates PM, Mestriner MA, Hopkinson DA. A preliminary genetic interpretation of the esterase isozymes of human tissues. *Ann. Hum. Genet.* 1975;**39**:1–20.

437. Satoh T, Hosokawa M. The mammalian carboxylesterases: From molecules to functions. *Annu. Rev. Pharmacol. Toxicol.* 1998;**38**:257–288.

438. Sanghani SP, Quinney SK, Fredenburg TB, Davis WI, Murry DJ, Bosron WF. Hydrolysis of irinotecan and its oxidative metabolites, 7-ethyl-10-[4-N-(5-aminopentanoic acid)-1-piperidino] carbonyloxycamptothecin and 7-ethyl-10-[4-(1-piperidino)-1-amino]-carbonyloxycamptothecin, by human carboxylesterases CES1A1, CES2, and a newly expressed carboxylesterase isoenzyme, CES3. *Drug Metab. Dispos.* 2004;**32**:505–511.

439. Satoh T, Taylor P, Bosron WF, Sanghani SP, Hosokawa M, La Du BN. Current progress on esterases: From molecular structure to function. *Drug Metab. Dispos.* 2002; **30**:488–493.

440. Schiel MA, Green SL, Davis WI, Sanghani PC, Bosron WF, Sanghani SP. Expression and characterization of a human carboxylesterase 2 splice variant. *J. Pharmacol. Exp. Ther.* 2007;**323**:94–101.

441. Hosokawa M. Structure and catalytic properties of carboxylesterase isozymes involved in metabolic activation of prodrugs. *Molecules* 2008;**13**:412–431.

442. Takai S, Matsuda A, Usami Y, et al. Hydrolytic profile for ester- or amide-linkage by carboxylesterases pI 5.3 and 4.5 from human liver. *Biol. Pharm. Bull.* 1997;**20**:869–873.

443. Pindel EV, Kedishvili NY, Abraham TL, et al. Purification and cloning of a broad substrate specificity human liver carboxylesterase that catalyzes the hydrolysis of cocaine and heroin. *J. Biol. Chem.* 1997;**272**:14769–14775.

444. Geshi E, Kimura T, Yoshimura M, et al. A single nucleotide polymorphism in the carboxylesterase gene is associated with the responsiveness to imidapril medication and the promoter activity. *Hypertens. Res.* 2005;**28**:719–725.

445. Yoshimura M, Kimura T, Ishii M, et al. Functional polymorphisms in carboxylesterase1A2 (CES1A2) gene involves specific protein 1 (Sp1) binding sites. *Biochem. Biophys. Res. Commun.* 2008;**369**:939–942.

446. Zhu HJ, Patrick KS, Yuan HJ, et al. Two CES1 gene mutations lead to dysfunctional carboxylesterase 1 activity in man: Clinical significance and molecular basis. *Am. J. Hum. Genet.* 2008;**82**:1241–1248.

447. Zhu HJ, Appel DI, Johnson JA, Chavin KD, Markowitz JS. Role of carboxylesterase 1 and impact of natural genetic variants on the hydrolysis of trandolapril. *Biochem. Pharmacol.* 2009;**77**:1266–1272.

448. Zhu HJ, Markowitz JS. Activation of the antiviral prodrug oseltamivir is impaired by two newly identified carboxylesterase 1 variants. *Drug Metab. Dispos.* 2009;**37**: 264–267.

449. Ghosh S, Natarajan R. Cloning of the human cholesteryl ester hydrolase promoter: Identification of functional peroxisomal proliferator-activated receptor responsive elements. *Biochem. Biophys. Res. Commun.* 2001;**284**:1065–1070.

450. Crow JA, Middleton BL, Borazjani A, Hatfield MJ, Potter PM, Ross MK. Inhibition of carboxylesterase 1 is associated with cholesteryl ester retention in human THP-1 monocyte/macrophages. *Biochim. Biophys. Acta.* 2008;**1781**:643–654.

451. Kalow W, Gunn DR. Some statistical data on atypical cholinesterase of human serum. *Ann. Hum. Genet.* 1959;**23**:239–250.

452. Lockridge O. Genetic variants of human serum cholinesterase influence metabolism of the muscle relaxant succinylcholine. *Pharmacol. Ther.* 1990;**47**:35–60.

453. Gatke MR, Bundgaard JR, Viby-Mogensen J. Two novel mutations in the BCHE gene in patients with prolonged duration of action of mivacurium or succinylcholine during anaesthesia. *Pharmacogenet. Genomics* 2007;**17**:995–999.

454. Duysen EG, Li B, Lockridge O. The butyrylcholinesterase knockout mouse a research tool in the study of drug sensitivity, bio-distribution, obesity and Alzheimer's disease. *Expert Opin. Drug Metab. Toxicol.* 2009;**5**:523–528.

455. Ferris S, Nordberg A, Soininen H, Darreh-Shori T, Lane R. Progression from mild cognitive impairment to Alzheimer's disease: Effects of sex, butyrylcholinesterase genotype, and rivastigmine treatment. *Pharmacogenet Genomics* 2009;**19**:635–646.

456. O'Brien KK, Saxby BK, Ballard CG, et al. Regulation of attention and response to therapy in dementia by butyrylcholinesterase. *Pharmacogenetics* 2003;**13**:231–239.

457. Duysen EG, Li B, Darvesh S, Lockridge O. Sensitivity of butyrylcholinesterase knockout mice to (−)-huperzine A and donepezil suggests humans with butyrylcholinesterase deficiency may not tolerate these Alzheimer's disease drugs and indicates butyrylcholinesterase function in neurotransmission. *Toxicology* 2007; **233**:60–69.

458. Primo-Parmo SL, Sorenson RC, Teiber J, La Du BN. The human serum paraoxonase/arylesterase gene (PON1) is one member of a multigene family. *Genomics* 1996;**33**:498–507.

459. Reddy ST, Wadleigh DJ, Grijalva V, et al. Human paraoxonase-3 is an HDL-associated enzyme with biological activity similar to paraoxonase-1 protein but is not regulated by oxidized lipids. *Arterioscler. Thromb. Vasc. Biol.* 2001;**21**:542–547.

460. Mochizuki H, Scherer SW, Xi T, et al. Human PON2 gene at 7q21.3: Cloning, multiple mRNA forms, and missense polymorphisms in the coding sequence. *Gene* 1998;**213**: 149–157.

461. Eckerson HW, Wyte CM, La Du BN. The human serum paraoxonase/arylesterase polymorphism. *Am. J. Hum. Genet.* 1983;**35**:1126–1138.

462. Draganov DI, Teiber JF, Speelman A, Osawa Y, Sunahara R, La Du BN. Human paraoxonases (PON1, PON2, and PON3) are lactonases with overlapping and distinct substrate specificities. *J. Lipid. Res.* 2005;**46**:1239–1247.

463. Leviev I, James RW. Promoter polymorphisms of human paraoxonase PON1 gene and serum paraoxonase activities and concentrations. *Arterioscler. Thromb. Vasc. Biol.* 2000;**20**:516–521.

464. Brophy VH, Jampsa RL, Clendenning JB, McKinstry LA, Jarvik GP, Furlong CE. Effects of 5′ regulatory-region polymorphisms on paraoxonase-gene (PON1) expression. *Am. J. Hum. Genet.* 2001;**68**:1428–1436.

465. Costa LG, Li WF, Richter RJ, Shih DM, Lusis A, Furlong CE. The role of paraoxonase (PON1) in the detoxication of organophosphates and its human polymorphism. *Chem. Biol. Interact.* 1999, **119–120**:429–438.

466. van Himbergen TM, van Tits LJ, Roest M, Stalenhoef AF. The story of PON1: How an organophosphate-hydrolysing enzyme is becoming a player in cardiovascular medicine. *Neth. J. Med.* 2006;**64**:34–38.

467. Liu C, Batliwalla F, Li W, et al. Genome-wide association scan identifies candidate polymorphisms associated with differential response to anti-TNF treatment in rheumatoid arthritis. *Mol. Med.* 2008;**14**:575–581.

468. Wheeler JG, Keavney BD, Watkins H, Collins R, Danesh J. Four paraoxonase gene polymorphisms in 11212 cases of coronary heart disease and 12786 controls: Meta-analysis of 43 studies. *Lancet* 2004;**363**:689–695.

469. Hofer SE, Bennetts B, Chan AK, et al. Association between PON 1 polymorphisms, PON activity and diabetes complications. *J. Diab. Complic.* 2006;**20**:322–328.

470. Ishii Y, Takeda S, Yamada H, Oguri K. Functional protein-protein interaction of drug metabolizing enzymes. *Front. Biosci.* 2005;**10**:887–895.

471. Fretland AJ, Omiecinski CJ. Epoxide hydrolases: Biochemistry and molecular biology. *Chem. Biol. Interact.* 2000;**129**:41–59.

472. Oesch F. Mammalian epoxide hydrases: Inducible enzymes catalysing the inactivation of carcinogenic and cytotoxic metabolites derived from aromatic and olefinic compounds. *Xenobiotica* 1973;**3**:305–340.

473. Omiecinski CJ, Hassett C, Hosagrahara V. Epoxide hydrolase–polymorphism and role in toxicology. *Toxicol. Lett.* 2000, **112–113**:365–370.

474. Coller JK, Fritz P, Zanger UM, et al. Distribution of microsomal epoxide hydrolase in humans: An immunohistochemical study in normal tissues, and benign and malignant tumours. *Histochem. J.* 2001;**33**:329–336.

475. Mertes I, Fleischmann R, Glatt HR, Oesch F. Interindividual variations in the activities of cytosolic and microsomal epoxide hydrolase in human liver. *Carcinogenesis* 1985; **6**:219–223.

476. Hassett C, Aicher L, Sidhu JS, Omiecinski CJ. Human microsomal epoxide hydrolase: Genetic polymorphism and functional expression in vitro of amino acid variants. *Hum. Mol. Genet.* 1994;**3**:421–428.

477. Makmor-Bakry M, Sills GJ, Hitiris N, Butler E, Wilson EA, Brodie MJ. Genetic variants in microsomal epoxide hydrolase influence carbamazepine dosing. *Clin. Neuropharmacol.* 2009;**32**:205–212.

478. Gaedigk A, Spielberg SP, Grant DM. Characterization of the microsomal epoxide hydrolase gene in patients with anticonvulsant adverse drug reactions. *Pharmacogenetics* 1994;**4**:142–153.

479. Green VJ, Pirmohamed M, Kitteringham NR, et al. Genetic analysis of microsomal epoxide hydrolase in patients with carbamazepine hypersensitivity. *Biochem. Pharmacol.* 1995;**50**:1353–1359.

480. Loebstein R, Vecsler M, Kurnik D, et al. Common genetic variants of microsomal epoxide hydrolase affect warfarin dose requirements beyond the effect of cytochrome P450 2C9. *Clin. Pharmacol. Ther.* 2005;**77**:365–372.

481. Lin TS, Huang HH, Fan YH, Chiou SH, Chow KC. Genetic polymorphism and gene expression of microsomal epoxide hydrolase in non-small cell lung cancer. *Oncol. Rep.* 2007;**17**:565–572.

482. Zhu QS, Xing W, Qian B, et al. Inhibition of human m-epoxide hydrolase gene expression in a case of hypercholanemia. *Biochim. Biophys. Acta* 2003;**1638**:208–216.

483. Zeldin DC, Wei S, Falck JR, Hammock BD, Snapper JR, Capdevila JH. Metabolism of epoxyeicosatrienoic acids by cytosolic epoxide hydrolase: Substrate structural determinants of asymmetric catalysis. *Arch. Biochem. Biophys.* 1995;**316**: 443–451.

484. Norris KK, DeAngelo TM, Vesell ES. Genetic and environmental factors that regulate cytosolic epoxide hydrolase activity in normal human lymphocytes. *J. Clin. Invest.* 1989;**84**:1749–1756.

485. Sandberg M, Meijer J. Structural characterization of the human soluble epoxide hydrolase gene (EPHX2). *Biochem. Biophys. Res. Commun.* 1996;**221**:333–339.

486. Sandberg M, Hassett C, Adman ET, Meijer J, Omiecinski CJ. Identification and functional characterization of human soluble epoxide hydrolase genetic polymorphisms. *J. Biol. Chem.* 2000;**275**:28873–28881.

487. Przybyla-Zawislak BD, Srivastava PK, Vazquez-Matias J, et al. Polymorphisms in human soluble epoxide hydrolase. *Mol. Pharmacol.* 2003;**64**:482–490.

488. Koerner IP, Jacks R, DeBarber AE, et al. Polymorphisms in the human soluble epoxide hydrolase gene EPHX2 linked to neuronal survival after ischemic injury. *J. Neurosci.* 2007;**27**:4642–4649.

489. Fornage M, Lee CR, Doris PA, et al. The soluble epoxide hydrolase gene harbors sequence variation associated with susceptibility to and protection from incident ischemic stroke. *Hum. Mol. Genet.* 2005;**14**:2829–2837.

490. Fornage M, Boerwinkle E, Doris PA, Jacobs D, Liu K, Wong ND. Polymorphism of the soluble epoxide hydrolase is associated with coronary artery calcification in African-American subjects: The coronary artery risk development in young adults (CARDIA) study. *Circulation* 2004;**109**:335–339.

491. Ohtoshi K, Kaneto H, Node K, et al. Association of soluble epoxide hydrolase gene polymorphism with insulin resistance in type 2 diabetic patients. *Biochem. Biophys. Res. Commun.* 2005;**331**:347–350.

CHAPTER 3

Pharmacogenetics of Phase II Drug Metabolizing Enzymes

INGOLF CASCORBI
University Hospital Schleswig–Holstein, Kiel, Germany

3.1 INTRODUCTION

Drug effects are subject to substantial interindividual variability. Polymorphic phase II enzymes facilitate the excretion of endogenous and foreign compounds by conjugating hydrophilic side groups (Fig. 3.1). Many substrates are activated beforehand by phase I enzymes, particularly by oxidation through cytochrome P450 enzymes. Some phase II enzymes exhibit genetically determined strong interindividual different phenotypes, thus contributing to variability in drug response, but also act as susceptibility factors for malignant diseases such as bladder or lung cancer, by modulating an individual's cancer risk according to the extent of environmental exposure (Table 3.1). The polymorphic character of NAT and GST, and particularly their functions with respect to malignancies, was extensively investigated, and the role of TPMT for azathioprine toxicity is well established. The UGT family provides certain polymorphic traits, hereditary defects may lead to mild or severe hyperbilirubinemia, and there is increasing evidence that genetic variants may have an important pharmacological impact on, for example, anticancer therapy with irinotecan [1,2]. The impact of polymorphisms of sulfotransferases is much more difficult to consider, since the different isoforms of sulfotransferases are involved in not only detoxification but also toxification pathways, leading to partly contradictory results [3]. Also, the phase II enzyme catecholamine-*S*-methyltransferase COMT is polymorphic and is related to neuropsychiatric disorders [4,5] or malignancies [6]. The associations with drug therapy, however, are weak or need confirmation. This chapter focuses on the role of the polymorphic phase II enzymes arylamine *N*-acetyltransferases, glutathione *S*-transferases, thiopurine *S*-methyltran-

Pharmacogenetics and Individualized Therapy, First Edition.
Edited by Anke-Hilse Maitland-van der Zee and Ann K. Daly.

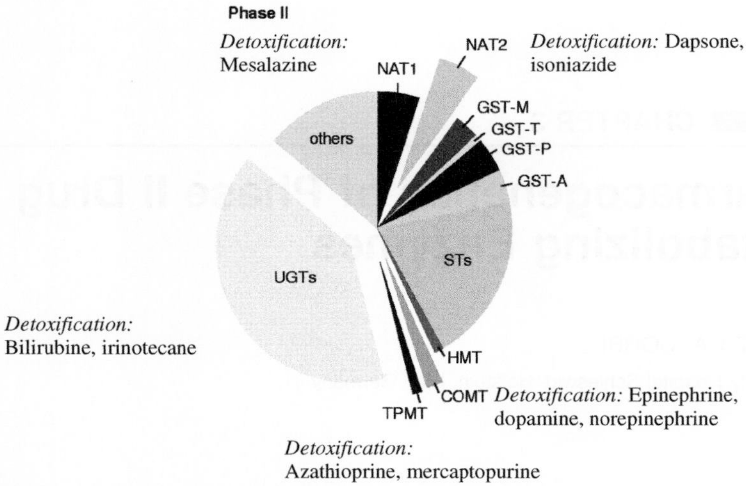

FIGURE 3.1 Phase II enzymes, involved in drug and xenobiotic metabolism (NAT – arylamine *N*-acetyltransferase; GST – glutathione *S*-transferases; ST – sulfotransferases; COMT – catecholamine *O*-methyltransferases; TPMT – thiopurine *S*-methyltransferases, UGT – UDP-glucuronosyltransferases). [From Evans WE, Relling MV. Pharmacogenomics: Translating functional genomics into rational therapeutics. *Science* 1999;**286**(5439):487–491. Reprinted with permission from AAAS.]

ferases, UDP glucuronosyltransferases, and sulfotransferases as detoxifying but also toxifying factors, modulating pharmacokinetics and disease susceptibility.

3.2 ARYLAMINE *N*-ACETYLTRANSFERASES

Only a short time after the introduction of isoniazid into clinical treatment of tuberculosis in the early 1950s, it was recognized that there exist considerable interindividual differences of urinary excretion of the acetylated metabolite [8] (see also Chapter 1). Because of this observation, Mitchel and Bell [9] inaugurated the terms *rapid* and *slow acetylator*. Arylamine *N*-acetyltransferase (EC 2.3.1.5),

TABLE 3.1 Polymorphic Phase II Enzymes Relevant for Drug Therapy or Cancer Susceptibility

Pharmacotherapy (Drugs)	Cancer Susceptibility
Arylamine *N*-acetyltransferase 2 (dapsone, hydralazine, isoniazid, procainamide, sulfamethazine, sulfapyridine)	Arylamine *N*-acetyltransferase 2 (bladder cancer)
Thiopurine *S*-methyltransferase (azathioprine, 6-mercaptopurine)	Glutathione *S*-transferases (bladder cancer, lung cancer, acute lymphatic leukemia)
UDP-glucuronosyltransferases (irinotecan, morphine, mycophenolate mofetil	Sulfotransferases

which is responsible for this conjugation reaction, consists of two isoenzymes, NAT1 and NAT2, which were shown to be independently expressed in different liver samples [10]. NAT2 catalyzes the acetylation of certain drugs such as sulfamethazine, whereas NAT1 acetylates arylamines such as *p*-aminosalicylic acid and *p*-aminobenzoic acid. The apparent interindividual differences of isoniazid or sulfamethazine acetylation were identified as being caused by genetic polymorphisms in *NAT2*. Slow acetylation in humans was shown to be based on a reduced activity of enzymes with aminoacid variants rather than lower expression rates. In rabbits, however, a complete deletion of the *NAT2* gene causes the slow acetylators phenotype [11]. NAT2 is expressed preferably in the human liver, whereas NAT1 can be determined in a wide variety of different tissues.

Before elucidation of the genetic basis of the NAT2 polymorphism, the acetylator status was determined by probe drugs such as isoniazid, dapsone, and sulfamethazine [12]. With these probe drugs, a large number of studies were conducted to investigate associations between the acetylator polymorphism and a variety of diseases, particularly cancer. The advantages of these probe drugs are chemical stability of the substrate and acetylated metabolite facilitating a reliable and sensitive detection; however, in some cases, side effects cannot be excluded. Grant et al. [13] introduced the caffeine test, which became a well-accepted and well-tolerated *in vivo* probe, by calculating the ratio of concentrations of the secondary metabolites 5-acetylamino-6-formylamino-3-methyluracil (AFMU) and 1-methylxanthine (1X) in urine. The caffeine test is also appropriate for determining the activity of cytochrome P450 1A2 (CYP1A2) [14].

Human arylamine *N*-acetyltransferases are encoded by different genes: the so-called polymorphic *NAT2* and the (formerly believed) monomorphic *NAT1*. Both genes are located on chromosome 8p21.3–23.1 and provide a relatively short distance of approximately 170–360 kb [15]. *NAT1* and *NAT2* consist of a 870-bp coding sequence. In contrast to *NAT1*, *NAT2* provides a noncoding exon approximately 800 bp upstream. Additionally, there is a pseudogene *pNAT* on chromosome 8, which does not code for a functional protein [16].

3.2.1 Genetic Basis and Functional Effect of NAT1 Polymorphisms

Until now (2011) more than 26 different alleles have been discovered. There is consensus to consider *NAT1*4* as the wild type (frequency in Caucasians approximately 75%). The most frequent variant is *NAT1*10* (allele frequency in Caucasians approximately 20%) [17]. It consists of a 1088T > A and a 1095C > A exchange in the 3′-untranslated region. The functional properties are not fully characterized; however, some haplotypes showed clearly diminished *in vitro* or *ex vivo* activity. Investigating the distribution of *NAT1* genotypes and *in vitro* activity in bladder and colon cancer patients, Bell et al. reported an increased frequency and an elevated activity of the *NAT1*10* allele in bladder and colon cancer patients [18]. It was suggested that the alteration of the polyadenylation signal possibly led to an increased activity toward *O*-acetylation in the urinary bladder or colon epithelium. The results were supported by the observation of raised DNA adducts among carriers of *NAT1*10* in bladder cancer tissue [19]. In clinical studies in humans, characterization of the specific activity of NAT1 is difficult to perform, since there are no NAT1-specific nontoxic substrates, which can be administered systemically. With the use of *p*-amino salicylic in an *in vitro*-assay of recombinantly expressed NAT1 in *Escherichia coli* as well as in *ex vivo*-tests in red blood cells, *NAT1*4* provided highest acetylation capacity. *NAT1*15* (559C > T) had no activity, due to a premature stop in codon 187, and *NAT1*14* (560G > A) presented a low activity as mirrored by a low V_{max} and increased K_M [20]. In *ex vivo* studies with *p*-aminosalicylic acid, *NAT1*10* showed no different kinetics to the wild-type *NAT1*4* but confirmed the finding on *NAT1*14* and **15* [21].

Since both NAT1 and NAT2 are located relatively close to each other, with a distance of only 170–360 kb on the same chromosome 8p21.3–23, it is not surprising that the SNPs of both genes are in linkage disequilibrium. *NAT1*10* was found linked to the rapid *NAT2*4* haplotype in two studies [22,23].

3.2.2 Genetic Basis of NAT2 Polymorphism

Although a number of SNPs have been identified in NAT1 and NAT2, seven SNPs in NAT2 form the most important haplotypes. Five of these nucleotide transitions lead to aminoacid exchanges: 191G > A (Arg63Glu), occurring preferentially among African blacks; 341T > C (Ile114Thr); 590G > A (Arg197Gln); 803A > G (Lys268Arg); and 857G > A (Gly286Glu). The remaining two SNPs 282C > T and 481C > T are silent mutations in wobble base positions. These mutations provided the basis for a large number of genotyping studies on the ethnic distribution of *NAT2* polymorphism or their association with different diseases. Beside these frequently described SNPs, there exist further SNPs, partly observed only in single individuals. Variants in regulatory or untranslated regions have not been reported so far.

Most *NAT2* variants are in linkage disequilibrium. There was initial consensus on the nomenclature in 1995 [24]. In 2008 an update considering, in particular, a new nomenclature on NAT in mammals was published [25]. The current known haplotypes are listed on the Internet [26].

In vivo studies using caffeine [27] or sulfamethazine [28] as probe drugs demonstrated concordance of the acetylator phenotype with *NAT2* genotypes of about 95%. However, in HIV patients, reportedly some individuals with rapid genotypes exhibited a slow phenotype [29]. In a *Schizosaccharomyces pombe* recombinant expression system, the silent SNPs 111T > C, 282C > T, 481C > T, and 759C > T showed no significant reductions in either sulfamethazine or aminofluorene metabolism compared to the wild-type *NAT2*4* [30]. Interestingly, the missense variant 803A > G, causing a Lys268Arg exchange, showed no altered activity, RNA or protein expression, or heat inactivation rates, confirming the *in vivo* data of a single family [31]. Considering *in vitro* data, besides *NAT2*4*, all *NAT2* haplotypes consisting exclusively of the abovementioned variants in haploytpes **11*, **12*, **13*, as well as **18* (845A > C) should be considered rapid acetylators. In contrast, alleles possessing 191G > A, 341T > C, or 434A > C exert a strongly reduced activity, whereas modest decreases are observed for 590G > A, 845A > C, or 857G > A. The low *in vivo* activity of haplotypes **6A* or **7B*, consisting of 590G>A or 857G>A can be explained by the 20-fold reductions in intrinsic protein stability. An important question arises as to whether the different slow NAT2 genotypes have different substrate specificities. Using caffeine as phenotyping substrate, *6A was less active *in vivo* than *5B [27]. In *in vitro* expression systems, however, *7B exhibited a higher affinity for 5-aminofluorene, for example, resulting in elevated clearances compared to the wild-type NAT2*4 [32].

In general, in order to predict the NAT2 phenotype from the genotype, it is sufficient to genotype only three SNPs, namely, SNPs 282C>T, 341T>C, and 857G>A for studies in subjects of Caucasians or Oriental descent. In Africans, however, 191G>A should also be considered [33].

3.2.3 Ethnic Distribution

Phenotyping studies in since the 1960s have disclosed distinct ethnic differences of slow acetylator frequencies. Extremes can be found between northern Africa with a frequency of genetically predicted phenotypes for slow acetylation of 95% and the Far East Pacific region with a frequency of only 11% (Fig. 3.2). Genotype revealed that the allelic pattern differs significantly between Caucasians, Asians, Aborigines, and in particular blacks. In Caucasians the predominant alleles are the slow *NAT2*5B* (40.9%) and **6A* (28.4%) and the rapid **4* (23.4%) [17]. All other alleles have a frequency lower than 3%. In Asians, within the slow acetylators, *NAT2*6A* is more common than **5B* (e.g., 23% vs. 19% in Japan). In Australian Aborigines, the highest frequency (25%) of the low stable variant *NAT2*7B* was observed [34]. In Africa, aside from the frequently observed G191A mutations, a large diversity of haplotypes can be observed; the rapid **4* allele, **12A,* and **13* occur in many samples obtained from different tribes [35].

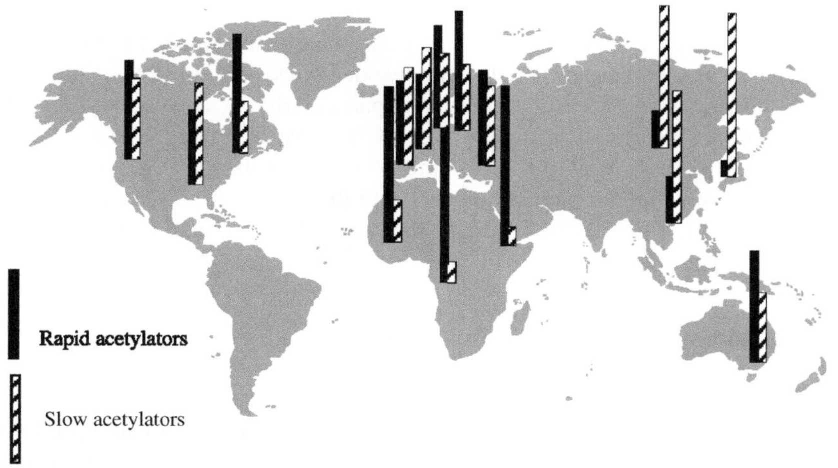

FIGURE 3.2 Ethnic distribution of rapid and slow NAT2 acetylators. The reference bars indicate a frequency of 10%.

TABLE 3.2 Substrates of Arylamine *N*-Acetyltransferases (NAT) 1 and 2

NAT1 Drugs	NAT1 and NAT2 Precarcinogens	NAT2 Drugs
p-Aminobenzoic acid	4-Aminobiphenyl	Amrinone
p-Aminosalicylic acid	2-Aminofluorene	Caffeine metabolite
	Benzidine	Clonazepam metabolite
	3,4-Dichloroaniline	Dapsone
	ß-Naphthylamine	Hydralazine
		Isoniazid
		Nitrazepam metabolite
		Procainamide
		Sulfamethazine
		Sulfapyridine

3.2.4 Involvement of NAT2 in Drug Therapy

Arylamine *N*-acetyltransferase 2 is responsible for the conjugation of drugs such as isoniazid, dapsone, procainamide, and many others (Table 3.2). There is a body of literature on the role of polymorphic *N*-acetyltransferase and the clinical outcome of isoniazid therapy in tuberculosis treatment. Some studies reported an increased rate of isoniazid-induced hepatotoxicity among slow acetylators [36,37], while others showed conflicting results [38–40]. This is possibly due to a complex situation of isoniazid metabolism. Isoniazid is metabolized to acetylisoniazid, acetylhydrazine, and diacetylhydrazine. Among rapid acetylators, the area under the plasma concentration–time curve (AUC) of acetylisoniazid and diacetylhydrazine is elevated, whereas the AUC of acetylhydrazine, the postulated precursor of a toxic metabolite formed from isoniazid, is increased in slow acetylators, probably caused by a lower acetylhydrazine clearance [41]. In summary, the rate of acetylation of isoniazid seems to influence the exposure to acetylhydrazine only moderately. Plasma levels of the anti-leprosy drug dapsone are clearly dependent on acetylator status. Side effects such as allergic skin reaction were found particularly in slow acetylators [42], possibly due to increased formation rates of *N*-hydroxylamines. These examples show that consideration of the arylamine *N*-acetyltransferase 2 genotype would possibly be beneficial for patients treated with drugs, which are *N*-acetylated and undergo further toxification by oxidative pathways. The results of large prospective studies, however are lacking.

3.2.5 Modulation of Disease Susceptibility

3.2.5.1 Bladder Cancer

Both oxidative metabolism by cytochrome P450s and conjugation with acetyl-CoA also play a major role in an individual's risk for suffering from certain diseases related to environmental toxicants, particular cancer. Phenotyping studies in the late 1960s provided evidence that slow acetylators are at increased risk for bladder cancer.

After elucidation of the genetic background of acetylation polymorphism, a huge number of studies have been performed since the 1980s which could in principle confirm these early findings [43]. It is hypothesized that in rapid acetylators arylamines, as contained in aniline dyes or cigarette smoke (e.g., 4-aminobiphenyl), are detoxified by *N*-acetylation in the liver and excreted in the urine. In contrast, low *N*-acetylation activity leads to increased formation of *N*-hydroxylated products. In case of bladder cancer, hydroxylamines may undergo further *O*-acetylation in the urinary bladder preferentially by arylamine *N*-acetyltransferase 1 (NAT1), which was found to be expressed in the urinary epithelium. The product, arylamine acetoxyesters, are unstable in the acid environment and disintegrate spontaneously to highly reactive arynitrenium ion radicals that may well interact with proteins and DNA of bladder epithelial cells forming adducts [44].

A number of *in vitro* studies provided evidence for this theory. Most carcinogenic compounds activated by acetyltransferases are heterocyclic aromatic amines, such as 2-amino-3-methylimidazo[4,5-*f*]quinoline (IQ) or 2-amino-1-methyl-6-phenylimidazo[4,5-*b*]pyridine (PhiP), which lead to dose-dependent effects in mutagenicity tests. However, to date, occupational exposure is fortunately decreasing. A meta-analysis comprising a total of 2496 cases and 3340 controls in different populations revealed that slow acetylators had a 40% increased risk compared to rapid acetylators (odds ratio 1.4) [45], and there is a clear gene–environment interaction. Slow acetylators with a smoking history of more than 50 pack years had a 2-fold higher risk of bladder cancer, as did subjects with typical risk occupations. Subjects meeting both criteria showed the highest risk. Aside from the unequivocal role of NAT2, discovery of the polymorphic nature of NAT1 raised the question as to whether different NAT1 genotypes may additionally modulate bladder cancer susceptibility. As mentioned above, NAT1*10 was found to provide elevated activity in bladder tissue compared to NAT1*4; however, *ex vivo* studies using *p*-aminosalicylic acid showed that NAT1*10 does not alter enzyme activity. In contrast, *NAT1*10* genotypes were significantly underrepresented among bladder cancer patients [46]. Moreover, individuals with *NAT2*4* and *NAT1*10* alleles are at a significantly lower risk for bladder cancer, particularly when exposed to environmental risk factors. More recent large-scale studies confirmed the NAT2 slow acetylator status as a risk factor for bladder cancer in individuals exposed to arylamines, whereas NAT1 genotypes exhibited weak associations [47–49].

3.2.5.2 Colon Cancer

Similar to bladder cancer, colon cancer is the result of a number of subsequent processes after initiation of a cascade of malfunctions of tumor suppressor genes, protooncogenes and cell cycle controlling factors. It was suggested that food-derived heterocylic amines are hydroxylated in a first step by locally expressed CYP1A2, moreover, it is well established that NAT1 as well as NAT2 are expressed in colon tissue. Enhanced *O*-acetylation in the colon mucosa could therefore contribute to the formation of adducts. However, findings on NAT1 and NAT2 as a susceptibility factor of colon cancer is not consistent or is less pronounced in several other large molecular–epidemiological studies [50–53]. A more recent meta-analysis revealed lack of evidence of an association of NAT2 genotypes with colon cancer, although there was loss of heterozygosity in colon cancer tissue [54].

3.2.5.3 Lung Cancer

A survey of the literature revealed no clear association of *NAT2* genotype with lung cancer. An increased risk was described for slow acetylators among individuals who never smoked but an increased risk for rapid acetylators among smokers [55]. Rapid acetylators were also reported to be at risk for lung cancer; in particular, homozygous rapid *NAT2*4/*4* carriers were found to be significantly overrepresented in a German sample (odds ratio 2.36) [56].

Interestingly, in another German sample *NAT1*10* carriers had a significantly increased risk of adenocarcinomas (odds ratio 1.92), and combined analysis with NAT2 revealed an odds ratio for *NAT1*10/NAT2*slow* carriers of 2.22 [57]. However, in large-scale studies, phenotypes reconstructed after haplotype analyses showed the carriers of the combined NAT1 rapid/NAT2 rapid phenotypes to be at lower risk when compared to those with the combined NAT1 slow/NAT2 slow acetylator phenotypes [58].

3.2.5.4 Association with Immunological Diseases

The role of acetylator genotype or phenotype in determination of susceptibility to idiopathic systemic lupus erythematosus (SLE) has been discussed often in the past. Some reports have indicated an increased frequency of slow acetylator phenotype in idiopathic SLE patients, while others found no association. A large study in a German sample revealed lack of evidence for an association of *NAT2* genotypes with SLE, making it unlikely that further attempts will lead to other results [59].

3.2.5.5 Summary

NAT2 plays a significant role in the susceptibility to bladder cancer; the evidence of application in individualized medicine is currently weak.

3.3 THIOPURINE-*S*-METHYLTRANSFERASE (TPMT)

A rare but serious side effect in treatment with the antimetabolites azathioprine or its metabolite 6-mercatopurine is a severe bone marrow depression, which may result in lethal side effects [60]. Detoxification takes place by TPMT, which was believed to be homozygously deficient in one of 300 individuals [61] (Fig. 3.3).

Later comprehensive studies on phenotype–genotype correlation in 1214 healthy German blood donors clearly defined a trimodal frequency distribution of TPMT activity: 0.6% were deficient, 9.9% were intermediate, and 89.5% were normal to high methylators [62]. The frequencies of the mutant alleles were 4.4% (*3A), 0.4% (*3C), and 0.2% (*2). Lack of activity was strictly associated with the homozygous deficient genotype. The overall concordance rate between TPMT genotypes and phenotypes was 98.4%. In a study on adverse effects of azathioprine in patients with inflammatory bowel disease (IBD), thiopurine-related adverse drug reactions are

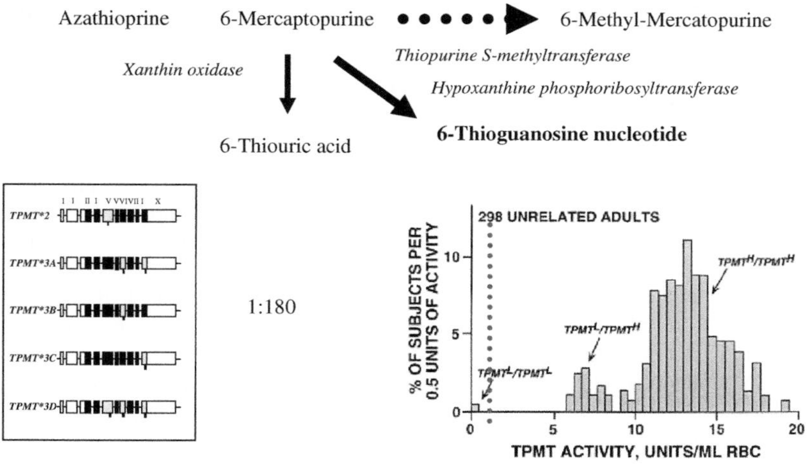

FIGURE 3.3 Metabolism of thiopurine drugs. In case of TPMT deficiency, the generation of 6-thioguanosines by hypoxanthine phosphoribosyltransferase is substantially enhanced. Adapted from [61]. Reproduced with permission from Informa healthcare.

frequent, ranging from 5% to 40%, in either a dose-dependent or dose-independent manner. Hematologic side effects were related to TPMT genotype, but intestinal adverse events occurred independent of the genotype. TPMT [63]. On the basis of several cost–benefit analyses, it was concluded that assessment of TPMT activity is recommended prior to thiopurine therapy in patients with IBD. It should be noted, however, that the concomitant use of allopurinol without dosage adjustment of azathioprine/mercaptopurine may lead to clinically relevant severe haematotoxicity due to inhibition of TPMT and subsequent elevated thiopurine levels [64]. Among TPMT-deficient patients, metabolism takes place by an alternative pathway to the 6-thioguanin nucleotide (6-TGN). The plasma concentration of 6-TGN correlates with the severity of the medication's side effects. However, a problem arises, since TPMT exhibits a high number of variants, which allows genotyping to only a limited degree. Many clinics still routinely prefer *ex vivo* phenotyping procedures to date, but increasing knowledge about rare variations and application of modern genotyping technologies allow a reliable prediction of TMPT status by means of genotyping [62]. The clinical importance was shown in a large study in pediatric acute lymphoblastic leukemia patients, showing that TPMT-poor metabolizers are at clear risk for severe azathioprine side effects, making a significant dose reduction necessary [65]. Much more recently it was shown, however, that TPMT genetics is not a major risk factor for secondary malignant neoplasms after treatment of childhood acute lymphoblastic leukaemia with purine analogs [66].

In summary, TPMT genotyping is recommended by FDA prior to treatment with irinotecan, and TPMT intermediate metabolizers (10%) have a higher risk for side effects. Poor metabolizers (0.6%) have a 100% chance of developing severe side effects. A reduction to 5–10% of the standard dose is recommended for such individuals.

TABLE 3.3 Classes of Glutathione *S*-Transferases, Chromosomal Location, and Major Substrates

Class	Gene	Chromosome Location	Substrate
Alpha (α)	GSTA1, GSTA2, GSTA3, GSTA4, GSTA5	6p12.1	Bilirubin, cyclophosphamide
Kappa (κ)	GSTK1	7q35	1-Chloro-2,4-dinitrobenzene (model substrate)
Mu (μ)	GSTM1, GSTM1L, GSTM2, GSTM3, GSTM4, GSTM5	1p13.3	Organic hydrocarbons and many other xenobiotics
Omega (ω)	GSTO1, GSTO2	10q24.3	Modulation of the activity of interleukin 1β
Pi (π)	GSTP1	11q13.2	Ifosfamide, busulfan, chlorambucil
Theta (θ)	GSTT1, GSTT2	22q11.23	Small aliphates
Zeta (ζ)	GSTZ1	14q24.3	Dichloroacetic acid
Microsomal	MGST1, MGST2, MGST3	12p12.3, 4q28.3, 1q23	Lipid peroxidation and others

3.4 GLUTATHIONE *S*-TRANSFERASES

Glutathione *S*-transferases (GSTs, EC 2.5.1.18) are a large family of cytosolic enzymes of classes GSTA, -M, -P, -T, and -Z that conjugate a variety of exogenous and endogenous compounds, including several cytostatics (Table 3.3). Most significant is the detoxification of electrophilic metabolites, including benzo[α]pyrene and other polycyclic aromatic hydrocarbons as present in tobacco smoke, forming soluble, nontoxic peptide derivatives. All are polymorphic, but widely most investigated are GSTM1 (50% in Caucasians) and GSTT1 (20%) deletions, which are recessive variants for which homozygous deletions result in null activity of their respective enzymes. GSTP1 Ile105Val is a nonsynonymous A>G SNP resulting in alterations in the substrate binding site and enzyme activity. The α-class genes, located in a cluster mapped to chromosome 6p12.1, are the most abundantly expressed glutathione *S*-transferases in liver. In addition to binding or metabolizing bilirubin and certain anticancer drugs in the liver, the α class of these enzymes exhibit glutathione peroxidase activity, thereby protecting the cells from reactive-oxygen species and the products of peroxidation.

Since glutathione conjugation represents a detoxification pathway, it becomes rapidly clear that the total absence of GSTM1 activity (genotype *GSTM1*0/*0*) may be linked to increased drug toxicity or cancer susceptibility. Indeed, some years ago GSTM1 deficiency was shown by several studies to be a risk factor for lung [67], laryngeal [68], and urinary bladder cancer [69,70], comprehensively reviewed by Parl et al. [71]. However, there is a clear lack of association between GSTM1,

GSTT1, and GSTP1 and breast cancer [72], although an increased risk of breast cancer was found among women with lower consumption of cruciferous vegetables and among current smokers who carry the GSTA1 B genotype. Interestingly, GSTM1 deficiency was also reportedly associated with other smoking-related diseases such as atherosclerosis [73].

These findings may be partly explained by the fact that glutathione *S*-transferase deficiency prevents detoxification of diepoxides from, for example, benzo(a)pyrene. Thus several studies could show elevated levels of DNA and protein adducts in carriers of GSTM1 and GSTT1 [74,75]. Independent meta-analyses for *GSTM1* deletion and lung cancer revealed a significant associations of GSTM1*0/0 with lung cancer with odds ratio ranging up to 1.34 [68,76,77]. Meta-analyses of the risk for bladder cancer calculated a significant risk for deletion carriers of 1.53 [78] or 1.44 [70]. Considering separately the loss of one or two GSTM1 copies, the odds ratios for individuals with deletion of one copy was 1.2 (95% CI 0.8–1.7) and 1.9 (1.4–2.7) for deletion of two copies [79]. More recently, data on the association of GSTM1 and GSTT1 on the risk for different types of leukaemia have been reported. For example, meta-analyses on acute lymphatic leukemia demonstrated a significant overrepresentation of carriers of the nonactive variant of GSTM1 (odds ratio = 1.20) [80].

In summary, among populations studied to date, there is evidence that GSTM1 null status is associated with a modest increase in the risk for lung and bladder cancer, as well as leukemia, but there is currently no application in individualized medicine.

3.5 UDP GLUCURONOSYLTRANSFERASES

Uridine diphosphate (UDP) glucuronosyltransferases (UGTs) are a superfamily of enzymes located primarily in the endoplasmic reticulum of cells that detoxify a diverse range of xenobiotics, as well as endogenous compounds, through their conjugation to glucuronic acid, generating more hydrophilic compounds that may be excreted via efflux transporters in kidney or bile. Moreover, the conjugates alter the biological properties into less pharmacologically active products. Glucuronidation plays a major role in a number of drugs, with specific UGT enzymes performing either *N*- or *O*-glucuronidation. A well-known substrate is the hemoglobin degradation product bilirubin. It is conjugated through a UGT1A1 to bilirubin–glucuronide that may be excreted after efflux transport by ABCC2 into the urine; additional drugs metabolized by UGT1A1 are the cytostatic irinotecan and the immunosuppressant mycophenolate mofetil.

The UGT superfamily is classified into UGT1 and UGT2 families on the basis of aminoacid sequence homology. Seventeen human enzymes have been identified thus far, each with high homology at their carboxy termini; some of them are expressed only in extrahepatic tissues (UGT1A and 2B subfamilies), whereas others have a more ubiquitous tissue distribution (UGTs 1A7, 1A8, and 1A10). UGT2 enzymes are coded by individual genes clustered in chromosome 4 (4q13), the nine functional

UGT1A isoforms are coded by a single gene (*UGT1A*) located on chromosome 2q37 and spanning approximately 290 kilobases. It consists of multiple isoform-specific exons that are expressed by alternate splicing of one unique exon (exon 1) to a domain consisting of four common exons (exons 2–5). The UGT2A enzymes are found mainly in olfactory tissues, with UGT2A1 active against odorants, steroid hormones, and some drugs [81]; to date, the only substrates shown to be glucuronidated by UGT2A2 are β-estradiol and epiestradiol. There are at least six members of the UGT2B family with unique genes clustered on chromosome 4 in humans. Interestingly, a considerable number of prevalent, functional polymorphisms were previously identified in several UGT genes, including 1A1, 1A3, 1A4, 1A6, 1A7, 1A8, 1A10, 2B4, 2B7, 2B15, and 2B17 with several implicated as determinants of cancer risk or response to different pharmacotherapies [82].

A TA tandem repeat polymorphism in the promoter region of UGT1A1 leads to the well-known clinical feature of Gilbert's syndrome. The presence of 7 TA repeats (allele UGT1A1*28) significantly lowers the transcription rate compared to the wild type with six TA repeats. Further studies, however, showed that the frequency is 40% in Caucasians, but few ever develop UGT1A1-associated hyperbilirubinemia. Thus the variant is necessary but not sufficient for developing Gilbert's syndrome. In contrast, the Crigler–Najjar syndrome type I is associated with mutations that result in a complete absence of normal UGT1A1 enzyme activity, causing severe hyperbilirubinemia with total serum bilirubin levels ranging from 20 to 45 mg/dL. Crigler–Najjar syndrome type II is associated with reduced activity of mutated UGT1A1, which causes elevated total serum bilirubin from 6 to 20 mg/dl.

Irinotecan is a topoisomerase I inhibitor approved worldwide for the treatment of metastatic colorectal cancer. It is metabolized by CYP3A enzymes and esterases to its active metabolite SN38, which is detoxified by conjugation with glutathione and extreceted preferentially via ABCC2 back into the intestine or into urine (Fig. 3.4). The genetic polymorphism in *UGT1A1* increases the risk of irinotecan toxicity, particularly when administered as a single agent in a dose-dependent manner [83]. Accordingly, in 2007 the US FDA changed the drug label for irinotecan to include the *UGT1A1*28* genotype as a risk factor for severe neutropenia, since irinotecan-treated patients who were homozygous for the *UGT1A1*28* allele had a greater risk of hematologic toxic effects than did patients who had one or two copies of the wild-type allele (*UGT1A1*1*) (see Fig. 3.5).

It appears that UGT2B7 is the most active hepatic UGT. Additionally, UGT2B7 expression has been detected in a variety of tissues, including liver, gastrointestinal tract, and breast; therefore, variations in UGT2B7 function or expression could potentially significantly impact individual response to drugs [84]. UGT2B7 is the major enzyme isoform for the metabolism of morphine to the main metabolites, morphine-3-glucuronide and morphine-6-glucuronide. Also, for tamoxifen it could be shown that *O*-glucuronidation of both *trans*-4-OH-tamoxifen and *trans*-endoxifen was significantly associated with UGT2B7 genotype, with lower activities correlated with increasing numbers of the UGT2B7 268Tyr allele [85]. These results are in line with observation for other substrates, including tobacco carcinogen metabolites.

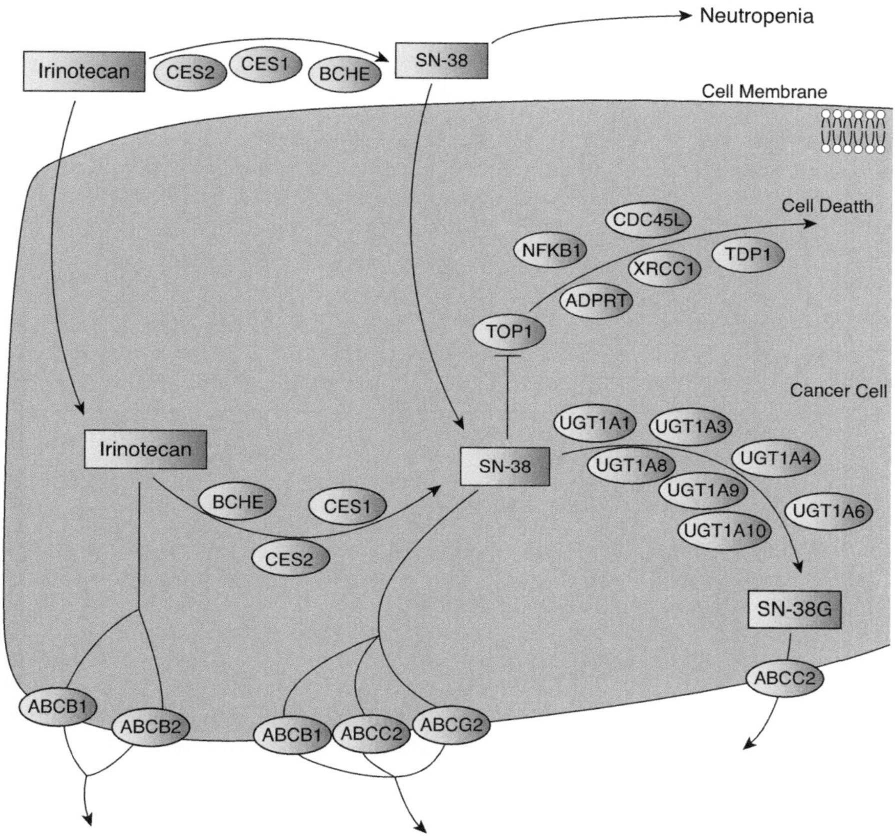

FIGURE 3.4 Pathway of irinotecan in the human liver. Irinotecan is transformed into its active metabolite SN38 by cytoplasmatic esterases. SN38, a topoisomerase inhibitor, is conjugated with glucuronic acid catalyzed by UGTs. UGT1A1 was proved to significantly modulate toxicity. [Figure adapted from the PharmGKB database (`www.pharmgkb.org`).]

3.6 SULFOTRANSFERASES

Sulfotransferase enzymes catalyze the transfer of a sulfo group from the cofactor 5′-phosphoadenosine-3′-phosphosulfate (PAPS) to relatively small acceptor molecules. Thus they conjugate sulfate to many hormones, neurotransmitters, drugs, and xenobiotic compounds. Within the SULT superfamily, 10 distinct human SULT forms are known so far, differing in their tissue distributions and substrate specificities. A total of 11 human SULT forms have been characterized at the gene, message, and protein levels. Two additional possible *SULT* genes (*SULT1C3* and *6B1*) were identified in the human genome [86]. Common functional polymorphisms of the transcribed region are known for many of them. The best described is the SULT1A family, consisting of SULT1A1, 1A2, 1A3 in human tissue [3]. SULT1A1

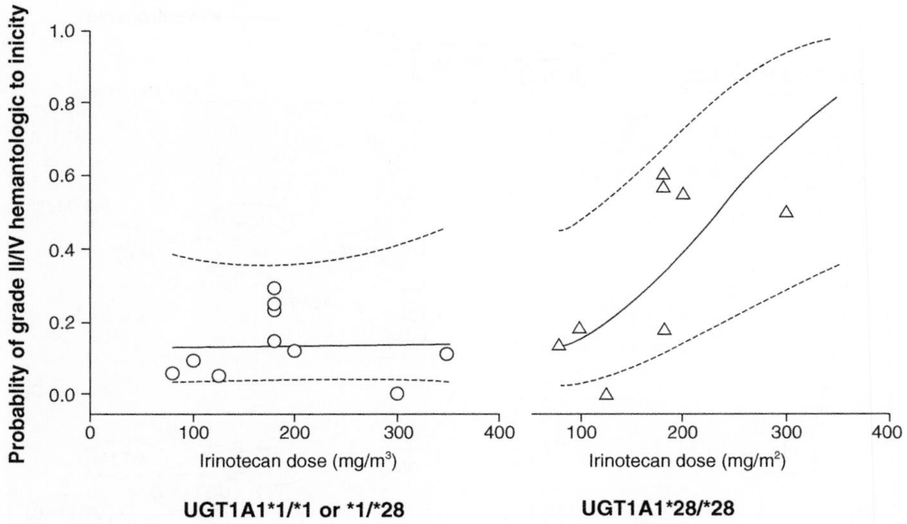

FIGURE 3.5 Dose-dependent irinotecan-mediated probability of hematologic toxicity and UGT1A1 genotype (solid lines indicate predicted values, dotted lines indicate 95% confidence limits). (Figure adapted from Hoskins et al. [83].)

metabolizes phenolic compounds such as 4-nitrophenol, a typical probe drug, medications such as acetaminophen and minoxidil; and endogenous and synthetic hormones such as estrone, estradiol, 2-hydoxyestrone, 2-hydroxyestradiol, 4-hydroxyestrone, 4-hydroxyestradiol, or diethylstilbestriol, *trans*-4-hydroxytamoxifen, and 2-methoxy estradiol. The SULT1B and SULT1E genes are located on chromosome 4q13, SULT1C on 2q11.2, and SULT2 on 19q13.3 [87]. The SULT1A genes are located on chromosome 16. SULT1A1 has a 885-nucleotide open reading frame, consists of seven cosing exons and two alternatively spliced noncoding exons upstream. It codes for a 295-aminoacid protein that is expressed cytosolic in certain organs such as liver and kidney and also in platelets. The presence in platelet allows investigation of its activity *ex vivo*. Such attempts revealed more than 50-fold interindividual differences in a large sample [88]. Besides a large number of SNPs, SULT1A1 is known to have copy number variations (CNVs) of up to five genes. In one study, 5% of Caucasian subjects contained a single copy of the gene and 26% had three or more copies, while 63% of African-American subjects had three or more copies [89]. The presence of CNVs is believed to have a stronger impact on interindividual SULT1A1 activity than single-nucleotide polymorphisms. The major SNPs are 638G>A, more recently addressed as *SULT1A1*2*, 667G>A (*SULT1A1*3*), –624G>C, and –396G>A (Table 3.4).

The analgesic drug acetaminophen (paracetamol) is excreted to a major extent as sulfo and glucuronic acid conjugates in the urine. In several studies, the ratio of these conjugates in 8-h or 24-h urine showed an approximately 6-fold variation among

TABLE 3.4 Functional Significance and Frequencies of Selected SULT1A1 SNPs

					Frequency		
Allele	SNP	rs Number	Location	Activity	Caucasians	Chinese	Africans
	−624G>C	rs3760091	Intron 1	↑	0.48	0.42	0.63
	−396G>A	rs750155	Intron 1	↓	—	—	—
SULT1A1*2	638G>A	rs9282861	Arg213His	↓	0.33	0.08	0.29
SULT1A1*3	667G>A	rs1801030	Val223Met	(↑)	0.012	0.006	0.23

healthy adult subjects [90]. The extent to which extent this variation is due to differences in the levels and properties of SULTs, UDP glucuronosyltransferases, or other factors, and whether genetic or environmental factors are more important, has not yet been elucidated. The genetic contribution to the total interindividual variation however, appears to be low.

Due to the role of sulfotransferases in the detoxification – and partly in the activation – of carcinogens, a number of studies have been performed to elucidate the significance of SULT gene polymorphisms to the risk of certain malignancies. Statistically significant associations were observed between presence of the *SULT1A1*2* genotype and age; obesity; and mammary, pulmonary, esophageal, and urothelial cancer [3].

REFERENCES

1. Ando Y, Saka H, Ando M, et al. Polymorphisms of UDP-glucuronosyltransferase gene and irinotecan toxicity: A pharmacogenetic analysis. *Cancer Res.* 2000;**60**(24):6921–6926.
2. Burchell B. Genetic variation of human UDP-glucuronosyltransferase: Implications in disease and drug glucuronidation. *Am. J. Pharmacogenomics* 2003;**3**(1):37–52.
3. Glatt H, Meinl W. Pharmacogenetics of soluble sulfotransferases (SULTs). *Naunyn. Schmiedebergs Arch. Pharmacol.* 2004;**369**(1):55–68.
4. Glatt SJ, Faraone SV, Tsuang MT. Association between a functional catechol O-methyltransferase gene polymorphism and schizophrenia: Meta-analysis of case-control and family-based studies. *Am. J. Psychiatry* 2003;**160**(3):469–476.
5. Redden DT, Shields PG, Epstein L, et al. Catechol-O-methyl-transferase functional polymorphism and nicotine dependence: An evaluation of nonreplicated results. *Cancer Epidemiol. Biomarkers Prev.* 2005;**14**(6):1384–1389.
6. Mitrunen K, Hirvonen A. Molecular epidemiology of sporadic breast cancer. The role of polymorphic genes involved in oestrogen biosynthesis and metabolism. *Mutat. Res.* 2003;**544**(1):9–41.
7. Evans WE, Relling MV. Pharmacogenomics: Translating functional genomics into rational therapeutics. *Science* 1999;**286**(5439):487–491.
8. Bönicke R, Reif W. Enzymatische Inaktivierung von Isonikotinsäurehydrazid im menschlichen und tierischen Organismus. *Arch. Exp. Pathol. Pharmak.* 1953;**220**:321–333.
9. Mitchell R, Bell J. Clinical implications of isoniazid PAS and streptomycin blood levels in pulmonary tuberculosis. *Trans. Am. Clin. Assoc.* 1957;**69**:98–105.

10. Grant DM, Möricke K, Eichelbaum M, Meyer UA. Acetylation pharmacogenetics. The slow acetylator phenotype is caused by decreased or absent arylamine *N*-acetyltransferase in human liver. *J. Clin. Invest.* 1990;**85**:968–972.

11. Blum M, Grant DM, Demierre A, Meyer UA. N-acetylation pharmacogenetics: A gene deletion causes absence of arylamine N-acetyltransferase in liver of slow acetylator rabbits. *Proc. Natl. Acad. Sci. USA* 1989;**86**(23):9554–9557.

12. Evans DAP, White TA. Human acetylation polymorphism. *J. Lab. Clin. Med.* 1963;**63**:394–403.

13. Grant DM, Tang BK, Kalow W. A simple test for acetylator phenotype using caffeine. *Br. J. Clin. Pharmacol.* 1984;**17**:459–464.

14. Fuhr U, Rost KL. Simple and reliable CYP1A2 phenotyping by the paraxanthine/caffeine ratio in plasma and in saliva. *Pharmacogenetics* 1994;**4**:109–116.

15. Matas N, Thygesen P, Stacey M, Risch A, Sim E. Mapping AAC1, AAC2 and AACP, the genes for arylamine *N*-acetyltransferases, carcinogen metabolising enzymes on human chromosome 8p22, a region frequently deleted in tumours. *Cytogenet. Cell. Genet.* 1997;**77**:290–295.

16. Sim E, Lack N, Wang CJ, et al. Arylamine N-acetyltransferases: Structural and functional implications of polymorphisms. *Toxicology* 2008;**254**(3):170–183.

17. Cascorbi I, Brockmöller J, Mrozikiewicz PM, Müller A, Roots I. Arylamine *N*-acetyltransferase activity in man. *Drug Metab. Rev.* 1999;**31**(2):489–502.

18. Bell DA, Badawi AF, Lang NP, Ilett KF, Kadlubar FF, Hirvonen A. Polymorphism in the *N*-acetyltransferase 1 (*NAT1*) polyadenylation signal association of *NAT1*10* allele with higher *N*-acetylation activity in bladder and colon tissue. *Cancer Res.* 1995;**55**:5226–5229.

19. Ward A, Hickman D, Gordon JW, Sim E. Arylamine N-acetyltransferase in human red blood cells. *Biochem. Pharmacol.* 1992;**44**:1099–1104.

20. Hughes NC, Janezic SA, McQueen KL, et al. Identification and characterization of variant alleles of human acetyltransferase NAT1 with defective function using *p*-aminosalicylate as an *in-vivo* and *in-vitro* probe. *Pharmacogenetics* 1998;**8**:55–66.

21. Bruhn C, Brockmöller J, Cascorbi I, Roots I, Borchert H. Correlation between genotype and phenotype of the human arylamine *N*-acetyltransferase type 1 (NAT1). *Biochem. Pharmacol.* 1999;**58**(11):1759–1764.

22. Henning S, Cascorbi I, Münchow B, Jahnke V, Roots I. Association of arylamine *N*-acetyltransferases *NAT1* and *NAT2* genotypes to laryngeal cancer risk. *Pharmacogenetics* 1999;**9**:103–111.

23. Smelt V, Mardon H, Sim E. Placental expression of arylamine *N*-acetyltransferases: Evidence for linkage disequilibrium between *NAT1*10* and *NAT2*4* alleles of the two human arylamine *N*-acetyltransferase loci *NAT1* and *NAT2*. *Pharmacol. Toxicol.* 1998;**83**(4):149–157.

24. Vatsis KP, Weber WW, Bell DA, et al. Nomenclature for *N*-acetyltransferases. *Pharmacogenetics* 1995;**5**(1):1–17.

25. Hein DW, Boukouvala S, Grant DM, Minchin RF, Sim E. Changes in consensus arylamine N-acetyltransferase gene nomenclature. *Pharmacogenet. Genomics* 2008;**18**(4):367–368.

26. Hein DW, Boukouvala S, Grant DM, Minchin RF, Sim E.Consensus Human Arylamine *N-Acetyltransferase Gene Nomenclature* (available at `http://louisville.edu/`

medschool/pharmacology/consensus-human-arylamine-n-acetyltransferase-gene-nomenclature/; accessed 2009).

27. Cascorbi I, Drakoulis N, Brockmöller J, Maurer A, Sperling K, Roots I. Arylamine *N*-acetyltransferase (*NAT2*) mutations and their allelic linkage in unrelated Caucasian individuals: Correlation with phenotypic activity. *Am. J. Hum. Genet.* 1995;**57**(3): 581–592.
28. Mrozikiewicz PM, Cascorbi I, Brockmöller J, Roots I. Determination and alleleic allocation of seven nucleotide transitions within the arylamine *N*-acetyltransferase gene in the Polish population. *Clin. Pharmacol. Ther.* 1996;**59**:376–382.
29. O'Neil WM, Drobitch RK, MacArthur RD, et al. Acetylator phenotype and genotype in patients infected with HIV: Discordance between methods for phenotype determination and genotype. *Pharmacogenetics* 2000;**10**(2):171–182.
30. Fretland AJ, Leff MA, Doll MA, Hein DW. Functional characterization of human N-acetyltransferase 2 (NAT2) single nucleotide polymorphisms. *Pharmacogenetics* 2001;**11**(3):207–215.
31. Cascorbi I, Brockmöller J, Bauer S, Reum T, I R. *NAT2**12A* 803A/G codes for rapid arylamine *N*-acetylation in humans. *Pharmacogenetics* 1996;**6**:257–260.
32. Hickman D, Sim E. *N*-acetyltransferase polymorphism. Comparison of phenotype and genotype in humans. *Biochem. Pharmacol.* 1991;**42**:1007–1014.
33. Patin E, Barreiro LB, Sabeti PC, et al. Deciphering the ancient and complex evolutionary history of human arylamine N-acetyltransferase genes. *Am. J. Hum. Genet.* 2006;**78** (3):423–436.
34. Ilett KF, Chiswell GM, Spargo RM, Platt E, Minchin RF. Acetylation phenotype and genotype in aboriginal leprosy patients from the north-west region of Western Australia. *Pharmacogenetics* 1993;**3**:264–269.
35. Deloménie C, Sica L, Grant DM, Krishnamoorthy R, Dupret JM. Genotyping of the polymorphic *N*-acetyltransferase (*NAT2**) gene locus in two native African populations. *Pharmacogenetics* 1996;**6**:177–185.
36. Ohno M, Yamaguchi I, Yamamoto I, et al. Slow N-acetyltransferase 2 genotype affects the incidence of isoniazid and rifampicin-induced hepatotoxicity. *Int. J. Tuberc. Lung. Dis.* 2000;**4**(3):256–261.
37. Pande JN, Singh SP, Khilnani GC, Khilnani S, Tandon RK. Risk factors for hepatotoxicity from antituberculosis drugs: A case-control study. *Thorax* 1996;**51**(2):132–136.
38. Gronhagen-Riska C, Hellstrom PE, Froseth B. Predisposing factors in hepatitis induced by isoniazid-rifampin treatment of tuberculosis. *Am. Rev. Respir. Dis.* 1978;**118**(3):461–466.
39. Gurumurthy P, Krishnamurthy MS, Nazareth O, et al. Lack of relationship between hepatic toxicity and acetylator phenotype in three thousand South Indian patients during treatment with isoniazid for tuberculosis. *Am. Rev. Respir. Dis.* 1984;**129**(1):58–61.
40. Singh J, Garg PK, Thakur VS, Tandon RK. Anti tubercular treatment induced hepatotoxicity: Does acetylator status matter? *Indian J. Physiol. Pharmacol.* 1995;**39**(1):43–46.
41. Lauterburg BH, Smith CV, Todd EL, Mitchell JR. Pharmacokinetics of the toxic hydrazino metabolites formed from isoniazid in humans. *J. Pharmacol. Exp. Ther.* 1985;**235** (3):566–570.
42. Bluhm RE, Adedoyin A, McCarver DG, Branch RA. Development of dapsone toxicity in patients with inflammatory dermatoses: Activity of acetylation and hydroxylation of dapsone as risk factors. *Clin. Pharmacol. Ther.* 1999;**65**(6):598–605.

43. Risch A, Wallace DMA, Bathers S, Sim E. Slow *N*-acetylation genotype is a susceptibility factor in occupational and smoking related bladder cancer. *Hum. Mol. Genet.* 1995;**4**:231–236.

44. Hein DW, Doll MA, Rustan TD, Gray K, Feng Y, Grant DM. Metabolic activation and deactivation of arylamine carcinogens by recombinant human NAT1 and polymorphic NAT2 acetyltransferases. *Carcinogenesis* 1993;**14**:1633–1638.

45. Marcus PM, Vineis P, Rothman N. NAT2 slow acetylation and bladder cancer risk: A meta-analysis of 22 case-control studies conducted in the general population. *Pharmacogenetics* 2000;**10**(2):115–122.

46. Cascorbi I, Roots I, Brockmöller J. Association of *NAT1* and *NAT2* polymorphisms to urinary bladder cancer: Significantly reduced risk in subjects with *NAT1*10*. *Cancer Res.* 2001;**61**(13):5051–5056.

47. Guey LT, Garcia-Closas M, Murta-Nascimento C, et al. Genetic susceptibility to distinct bladder cancer subphenotypes. *Eur. Urol.* 2009.

48. Malats N. Genetic epidemiology of bladder cancer: Scaling up in the identification of low-penetrance genetic markers of bladder cancer risk and progression. *Scand. J. Urol. Nephrol. Suppl.* 2008; (218):131–140.

49. Yuan JM, Chan KK, Coetzee GA, et al. Genetic determinants in the metabolism of bladder carcinogens in relation to risk of bladder cancer. *Carcinogenesis* 2008;**29**(7):1386–1393.

50. Chen J, Stampfer MJ, Hough HL, et al. A prospective study of *N*-acetyltransferase genotype, red meat intake, and risk of colorectal cancer. *Cancer Res.* 1998;**58**(15):3307–3311.

51. Welfare MR, Cooper J, Bassendine MF, Daly AK. Relationship between acetylator status, smoking, and diet and colorectal cancer risk in the north-east of England. *Carcinogenesis* 1997;**18**(7):1351–1354.

52. Slattery ML, Potter JD, Samowitz W, Bigler J, Caan B, Leppert M. NAT2, GSTM-1, cigarette smoking, and risk of colon cancer. *Cancer Epidemiol. Biomarkers Prev.* 1998;**7**(12):1079–1084.

53. Butler LM, Millikan RC, Sinha R, et al. Modification by N-acetyltransferase 1 genotype on the association between dietary heterocyclic amines and colon cancer in a multiethnic study. *Mutat. Res.* 2008;**638**(1–2):162–174.

54. Borlak J, Reamon-Buettner SM. N-acetyltransferase 2 (NAT2) gene polymorphisms in colon and lung cancer patients. *BMC Med. Genet.* 2006;**7**:58.

55. Nyberg F, Hou SM, Hemminki K, Lambert B, Pershagen G. Glutathione S-transferase mu1 and N-acetyltransferase 2 genetic polymorphisms and exposure to tobacco smoke in nonsmoking and smoking lung cancer patients and population controls. *Cancer Epidemiol. Biomarkers Prev.* 1998;**7**(10):875–883.

56. Cascorbi I, Brockmöller J, Mrozikiewicz PM, Bauer S, Loddenkemper R, Roots I. Homozygous rapid arylamine *N*-acetyltransferase *NAT2* genotype as susceptibility factor for lung cancer. *Cancer Res.* 1996;**56**:3961–3966.

57. Wikman H, Thiel S, Jager B, et al. Relevance of N-acetyltransferase 1 and 2 (NAT1, NAT2) genetic polymorphisms in non-small cell lung cancer susceptibility. *Pharmacogenetics* 2001;**11**(2):157–168.

58. Gemignani F, Landi S, Szeszenia-Dabrowska N, et al. Development of lung cancer before the age of 50: The role of xenobiotic metabolizing genes. *Carcinogenesis* 2007;**28**(6):1287–1293.

59. Zschieschang P, Hiepe F, Gromnica-Ihle E, Roots I, Cascorbi I. Lack of association between arylamine N-acetyltransferase 2 (NAT2) polymorphism and systemic lupus erythematosus. *Pharmacogenetics* 2002;**12**(7):559–563.

60. Krynetski EY, Evans WE. Genetic polymorphism of thiopurine S-methyltransferase: Molecular mechanisms and clinical importance. *Pharmacology* 2000;**61**(3):136–146.

61. Weinshilboum RM. Methylation pharmacogenetics: Thiopurine methyltransferase as a model system. *Xenobiotica* 1992;**22**(9–10):1055–1071.

62. Schaeffeler E, Fischer C, Brockmeier D, et al. Comprehensive analysis of thiopurine S-methyltransferase phenotype-genotype correlation in a large population of German-Caucasians and identification of novel TPMT variants. *Pharmacogenetics* 2004;**14** (7):407–417.

63. Schwab M, Schaffeler E, Marx C, et al. Azathioprine therapy and adverse drug reactions in patients with inflammatory bowel disease: Impact of thiopurine S-methyltransferase polymorphism. *Pharmacogenetics* 2002;**12**(6):429–436.

64. Teml A, Schaeffeler E, Herrlinger KR, Klotz U, Schwab M. Thiopurine treatment in inflammatory bowel disease: Clinical pharmacology and implication of pharmacogenetically guided dosing. *Clin. Pharmacokinet.* 2007;**46**(3):187–208.

65. Stanulla M, Schaeffeler E, Flohr T, et al. Thiopurine methyltransferase (TPMT) genotype and early treatment response to mercaptopurine in childhood acute lymphoblastic leukemia. *JAMA* 2005;**293**(12):1485–1489.

66. Stanulla M, Schaeffeler E, Moricke A, et al. Thiopurine methyltransferase genetics is not a major risk factor for secondary malignant neoplasms after treatment of childhood acute lymphoblastic leukemia on Berlin-Frankfurt-Munster protocols. *Blood* 2009;**114** (7):1314–1318.

67. Houlston RS. Glutathione S-transferase M1 status and lung cancer risk: A meta-analysis. *Cancer Epidemiol. Biomarkers Prev.* 1999;**8**(8):675–682.

68. Hashibe M, Brennan P, Strange RC, et al. Meta- and pooled analyses of GSTM1, GSTT1, GSTP1, and CYP1A1 genotypes and risk of head and neck cancer. *Cancer Epidemiol. Biomarkers Prev.* 2003;**12**(12):1509–1517.

69. Brockmöller J, Cascorbi I, Kerb R, Roots I. Combined analysis of inherited polymorphisms in arylamine *N*-acetyltransferase 2, glutathione *S*-transferase M1 and T1, microsomal epoxide hydrolase, and cytochrome P450 enzymes as modulators of bladder cancer risk. *Cancer Res.* 1996;**56**:3915–3925.

70. Engel LS, Taioli E, Pfeiffer R, et al. Pooled analysis and meta-analysis of glutathione S-transferase M1 and bladder cancer: A HuGE review. *Am. J. Epidemiol.* 2002;**156** (2):95–109.

71. Parl FF. Glutathione S-transferase genotypes and cancer risk. *Cancer Lett.* 2005;**221** (2):123–129.

72. Vogl FD, Taioli E, Maugard C, et al. Glutathione S-transferases M1, T1, and P1 and breast cancer: A pooled analysis. *Cancer Epidemiol. Biomarkers Prev.* 2004;**13** (9):1473–1479.

73. Olshan AF, Li R, Pankow JS, et al. Risk of atherosclerosis: Interaction of smoking and glutathione S-transferase genes. *Epidemiology* 2003;**14**(3):321–327.

74. Alexandrov K, Cascorbi I, Rojas M, Bouvier G, Kriek E, Bartsch H. CYP1A1 and GSTM1 genotypes affect benzo[a]pyrene DNA adducts in smokers' lung: Comparison with aromatic/hydrophobic adduct formation. *Carcinogenesis* 2002;**23**(12):1969–1977.

75. Bartsch H, Rojas M, Nair U, Nair J, Alexandrov K. Genetic cancer susceptibility and DNA adducts: Studies in smokers, tobacco chewers, and coke oven workers. *Cancer Detect. Prev.* 1999;**23**(6):445–453.

76. Carlsten C, Sagoo GS, Frodsham AJ, Burke W, Higgins JP. Glutathione S-transferase M1 (GSTM1) polymorphisms and lung cancer: A literature-based systematic HuGE review and meta-analysis. *Am. J. Epidemiol.* 2008;**167**(7):759–774.

77. Ye Z, Song H, Higgins JP, Pharoah P, Danesh J. Five glutathione s-transferase gene variants in 23,452 cases of lung cancer and 30, 397 controls: Meta-analysis of 130 studies. *PLoS Med* 2006;**3**(4):e91.

78. Johns LE, Houlston RS. Glutathione S-transferase mu1 (GSTM1) status and bladder cancer risk: A meta-analysis. *Mutagenesis* 2000;**15**(5):399–404.

79. Garcia-Closas M, Malats N, Silverman D, et al. NAT2 slow acetylation, GSTM1 null genotype, and risk of bladder cancer: Results from the Spanish bladder cancer study and meta-analyses. *Lancet* 2005;**366**(9486):649–659.

80. Dong LM, Potter JD, White E, Ulrich CM, Cardon LR, Peters U. Genetic susceptibility to cancer: The role of polymorphisms in candidate genes. *JAMA* 2008;**299**(20):2423–2436.

81. Jedlitschky G, Cassidy AJ, Sales M, Pratt N, Burchell B. Cloning and characterization of a novel human olfactory UDP-glucuronosyltransferase. *Biochem. J.* 1999;**340**(Pt. 3): 837–843.

82. Court MH. Isoform-selective probe substrates for in vitro studies of human UDP-glucuronosyltransferases. *Methods Enzymol.* 2005;**400**:104–116.

83. Hoskins JM, Goldberg RM, Qu P, Ibrahim JG, McLeod HL. UGT1A1*28 genotype and irinotecan-induced neutropenia: Dose matters. *J. Natl. Cancer Inst.* 2007;**99** (17):1290–1295.

84. Innocenti F, Liu W, Fackenthal D, et al. Single nucleotide polymorphism discovery and functional assessment of variation in the UDP-glucuronosyltransferase 2B7 gene. *Pharmacogenet. Genomics* 2008;**18**(8):683–697.

85. Blevins-Primeau AS, Sun D, Chen G, et al. Functional significance of UDP-glucuronosyltransferase variants in the metabolism of active tamoxifen metabolites. *Cancer Res.* 2009;**69**(5):1892–1900.

86. Freimuth RR, Wiepert M, Chute CG, Wieben ED, Weinshilboum RM. Human cytosolic sulfotransferase database mining: Identification of seven novel genes and pseudogenes. *Pharmacogenomics J.* 2004;**4**(1):54–65.

87. Freimuth RR, Raftogianis RB, Wood TC, et al. Human sulfotransferases SULT1C1 and SULT1C2: cDNA characterization, gene cloning, and chromosomal localization. *Genomics* 2000;**65**(2):157–165.

88. Raftogianis RB, Wood TC, Otterness DM, Van Loon JA, Weinshilboum RM. Phenol sulfotransferase pharmacogenetics in humans: Association of common SULT1A1 alleles with TS PST phenotype. *Biochem. Biophys. Res. Commun.* 1997;**239**(1):298–304.

89. Hebbring SJ, Adjei AA, Baer JL, et al. Human SULT1A1 gene: Copy number differences and functional implications. *Hum. Mol. Genet.* 2007;**16**(5):463–470.

90. Esteban A, Calvo R, Perez-Mateo M. Paracetamol metabolism in two ethnically different Spanish populations. *Eur. J. Drug Metab. Pharmacokinet.* 1996;**21**(3):233–239.

CHAPTER 4

Pharmacogenetics of Drug Transporters

HENRIETTE E. MEYER ZU SCHWABEDISSEN, MARKUS GRUBE, and HEYO K. KROEMER

Ernst Moritz Arndt-University of Greifswald, Greifswald, Germany

4.1 INTRODUCTION

Pharmacogenetics is a field of clinical pharmacology focusing on the impact of genetic variations of interindividual differences in drug disposition, toxicity, and efficacy. The extent of intersubject variation determined by inherited factors is currently assumed to account for 15–30% of interindividual differences in drug disposition and response, although for some drugs it can be as high as 95% [1]. Initially the influence of genetic variations on drug disposition was studied looking mostly into phase I and phase II metabolizing enzymes [1,2].

Membrane–bound carrier-mediated processes and their contribution to drug disposition is an emerging aspect of pharmacogenetics. Thus far several transporters mediating cellular uptake or elimination of endogenous and exogenous compounds have been identified. Particularly transporters, which are highly expressed in organs such as the liver, intestine, and kidney (see Fig. 4.1), seem to play a major role in drug disposition and are described in detail below. In the following chapter we will focus on drug transporters for which a significant impact on drug disposition and/or drug efficacy has been discussed in association with inherited variability of the encoding gene.

4.2 PHARMACOGENETICS OF UPTAKE TRANSPORTERS

Cellular entry of a variety of compounds has been shown to be facilitated by transport mediating carrier proteins located in the cellular membrane. Until the present, a

Pharmacogenetics and Individualized Therapy, First Edition.
Edited by Anke-Hilse Maitland-van der Zee and Ann K. Daly.

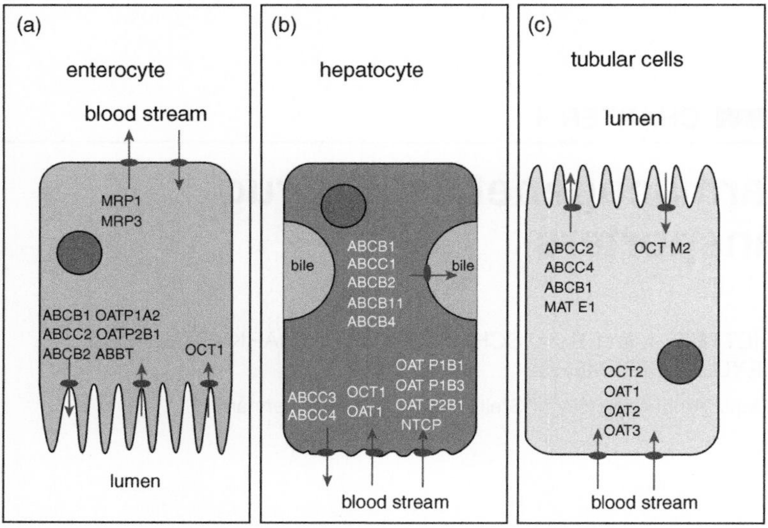

FIGURE 4.1 Schematic summary of drug transporters described in intestine, kidney, and liver. In enterocytes (a) several efflux and uptake transporters have been detected and studied for their involvement in drug disposition. An important aspect for pharmacology is the polarized distribution of drug transporters, thereby mediating directed transport in elimination organs such as liver (b) and kidney (c).

number of these transport proteins have been identified and characterized for their expression profile in humans. However, not all transporters have been screened for genetic variants, and not every transporter exhibits genetic variability that has been associated with changes in drug disposition. In fact, substrate overlap and regulative processes have been assumed to limit the effect of function impairing mutations. However, in general uptake transporters significantly influence cellular accumulation of their substrates and therefore are assumed to function as a rate limiting step for intracellular processes, including binding to the drug target, drug metabolism, or even elimination of parent compound.

4.2.1 Organic Anion Transporting Polypeptides (OATPs)

Organic anion transporting polypeptides (OATPs) are classified within the solute carrier class (SLC) superfamily, referred to as *solute carrier organic anion transporter family* (SLCO) [3]. This subfamily summarizes membrane proteins shown to be involved in sodium-independent cellular uptake. Thus far, in particular OATP1B1 and OATP1B3, members of the human OATP1B subfamily, have been studied for their implication in drug disposition. Both transporters have been noted to be liver-enriched and located in the sinusoidal membrane of hepatocytes [4–6]. In addition, OATP1B transporters exhibit a remarkably broad substrate specificity (for summary, see Table 4.1), including many drugs of clinical relevance.

TABLE 4.1 Summary of Exogenous Substrates of Uptake and Efflux Transporters

Uptake Transporters
OATP1B1
ACU154[a] [256], arsenic (arsenite, arsenate) [257], atorvastatin [8,9,258], atrasentan [259], Bamet-R2[a] [69], Bamet-UD2[a] [69], benzylpenicillin [75], bosentan [260,261] BQ123 [46], bromosulfophthalein [BSP] [41,46], caspofungin [262], cerivastatin [263], demethylphalloin [264], enalapril [265], ezetimibe-G [266], fluvastatin [10,11], methotrexate [6], olmesartan [267,268], phalloidin [264,269], pitavastatin [270,271], pravastatin [8,272,273], rifampin [274,275], RO48-5033 [260], rosuvastatin [7,276], SN-38 [39], S-8921G [277,278], temocaprilat [26], TR14035 [279], troglitazone-*S* [280], valsartan [26,281]
OATP1B3
Amanitin[a] [282], atrasentan [259], bosentan [260,261], BQ123 [46], bromosulfophthalein (BSP) [46,47,283], deltorphin II [46], demethylphalloin [264], digoxin[a] [46], docetaxel [51] D-[penicillamine-2,5]enkephalin [46], enalapril [265], erythromycin [54], fexofenadine [284], fluvastatin [10], fluo-3 [285], methotrexate [6], microcystin [286,287], olmesartan [267,268], ouabain[a] [46], paclitaxel [51], phalloidin [264], pitavastatin [270,271], rifampin [274], RO 48-5033 [260], rosuvastatin [7] SN38 [58], S-8921G [277,278], telmisartan [48], TR14035 [279], valsartan [281]
OCT1
Aciclovir [288] Bamet-R2 [69], Bamet-UD2 [69], berberine [289], cimetidine [290], famotidine [290], furamidine[a] [291], ganciclovir [288], HPP^{+}[b][292], imatinib [101,102], lamivudine [111,293], 1-methyl-4-phenylpyridinium [84,142], pentamidine[a] [291], procainamide [294], quinidine[a] [294], ranitidine [295], RHPP^{+}[c] [292]
OCT2
Amantadine [296], amilorid [297], Bamet-R2 [69], Bamet-UD2 [69], berberine [289], cimetidine [290], famotidine [290], HPP^{+}[b] [292], lamivudine [111,293], memantine [296], 1-methyl-4-phenylpyridinium [113], paraquat[a] [298], procainamide [294], ranitidine [290], RHPP^{+}[c] [292]
Efflux Transporters
ABCB1[d]
Actinomycin D, amitryptiline, amprenavir, atovastatin, bunitrolol, celipolol, chlorpromazine, cimetidine, citalopram, cyclosporine, daunorubicin, dexamethasone, digitoxin, digoxin, diltiazem, docetaxel, domperidon, doxepine, doxorubicin, erythromycin, etoposide, etoposide, FK506, indinavir, irinotecan, itraconazole, levofloxacin, loperamide, losartan, lovastatin, methotrexate, mibefradil, mitoxantrone, mitoycin C, morphine, nelfinavir, nortriptyline, ondansetron, paclitaxel, paroxetine, phenobarbital, phenytoin, quetiapine, quinidine, ranitidine, rifampin, risperidon, ritonavir, saquinavir, sparfloxacin, tacrolismus, talinolol, teniposide, terfenadine, tetracycline, topotecan, trimipramine, venlafaxine, verapamil, vinblastine, vincristine
ABCC1[d]
Daunorubicin, difloxacin, DNP-SG, doxorubicin, etoposide, etoposide-G, geprafloxacin, imatinib, irinotecan, methotrexate, ritonavir, saquinvir, SN38, teniposide, topotecan, vinblastine, vincristine
ABCC2[d]
Acetaminophen-G, ampicillin, cisplatin, daunorubicin, diclofenac-G, DNP-SG, doxorubicin, epirubicin, etoposide, grepafloxacin-G, imatinib, indinavir, indomethacin-G, irinotecan, methotrexate, pravastatin, ritonavir, saquinavir, SN38, SN38-G, teniposide, topotecan, vinblastine, vincristine

(*Continued*)

TABLE 4.1 (*Continued*)

Efflux Transporters
ABCC3[d]
MTX, etoposide, morphine-3-glucuronide, vincristine
ABCC4[d]
3TC [2′,3′-dideoxy-3′thiacytidine], 6-mercaptopurine, AZT, camptothecins, ganciclovir, methotrexate, PMEA, PMEG, thioguanine
ABCC5[d]
5FU, 6-mercaptopurine, cladarabine, cladribine, cytarabine, gemcitabine, methotrexate, PMEA, PMEG, thioguanine
ABCG2[d]
Cerivastatin, cimetidine, ciprofloxacin, cyclosporine, DNP-SG, diflomotecan, flavopiridol, gefitinib, imantinib, irinotecan [SN38], lamivudine, methotrexate, mitoxantrone, nelfinavir, norfloxacin, oflaxacin, omeprazole, pantoprazole, resveratol, ritonavir, rosuvastatin, saquinavir, sirolimus, tacrolimus, topotecan, UCN01, zidovudine

[a]Substrates that are assumed to be transported by only one member of the OATP1B subfamily or one member of organic cation transporters.

[b]HPP^+ is 4-[4-chlorophenyl]-1-[4-[4-fluorophenyl]-4-oxybutyl]pyridinium ion, a pyridium metabolite of haloperidol.

[c]$RHPP^+$ is a reduced form of HPP^+.

[d]Adopted from References 195,200, and 299–301.

G glucuronide.

4.2.1.1 OATP1B1 Substrates and Polymorphisms

The notion that hepatic uptake transporters act as a rate limiting step in drug elimination and drug efficacy has been strongly supported by studies on the influence of OATP1B1 transport activity on pharmacokinetics and pharmacodynamics of statins. Statins inhibit 3-hydroxy-3-methylglutaryl coenzyme A (HMG-CoA) reductase, the rate limiting enzyme of endogenous cholesterol synthesis, and are therefore used to treat hypercholesterolemia. The hepatic route of elimination, in addition to the hepatocellular drug target, made statins an excellent probe to study the effect of genetic variants in liver-enriched OATP1Bs on drug disposition and efficacy.

Initially, *in vitro* studies suggested that OATP1B transporters, especially OATP1B1, determine the cellular uptake of rosuvastatin [7], pravastatin [8,9], atorvastatin [9], cerivastatin [9], and fluvastatin [10,11]. Identification of frequent, naturally occurring-single nucleotide polymorphisms of *SLCO1B1* by Tirona and colleagues in 2001 [12] and demonstration of their functional impact proved to be an important milestone setting the stage for determining the *in vivo* relevance of *SLCO1B1* SNPs [13]. A number of variant alleles were identified, of which *SLCO1B1**2* (c.217T>C), *SLCO1B1**3 (c.245T>C and c.467A>G), *SLCO1B1**5 (c.521T>C), *SLCO1B1**9 (c.1463G>C), *SLCO1B1**10 (c.1964A>G), and *SLCO1B1**12 (c.217T>C and c.1964A>G) exhibited reduced transport activity *in vitro*. Most of these variants are rather rare; however, one, namely, the c.521T>C (p.174V>A), proved to be relatively common. Subsequent studies identified several *SLCO1B1* haplotypes, which include the c.521T>C SNP such as *SLCO1B1**15 (c.388A>G + c.512T>C) [14,15], and *SLCO1B1**17 (−11187G>A + c.388A>G + c.521T>C) [16].

Subsequently, the *in vitro* findings on *SLCO1B1* variants were translated into humans (see Table 4.2), revealing pronounced changes in pharmacokinetic parameters for pravastatin [16–19], pitavastatin [20,21], simvastatin [22], rosuvastatin [23,24], and atorvastatin [24,25]. Closer studies revealed that subjects harboring the *SLCO1B1**15 allele exhibited elevated systemic exposure of pravastatin as compared to subjects lacking this allele [16,18]. Some reports indicated that the *SLCO1B1**1b allele (c.388A>G) may have enhanced transport activity as compared to the wild-type allele (*SLCO1B1**1a) [17,19,26]. In fact, this is supported by a more recent report on the efficacy of fluvastatin [27].

Regarding statins with their intrahepatocellular drug target and resultant extrahepatic side effects, reduced hepatic uptake would lead not only to significantly lower efficacy but also to an increased risk for side effects due to higher systemic exposure. However, an effect of the functional impaired alleles on the short-term efficacy of fluvastatin, rosuvastatin, atorvastatin, and simvastatin has not been detected in healthy volunteers [28–30]. An attenuated pharmacodynamic effect was reported in patients receiving pravastatin in secondary prevention of coronary heart disease [31]. Concerning the adverse events, it is assumed that carrying impaired function alleles is associated with an increased risk for myotoxic side effects [31–33] (see chapter 6).

Various other drugs have been studied for their susceptibility to changes in OATP1B1 activity revealing an impact on the pharmacokinetic profile of torasemide [34], repaglinide [35,36], fexofenadine [37], and nateglinide [38]. However, changes in drug efficacy or the incidence of side effects have not been described for these substances yet. OATP1B1 also appears to play a role in the hepatic uptake of anticancer drugs, such as SN-38 (the active metabolite of irinotecan) [39], a drug widely used to treat colon cancer. Here, most studies to date have focused on the role of the promoter polymorphism in the drug conjugating enzyme UGT1A1 as the main determinant of unexpected toxicity from SN38 therapy. However, the observed toxicities may be the result of synergistic or additive effects of low metabolic (*UGT1A1**6/*28) and transport (*SLCO1B1**15/*15) capabilities [40].

In summary, OATP1B1 is the best clinically characterized uptake transporter. Frequently occurring SNPs are associated with impaired function *in vitro,* and this translates into changes in pharmacokinetics and dynamics *in vivo.*

4.2.1.2 OATP1B3 Substrates and Polymorphisms

OATP1B3 is the second member of the liver-enriched human OATP1B subfamily [4,41]. However, expression has also been detected in other tissues, including placenta [42], prostate [43], and colon [44]. In general, OATP1B3 shares a variety of substrates with OATP1B1, but in most cases transports with lower affinity (Table 4.1). Only a few substrates have been shown to be exclusively transported by OATP1B3 such as the gastrointestinal peptide hormone CCK8 [45] and the cardiac glycoside digoxin [46]. Similar to OATP1B1, several naturally occurring SNPs have been identified in the *SLCO1B3* gene. Specifically, the c.334T>G (p.112S>A) and the c.699G>A (p.233M>I) variant have been shown to occur with relative high allele

TABLE 4.2 Overview of *in vivo* Studies Testing the Pharmacokinetic Impact of Genetic Variants of SLC Transporters, Including OATP1B1 (SLCO1B1), OCT1 (SLO22A1), and OCT2 (SLO22A2)

Study	Studied Substrate	SNP	Effect
		OATP1B1	
Choi et al. [23]	Rosuvastatin	521T>C, 388G>A	AUC↑, C_{max}↑
Chung et al. [20]	Pitavastatin	521T>C, 388G>A	AUC↑, C_{max} ↑, no effect on pitavastatin lactone
Couvert et al. [27]	Fluvastatin	c.463C>A	Lower efficacy LDL reduction
Deng et al. [302]	Pravastatin, pitavastatin	521T>C, 388G>A	CL(t)/F↓, AUC↑, C_{max}↑
Han et al. [303]	Irinotecan	−11187G>A, 388A>G, 521T>C	SN38 AUC↑, hematopoetic toxicity (neutropenia) associated with 521C and GIT toxicity associated with 388G
He et al. [304]	Atorvastatin (and rifampin)	521T>C	AUC↑, C_{max}↑
Hedmann et al. [325]	Pravastatin (heart transplant recipients treated concomitantly with immunosuppressants)	521T>C	AUC↓, C_{max}↓, lower LDL reduction, greater HDL increase
Ho et al. [17]	Pravastatin	521T>C, 388G>A	AUC↑, C_{max}↑
Ieri et al. [21]	Pitavastatin	521T>C, 388G>A	AUC↑
Igel et al. [30]	Pravastatin	521C>T	AUC↑, C_{max}↑, no effect on LDL lowering efficacy
Kalliokoski et al. [25]	Repaglindine (gemfibrozil)	521T>C	Higher sensitivity in gemfibrozil inhibition AUC
Kalliokoski et al. [36]	Repaglindine	521T>C	AUC ↑, C_{max}↑
Kalliokoski et al. [305]	Nateglindine	521T>C	No effect on nateglindine
Kalliokoski et al. [305]	Repaglinidine	521T>C	AUC ↑, C_{max}↑ of repaglindine and metabolites M2 and M4, no effect on M1

Kalliokoski et al. [306]	Rosiglitazone	521T > C	No effect
Kalliokoski et al. [306]	Pioglitazone	521T > C	No effect
Kajosaari et al. [307]	Ciclosporine, repaglindine	521T > C	Lower increase of repaglinidne AUC
Maeda et al. [26]	Valsartan, temocapril, pravastatin	388G > A	Lower AUC in individuals carrying the 388G variant for all drugs tested
Mwinyi et al. [19]	Pravastatin	521T > C, 388A > G	521C AUC↑, 388G AUC↓
Niemi et al. [308]	Rifampin induction of CYP3A4	521C > T, –11187G > A	No effect on CYP3A4 induction (4β-hydroxycholesterol)
Niemi et al. [37]	Fexofenadine	521T > C	AUC ↑
Niemi et al. [309]	Pravastatin	11187G > A, 388A > G, 521T > C	Smaller effect on lathosterol and lathosterol/cholesterol ratio
Niemi et al. [310]	Fluvastatin	521T > C	No effect on pharmacokinetics
Niemi et al. [16]	Pravastatin	521T > C	AUC↑
Nishizato et al. [18]	Pravastatin	521T > C, 388A > G	Reduced total and nonrenal clearance
Oswald et al. [266]	Ezetimibe	521T > C	AUC ezetimibe ↓ Ae fecal ↓
Pasanen et al. [24]	Atorvastatin	521T > C	AUC↑, C_{max}↑ (atorvastatin, 2-OH atorvastatin)
Pasanen et al. [22]	Simvastatin	521T > C	Simvastatin acid AUC↑, C_{max}↑
Pasanen et al. [24]	Rosuvastatin	521T > C	AUC↑, C_{max}↑
Suwannakul et al. [311]	Olmesartan, Pravastatin	521T > C	CL(t)/F ↓, tendency toward higher C_{max}, no influence on pravastatin
Takane et al. [312] (case report)	Irinotecan	521T > C, 388A > G	Irinotecan toxicity
Zhang et al. [38]	Nateglinidne	521T > C	AUC↑, C_{max}↑

(Continued)

TABLE 4.2 (*Continued*)

Study	Studied Substrate	SNP	Effect
Zhang et al. [31]	Pravastatin	521T>C	Lower cholesterol reducing efficacy in CHD patients
Zhang et al. [313]	Rifampine	521T>C	Effect on bilirubin induction
		OCT1	
Tzvetkov et al. [314]	Metformin	181C>T, 1201G>A, 1256delATG, 1489G>A	Renal CL↓
Shu et al. [145]	Metformin	181C>T, 1201G>A, 1256delATG, 1489G>A	AUC↑, C_{max}↑
Shu et al. [94]	Metformin	181C>T, 1201G>A, 1256delATG, 1489G>A	Lower metformin efficacy in oGTT
Zhou et al. [154]	Metformin	181C>T, 1256delATG	No effect on efficacy (Hb1Ac)
Becker et al. [315]	Metformin	rs622342 (intronic, A>C)	Effect on efficacy (Hb1Ac reduction)
		OCT2	
Filipski et al. [135]	Cisplatin	808G>T	No influence on PK
Filipski et al. [135]	Cisplatin	808G>T	(08G genotype associated with higher cisplatin-induced nephrotoxicity but no change in PK
Wang et al. [87]	Metformin	808G>T	Lower clearance, lower sensitivity to cimetidine inhibition

frequencies. *In vitro* assessments of the impact in terms of transport activity have been inconclusive, and the understanding seems still rather vague, although these SNPs have been reported to result in altered transport of prototypical substrates *in vitro* [47].

Various studies focused on the impact of these OATP1B3 variants on the pharmacokinetic parameters of telmisartan, a drug initially thought to be a substrate of only OATP1B3 and not OATP1B1, revealing no differences in exposure or clearance [48–50]. Similar results were seen for paclitaxel and docetaxel [51–53], suggesting that OATP1B3 variants play a minor role in the interindividual variability of pharmacokinetics. However, there are more recent reports that the OATP1B3 genotype influences hepatic accumulation of erythromycin as assessed using the erythromycin breath test (ERMBT). This was unexpected given that the ERMBT is commonly used as a marker of hepatic CYP3A4 activity. Franke et al. were able to show that individuals carrying two copies of the T allele at the 334 locus had a 2.4-fold lower value for ERMBT $1/T_{\max}$, suggesting a more rapid hepatic uptake [54]. In summary, the role of OATP1B3 in terms of drug elimination and therefore classical pharmacokinetic parameters seems rather negligible.

However, more recent findings suggest that OATP1B3 might participate in cancer biology. In fact, OATP1B3 has been detected in several tumor entities, including gastric, colon, pancreatic, and breast cancer [6,55,56]. The function of OATP1B3-mediated transport is seen differently in tumor progression. In breast cancer, for example, the expression level of the transporter has been described as an important prognostic factor, showing that higher levels of the transporter are associated with smaller tumor size, with lower risk of recurrence, and with improved prognosis [55]. In contrast, in prostate cancer, OATP1B3 function is noted to be a risk factor for androgen insensitivity as reduced function variants are beneficial for the outcome [43,57]. Similarly, in colon cancer OATP1B3 is assumed to function as an anti-apoptotic factor and is therefore assumed to be associated with higher tumor growth [56]. The role of OATP1B3 in tumor progression and therapy needs to be further elucidated, especially considering the findings of OATP1B3 mediating the transport of various anticancer agents, including taxanes such as docetaxel and paclitaxel [51,53] or the camptothecin derivate SN38 [58].

4.2.1.3 The Other OATPs

The huge family of OATP transporters summarizes several other transporters shown to mediate sodium-independent uptake. However, few of these transporters have been studied in detail for their role in pharmacokinetics and -genetics.

As summarized by Franke and Sparreboom, it seems worthwhile to mention OATP1A2 as another candidate gene for pharmacogenetic analyses *in vivo* [59]. The expression and localization of this transporter have been object of expert discussions, however, the transporter is expressed in a variety of tissues [60–62]. Moreover, its localization in intestine and kidney might result in effects on oral drug absorption and renal elimination. The high expression in the blood–brain barrier suggests a potential role of OATP1A2 in brain penetration of therapeutic agents [63]. Several drugs have been shown to be transported by OATP1A2, including fexofenadine [64], mitoxantrone [65], imatinib [66], ouabain [67], rocuronium [68], and Bamet-UD2 and Bamet-R2 [69]. Even if frequently occurring nonsynonymous SNPs have been identified in the gene encoding OATP1A2, such as c.516A>C (p.172E>D) and *c*.38T>C (p.13I>T), the influence on *in vivo* pharmacokinetics has not been studied yet [59,63,65].

Moreover, OATP2B1, which is the only member of the human OATP2B subfamily of solute carriers should be included at this point [70]. In contrast to other previously described members of the family of OATPs, the substrate specificity of OATP2B1 is much more restricted, whereas the expression pattern is less confined. In fact, OATP2B1 expression has been demonstrated in small intestine, colon, liver, pancreas, heart, testis, mammary gland, thrombocytes, and placenta [14,71–75]. More recent findings suggest that OATP2B1 might be involved in oral drug disposition, as a reduced function variant was associated with significantly reduced oral bioavailability of the leukotriene inhibitor montelucast [76]. OATP2B1 is implicated in the transport of several substances, including aliskiren (K_m 72 μM) [77], atorvastatin (K_m 0.2 μM) [72], amiodarone [78], rosuvastatin (K_m 2–6 μM) [7,79], fluvastatin (K_m 0.7 μM) [11], pravastatin [80,81], and glibenclamide (K_m 6.24 μM) [82].

Even if a few genetic variants have been identified as being located in the *SLCO2B1* gene locus, the impact of those on drug disposition needs to be further elucidated. *In vitro* experiments suggested reduced transport activity of the frequently occurring c.1457C>T variant that results in an aminoacid exchange in position 486 (p.486S>P also referred to as *SLCO2B1**3) [14]. However this variant was also detected in one individual, which aroused attention because this variant was an outlier in an analysis of the effect of OATP1B1 variants on pravastatin [16]. No effect of the *SLCO2B1**3 variant was seen on the disposition of montelukast; however, the same study reported a significant effect of the *SLCO2B1* variant c.935A>G (p.312R>G) on disposition and efficacy of this leukotriene receptor antagonist [76].

4.2.2 Organic Cation Transporters

The polyspecific organic cation transporters OCT1–3 (*SLC22A1–3*) are members of the solute carrier subfamily 22A (*SLC22A*), a part of the major facilitator superfamily (MFS) that comprises transporters from bacteria, plants, animals, and humans in 18 transporter families [83]. Members of the SLC22A family facilitate the transport of a variety of structurally diverse organic cations, including many drugs, toxins, and endogenous compounds. The distinctive tissue distribution of the OCTs suggests that even if there are wide substrate overlaps, changes in transport activity might translate into rather unique differences in pharmacokinetics.

4.2.2.1 Organic Cation Transporter 1 (OCT1) Substrates and Polymorphisms

OCT1 (*SLC22A1*) is located mainly in the sinusoidal membrane of hepatocytes and is thus assumed to facilitate the hepatocellular accumulation of its substrates [84]. In addition, OCT1 has been detected in the basolateral membrane of enterocytes, where it might function as modulator of direct intestinal secretion [83,85]. Findings using mice harboring a deletion of *Slc22a1* ($Oct1^{-/-}$mice) showing reduced hepatic accumulation and decreased intestinal secretion support this assumption [86–90]. Genetic variations with impaired transport function in humans might therefore be expected to result in reduced efficacy of drugs that exert the desired pharmacodynamic action (or metabolic activation) in the liver or in reduced adverse events for drugs that induce their adverse side effects in hepatocytes.

Several genetic variants have been identified in the *SLC22A1* gene [91–95]. Most of those currently known nonsynonymous variants of *SLC22A1* are rare; however, the polymorphisms p.61R>C (c.181C>T), p.341P>L (c.1022C>T), p.420del (c.1256delATG), and p.465G>R (c.1489G>A) are of higher frequency, with pronounced variation in populations of different ethnic backgrounds [96]. These latter SNPs have been consistently linked to reduced transport activity *in vitro* [91,94,97]. Various of compounds have been described to interact with the hepatic uptake transporter (summarized by Koepsell et al. [83] and Ciarimboli [98]). However, as summarized in Table 4.1, only a small number of drugs have actually been shown to be transported by OCT1.

Imatinib, a specific abl-tyrosine kinase inhibitor (TKI), has been successfully used in the treatment of patients with Philadelphia chromosome–positive chronic myeloid leukemia (CML). More than 95% of patients achieve a complete hematologic response and more than 80%, a complete cytogenetic response. However, a proportion of patients demonstrate resistance or suboptimal response; in many cases the mechanism is unknown [99]. More recent findings suggest a possible role for OCT1 (SLC22A1) in the uptake of imatinib into leukemic cells [100]. This translates into a lower probability of achieving a cytogenetic or molecular remission in patients harboring functional impaired variants of this transporter [101,102]. Even if those data have to be further validated, especially as more recent reports deny a predictive value of OCT1 [103,104], it is hypothesized that patients in whom impaired response is associated with OCT1 might profit from a treatment with desatinib, as this TKI exhibits a lower dependence on OCT1 for cellular accumulation [102,105]. As mentioned above, it had been hypothesized that OCT1 might be involved in direct intestinal secretion; therefore, it seems noteworthy that no relevance of OCT1 genotype (p.61R>C, p.465G>R) was seen in the oral clearance of imatinib [106]. However, the same study was able to show that OCT1 expression interrelates with several efflux transporters that were implicated in the transport of imatinib before, such as ABCB1, ABCC4, and ABCG2.

In conclusion, it seems worthwhile to include genetic variants of OCT1 in pharmacogenomic approaches. However, especially in the case of imatinib, several other genetically variable transporters [66,107,108] have been assumed to be implicated in drug disposition; therefore, a multigenic approach seems inevitable.

More recent findings suggest a role of OCT1 in the uptake of cationic compounds into HIV target cells. OCT1 has been detected not only in several peripheral blood cells, including $CD4^+$ T lymphocytes, but also in lymph nodes [109–111]. Of particular interest seems the finding that mononuclear cells of the lymph nodes of

HIV-infected individuals exhibited significantly higher levels of OCT1 compared to HIV-negative controls [111]. The antiretroviral drugs lamivudine and zalcitabine have been reported to be transported by organic cation transporters including OCT1 and OCT2 [111]. It would be of interest to determine whether genetic variants are associated with differences in drug therapy outcome. Other compounds used in antiretroviral drug therapy have been shown to interact with OCT1, but are not transported [112].

4.2.2.2 OCT2 Drug Substrates and Polymorphisms

The majority of the polyspecific cation transporter 2 (OCT2/gene name *SLC22A2*) is expressed in the renal proximal tubule epithelial cells [113,114], mediating the pH-sensitive cellular uptake of cationic compounds [115,116]. Because of the localization in the basolateral membrane and the high abundance in kidney, OCT2 is assumed to be the first and rate limiting step in renal elimination of its substrate compounds. Previously, several drugs in clinical use have been shown to interact with OCT2, including NSAIDs [117], oral antidiabetics [118], class Ia antiarrhythmics [119], α-receptor antagonists [120], H_2-receptor antagonists [121,122] and platinum drugs [123,124]. However, even if interactions have been shown for a variety of compounds, the influence of OCT2 facilitated transmembrane transport on actual cellular uptake has been demonstrated only for a few drugs in clinical use (Table 4.1).

To date several genetic polymorphisms of the OCT2 transporter have been reported. Leabman et al. screened 247 ethnically diverse individuals for polymorphisms in the gene locus of *SLC22A2* and identified eight nonsynonymous SNPs; however, only 2 of these, namely, p.165M>I (c.493A>G) and p.400R>C (c.1198C>T), were identified with allele frequency $\geq$ 1% [119]. Subsequently, the nonsynonymous variants p.199T>I (c.596C>T) and p.201T>M (c.602C>T) of OCT2 were found in studies of Asian populations, again exhibiting low allele frequency ($\leq$1%) [95,125,126]. The only frequently occurring variant of OCT2 seems to be the p.270A>S (c.808G>T) variant, which has been identified in all ethnic groups examined so far [95,119,125,127]. *In vitro* data suggest significant changes in transport mediated by the OCT2 variants p.165M>I, p.199T>I and p.201T>M, p.270A>S, p.400R>C [95,119,128–130].

Platinum drugs are widely used in anticancer therapy; in particular, *cis*-dichlorodiammine platinum [II] (cisplatin), has emerged as a principal chemotherapeutic agent in the treatment of otherwise resistant solid tumors and is currently among the most widely used agents in the chemotherapy of cancer [131]. The major limitation to its use is the induction of nephrotoxicity [132]. The major site of renal damage is assumed to be located in the proximal tubule of the nephron [133], and more recent findings suggest that a basolateral cationic uptake mechanism might be implicated in the mechanism [134].

Organic cation transporters, especially OCT2, have been demonstrated to facilitate the uptake of cisplatin, thereby inducing cytotoxic effects [123,135,136]. Functional impaired variants of the renal organic cation transporter would therefore be expected to display benefits in the outcome of patients receiving cisplatin. This assumption is supported by findings in male rats, where gender-related expression levels of OCT2 have been shown to result in changes in susceptibility of cisplatin-induced nephrotoxicity [124].

In accordance with those findings, Ciarimboli et al. provided convincing evidence that human OCT2 expression and cisplatin-induced nephrotoxicity might be associated. On one hand, they were able to demonstrate that cimetidine, a well-documented OCT inhibitor, was able to decrease cisplatin uptake in freshly isolated human proximal tubular cells. On the other hand, they also demonstrated that proximal tubular cells isolated from a human diabetic kidney showed reduced cisplatin uptake, which is attributed to the well-documented lower expression of OCT2 in diabetic kidneys [137,138]. However, Zhang et al. noted a minor contribution of OCT transporters in general to cisplatin-induced cytotoxicity using a heterologous expression system [139]. A more recent study conducted in 106 patients treated with cisplatin was not able to demonstrate any changes in cisplatin clearance associated with genetic variant *SLC22A2* [135]. However, this does not exclude the possibility that OCT2 might be involved in the development of cytotoxic side effects. It should be mentioned at this point that Ctr1, a renally expressed copper transporter, has been reported to also facilitate tubular accumulation of cisplatin [140]. In summary, it is hypothesized that OCT2 plays a role in cisplatin-induced renal toxicity; however, the impact of genetic variants needs to be further evaluated in clinical studies.

In addition, OCT2 has been implicated in physiological and pathophysiological processes. Indeed, testing the influence of genetic variants in the transporter revealed a higher prevalence of the p.270A > S variant in patients diagnosed with essential hypertension [141]. It is hypothesized that this might be associated with OCT2 functioning as an extraneuronal transporter of neurotransmitters such as dopamine, norepinephrine, and epinephrine [142]. Another study suggests a role of this transporter in the development of Parkinson disease, which is hypothesized to be associated with the dopaminergic neuromodulators histidylproline diketopiperazine [cyclo(HisPro)] and salsolinol [143].

4.2.2.3 Organic Cation Transporters and Metformin Pharmacokinetics

Interindividual differences in pharmacokinetics and dynamics are an important part of the approach of individualized medicine. Because of easy accessibility and high sensitivity, analysis of blood glucose levels as an index of the efficacy of antidiabetic drug therapy is often applied used to exemplify the potential of genetics in future concepts of pharmacology. Metformin is an antidiabetic drug that has been proved to exert beneficial effects in the prevention of secondary macro- and microvascular complications of diabetes mellitus, especially in overweight patients [144]. In general, it is assumed that the glucose lowering efficacy of metformin is governed by its pharmacokinetics. Plasma concentration and tissue distribution are of particular importance for the interindividual response to metformin [145]. Among various pharmacokinetically related genes, drug transporters governing renal tubular secretion and/or hepatic uptake are of particular interest concerning the evaluation of the influence of genetics on metformin disposition and efficacy. Renal secretion is the major elimination route, whereas hepatic uptake facilitates the drug response as the drug target is located in hepatocytes [146]. This was first reported using knockout mouse models showing that the lack of OCT1 results in significant changes in hepatic accumulation and the development of lactacidosis, the feared serious side effect of metformin treatment [87,88]. In accordance with those findings are more recent reports on the influence of OCT1 variants (p.R61R>C,p.401G>S, p.420del and p.465G>R) on the pharmacodynamic effects of metformin in healthy volunteers [94]. Surprisingly, it has been noted that OCT1 variants also affect metformin disposition [145], even if it has been suggested that active renal secretion is the major metformin elimination route. In fact, in humans approximately 79–86% of an intravenous dose of the biguanide is recovered in urine unmetabolized [147,148]. Previously it was estimated that 93% of the interindividual variability of metformin clearance is determined by genetic factors [149,150], and OCT2, the kidney-enriched transporter, has been suggested to play a pivotal role in this process [118,151,152]. Subsequent studies testing the influence of variants of *SLC22A2* revealed significant decreased renal and total clearance of metformin in individuals harboring the functionally impaired transporter [127,129]. Attempts to translate those findings into response to metformin of diabetes patients are rather disappointing [153,154].

In conclusion, although several groups reported changes in metformin disposition and efficacy associated with genetic variants of OCTs (Table 4.2), additional studies are needed to elucidate the role of function impairing SNPs in clinical practice. However, it seems inevitable to include these transporters in consideration of a pharmacogenomic approach for metformin treatment.

4.3 PHARMACOGENETICS OF EFFLUX TRANSPORTERS

In addition to the above mentioned uptake transporters, cellular accumulation and therefore efficacy of exogenous and endogenous compounds are assumed to be significantly modulated by transporters facilitating cellular efflux. The family of ATP binding cassette (ABC) transporters summarizes a variety of phylogenic conserved membrane proteins that mediate ATP-dependent processes. In total, the ABC transporter family consists of about 50 human members that have been shown to be involved in a variety of cellular processes. With regard to drug transport processes, the most frequently studied ABC transporters are P-glycoprotein (P-gp, MDR1, ABCB1), the multidrug resistance related transporters (MRP, ABCC), and the breast cancer resistance protein (BCRP, MXR, ABCG2). Since all of those proteins transport various structurally and functionally unrelated drugs, it was not surprising that drug–drug interactions on the level of transport processes influence drug efficacy and bioavailability. But not only coadministration of a second transporter substrate or an inhibitor can affect this processes, there is also evidence that genetic variations within transporter genes can affect transport function and therefore influence drug disposition and efficacy.

In this context, the most interesting and best studied ABC transporters are ABCB1, ABCC2, and ABCG2, as they are highly expressed in tissues that are assumed to play a pivotal role in drug disposition such as intestine, liver, and kidney. Genetic variants have been described for all of these transporters that affect expression and/or function of these proteins and in turn modulate bioavailability and distribution of drugs transported by them and hence that might alter efficacy.

4.3.1 ABCB1 (P-gp, MDR1) Substrates and Pharmacogenetics

P-glycoprotein (*ABCB1*) is the best characterized ABC transporter and has been demonstrated to facilitate the export of a variety of compounds including several drugs in clinical use (summarized in Table 4.1). Because of its broad substrate specificity, and its expression in tissues such as intestine, liver, kidney, or the blood–brain barrier, its impact on pharmacokinetic parameters has been addressed in a multitude of studies. One aspect of those studies was the influence of genetic variances. Indeed, a variety of single-nucleotide polymorphisms has been identified within the *ABCB1* gene locus [155]; however, only a few of these have been shown to affect ABCB1 function.

For position 2677, two nonsynonymous variants, c.2677G > T and c.2677G > A (p.893A > S and p.893A >T, respectively), have been identified. The frequency of the respective alleles, however, was different and exhibits interethnic differences. While these polymorphisms do not affect ABCB1 expression [156], the majority of *in vitro* reports indicate an enhanced transport activity for the p.893S/T variant [157–159], while only one failed to show any difference [160].

In contrast, the c.3435C > T polymorphism in exon 26 is a synonymous exchange; however, there is convincing evidence that this SNP might result in reduced expression of the transporter [161,162] explained by reduced stability of transcripts, prolonged translational processes due to altered protein conformation, or linkage to functional impairing polymorphisms such as c.2677G > T and c.1236C > T [159,163–166]. However, it should be noted that the data concerning the impact of this polymorphism are not consistent [167–171]. Current knowledge regarding ABCB1 polymorphisms and their influence on ABCB1 mRNA and protein expression has been summarized by Leschziner et al. [172].

Functional findings may therefore be a consequence of haplotypes rather than that of the isolated SNP. In this context, it should be noted that the haplotype frequency for the positions 1236–2677–3435 significantly differs between ethnicities. While the dominant haplotypes for Caucasians were TTT and CGC, the majority of African-Americans had CGC, and in the Japanese population three (CAC, CGC, and TTT) common haplotypes were described [159,163,173]. Taken together, *in vitro* results indicate an enhanced transport activity for p.893A > S and p.893A >T, whereas the c.3435C > T might affect ABCB1 expression.

Besides these *in vitro* and expression data, ABCB1 polymorphisms have been widely addressed in clinical studies regarding their pharmacokinetic impact and treatment outcome. One of the most intensively studied drugs in association with ABCB1 polymorphisms is the cardiac glycoside digoxin. It has been demonstrated that the c.3435C > T variant results in enhanced digoxin plasma levels [162,174,175], which has been explained by lower intestinal ABCB1 activity. However, several studies failed to reproduce this association [176,177]. A more recent meta-analysis concluded that the c.3435C > T SNP alone has no influence on digoxin pharmacokinetics [178]. The most likely explanations for the controversial results could be the fact that the study populations exhibited different haplotypes. An association between ABCB1 haplotypes and pharmacokinetics of digoxin has been reported [175]. This is in accordance with a Japanese study focusing on c.2677G > T/A and c.3435C > T, demonstrating a dominant effect of the 2677 polymorphism [166]. However, a more recent study focusing on the influence of c.1236C > T, c.2677G > T/A and c.3435C > T on digoxin plasma levels of European digoxin users described elevated digoxin concentrations for each T allele and an even more pronounced effect for the TTT haplotype [173]. In addition, it is now increasingly accepted that polymorphic uptake transporters might also be involved in disposition of digoxin.

In addition to digoxin, the antihistaminic agent fexofenadine has often been used as a probe drug for ABCB1 function. As for digoxin, the results for fexofenadine are not consistent. While it has been proposed that the c.2677C > T/A SNP is the most important [159], there are also convincing data on the relevance of c.3435C > T [179] in fexofenadine kinetics. From these results, it is not surprising that there are also studies that failed to show any effect of ABCB1 genetics on fexofenadine kinetics [180], or that the effect was present only after pretreatment with an ABCB1 inhibitor [181].

A multitude of clinical studies are also available on interaction of ABCB1 with the immunosuppressant cyclosporine A (CsA). In contrast to digoxin and fexofenadine studies, these studies were performed mostly in (transplant) patients. The results are in line with the findings described above, while some studies demonstrate a reduced absorption or enhanced elimination of CsA in association with the 2677 and 3435 T alleles [182–184]. Other groups found an opposite effect or even no effect of these polymorphisms [185–190]. Interestingly, one study in pediatric patients described an age-dependent effect of ABCB1 polymorphisms on the CsA kinetics [191]. In view of these conflicting results, it is unlikely that ABCB1 polymorphisms by themselves play an important role in CsA disposition, and this is supported by a meta-analysis that failed to demonstrate a definitive correlation between CsA kinetics and c.3435C > T [192]. Interestingly, the same study indicated an association of the T allele with an elevated CsA AUC [192].

Besides digoxin, fexofenadine, and CsA, several other ABCB1 substrates have been studied for a genetic influence on their pharmacokinetic characteristics. The results are as contradictory as the studies described in detail above (for summary, see Table 4.3).

In addition to pharmacokinetics, there are a vast amount of data focusing on the possible impact of ABCB1 polymorphisms on pharmacodynamic effects. This relationship was especially studied for anticancer and retroviral drugs, which are often transported by ABCB1. Because this field is beyond the scope of this chapter, it is not discussed in detail.

In summary, many efforts have been made to investigate the influence of genetic variants on disposition and efficacy of P-gp substrates. However, various studies

TABLE 4.3 Overview of *in vivo* Studies Testing Pharmacokinetic Impact of Genetic Variants of ABC Transporters, Including ABCB1, ABCC2, ABCC4, and ABCG2

Study	Studied Substrate	SNP	Effect
		ABCB1 (also summarized in Ref. 172)	
Aarnoudse et al. [173]	Digoxin	1236C>T	Serum conc. ↑
		2677G>T	Serum conc. ↑
		3435C>T	Serum conc. ↑
Ahsen et al. [189]	Cyclosporine A	3435C>T	No significant association
Anderson et al. [211]	IDV, lamivudine, ZDV	2677G>T	GT and TT had a greater reduction in HIV RNA; GG vs. TT had a faster CL/F for IDV
		3435C>T	No significant association
Anglicheau et al. [190]	CsA	−129T>C	—
		1236C>T	Dose adjusted AUC_{0-4}↑ for T allele carriers
		2677G>T	
		3435C>T	
Azarpira et al. [246]	CsA	3435C>T	CsA blood conc./dose was higher for TT carriers
Bernsdorf et al. [316]	Simvastatin and talinolol	2677G>T/A	No significant association
		3435C>T	No significant association
Drescher et al. [180]	Fexofenadine	3435C>T	No significant association
Foote et al. [183]	CsA	2677G>T/A	The dose corrected AUC_{0-4} was reduced in 3435T allele carriers
		3435C>T	
Foote et al. [182]	CsA	2677G>T/A	Enhanced AUC in association with GC haplotype
		3435C>T	
Gardner et al. [317]	Imatinib	3435C>T	No significant association
Gerloff et al. [176]	Digoxin	2677G>T/A	No significant association
		3435C>T	No significant association
Han et al. [208]	Irinotecan	1236C>T	No significant association
		2677G>T	No significant association
		3435C>T	AUC↓, CL↑ (only for SN-38G)

(*Continued*)

TABLE 4.3 (*Continued*)

Study	Studied Substrate	SNP	Effect
Hoffmeyer et al. [162]	Digoxin		
(Rifampin pretreatment)	3435C > T	$C_{max}\uparrow$	
Hu et al. [185]	CsA	1236C > T	Lower blood conc. (dose adjusted) in T allele carriers
		2677G > T/A	Higher blood conc. (dose adjusted) in T and A allele carriers
		3435C > T	No significant association
Johne et al. [175]	Digoxin	2677G > T/A	$AUC_{0-4}\uparrow$, $C_{max}\uparrow$ for 3435C > T; haplotype effects
		3435C > T	No significant association
Kim et al. [159]	Fexofenadine	2677G > T/A	Lower plasma levels for TT carriers (only in European Amercians)
		3435C > T	AUC [CC vs.TT]
Li et al. [241]	Gefitinib	3435C > T	No association
Min et al. [188]	CsA	3435C > T	No significant association
Sakaeda et al. [177]	Digoxin	3435C > T	$AUC_{0-4}\downarrow$
Siegmund et al. [168]	Talinolol	2677G > T/A	AUC↑ for carriers of TT/TA
		3435C > T	No significant association
Shon et al. [181]	Fexofenadine		
±Itraconazole pretreatment	2677G > T/A/—3435C > T		
(Haplotype)	GG/CC vs.TT/TT: AUC↑, $C_{max}\uparrow$, CL/F↓ (only in the pretreatment group)		
	Itraconazole		No significant association
Verstuyft et al. [174]	Digoxin	2677G > T/A	No significant association
		3435C > T	AUC ↑
Weiss et al. [318]	Voriconazole	2677G > T	No significant association
		3435C > T	Oral and nonrenal CL↓ (CC vs. TT)

Xu et al. [163]	Digoxin	1236C > T 2677G > T/A 3435C > T haplotype	AUC↑, C_{max}↑ (TGC-CGC vs. TTT-TTT)
Yamaguchi et al. [319]	Paclitaxel	−129T > C	AUC was reduced in association with —129T > C, 1236C > T, and 2677G > T but not with 3435C > T
		1236C > T	
		2677G > T	
		3435C > T	
Yates et al. [184]	CsA	3435C > T	Oral CL↑ in T allele carriers
Yi et al. [179]	Fexofenadine	1236C > T	AUC↑, C_{max}↑ for 3435 CC vs. TT; AUC for AA/CC haplotype
		↑2677G > T	
		−3435C > T	
Zhou et al. [196]	Irinotecan (SN38)	1236C > T	No significant association
		2677G > T	No significant association
		3435C > T	C_{max}↑ for CPT-11 (CC vs. CT and TT)
		ABCC2	
Anderson et al. [211]	IDV, lamivudine, ZDV	−24C > T	TT carriers had a faster CL/F for IDV (after adjustment for African-Amercian)
		1249G > A	No significant association
Bernsdorf et al. [316]	Simvastatin, talinolol	−24C > T	No significant association
Fujita et al. [207]	Irinotecan and metabolites (plus infusional 5-FU/leukovorin)	−1549G > A	
		−1023G > A	SN38 AUC↓ for GA and AA carriers
		−1019A > G	
		−24C > T	
		1249G > A	AUC↓ for GA and AA carriers
		3972C > T	

(Continued)

TABLE 4.3 (*Continued*)

Study	Studied Substrate	SNP	Effect
Haenisch et al. [203]	Talinolol (‡rifampin induction)	1249G>A	Lower bioavailability and higher residual CL for A allele carriers
Han et al. [208]	Irinotecan	−24C>T	Higher AUC ratio (SN38 + SN38-G)/irinotecan; higher tumor response
		1249G>A	No significant association
		3976C>T	Higher tumor response
Ho et al. [17]	Pravastatin	1249G>A 3563T>A 4544G>A	No significant association
Kiser et al. [231]	Tenofovir	−24C>T	CT carriers had an enhanced excretion
		1249G>A	No significant association
Miura et al. [50]	Telmisartan	−24C>T	AUC↑ and C_{max}↑ for CC vs. CT
Miura et al. [209]	Mycophenolic acid	−24 C>T	No significant association
Naesen et al. [320]	Mycophenolic acid	−24C>T	AUC↑ and C↑ for T allele carriers
Niemi et al. [321]	Pravastatin	1446C>G	AUC↑ and C↑
Rau et al. [210]	Methotrexate	−24C>T	$AUC_{36—48}$↑ for T allele carriers, but only in female patients
Zhou et al. [196]	Irinotecan (SN38)	−24C>T C334-49T	No significant association
		ABCC4	
Anderson et al. [211]	IDV, lamivudine, ZDV	1612C>T	No significant association
		3463G>A	No significant association
		3724G>A	Variants vs. GG had an enhanced ZDV—triphosphate concentration
		4131T>G	GT and GG carriers had higher lamivudine—triphosphate concentrations

Kiser et al. [231]	Tenofovir	3463A > G	CL↓, AUC↑
		4131T > G	No significant association
		ABCG2 (BCRP)	
Adkison et al. [247]	Nitrofurantoin	421C > A	No effect
Anderson et al. [211]	IDV, lamivudine, ZDV	34G > A	No significant association
		421C > A	No significant association
Gardner et al. [317]	Imatinib	421C > A	No significant association
Han et al. [208]	Irinotecan	34G > A	No significant association
		421C > A	No significant association
Ho et al. [17]	Pravastatin	34G > A	No significant association
		421C > A	
Ieiri et al. [21]	Pitavastatin	421C > A	No effect
Jada et al. [322]	Irinotecan (SN38)	421C > A	AUC ratio of SN38G to SN38↑ (CC vs. CA)
Li et al. [241]	Gefitinib	421C > A	Steady-state accumulation↑
Sparreboom et al. [323]	Diflomotecan	421C > A	AUC↑, C_{max}↑ (only after IV); F↓ (CC vs. CA)
Sparreboom et al. [324]	Topotecan	421C > A	F↑ (CC vs. CA)
Urquhart et al. [245]	Sulfasalazine	421C > A	AUC↑, C_{max}↑ (CA vs. CC)
Yamasaki et al. [244]	Sulfasalazine	421C > A	AUC↑, C_{max}↑
Zhang et al. [243]	Rosuvastatin	421C > A	AUC↑, C_{max}↑
Zhou et al. [196]	Irinotecan (SN38)	−19572—19569 CTCA del	Higher REC (AUC_{SN38}/AUC_{CPT11})
		−19202G > C	No significant association
		−18604A del	No significant association
		34G > A	No significant association
		376C > T	No significant association
		421C > A	No significant association
		1244A > G	No significant association
		1245G > C	No significant association

IDV indinavir, ZDV zidovudin.

focusing on the same issue yielded different results, and available meta-analyses for compounds such as digoxin or CsA revealed no significant associations. The most likely explanations for the differing results in this field may be the presence of different haplotypes. Lack of haplotype identification could explain at least some of the observed differences. This may be of particular relevance since *in vitro* data suggest enhanced transport activity for c.2677C > T/A, and reduced expression for c.3435C > T. In addition, the effect of ABCB1 polymorphisms on pharmacokinetics seems to be minimal for drugs such as digoxin, fexofenadine, or CsA and much less important compared to genetic variations in metabolizing enzymes, which could be explained by the fact that drug transport is often mediated by several transporters. Moreover, the transporter expression is influenced by a variety of other parameters (e.g., environmental factors or other drugs), which may enhance the interindividual variability and may be more important than genetic factors (for further reading on the relationship between ABCB1 polymorphisms and pharmacokinetic, see Ref. 193).

4.3.2 Multidrug Resistance Protein (MRP) Transporters

Multidrug resistance protein transporters belong to the C branch of the ABC-transporter superfamily, which consists of 12 members. Among these, only nine are transporters (MPR1–9), while the other members are ion channels (ABCC7/CFTR) or sulfonylurea receptors (ABCC8/SUR1 and ABCC9/SUR2). Structurally, MRP1–3, 6, 7 contain an additional *N*-terminal transmembrane domain of five transmembrane helices (TMD_0), which make these proteins larger (around 1500 amino acids) compared to MRP4, 5, 8, 9 (MRP4, 1325 amino acids; MRP5, 1437 amino acids). Like most other ABC transporters, MRPs are expressed in various tissues.

4.3.2.1 ABCC1 (MRP1) Substrates and Pharmacogenetics

In 1992, ABCC1 was first identified as multidrug resistance factor in a doxorubicin-resistant lung cancer cell line [194]. This transporter is ubiquitously expressed with high amounts in heart, kidney, placenta, and testis, whereas only modest levels are found in intestine, liver, and brain. ABCC1 is distributed mainly to the basolateral membrane of polarized cells [195]. Like other members of the ABC transporter family, the gene encoding this transporter has been screened for single-nucleotide polymorphisms [155,196]; however, because of its expression and localization, its impact on general oral drug disposition or hepatic elimination seems rather limited. Nevertheless, ABCC1 polymorphisms may be relevant for drug efficiency, local drug concentrations, or unwanted side effects [197]. It seems noteworthy that the c.2012G > T (p.671G > V) variant has been associated with acute cardiac toxicity of doxorubicin [198], a well-known substrate of this transporter.

4.3.2.2 ABCC2 (MRP1) Substrates and Pharmacogenetics

As ABCC2 (MRP2) is localized in the apical membrane of polarized cells, it is assumed to play a pivotal role in the final excretion for substances where the major route of elimination is the kidney or the liver. Moreover, ABCC2 is highly expressed in intestine, indicating an impact on intestinal absorption [199]. As demonstrated by *loss of function* mutations of MRP2 leading to the rare Dubin–Johnson syndrome (DJS), one major physiological function of this transporter is the hepatic elimination of bilirubin conjugates as DJS patients present with conjugated hyperbilirubinemia [200]. In addition to these disease-associated variants, several other genetic variants have been identified within the *ABCC2* gene [199,201], some of which have already been tested for pharmacogenetic relevance. Among those, there has been substantial interest in –24C > T polymorphism, which occurs with a frequency of around 20%. While this polymorphism is unlikely to affect ABCC2 protein stability or functional activity, it is assumed to influence ABCC2 transcription. Indeed, decreased renal mRNA amounts have been described [202]; however, this finding has not been reproduced for intestinal or placental ABCC2 expression, respectively [169,203,204]. Other candidate SNPs with potential clinical importance have been described at positions c.3563T > A (p.1188V > E) and c.4544G > A (p.1515C > Y), which occurred with 5–10% frequency in the Caucasian population and are associated with a reduced hepatic protein expression [205]. Other variants, such as the frequent (10–20% with little ethnic differences) p.417V > I, did not affect ABCC2 function *in vitro* or are rare, such as p.789S > F and p.1450A > T, which also exhibit a reduced *in vitro* function [206].

The *in vivo* relevance of ABCC2 polymorphisms has been addressed in numerous studies (see Table 4.3). For example, the topoisomerase inhibitor irinotecan and its active metabolite SN38 themselves, which are also studied for ABCB1 and ABCG2 polymorphisms, have been tested in several independent studies. While Fujita et al. were able to demonstrate an association between irinotecan AUC and c.1249G > A, as well as for the irinotecan metabolite SN38 and -1023G > A [207], other studies failed to show any impact. One group observed at least a trend toward a higher AUC in association with –24TT [196], and in another study an elevated AUC ratio of the combination of SN38 and SN38 glucuronide against irinotecan in association with –24C > T indicated a reduced elimination. In addition, the same study clearly demonstrated a relationship between –24C > T as well as c.3972C > T and progression-free survival and tumor response rate [208]. Taken together, these data provide strong evidence for an influence of ABCC2 polymorphisms and the kinetic and dynamic of irinotecan and its metabolites.

In the same way as for irinotecan, similar results were reported for the –24C > T SNP and telmisartan [50], mycophenolic acid [209], and methotrexate [210], indicating a reduced expression or function of ABCC2. However, in the cases of retroviral drugs this genotype was also associated with the opposite effect [211]. Further studies focusing on pharmacodynamic parameters provide indirect evidence of an influence of ABCC2 genotypes on pharmacokinetics. For example, the presence of the –24C > T variant was identified as a risk factor for diclofenac-induced hepatotoxicity, which may be explained by higher hepatic diclofenac and especially diclofenac–metabolite concentrations due to lower ABCC2-mediated billary elimination [212].

In summary, for ABCC2, the –24C > T variant seems to be of special relevance and should be included in pharmacogenetic analyses. In addition, some unexpected results may be explained by linkage to other SNPs and the presence of certain haplotypes [207,213].

4.3.2.3 The Other MRPs

From the current perspective, other ABCC transporters may also impact pharmacokinetic, such as ABCC3 (MRP3), ABCC4 (MRP4), and ABCC5 (MRP5). While ABCC3 is structurally closely related to ABCC1, its mRNA is highly expressed in liver and tissues such as adrenal gland or small intestine. In polarized cells such as hepatocytes or enterocytes, ABCC3 is expressed mainly in the basolateral membrane; however, the main hepatic ABCC3 expression is located in cholangiocytes [214]. Compared to studies of other ABC transporters, not much effort has been exerted to identify polymorphisms within the ABCC3 gene; however, some general data are available [215–218]. Functional studies have been performed for some variants indicating that the p.1381R > S is associated with a distribution defect, while p.346S > F and p.670S > N led to a reduced transport activity *in vitro* [219]. Another polymorphism (−211C > T) in the ABCC3 promotor region was initially associated with a reduced hepatic ABCC3 mRNA expression probably by affecting a transcription factor binding site [216]; however, this finding was not present in leukocytes [220]. Moreover, a further study performing reporter gene assays could not demonstrate any impact of the –211C > T on promoter activity [221]. The *in vivo* relevance of this polymorphism is still unclear; however, in one study the −211C > T SNP was associated with the clinical outcome of lung cancer patients indicating at least an impact on drug disposition to microcompartments [222].

The last two MRPs that are discussed here are ABCC4 and ABCC5. Both transporters have a broad tissue distribution, including liver, brain, and kidney (ABCC4) and brain, lung, heart, or skeletal muscle (ABCC5) [223]. In addition, ABCC4 has also been detected in anuclear structures such as human platelets, where it is discussed to be involved in ADP storage [224]. ABCC4 is of further interest because of its apical localization in kidney (in contrast to other tissues such as liver [225], indicating a possible involvement in renal secretion of drugs transported by ABCC4 [226]. Physiological substrates of these transporters are cyclic nucleotides such as cGMP and cAMP [227,228], but several drugs have also been shown to be transported (see Table 4.1). Compared to other ABC transporters, ABCC4 is highly polymorphic; for example, in a Japanese study on 48 individuals 257 variations were detected (cf. 95 for ABCC1 and 41 for ABCC2) [218]. While few of these SNPs have been studied in detail, some have already been tested *in vitro,* indicating a reduced function for c.1460G > A (p.487G > E) and an enhanced activity for c.2867G > C (p.956C > S) [229]. For c.2269G > A (p.757E > A), which is especially common within the Japanese population, an altered cell surface expression has been demonstrated [191].

To date, only a limited number of studies focused on ABCC4 polymorphisms and the impact on transport activity *in vivo*. However, the p.757E > A variation has been identified as a risk factor for the thiopurine-induced hematopoietic toxicity, which could be explained by an enhanced intracellular accumulation [191], and in HIV patients the c.4131T > G polymorphism was associated with elevated lamivudine–triphosphate concentrations in PBMC [211]. Similar findings were also made for tenofovir diphosphonate (TFV-DP) and the c.3463A > G on PBMC level (enhanced intracellular levels) [230] and for renal elimination of tenofovir (reduced CL) [231]. Since c.3463A > G and c.4131T > G are synonymous variations or located in the 3′UTR, it is unlikely that they affect the function and distribution of ABCC4, while a reduced mRNA stability or an altered splicing process may be an explanation.

4.3.3 ABCG2 Substrates and Pharmacogenetics

The breast cancer resistant protein (BCRP/ABCG2) was first identified in a mitoxantrone-resistant cell line, which did not express the previously described multidrug resistance factors P-gp and MRP1 [232]. In contrast to the ABC transporters described above ABCG2 belongs to the so-called subfamily of half-transporters. Members of this family consist of only one transmembrane domain (TMD) and one nucleotide binding fold (NBF). To achieve functional activity, ABCG2 has to form homodimers [233]. ABCG2 is expressed in a variety of different tissues such as intestine, liver, kidney, blood–brain barrier, placenta, or stem cells [234]. In addition, several single-nucleotide polymorphisms have been described and characterized for this protein [235]. Some *ABCG2* variants have been reported to result in impaired transport function associated with increased susceptibility to cytotoxic effects of cells expressing genetic variants of *ABCG2*. In particular, the variants c.34G > A (p.12V > M, allele frequency 2–45%), c.421C > A (p.141Q > K, allele frequency 8–35%), c.1465T > C (p.489F > L, allele frequency < 1%), and c.1291T > C (p.441S > N, allele frequency < 1%) are assumed to exhibit changes in transport capacity [236–238]. However, many of those reported SNPs are rather rare, and interethnic differences in allele frequency might be fundamental. ABCG2 substrates are mostly cytotoxic compounds clinically used as anticancer drugs; therefore, translations of *in vitro* findings on functional impairing SNPs are limited. However, the p.141Q > K variant exhibits relative high frequency in Caucasians and especially Asians and has therefore been subject of several pharmacogenetic association studies.

Because of its localization in the apical membrane of enterocytes, ABCG2 is assumed to function as a limiting factor in the intestinal absorption of orally administered drugs [239,240]. This assumption is supported by findings showing enhanced steady-state plasma concentrations associated with an increased risk for developing intestinal side effects in individuals treated with gefitinib and harboring the impaired function allele (p.141Q > K) [241,242]. Similar results were obtained testing the influence of this ABCG2 variant on disposition of rosuvastatin and sulfasalazine [243–245]. Because of the lack of cytotoxicity and the finding that ABCG2 might be the major contributor to sulfasalazine disposition [246], this compound has been proposed as a potential probe drug for genotype–phenotype analyses of ABCG2 [245].

It seems noteworthy that several studies failed to show an association between c.421C > A of known ABCG2 substrates, including nitrofurantoin [247], lamidvudine, indinavir, and zidovudine [211]. Regarding the impact of ABCG2 polymorphisms on the disposition and efficacy of anticancer drugs, prospective pharmacokinetic analyses are rather limited. However, it has been shown that the p.141Q > K variant is associated with enhanced response and survival of hormone-refractory prostate cancer patients, suggesting an influence at least on the intracellular docetaxel accumulation [248]. In addition, a retrospective Hungarian study reported that in children with acute lymphoblastic leukemia (ALL) treated with ABCG2 and ABCB1 substrates (vincristine, doxorubicin, daunorubicin, or MTX), the combination of the 3435TT and 421AA/AC genotype was most predictive for the development of toxic encephalopathy [249]. Most of these described clinical data are in line with *in vitro* studies demonstrating reduced activity (e.g. lower resistance against drugs such as SN38, mitoxantrone, or toptecan and higher intracellular accumulation for c.421C > A) (see discussion below and Ref. 237). The underlying mechanisms, however, remain unclear. While there are some indications for an altered transport activity [250,251], other studies indicate an effect on protein stability, possibly due to enhanced proteosomal and lysosomal degradation [237,238,252,253]. In addition, reduced protein expression of the p.141Q > K variant was observed at least in placenta; however, this finding could not be reproduced for intestinal ABCG2 protein expression [245,254,255].

For the other frequent mutation c.34G > A, although, initial *in vitro* findings indicated a decreased expression of ABCG2 at the apical plasma membrane and increased intracellular accumulation of ABCG2 substrates [251], *in vivo* studies failed to demonstrate an association with pharmacokinetic parameters. This is in accordance with further *in vivo* studies that could neither reproduce altered localization of the p.12V > M variant [252], nor show an effect on protein expression, sensitivity toward chemotherapeutic drugs, and transport activity [237,252].

Taken together, the c.421C > A polymorphism within the ABCG2 gene should be considered as a modulating factor for pharmacokinetics of ABCG2 substrates, while the c.34G > A variation seems to have no functional consequences *in vivo*. In addition, for studies on drugs transported by several transporters, it might be critical to not only focus on the genetics of one transporter, but also to consider all (uptake and efflux) transporters (and metabolizing enzymes) involved in the transport of the investigated drug.

4.4 CONCLUSION

In conclusion, there is growing evidence that transporters are of importance for drug disposition and efficacy. In addition to being subject of drug–drug interactions, transporters are assumed to function as a rate limiting step in absorption, elimination, and tissue distribution of clinically used compounds. Even if several genetic variants have been identified and functionally characterized, it seems noteworthy that, considering the broad substrate overlap, or even if not discussed in detail in this chapter, regulative processes are factors that significantly influence the effect of those genetic variants. In general, haplotype analysis and multiple gene approaches that also account for drug metabolizing enzymes seem mandatory in order to evaluate the overall impact of transport mechanisms in clinical studies.

REFERENCES

1. Eichelbaum M, Ingelman-Sundberg M, Evans WE. Pharmacogenomics and individualized drug therapy. *Annu. Rev. Med.* 2006;**57**:119–137.
2. Wilkinson GR. Drug metabolism and variability among patients in drug response. *N. Engl. J. Med.* 2005;**352**(21):2211–2221.
3. Hagenbuch B, Meier PJ. Organic anion transporting polypeptides of the OATP/SLC21 family: Phylogenetic classification as OATP/SLCO superfamily, new nomenclature and molecular/functional properties. *Pflugers Arch.* 2004;**447**(5):653–665.
4. Abe T, Kakyo M, Tokui T, Nakagomi R, Nishio T, Nakai D, et al. Identification of a novel gene family encoding human liver-specific organic anion transporter LST-1. *J. Biol. Chem.* 1999;**274**(24):17159–17163.
5. Konig J, Cui Y, Nies AT, Keppler D. A novel human organic anion transporting polypeptide localized to the basolateral hepatocyte membrane. *Am. J. Physiol. Gastrointest. Liver Physiol.* 2000;**278**(1):G156–G164.
6. Abe T, Unno M, Onogawa T, Tokui T, Kondo TN, Nakagomi R, et al. LST-2, a human liver-specific organic anion transporter, determines methotrexate sensitivity in gastrointestinal cancers. *Gastroenterology* 2001;**120**(7):1689–1699.
7. Ho RH, Tirona RG, Leake BF, Glaeser H, Lee W, Lemke CJ, et al. Drug and bile acid transporters in rosuvastatin hepatic uptake: Function, expression, and pharmacogenetics. *Gastroenterology* 2006;**130**(6):1793–1806.
8. Hsiang B, Zhu Y, Wang Z, Wu Y, Sasseville V, Yang WP, et al. A novel human hepatic organic anion transporting polypeptide (OATP2). Identification of a liver-specific human organic anion transporting polypeptide and identification of rat and human hydroxymethylglutaryl-CoA reductase inhibitor transporters. *J. Biol. Chem.* 1999;**274**(52):37161–37168.
9. Kameyama Y, Yamashita K, Kobayashi K, Hosokawa M, Chiba K. Functional characterization of SLCO1B1 (OATP-C) variants, SLCO1B1*5, SLCO1B1*15 and SLCO1B1*15+C1007G, by using transient expression systems of HeLa and HEK293 cells. *Pharmacogenet. Genomics* 2005;**15**(7):513–522.
10. Kopplow K, Letschert K, Konig J, Walter B, Keppler D. Human hepatobiliary transport of organic anions analyzed by quadruple-transfected cells. *Mol. Pharmacol.* 2005;**68**(4):1031–1038.
11. Noe J, Portmann R, Brun ME, Funk C. Substrate-dependent drug-drug interactions between gemfibrozil, fluvastatin and other organic anion-transporting peptide (OATP) substrates on OATP1B1, OATP2B1, and OATP1B3. *Drug Metab. Dispos.* 2007;**35**(8):1308–1314.
12. Tirona RG, Leake BF, Merino G, Kim RB. Polymorphisms in OATP-C: Identification of multiple allelic variants associated with altered transport activity among European- and African-Americans. *J. Biol. Chem.* 2001;**276**(38):35669–35675.
13. Tirona RG, Leake BF, Podust LM, Kim RB. Identification of amino acids in rat pregnane X receptor that determine species-specific activation. *Mol. Pharmacol.* 2004;**65**(1):36–44.
14. Nozawa T, Nakajima M, Tamai I, Noda K, Nezu J, Sai Y, et al. Genetic polymorphisms of human organic anion transporters OATP-C (SLC21A6) and OATP-B (SLC21A9): Allele frequencies in the Japanese population and functional analysis. *J. Pharmacol. Exp. Ther.* 2002;**302**(2):804–813.

15. Iwai M, Suzuki H, Ieiri I, Otsubo K, Sugiyama Y. Functional analysis of single nucleotide polymorphisms of hepatic organic anion transporter OATP1B1 (OATP-C). *Pharmacogenetics* 2004;**14**(11):749–757.
16. Niemi M, Schaeffeler E, Lang T, Fromm MF, Neuvonen M, Kyrklund C, et al. High plasma pravastatin concentrations are associated with single nucleotide polymorphisms and haplotypes of organic anion transporting polypeptide-C (OATP-C, SLCO1B1). *Pharmacogenetics* 2004;**14**(7):429–440.
17. Ho RH, Choi L, Lee W, Mayo G, Schwarz UI, Tirona RG, et al. Effect of drug transporter genotypes on pravastatin disposition in European- and African-American participants. *Pharmacogenet. Genomics* 2007;**17**(8):647–656.
18. Nishizato Y, Ieiri I, Suzuki H, Kimura M, Kawabata K, Hirota T, et al. Polymorphisms of OATP-C (SLC21A6) and OAT3 (SLC22A8) genes: Consequences for pravastatin pharmacokinetics. *Clin. Pharmacol. Ther.* 2003;**73**(6):554–565.
19. Mwinyi J, Johne A, Bauer S, Roots I, Gerloff T. Evidence for inverse effects of OATP-C (SLC21A6) 5 and 1b haplotypes on pravastatin kinetics. *Clin. Pharmacol. Ther.* 2004;**75**(5):415–421.
20. Chung JY, Cho JY, Yu KS, Kim JR, Oh DS, Jung HR, et al. Effect of OATP1B1 (SLCO1B1) variant alleles on the pharmacokinetics of pitavastatin in healthy volunteers. *Clin. Pharmacol. Ther.* 2005;**78**(4):342–350.
21. Ieiri I, Suwannakul S, Maeda K, Uchimaru H, Hashimoto K, Kimura M, et al. SLCO1B1 (OATP1B1, an uptake transporter) and ABCG2 (BCRP, an efflux transporter) variant alleles and pharmacokinetics of pitavastatin in healthy volunteers. *Clin. Pharmacol. Ther.* 2007;**82**(5):541–547.
22. Pasanen MK, Neuvonen M, Neuvonen PJ, Niemi M. SLCO1B1 polymorphism markedly affects the pharmacokinetics of simvastatin acid. *Pharmacogenet. Genomics* 2006;**16**(12):873–879.
23. Choi JH, Lee MG, Cho JY, Lee JE, Kim KH, Park K. Influence of OATP1B1 genotype on the pharmacokinetics of rosuvastatin in Koreans. *Clin. Pharmacol. Ther.* 2008;**83**(2):251–257.
24. Pasanen MK, Fredrikson H, Neuvonen PJ, Niemi M. Different effects of SLCO1B1 polymorphism on the pharmacokinetics of atorvastatin and rosuvastatin. *Clin. Pharmacol. Ther.* 2007;**82**(6):726–733.
25. Kalliokoski A, Backman J, Kurkinen K, Neuvonen P, Niemi M. Effects of Gemfibrozil and Atorvastatin on the Pharmacokinetics of Repaglinide in Relation to SLCO1B1 Polymorphism. *Clin. Pharmacol. Ther.* 2008;**84**(4):488–96.
26. Maeda K, Ieiri I, Yasuda K, Fujino A, Fujiwara H, Otsubo K, et al. Effects of organic anion transporting polypeptide 1B1 haplotype on pharmacokinetics of pravastatin, valsartan, and temocapril. *Clin. Pharmacol. Ther.* 2006;**79**(5):427–439.
27. Couvert P, Giral P, Dejager S, Gu J, Huby T, Chapman MJ, et al. Association between a frequent allele of the gene encoding OATP1B1 and enhanced LDL-lowering response to fluvastatin therapy. *Pharmacogenomics* 2008;**9**(9):1217–1227.
28. Pasanen MK, Neuvonen PJ, Niemi M. Global analysis of genetic variation in SLCO1B1. *Pharmacogenomics* 2008;**9**(1):19–33.
29. Gerloff T, Schaefer M, Mwinyi J, Johne A, Sudhop T, Lutjohann D, et al. Influence of the SLCO1B1*1b and *5 haplotypes on pravastatin's cholesterol lowering capabilities and basal sterol serum levels. *Naunyn. Schmiedebergs Arch. Pharmacol.* 2006;**373**(1):45–50.

30. Igel M, Arnold KA, Niemi M, Hofmann U, Schwab M, Lutjohann D, et al. Impact of the SLCO1B1 polymorphism on the pharmacokinetics and lipid-lowering efficacy of multiple-dose pravastatin. *Clin. Pharmacol. Ther.* 2006;**79**(5):419–426.

31. Zhang W, Chen BL, Ozdemir V, He YJ, Zhou G, Peng DD, et al. SLCO1B1 521T-- > C functional genetic polymorphism and lipid-lowering efficacy of multiple-dose pravastatin in Chinese coronary heart disease patients. *Br. J. Clin. Pharmacol.* 2007;**64**(3):346–352.

32. Link E, Parish S, Armitage J, Bowman L, Heath S, Matsuda F, et al. SLCO1B1 variants and statin-induced myopathy - a genomewide study. *New Engl. J. Med.* 2008;**359**(8):789–799.

33. Furihata T, Satoh N, Ohishi T, Ugajin M, Kameyama Y, Morimoto K, et al. Functional analysis of a mutation in the SLCO1B1 gene (c.1628T>G) identified in a Japanese patient with pravastatin-induced myopathy. *Pharmacogenomics J.* 2009;**9**(3):185–193.

34. Werner D, Werner U, Meybaum A, Schmidt B, Umbreen S, Grosch A, et al. Determinants of steady-state torasemide pharmacokinetics: Impact of pharmacogenetic factors, gender and angiotensin II receptor blockers. *Clin. Pharmacokinet.* 2008;**47**(5):323–332.

35. Niemi M, Backman JT, Kajosaari LI, Leathart JB, Neuvonen M, Daly AK, et al. Polymorphic organic anion transporting polypeptide 1B1 is a major determinant of repaglinide pharmacokinetics. *Clin. Pharmacol. Ther.* 2005;**77**(6):468–478.

36. Kalliokoski A, Neuvonen M, Neuvonen PJ, Niemi M. The effect of SLCO1B1 polymorphism on repaglinide pharmacokinetics persists over a wide dose range. *Br. J. Clin. Pharmacol.* 2008;**66**(6):818–825.

37. Niemi M, Kivisto KT, Hofmann U, Schwab M, Eichelbaum M, Fromm MF. Fexofenadine pharmacokinetics are associated with a polymorphism of the SLCO1B1 gene (encoding OATP1B1). *Br. J. Clin. Pharmacol.* 2005;**59**(5):602–604.

38. Zhang W, He YJ, Han CT, Liu ZQ, Li Q, Fan L, et al. Effect of SLCO1B1 genetic polymorphism on the pharmacokinetics of nateglinide. *Br. J. Clin. Pharmacol.* 2006;**62**(5):567–572.

39. Nozawa T, Minami H, Sugiura S, Tsuji A, Tamai I. Role of organic anion transporter OATP1B1 (OATP-C) in hepatic uptake of irinotecan and its active metabolite, 7-ethyl-10-hydroxycamptothecin: In vitro evidence and effect of single nucleotide polymorphisms. *Drug Metab. Dispos.* 2005;**33**(3):434–439.

40. Takane H, Kawamoto K, Sasaki T, Moriki K, Moriki K, Kitano H, et al. Life-threatening toxicities in a patient with UGT1A1*6/*28 and SLCO1B1*15/*15 genotypes after irinotecan-based chemotherapy. *Cancer Chemother. Pharmacol.* 2000;**63**(6):1165–1169.

41. Cui Y, Konig J, Leier I, Buchholz U, Keppler D. Hepatic uptake of bilirubin and its conjugates by the human organic anion transporter SLC21A6. *J. Biol. Chem.* 2001;**276**(13):9626–9630.

42. Briz O, Serrano MA, MacIas RI, Gonzalez-Gallego J, Marin JJ. Role of organic anion-transporting polypeptides, OATP-A, OATP-C and OATP-8, in the human placenta-maternal liver tandem excretory pathway for foetal bilirubin. *Biochem. J.* 2003;**371**(Pt 3):897–905.

43. Hamada A, Sissung T, Price DK, Danesi R, Chau CH, Sharifi N, et al. Effect of SLCO1B3 haplotype on testosterone transport and clinical outcome in caucasian patients with androgen-independent prostatic cancer. *Clin. Cancer Res.* 2008;**14**(11):3312–3318.

44. Ballestero MR, Monte MJ, Briz O, Jimenez F, Gonzalez-San Martin F, Marin JJ. Expression of transporters potentially involved in the targeting of cytostatic bile acid derivatives to colon cancer and polyps. *Biochem. Pharmacol.* 2006;**72**(6):729–738.
45. Ismair MG, Stieger B, Cattori V, Hagenbuch B, Fried M, Meier PJ, et al. Hepatic uptake of cholecystokinin octapeptide by organic anion-transporting polypeptides OATP4 and OATP8 of rat and human liver. *Gastroenterology* 2001;**121**(5):1185–1190.
46. Kullak-Ublick GA, Ismair MG, Stieger B, Landmann L, Huber R, Pizzagalli F, et al. Organic anion-transporting polypeptide B (OATP-B) and its functional comparison with three other OATPs of human liver. *Gastroenterology* 2001;**120**(2):525–533.
47. Letschert K, Keppler D, Konig J. Mutations in the SLCO1B3 gene affecting the substrate specificity of the hepatocellular uptake transporter OATP1B3 (OATP8). *Pharmacogenetics* 2004;**14**(7):441–452.
48. Ishiguro N, Maeda K, Kishimoto W, Saito A, Harada A, Ebner T, et al. Predominant contribution of OATP1B3 to the hepatic uptake of telmisartan, an angiotensin II receptor antagonist, in humans. *Drug Metab. Dispos.* 2006;**34**(7):1109–1115.
49. Ishiguro N, Maeda K, Saito A, Kishimoto W, Matsushima S, Ebner T, et al. Establishment of a set of double transfectants coexpressing organic anion transporting polypeptide 1B3 and hepatic efflux transporters for the characterization of the hepatobiliary transport of telmisartan acylglucuronide. *Drug Metab. Dispos.* 2008;**36**(4):796–805.
50. Miura M, Satoh S, Inoue K, Saito M, Habuchi T, Suzuki T. Telmisartan pharmacokinetics in Japanese renal transplant recipients. *Clin. Chim. Acta.* 2009;**399**(1–2):83–87.
51. Smith NF, Acharya MR, Desai N, Figg WD, Sparreboom A. Identification of OATP1B3 as a high-affinity hepatocellular transporter of paclitaxel. *Cancer Biol. Ther.* 2005; **4**(8):815–818.
52. Smith NF, Marsh S, Scott-Horton TJ, Hamada A, Mielke S, Mross K, et al. Variants in the SLCO1B3 gene: Interethnic distribution and association with paclitaxel pharmacokinetics. *Clin. Pharmacol. Ther.* 2007;**81**(1):76–82.
53. Baker S, Verweij J, Cusatis G, van Schaik R, Marsh S, Orwick S, et al. Pharmacogenetic pathway analysis of docetaxel elimination. *Clin. Pharmacol. Ther.* 2009;**85**(5):155–163.
54. Franke RM, Baker SD, Mathijssen RH, Schuetz EG, Sparreboom A. Influence of solute carriers on the pharmacokinetics of CYP3A4 probes. *Clin. Pharmacol. Ther.* 2008; **84**(6):704–709.
55. Muto M, Onogawa T, Suzuki T, Ishida T, Rikiyama T, Katayose Y, et al. Human liver-specific organic anion transporter-2 is a potent prognostic factor for human breast carcinoma. *Cancer Sci.* 2007;**98**(10):1570–1576.
56. Lee W, Belkhiri A, Lockhart AC, Merchant N, Glaeser H, Harris EI, et al. Overexpression of OATP1B3 confers apoptotic resistance in colon cancer. *Cancer Res.* 2008; **68**(24):10315–10323.
57. Sharifi N, Hamada A, Sissung T, Danesi R, Venzon D, Baum C, et al. A polymorphism in a transporter of testosterone is a determinant of androgen independence in prostate cancer. *British Journal of Urology International* 2008;**102**(5):617–621.
58. Yamaguchi H, Kobayashi M, Okada M, Takeuchi T, Unno M, Abe T, et al. Rapid screening of antineoplastic candidates for the human organic anion transporter OATP1B3 substrates using fluorescent probes. *Cancer Lett.* 2008;**260**(1–2):163–169.
59. Franke RM, Scherkenbach LA, Sparreboom A. Pharmacogenetics of the organic anion transporting polypeptide 1A2. *Pharmacogenomics* 2009;**10**(3):339–344.

60. Kullak-Ublick GA, Fisch T, Oswald M, Hagenbuch B, Meier PJ, Beuers U, et al. Dehydroepiandrosterone sulfate (DHEAS): Identification of a carrier protein in human liver and brain. *FEBS Lett.* 1998;**424**(3):173–176.

61. Kullak-Ublick GA, Hagenbuch B, Stieger B, Schteingart CD, Hofmann AF, Wolkoff AW, et al. Molecular and functional characterization of an organic anion transporting polypeptide cloned from human liver. *Gastroenterology* 1995;**109**(4):1274–1282.

62. Glaeser H, Bailey DG, Dresser GK, Gregor JC, Schwarz UI, McGrath JS, et al. Intestinal drug transporter expression and the impact of grapefruit juice in humans. *Clin. Pharmacol. Ther.* 2007;**81**(3):362–370.

63. Lee W, Glaeser H, Smith LH, Roberts RL, Moeckel GW, Gervasini G, et al. Polymorphisms in human organic anion-transporting polypeptide 1A2 (OATP1A2): Implications for altered drug disposition and central nervous system drug entry. *J. Biol. Chem.* 2005;**280**(10):9610–9617.

64. Cvetkovic M, Leake B, Fromm MF, Wilkinson GR, Kim RB. OATP and P-glycoprotein transporters mediate the cellular uptake and excretion of fexofenadine. *Drug Metab. Dispos.* 1999;**27**(8):866–871.

65. Badagnani I, Castro RA, Taylor TR, Brett CM, Huang CC, Stryke D, et al. Interaction of methotrexate with organic-anion transporting polypeptide 1A2 and its genetic variants. *J. Pharmacol. Exp. Ther.* 2006;**318**(2):521–529.

66. Franke RM, Sparreboom A. Inhibition of imatinib transport by uremic toxins during renal failure. *J. Clin. Oncol.* 2008;**26**(25):4226–4227.

67. Bossuyt X, Muller M, Meier PJ. Multispecific amphipathic substrate transport by an organic anion transporter of human liver. *J. Hepatol.* 1996;**25**(5):733–738.

68. van Montfoort JE, Hagenbuch B, Fattinger KE, Muller M, Groothuis GM, Meijer DK, et al. Polyspecific organic anion transporting polypeptides mediate hepatic uptake of amphipathic type II organic cations. *J. Pharmacol. Exp. Ther.* 1999;**291**(1): 147–152.

69. Briz O, Serrano MA, Rebollo N, Hagenbuch B, Meier PJ, Koepsell H, et al. Carriers involved in targeting the cytostatic bile acid-cisplatin derivatives cis-diammine-chloro-cholylglycinate-platinum (II) and cis-diammine-bisursodeoxycholate-platinum (II) toward liver cells. *Mol. Pharmacol.* 2002;**61**(4):853–860.

70. Hagenbuch B, Gui C. Xenobiotic transporters of the human organic anion transporting polypeptides (OATP) family. *Xenobiotica* 2008;**38**(7–8):778–801.

71. Tamai I, Nozawa T, Koshida M, Nezu J, Sai Y, Tsuji A. Functional characterization of human organic anion transporting polypeptide B (OATP-B) in comparison with liver-specific OATP-C. *Pharm. Res.* 2001;**18**(9):1262–1269.

72. Grube M, Kock K, Oswald S, Draber K, Meissner K, Eckel L, et al. Organic anion transporting polypeptide 2B1 is a high-affinity transporter for atorvastatin and is expressed in the human heart. *Clin. Pharmacol. Ther.* 2006;**80**(6):607–620.

73. Grube M, Reuther S, Meyer zu Schwabedissen HE, Kock K, Draber K, Ritter CA, et al. Organic anion transporting polypeptide 2B1 and breast cancer resistance protein interact in the transepithelial transport of steroid sulfates in human placenta. *Drug Metab. Dispos.* 2007;**35**(1):30–35.

74. Niessen J, Jedlitschky G, Grube M, Bien S, Schwertz H, Ohtsuki S, et al. Human platelets express OATP2B1, an uptake transporter for atorvastatin. *Drug Metab. Dispos.* 2009; **37**(5):1129–1137.

75. Tamai I, Nezu J, Uchino H, Sai Y, Oku A, Shimane M, et al. Molecular identification and characterization of novel members of the human organic anion transporter (OATP) family. *Biochem. Biophys. Res. Commun.* 2000;**273**(1):251–260.
76. Mougey EB, Feng H, Castro M, Irvin CG, Lima JJ. Absorption of montelukast is transporter mediated: A common variant of OATP2B1 is associated with reduced plasma concentrations and poor response. *Pharmacogenet. Genomics* 2009;**19**(2):129–138.
77. Vaidyanathan S, Camenisch G, Schuetz H, Reynolds C, Yeh CM, Bizot MN, et al. Pharmacokinetics of the oral direct renin inhibitor aliskiren in combination with digoxin, atorvastatin, and ketoconazole in healthy subjects: The role of P-glycoprotein in the disposition of aliskiren. *J. Clin. Pharmacol.* 2008;**48**(11):1323–1338.
78. Seki S, Kobayashi M, Itagaki S, Hirano T, Iseki K. Contribution of organic anion transporting polypeptide OATP2B1 to amiodarone accumulation in lung epithelial cells. *Biochim. Biophys. Acta* 2009;**1788**(5):911–917.
79. Kitamura S, Maeda K, Wang Y, Sugiyama Y. Involvement of multiple transporters in the hepatobiliary transport of rosuvastatin. *Drug Metab. Dispos.* 2008;**36**(10): 2014–2023.
80. Kobayashi D, Nozawa T, Imai K, Nezu J, Tsuji A, Tamai I. Involvement of human organic anion transporting polypeptide OATP-B (SLC21A9) in pH-dependent transport across intestinal apical membrane. *J. Pharmacol. Exp. Ther.* 2003;**306**(2):703–708.
81. Nozawa T, Imai K, Nezu J, Tsuji A, Tamai I. Functional characterization of pH-sensitive organic anion transporting polypeptide OATP-B in human. *J. Pharmacol. Exp. Ther.* 2004;**308**(2):438–445.
82. Satoh H, Yamashita F, Tsujimoto M, Murakami H, Koyabu N, Ohtani H, et al. Citrus juices inhibit the function of human organic anion-transporting polypeptide OATP-B. *Drug Metab. Dispos.* 2005;**33**(4):518–523.
83. Koepsell H, Lips K, Volk C. Polyspecific organic cation transporters: Structure, function, physiological roles, and biopharmaceutical implications. *Pharm. Res.* 2007; **24**(7):1227–1251.
84. Zhang L, Dresser MJ, Gray AT, Yost SC, Terashita S, Giacomini KM. Cloning and functional expression of a human liver organic cation transporter. *Mol. Pharmacol.* 1997;**51**(6):913–921.
85. Terada T, Inui K. Gene expression and regulation of drug transporters in the intestine and kidney. *Biochem. Pharmacol.* 2007;**73**(3):440–449.
86. Jonker JW, Wagenaar E, Mol CA, Buitelaar M, Koepsell H, Smit JW, et al. Reduced hepatic uptake and intestinal excretion of organic cations in mice with a targeted disruption of the organic cation transporter 1 (Oct1 [Slc22a1]) gene. *Mol. Cell. Biol.* 2001;**21**(16):5471–5477.
87. Wang DS, Jonker JW, Kato Y, Kusuhara H, Schinkel AH, Sugiyama Y. Involvement of organic cation transporter 1 in hepatic and intestinal distribution of metformin. *J. Pharmacol. Exp. Ther.* 2002;**302**(2):510–515.
88. Wang DS, Kusuhara H, Kato Y, Jonker JW, Schinkel AH, Sugiyama Y. Involvement of organic cation transporter 1 in the lactic acidosis caused by metformin. *Mol. Pharmacol.* 2003;**63**(4):844–848.
89. Jonker JW, Wagenaar E, Van Eijl S, Schinkel AH. Deficiency in the organic cation transporters 1 and 2 (Oct1/Oct2 [Slc22a1/Slc22a2]) in mice abolishes renal secretion of organic cations. *Mol. Cell. Biol.* 2003;**23**(21):7902–7908.

90. Jonker JW, Schinkel AH. Pharmacological and physiological functions of the polyspecific organic cation transporters: OCT1 2, and 3 (SLC22A1-3). *J. Pharmacol. Exp. Ther.* 2004;**308**(1):2–9.

91. Kerb R, Brinkmann U, Chatskaia N, Gorbunov D, Gorboulev V, Mornhinweg E, et al. Identification of genetic variations of the human organic cation transporter hOCT1 and their functional consequences. *Pharmacogenetics* 2002;**12**(8):591–595.

92. Saito S, Iida A, Sekine A, Ogawa C, Kawauchi S, Higuchi S, et al. Catalog of 238 variations among six human genes encoding solute carriers (hSLCs) in the Japanese population. *J. Hum. Genet.* 2002;**47**(11):576–584.

93. Itoda M, Saito Y, Maekawa K, Hichiya H, Komamura K, Kamakura S, et al. Seven novel single nucleotide polymorphisms in the human SLC22A1 gene encoding organic cation transporter 1 (OCT1). *Drug Metab. Pharmacokinet.* 2004;**19**(4):308–312.

94. Shu Y, Sheardown SA, Brown C, Owen RP, Zhang S, Castro RA, et al. Effect of genetic variation in the organic cation transporter 1 (OCT1) on metformin action. *J. Clin. Invest.* 2007;**117**(5):1422–1431.

95. Kang HJ, Song IS, Shin HJ, Kim WY, Lee CH, Shim JC, et al. Identification and functional characterization of genetic variants of human organic cation transporters in a Korean population. *Drug Metab. Dispos.* 2007;**35**(4):667–675.

96. Shu Y, Leabman MK, Feng B, Mangravite LM, Huang CC, Stryke D, et al. Evolutionary conservation predicts function of variants of the human organic cation transporter, *OCT1. Proc. Natl. Acad. Sci. USA* 2003;**100**(10):5902–5907.

97. Takeuchi A, Motohashi H, Okuda M, Inui K. Decreased function of genetic variants, Pro283Leu and Arg287Gly, in human organic cation transporter hOCT1. *Drug Metab. Pharmacokinet.* 2003;**18**(6):409–412.

98. Ciarimboli G. Organic cation transporters. *Xenobiotica* 2008;**38**(7–8):936–971.

99. Goldman JM. How I treat chronic myeloid leukemia in the imatinib era. *Blood* 2007; **110**(8):2828–2837.

100. Thomas J, Wang L, Clark RE, Pirmohamed M. Active transport of imatinib into and out of cells: Implications for drug resistance. *Blood* 2004;**104**(12):3739–3745.

101. Wang L, Giannoudis A, Lane S, Williamson P, Pirmohamed M, Clark RE. Expression of the uptake drug transporter hOCT1 is an important clinical determinant of the response to imatinib in chronic myeloid leukemia. *Clin. Pharmacol. Ther.* 2008;**83**(2):258–264.

102. Giannoudis A, Davies A, Lucas CM, Harris RJ, Pirmohamed M, Clark RE. Effective dasatinib uptake may occur without human organic cation transporter 1 (hOCT1): Implications for the treatment of imatinib-resistant chronic myeloid leukemia. *Blood* 2008;**112**(8):3348–3354.

103. Zach O, Krieger O, Foedermayr M, Zellhofer B, Lutz D. OCT1 (SLC22A1) R61C polymorphism and response to imatinib treatment in chronic myeloid leukemia patients. *Leuk. Lymphoma* 2008;**49**(11):2222–2223.

104. Hirayama C, Watanabe H, Nakashima R, Nanbu T, Hamada A, Kuniyasu A, et al. Constitutive overexpression of P-glycoprotein, rather than breast cancer resistance protein or organic cation transporter 1, contributes to acquisition of imatinib-resistance in K562 cells. *Pharm. Res.* 2008;**25**(4):827–835.

105. Hiwase DK, Saunders V, Hewett D, Frede A, Zrim S, Dang P, et al. Dasatinib cellular uptake and efflux in chronic myeloid leukemia cells: Therapeutic implications. *Clin. Cancer Res.* 2008;**14**(12):3881–3888.

106. Hu S, Franke RM, Filipski KK, Hu C, Orwick SJ, de Bruijn EA, et al. Interaction of imatinib with human organic ion carriers. *Clin. Cancer Res.* 2008;**14**(10):3141–3148.

107. Dulucq S, Bouchet S, Turcq B, Lippert E, Etienne G, Reiffers J, et al. Multidrug resistance gene (MDR1) polymorphisms are associated with major molecular responses to standard-dose imatinib in chronic myeloid leukemia. *Blood* 2008;**112**(5):2024–2027.

108. Ozvegy-Laczka C, Cserepes J, Elkind NB, Sarkadi B. Tyrosine kinase inhibitor resistance in cancer: Role of ABC multidrug transporters. *Drug Resist. Updat.* 2005; **8**(1–2):15–26.

109. Schneider E, Machavoine F, Pleau JM, Bertron AF, Thurmond RL, Ohtsu H, et al. Organic cation transporter 3 modulates murine basophil functions by controlling intracellular histamine levels. *J. Exp. Med.* 2005;**202**(3):387–393.

110. Minuesa G, Purcet S, Erkizia I, Molina-Arcas M, Bofill M, Izquierdo-Useros N, et al. Expression and functionality of anti-human immunodeficiency virus and anticancer drug uptake transporters in immune cells. *J. Pharmacol. Exp. Ther.* 2008;**324**(2):558–567.

111. Jung N, Lehmann C, Rubbert A, Knispel M, Hartmann P, van Lunzen J, et al. Relevance of the organic cation transporters 1 and 2 for antiretroviral drug therapy in human immunodeficiency virus infection. *Drug Metab. Dispos.* 2008;**36**(8):1616–1623.

112. Zhang L, Gorset W, Washington CB, Blaschke TF, Kroetz DL, Giacomini KM. Interactions of HIV protease inhibitors with a human organic cation transporter in a mammalian expression system. *Drug Metab. Dispos.* 2000;**28**(3):329–334.

113. Gorboulev V, Ulzheimer JC, Akhoundova A, Ulzheimer-Teuber I, Karbach U, Quester S, et al. Cloning and characterization of two human polyspecific organic cation transporters. *DNA Cell Biol.* 1997;**16**(7):871–881.

114. Grundemann D, Koster S, Kiefer N, Breidert T, Engelhardt M, Spitzenberger F, et al. Transport of monoamine transmitters by the organic cation transporter type 2, *OCT2*. *J. Biol. Chem.* 1998;**273**(47):30915–30920.

115. Urakami Y, Okuda M, Masuda S, Saito H, Inui KI. Functional characteristics and membrane localization of rat multispecific organic cation transporters, OCT1 and OCT2, mediating tubular secretion of cationic drugs. *J. Pharmacol. Exp. Ther.* 1998; **287**(2):800–805.

116. Motohashi H, Sakurai Y, Saito H, Masuda S, Urakami Y, Goto M, et al. Gene expression levels and immunolocalization of organic ion transporters in the human kidney. *J. Am. Soc. Nephrol.* 2002;**13**(4):866–874.

117. Khamdang S, Takeda M, Noshiro R, Narikawa S, Enomoto A, Anzai N, et al. Interactions of human organic anion transporters and human organic cation transporters with nonsteroidal anti-inflammatory drugs. *J. Pharmacol. Exp. Ther.* 2002;**303**(2): 534–539.

118. Dresser MJ, Xiao G, Leabman MK, Gray AT, Giacomini KM. Interactions of n-tetraalkylammonium compounds and biguanides with a human renal organic cation transporter (hOCT2). *Pharm. Res.* 2002;**19**(8):1244–1247.

119. Leabman MK, Huang CC, Kawamoto M, Johns SJ, Stryke D, Ferrin TE, et al. Polymorphisms in a human kidney xenobiotic transporter, OCT2, exhibit altered function. *Pharmacogenetics* 2002;**12**(5):395–405.

120. Hayer-Zillgen M, Bruss M, Bonisch H. Expression and pharmacological profile of the human organic cation transporters hOCT1, hOCT2 and hOCT3. *Br. J. Pharmacol.* 2002;**136**(6):829–836.

121. Urakami Y, Kimura N, Okuda M, Inui K. Creatinine transport by basolateral organic cation transporter hOCT2 in the human kidney. *Pharm. Res.* 2004;**21**(6):976–981.

122. Okuda M, Saito H, Urakami Y, Takano M, Inui K. cDNA cloning and functional expression of a novel rat kidney organic cation transporter, OCT2. *Biochem. Biophys. Res. Commun.* 1996;**224**(2):500–507.

123. Yokoo S, Yonezawa A, Masuda S, Fukatsu A, Katsura T, Inui K. Differential contribution of organic cation transporters, OCT2 and MATE1, in platinum agent-induced nephrotoxicity. *Biochem. Pharmacol.* 2007;**74**(3):477–487.

124. Yonezawa A, Masuda S, Nishihara K, Yano I, Katsura T, Inui K. Association between tubular toxicity of cisplatin and expression of organic cation transporter rOCT2 (Slc22a2) in the rat. *Biochem. Pharmacol.* 2005;**70**(12):1823–1831.

125. Fujita T, Urban TJ, Leabman MK, Fujita K, Giacomini KM. Transport of drugs in the kidney by the human organic cation transporter, OCT2 and its genetic variants. *J. Pharm. Sci.* 2006;**95**(1):25–36.

126. Fukushima-Uesaka H, Maekawa K, Ozawa S, Komamura K, Ueno K, Shibakawa M, et al. Fourteen novel single nucleotide polymorphisms in the SLC22A2 gene encoding human organic cation transporter (OCT2). *Drug Metab. Pharmacokinet.* 2004; **19**(3):239–244.

127. Wang ZJ, Yin OQ, Tomlinson B, Chow MS. OCT2 polymorphisms and in-vivo renal functional consequence: Studies with metformin and cimetidine. *Pharmacogenet. Genomics* 2008;**18**(7):637–645.

128. Song IS, Shin HJ, Shin JG. Genetic variants of organic cation transporter 2 (OCT2) significantly reduce metformin uptake in oocytes. *Xenobiotica* 2008;**38**(9):1252–1262.

129. Song IS, Shin HJ, Shim EJ, Jung IS, Kim WY, Shon JH, et al. Genetic variants of the organic cation transporter 2 influence the disposition of metformin. *Clin. Pharmacol. Ther.* 2008;**84**(5):559–562.

130. Zolk O, Solbach TF, Konig J, Fromm MF. Functional characterization of the human organic cation transporter 2 variant p.270Ala>Ser. *Drug Metab. Dispos.* 2009; **37**(6):1312–1318.

131. Launay-Vacher V, Rey JB, Isnard-Bagnis C, Deray G, Daouphars M. Prevention of cisplatin nephrotoxicity: State of the art and recommendations from the European Society of Clinical Pharmacy Special Interest Group on Cancer Care. *Cancer Chemother. Pharmacol.* 2008;**61**(6):903–909.

132. Pabla N, Dong Z. Cisplatin nephrotoxicity: Mechanisms and renoprotective strategies. *Kidney Int.* 2008;**73**(9):994–1007.

133. Safirstein R, Winston J, Moel D, Dikman S, Guttenplan J. Cisplatin nephrotoxicity: Insights into mechanism. *Int. J. Androl.* 1987;**10**(1):325–346.

134. Ludwig T, Riethmuller C, Gekle M, Schwerdt G, Oberleithner H. Nephrotoxicity of platinum complexes is related to basolateral organic cation transport. *Kidney Int.* 2004; **66**(1):196–202.

135. Filipski KK, Loos WJ, Verweij J, Sparreboom A. Interaction of cisplatin with the human organic cation transporter 2. *Clin. Cancer Res.* 2008;**14**(12):3875–3880.

136. Yonezawa A, Masuda S, Yokoo S, Katsura T, Inui K. Cisplatin and oxaliplatin, but not carboplatin and nedaplatin, are substrates for human organic cation transporters (SLC22A1-3 and multidrug and toxin extrusion family). *J. Pharmacol. Exp. Ther.* 2006;**319**(2):879–886.

137. Ciarimboli G, Ludwig T, Lang D, Pavenstadt H, Koepsell H, Piechota HJ, et al. Cisplatin nephrotoxicity is critically mediated via the human organic cation transporter 2. *Am. J. Pathol.* 2005;**167**(6):1477–1484.

138. Grover B, Buckley D, Buckley AR, Cacini W. Reduced expression of organic cation transporters rOCT1 and rOCT2 in experimental diabetes. *J. Pharmacol. Exp. Ther.* 2004;**308**(3):949–956.

139. Zhang S, Lovejoy KS, Shima JE, Lagpacan LL, Shu Y, Lapuk A, et al. Organic cation transporters are determinants of oxaliplatin cytotoxicity. *Cancer Res.* 2006; **66**(17):8847–8857.

140. Pabla N, Murphy RF, Liu K, Dong Z. The copper transporter Ctr1 contributes to cisplatin uptake by renal tubular cells during cisplatin nephrotoxicity. *Am. J. Physiol. Renal Physiol.* 2009;**296**(3):F505–F511.

141. Lazar A, Zimmermann T, Koch W, Grundemann D, Schomig A, Kastrati A, et al. Lower prevalence of the OCT2 Ser270 allele in patients with essential hypertension. *Clin. Exp. Hypertens.* 2006;**28**(7):645–653.

142. Schomig E, Lazar A, Grundemann D. Extraneuronal monoamine transporter and organic cation transporters 1 and 2: A review of transport efficiency. *Handbooks Exp. Pharmacol.* 2006;(175):151–180.

143. Taubert D, Grimberg G, Stenzel W, Schomig E. Identification of the endogenous key substrates of the human organic cation transporter OCT2 and their implication in function of dopaminergic neurons. *PLoS ONE* 2007;**2**(4):e385.

144. Holman RR, Paul SK, Bethel MA, Matthews DR, Neil HA. 10-year follow-up of intensive glucose control in type 2 diabetes. *New Engl. J. Med.* 2008;**359**(15):1577–1589.

145. Shu Y, Brown C, Castro RA, Shi RJ, Lin ET, Owen RP, et al. Effect of genetic variation in the organic cation transporter 1, OCT1, on metformin pharmacokinetics. *Clin. Pharmacol. Ther.* 2008;**83**(2):273–280.

146. Zhou G, Myers R, Li Y, Chen Y, Shen X, Fenyk-Melody J, et al. Role of AMP-activated protein kinase in mechanism of metformin action. *J. Clin. Invest.* 2001;**108**(8):1167–1174.

147. Sirtori CR, Franceschini G, Galli-Kienle M, Cighetti G, Galli G, Bondioli A, et al. Disposition of metformin (N, N-dimethylbiguanide) in man. *Clin. Pharmacol. Ther.* 1978;**24**(6):683–693.

148. Tucker GT, Casey C, Phillips PJ, Connor H, Ward JD, Woods HF. Metformin kinetics in healthy subjects and in patients with diabetes mellitus. *Br. J. Clin. Pharmacol.* 1981; **12**(2):235–246.

149. Leabman MK, Giacomini KM. Estimating the contribution of genes and environment to variation in renal drug clearance. *Pharmacogenetics* 2003;**13**(9):581–584.

150. Yin OQ, Tomlinson B, Chow MS. Variability in renal clearance of substrates for renal transporters in chinese subjects. *J. Clin. Pharmacol.* 2006;**46**(2):157–163.

151. Kimura N, Masuda S, Tanihara Y, Ueo H, Okuda M, Katsura T, et al. Metformin is a superior substrate for renal organic cation transporter OCT2 rather than hepatic OCT1. *Drug Metab. Pharmacokinet.* 2005;**20**(5):379–386.

152. Kimura N, Okuda M, Inui K. Metformin transport by renal basolateral organic cation transporter hOCT2. *Pharm. Res.* 2005;**22**(2):255–259.

153. Shikata E, Yamamoto R, Takane H, Shigemasa C, Ikeda T, Otsubo K, et al. Human organic cation transporter (OCT1 and OCT2) gene polymorphisms and therapeutic effects of metformin. *J. Hum. Genet.* 2007;**52**(2):117–122.

154. Zhou K, Donnelly LA, Kimber CH, Donnan PT, Doney AS, Leese G, et al. Reduced function SLC22A1 polymorphisms encoding Organic Cation Transporter 1 (OCT1) and glycaemic response to metformin: A Go-DARTS study. *Diabetes* 2009; **58**(6):1434–1439.

155. Cascorbi I. Role of pharmacogenetics of ATP-binding cassette transporters in the pharmacokinetics of drugs. *Pharmacol. Ther.* 2006;**112**(2):457–473.

156. Mickley LA, Lee JS, Weng Z, Zhan Z, Alvarez M, Wilson W, et al. Genetic polymorphism in MDR-1: A tool for examining allelic expression in normal cells, unselected and drug-selected cell lines, and human tumors. *Blood* 1998;**91**(5):1749–1756.

157. Schaefer M, Roots I, Gerloff T. In-vitro transport characteristics discriminate wild-type ABCB1 (MDR1) from ALA893SER and ALA893THR polymorphisms. *Pharmacogenet. Genomics* 2006;**16**(12):855–861.

158. Ishikawa T, Sakurai A, Kanamori Y, Nagakura M, Hirano H, Takarada Y, et al. High-speed screening of human ATP-binding cassette transporter function and genetic polymorphisms: New strategies in pharmacogenomics. *Methods Enzymol.* 2005;**400**:485–510.

159. Kim RB, Leake BF, Choo EF, Dresser GK, Kubba SV, Schwarz UI, et al. Identification of functionally variant MDR1 alleles among European Americans and African Americans. *Clin. Pharmacol. Ther.* 2001;**70**(2):189–199.

160. Kimchi-Sarfaty C, Gribar JJ, Gottesman MM. Functional characterization of coding polymorphisms in the human MDR1 gene using a vaccinia virus expression system. *Mol. Pharmacol.* 2002;**62**(1):1–6.

161. Fellay J, Marzolini C, Meaden ER, Back DJ, Buclin T, Chave JP, et al. Response to antiretroviral treatment in HIV-1-infected individuals with allelic variants of the multidrug resistance transporter 1: A pharmacogenetics study. *Lancet* 2002; **359**(9300):30–36.

162. Hoffmeyer S, Burk O, von Richter O, Arnold HP, Brockmoller J, Johne A, et al. Functional polymorphisms of the human multidrug-resistance gene: Multiple sequence variations and correlation of one allele with P-glycoprotein expression and activity in vivo. *Proc. Natl. Acad. Sci. USA* 2000;**97**(7):3473–3478.

163. Xu P, Jiang ZP, Zhang BK, Tu JY, Li HD. Impact of MDR1 haplotypes derived from C1236T, G2677T/A and C3435T on the pharmacokinetics of single-dose oral digoxin in healthy Chinese volunteers. *Pharmacology* 2008;**82**(3):221–227.

164. Kimchi-Sarfaty C, Oh JM, Kim IW, Sauna ZE, Calcagno AM, Ambudkar SV, et al. A "silent" polymorphism in the MDR1 gene changes substrate specificity. *Science* 2007;**315**(5811):525–528.

165. Wang D, Johnson AD, Papp AC, Kroetz DL, Sadee W. Multidrug resistance polypeptide 1 (MDR1, ABCB1) variant 3435C > T affects mRNA stability. *Pharmacogenet. Genomics* 2005;**15**(10):693–704.

166. Horinouchi M, Sakaeda T, Nakamura T, Morita Y, Tamura T, Aoyama N, et al. Significant genetic linkage of MDR1 polymorphisms at positions 3435 and 2677: Functional relevance to pharmacokinetics of digoxin. *Pharm. Res.* 2002;**19**(10):1581–1585.

167. Mosyagin I, Runge U, Schroeder HW, Dazert E, Vogelgesang S, Siegmund W, et al. Association of ABCB1 genetic variants 3435C > T and 2677G > T to ABCB1 mRNA and protein expression in brain tissue from refractory epilepsy patients. *Epilepsia* 2008;**49**(9):1555–1561.

168. Siegmund W, Ludwig K, Giessmann T, Dazert P, Schroeder E, Sperker B, et al. The effects of the human MDR1 genotype on the expression of duodenal P-glycoprotein and disposition of the probe drug talinolol. *Clin. Pharmacol. Ther.* 2002;**72**(5):572–583.

169. Moriya Y, Nakamura T, Horinouchi M, Sakaeda T, Tamura T, Aoyama N, et al. Effects of polymorphisms of MDR1, MRP1, and MRP2 genes on their mRNA expression levels in duodenal enterocytes of healthy Japanese subjects. *Biol. Pharm. Bull.* 2002; **25**(10):1356–1359.

170. Goto M, Masuda S, Saito H, Uemoto S, Kiuchi T, Tanaka K, et al. C3435T polymorphism in the MDR1 gene affects the enterocyte expression level of CYP3A4 rather than Pgp in recipients of living-donor liver transplantation. *Pharmacogenetics* 2002;**12**(6):451–457.

171. Nakamura T, Sakaeda T, Horinouchi M, Tamura T, Aoyama N, Shirakawa T, et al. Effect of the mutation (C3435T) at exon 26 of the MDR1 gene on expression level of MDR1 messenger ribonucleic acid in duodenal enterocytes of healthy Japanese subjects. *Clin. Pharmacol. Ther.* 2002;**71**(4):297–303.

172. Leschziner GD, Andrew T, Pirmohamed M, Johnson MR. ABCB1 genotype and PGP expression, function and therapeutic drug response: A critical review and recommendations for future research. *Pharmacogenomics J* 2007;**7**(3):154–179.

173. Aarnoudse AJ, Dieleman JP, Visser LE, Arp PP, van dH, I, van Schaik RH, et al. Common ATP-binding cassette B1 variants are associated with increased digoxin serum concentration. *Pharmacogenet. Genomics* 2008;**18**(4):299–305.

174. Verstuyft C, Schwab M, Schaeffeler E, Kerb R, Brinkmann U, Jaillon P, et al. Digoxin pharmacokinetics and MDR1 genetic polymorphisms. *Eur. J. Clin. Pharmacol.* 2003; **58**(12):809–812.

175. Johne A, Kopke K, Gerloff T, Mai I, Rietbrock S, Meisel C, et al. Modulation of steady-state kinetics of digoxin by haplotypes of the P-glycoprotein MDR1 gene. *Clin. Pharmacol. Ther.* 2002;**72**(5):584–594.

176. Gerloff T, Schaefer M, Johne A, Oselin K, Meisel C, Cascorbi I, et al. MDR1 genotypes do not influence the absorption of a single oral dose of 1 mg digoxin in healthy white males. *Br. J. Clin. Pharmacol.* 2002;**54**(6):610–616.

177. Sakaeda T, Nakamura T, Horinouchi M, Kakumoto M, Ohmoto N, Sakai T, et al. MDR1 genotype-related pharmacokinetics of digoxin after single oral administration in healthy Japanese subjects. *Pharm. Res.* 2001;**18**(10):1400–1404.

178. Chowbay B, Li H, David M, Cheung YB, Lee EJ. Meta-analysis of the influence of MDR1 C3435T polymorphism on digoxin pharmacokinetics and MDR1 gene expression. *Br. J. Clin. Pharmacol.* 2005;**60**(2):159–171.

179. Yi SY, Hong KS, Lim HS, Chung JY, Oh DS, Kim JR, et al. A variant 2677A allele of the MDR1 gene affects fexofenadine disposition. *Clin. Pharmacol. Ther.* 2004;**76**(5):418–427.

180. Drescher S, Schaeffeler E, Hitzl M, Hofmann U, Schwab M, Brinkmann U, et al. MDR1 gene polymorphisms and disposition of the P-glycoprotein substrate fexofenadine. *Br. J. Clin. Pharmacol.* 2002;**53**(5):526–534.

181. Shon JH, Yoon YR, Hong WS, Nguyen PM, Lee SS, Choi YG, et al. Effect of itraconazole on the pharmacokinetics and pharmacodynamics of fexofenadine in relation to the MDR1 genetic polymorphism. *Clin. Pharmacol. Ther.* 2005;**78**(2):191–201.

182. Foote CJ, Greer W, Kiberd B, Fraser A, Lawen J, Nashan B, et al. Polymorphisms of multidrug resistance gene (MDR1) and cyclosporine absorption in de novo renal transplant patients. *Transplantation* 2007;**83**(10):1380–1384.

183. Foote CJ, Greer W, Kiberd BA, Fraser A, Lawen J, Nashan B, et al. MDR1 C3435T polymorphisms correlate with cyclosporine levels in de novo renal recipients. *Transplant. Proc.* 2006;**38**(9):2847–2849.

184. Yates CR, Zhang W, Song P, Li S, Gaber AO, Kotb M, et al. The effect of CYP3A5 and MDR1 polymorphic expression on cyclosporine oral disposition in renal transplant patients. *J. Clin. Pharmacol.* 2003;**43**(6):555–564.

185. Hu YF, Qiu W, Liu ZQ, Zhu LJ, Liu ZQ, Tu JH, et al. Effects of genetic polymorphisms of CYP3A4, CYP3A5 and MDR1 on cyclosporine pharmacokinetics after renal transplantation. *Clin. Exp. Pharmacol. Physiol.* 2006;**33**(11):1093–1098.

186. Mai I, Stormer E, Goldammer M, Johne A, Kruger H, Budde K, et al. MDR1 haplotypes do not affect the steady-state pharmacokinetics of cyclosporine in renal transplant patients. *J. Clin. Pharmacol.* 2003;**43**(10):1101–1107.

187. Chowbay B, Cumaraswamy S, Cheung YB, Zhou Q, Lee EJ. Genetic polymorphisms in MDR1 and CYP3A4 genes in Asians and the influence of MDR1 haplotypes on cyclosporin disposition in heart transplant recipients. *Pharmacogenetics* 2003; **13**(2):89–95.

188. Min DI, Ellingrod VL. C3435T mutation in exon 26 of the human MDR1 gene and cyclosporine pharmacokinetics in healthy subjects. *Ther. Drug Monit.* 2002;**24**(3):400–404.

189. von Ahsen N, Richter M, Grupp C, Ringe B, Oellerich M, Armstrong VW. No influence of the MDR-1 C3435T polymorphism or a CYP3A4 promoter polymorphism (CYP3A4-V allele) on dose-adjusted cyclosporin A trough concentrations or rejection incidence in stable renal transplant recipients. *Clin. Chem.* 2001;**47**(6):1048–1052.

190. Anglicheau D, Thervet E, Etienne I, Hurault DL, Le Meur Y, Touchard G, et al. CYP3A5 and MDR1 genetic polymorphisms and cyclosporine pharmacokinetics after renal transplantation. *Clin. Pharmacol. Ther.* 2004;**75**(5):422–433.

191. Krishnamurthy P, Schwab M, Takenaka K, Nachagari D, Morgan J, Leslie M, et al. Transporter-mediated protection against thiopurine-induced hematopoietic toxicity. *Cancer Res.* 2008;**68**(13):4983–4989.

192. Jiang ZP, Wang YR, Xu P, Liu RR, Zhao XL, Chen FP. Meta-analysis of the effect of MDR1 C3435T polymorphism on cyclosporine pharmacokinetics. *Basic Clin. Pharmacol. Toxicol.* 2008;**103**(5):433–444.

193. Sakaeda T. MDR1 genotype-related pharmacokinetics: Fact or fiction? *Drug Metab. Pharmacokinet.* 2005;**20**(6):391–414.

194. Cole SP, Bhardwaj G, Gerlach JH, Mackie JE, Grant CE, Almquist KC, et al. Overexpression of a transporter gene in a multidrug-resistant human lung cancer cell line. *Science* 1992;**258**(5088):1650–1654.

195. Bakos E, Homolya L. Portrait of multifaceted transporter, the multidrug resistance-associated protein 1 (MRP1/ABCC1). *Pflugers Arch.* 2007;**453**(5):621–641.

196. Zhou Q, Sparreboom A, Tan EH, Cheung YB, Lee A, Poon D, et al. Pharmacogenetic profiling across the irinotecan pathway in Asian patients with cancer. *Br. J. Clin. Pharmacol.* 2005;**59**(4):415–424.

197. Sharom FJ. ABC multidrug transporters: Structure, function and role in chemoresistance. *Pharmacogenomics* 2008;**9**(1):105–127.

198. Wojnowski L, Kulle B, Schirmer M, Schluter G, Schmidt A, Rosenberger A, et al. NAD (P)H oxidase and multidrug resistance protein genetic polymorphisms are associated with doxorubicin-induced cardiotoxicity. *Circulation* 2005;**112**(24):3754–3762.

199. Nies AT, Keppler D. The apical conjugate efflux pump ABCC2 (MRP2). *Pflugers Arch.* 2007;**453**(5):643–659.
200. Choudhuri S, Klaassen CD. Structure, function, expression, genomic organization, and single nucleotide polymorphisms of human ABCB1 (MDR1), ABCC (MRP), and ABCG2 (BCRP) efflux transporters. *Int. J. Toxicol.* 2006;**25**(4):231–259.
201. Sai K, Saito Y, Itoda M, Fukushima-Uesaka H, Nishimaki-Mogami T, Ozawa S, et al. Genetic variations and haplotypes of ABCC2 encoding MRP2 in a Japanese population. *Drug Metab. Pharmacokinet.* 2008;**23**(2):139–147.
202. Haenisch S, Zimmermann U, Dazert E, Wruck CJ, Dazert P, Siegmund W, et al. Influence of polymorphisms of ABCB1 and ABCC2 on mRNA and protein expression in normal and cancerous kidney cortex. *Pharmacogenomics J.* 2007;**7**(1):56–65.
203. Haenisch S, May K, Wegner D, Caliebe A, Cascorbi I, Siegmund W. Influence of genetic polymorphisms on intestinal expression and rifampicin-type induction of ABCC2 and on bioavailability of talinolol. *Pharmacogenet. Genomics* 2008;**18**(4):357–365.
204. Meyer zu Schwabedissen HE, Jedlitschky G, Gratz M, Haenisch S, Linnemann K, Fusch C, et al. Variable expression of MRP2 (ABCC2) in human placenta: Influence of gestational age and cellular differentiation. *Drug Metab. Dispos.* 2005;**33**(7):896–904.
205. Meier Y, Pauli-Magnus C, Zanger UM, Klein K, Schaeffeler E, Nussler AK, et al. Interindividual variability of canalicular ATP-binding-cassette (ABC)-transporter expression in human liver. *Hepatology* 2006;**44**(1):62–74.
206. Hirouchi M, Suzuki H, Itoda M, Ozawa S, Sawada J, Ieiri I, et al. Characterization of the cellular localization, expression level, and function of SNP variants of MRP2/ABCC2. *Pharm. Res.* 2004;**21**(5):742–748.
207. Fujita K, Nagashima F, Yamamoto W, Endo H, Sunakawa Y, Yamashita K, et al. Association of ATP-binding cassette, sub-family C, number 2 (ABCC2) genotype with pharmacokinetics of irinotecan in Japanese patients with metastatic colorectal cancer treated with irinotecan plus infusional 5-fluorouracil/leucovorin (FOLFIRI). *Biol. Pharm. Bull.* 2008;**31**(11):2137–2142.
208. Han JY, Lim HS, Yoo YK, Shin ES, Park YH, Lee SY, et al. Associations of ABCB1, ABCC2, and ABCG2 polymorphisms with irinotecan-pharmacokinetics and clinical outcome in patients with advanced non-small cell lung cancer. *Cancer* 2007;**110**(1):138–147.
209. Miura M, Satoh S, Inoue K, Kagaya H, Saito M, Inoue T, et al. Influence of SLCO1B1, 1B3, 2B1 and ABCC2 genetic polymorphisms on mycophenolic acid pharmacokinetics in Japanese renal transplant recipients. *Eur J. Clin. Pharmacol.* 2007;**63**(12):1161–1169.
210. Rau T, Erney B, Gores R, Eschenhagen T, Beck J, Langer T. High-dose methotrexate in pediatric acute lymphoblastic leukemia: Impact of ABCC2 polymorphisms on plasma concentrations. *Clin. Pharmacol. Ther.* 2006;**80**(5):468–476.
211. Anderson PL, Lamba J, Aquilante CL, Schuetz E, Fletcher CV. Pharmacogenetic characteristics of indinavir, zidovudine, and lamivudine therapy in HIV-infected adults: A pilot study. *J. AIDS* 2006;**42**(4):441–449.
212. Daly AK, Aithal GP, Leathart JB, Swainsbury RA, Dang TS, Day CP. Genetic susceptibility to diclofenac-induced hepatotoxicity: Contribution of UGT2B7, CYP2C8, and ABCC2 genotypes. *Gastroenterology* 2007;**132**(1):272–281.
213. Choi JH, Ahn BM, Yi J, Lee JH, Lee JH, Nam SW, et al. MRP2 haplotypes confer differential susceptibility to toxic liver injury. *Pharmacogenet. Genomics* 2007;**17**(6):403–415.

214. Scheffer GL, Kool M, de Haas M, de Vree JM, Pijnenborg AC, Bosman DK, et al. Tissue distribution and induction of human multidrug resistant protein 3. *Lab. Invest.* 2002; **82**(2):193–201.

215. Fukushima-Uesaka H, Saito Y, Maekawa K, Hasegawa R, Suzuki K, Yanagawa T, et al. Genetic variations of the ABC transporter gene ABCC3 in a Japanese population. *Drug Metab. Pharmacokinet.* 2007;**22**(2):129–135.

216. Lang T, Hitzl M, Burk O, Mornhinweg E, Keil A, Kerb R, et al. Genetic polymorphisms in the multidrug resistance-associated protein 3 (ABCC3, MRP3) gene and relationship to its mRNA and protein expression in human liver. *Pharmacogenetics* 2004;**14** (3):155–164.

217. Lee YM, Cui Y, Konig J, Risch A, Jager B, Drings P, et al. Identification and functional characterization of the natural variant MRP3-Arg1297His of human multidrug resistance protein 3 (MRP3/ABCC3). *Pharmacogenetics* 2004;**14**(4):213–223.

218. Saito S, Iida A, Sekine A, Miura Y, Ogawa C, Kawauchi S, et al. Identification of 779 genetic variations in eight genes encoding members of the ATP-binding cassette, subfamily C (ABCC/MRP/CFTR. *J. Hum. Genet.* 2002;**47**(4):147–171.

219. Kobayashi K, Ito K, Takada T, Sugiyama Y, Suzuki H. Functional analysis of non-synonymous single nucleotide polymorphism type ATP-binding cassette transmembrane transporter subfamily C member 3. *Pharmacogenet. Genomics* 2008;**18**(9):823–833.

220. Doerfel C, Rump A, Sauerbrey A, Gruhn B, Zintl F, Steinbach D. In acute leukemia, the polymorphism -211C > T in the promoter region of the multidrug resistance-associated protein 3 (MRP3) does not determine the expression level of the gene. *Pharmacogenet. Genomics* 2006;**16**(2):149–150.

221. Gradhand U, Tegude H, Burk O, Eichelbaum M, Fromm MF, Konig J. Functional analysis of the polymorphism -211C > T in the regulatory region of the human ABCC3 gene. *Life Sci.* 2007;**80**(16):1490–1494.

222. Muller PJ, Dally H, Klappenecker CN, Edler L, Jager B, Gerst M, et al. Polymorphisms in ABCG2, ABCC3 and CNT1 genes and their possible impact on chemotherapy outcome of lung cancer patients. *Int. J. Cancer* 2009;**124**(7):1669–1674.

223. Ritter CA, Jedlitschky G, Meyer Zu SH, Grube M, Kock K, Kroemer HK. Cellular export of drugs and signaling molecules by the ATP-binding cassette transporters MRP4 (ABCC4) and MRP5 (ABCC5). *Drug Metab. Rev.* 2005;**37**(1):253–278.

224. Jedlitschky G, Tirschmann K, Lubenow LE, Nieuwenhuis HK, Akkerman JW, Greinacher A, et al. The nucleotide transporter MRP4 (ABCC4) is highly expressed in human platelets and present in dense granules, indicating a role in mediator storage. *Blood* 2004;**104**(12):3603–3610.

225. Rius M, Nies AT, Hummel-Eisenbeiss J, Jedlitschky G, Keppler D. Cotransport of reduced glutathione with bile salts by MRP4 (ABCC4) localized to the basolateral hepatocyte membrane. *Hepatology* 2003;**38**(2):374–384.

226. van Aubel RA, Smeets PH, Peters JG, Bindels RJ, Russel FG. The MRP4/ABCC4 gene encodes a novel apical organic anion transporter in human kidney proximal tubules: Putative efflux pump for urinary cAMP and cGMP. *J. Am. Soc. Nephrol.* 2002; **13**(3):595–603.

227. Chen ZS, Lee K, Kruh GD. Transport of cyclic nucleotides and estradiol 17-beta-D-glucuronide by multidrug resistance protein 4. Resistance to 6-mercaptopurine and 6-thioguanine. *J. Biol. Chem.* 2001;**276**(36):33747–33754.

228. Jedlitschky G, Burchell B, Keppler D. The multidrug resistance protein 5 functions as an ATP-dependent export pump for cyclic nucleotides. *J. Biol. Chem.* 2000; **275**(39):30069–30074.

229. Abla N, Chinn LW, Nakamura T, Liu L, Huang CC, Johns SJ, et al. The human multidrug resistance protein 4 (MRP4, ABCC4): Functional analysis of a highly polymorphic gene. *J. Pharmacol. Exp. Ther.* 2008;**325**(3):859–868.

230. Kiser JJ, Aquilante CL, Anderson PL, King TM, Carten ML, Fletcher CV. Clinical and genetic determinants of intracellular tenofovir diphosphate concentrations in HIV-infected patients. *J. AIDS* 2008;**47**(3):298–303.

231. Kiser JJ, Carten ML, Aquilante CL, Anderson PL, Wolfe P, King TM, et al. The effect of lopinavir/ritonavir on the renal clearance of tenofovir in HIV-infected patients. *Clin. Pharmacol. Ther.* 2008;**83**(2):265–272.

232. Doyle LA, Yang W, Abruzzo LV, Krogmann T, Gao Y, Rishi AK, et al. A multidrug resistance transporter from human MCF-7 breast cancer cells. *Proc. Natl. Acad. Sci. USA* 1998;**95**(26):15665–15670.

233. Kage K, Tsukahara S, Sugiyama T, Asada S, Ishikawa E, Tsuruo T, et al. Dominant-negative inhibition of breast cancer resistance protein as drug efflux pump through the inhibition of S-S dependent homodimerization. *Int. J. Cancer* 2002;**97**(5): 626–630.

234. Maeda K, Sugiyama Y. Impact of genetic polymorphisms of transporters on the pharmacokinetic, pharmacodynamic and toxicological properties of anionic drugs. *Drug Metab. Pharmacokinet.* 2008;**23**(4):223–235.

235. Gradhand U, Kim RB. Pharmacogenomics of MRP transporters (ABCC1-5) and BCRP (ABCG2). *Drug Metab. Rev.* 2008;**40**(2):317–354.

236. Honjo Y, Morisaki K, Huff LM, Robey RW, Hung J, Dean M, et al. Single-nucleotide polymorphism (SNP) analysis in the ABC half-transporter ABCG2 (MXR/BCRP/ABCP1). *Cancer Biol. Ther.* 2002;**1**(6):696–702.

237. Imai Y, Nakane M, Kage K, Tsukahara S, Ishikawa E, Tsuruo T, et al. C421A polymorphism in the human breast cancer resistance protein gene is associated with low expression of Q141K protein and low-level drug resistance. *Mol. Cancer Ther.* 2002;**1**(8):611–616.

238. Tamura A, Wakabayashi K, Onishi Y, Takeda M, Ikegami Y, Sawada S, et al. Re-evaluation and functional classification of non-synonymous single nucleotide polymorphisms of the human ATP-binding cassette transporter ABCG2. *Cancer Sci.* 2007;**98**(2):231–239.

239. Koshiba S, An R, Saito H, Wakabayashi K, Tamura A, Ishikawa T. Human ABC transporters ABCG2 (BCRP) and ABCG4. *Xenobiotica* 2008;**38**(7–8):863–888.

240. Hardwick LJ, Velamakanni S, van Veen HW. The emerging pharmacotherapeutic significance of the breast cancer resistance protein (ABCG2). *Br. J. Pharmacol.* 2007;**151**(2):163–174.

241. Li J, Cusatis G, Brahmer J, Sparreboom A, Robey RW, Bates SE, et al. Association of variant ABCG2 and the pharmacokinetics of epidermal growth factor receptor tyrosine kinase inhibitors in cancer patients. *Cancer Biol. Ther.* 2007;**6**(3):432–438.

242. Cusatis G, Gregorc V, Li J, Spreafico A, Ingersoll RG, Verweij J, et al. Pharmacogenetics of ABCG2 and adverse reactions to gefitinib. *J. Natl. Cancer. Inst.* 2006; **98**(23):1739–1742.

243. Zhang W, Yu BN, He YJ, Fan L, Li Q, Liu ZQ, et al. Role of BCRP 421C>A polymorphism on rosuvastatin pharmacokinetics in healthy Chinese males. *Clin. Chim. Acta.* 2006;**373**(1–2):99–103.

244. Yamasaki Y, Ieiri I, Kusuhara H, Sasaki T, Kimura M, Tabuchi H, et al. Pharmacogenetic characterization of sulfasalazine disposition based on NAT2 and ABCG2 (BCRP) gene polymorphisms in humans. *Clin. Pharmacol. Ther.* 2008;**84**(1):95–103.

245. Urquhart BL, Ware JA, Tirona RG, Ho RH, Leake BF, Schwarz UI, et al. Breast cancer resistance protein (ABCG2) and drug disposition: Intestinal expression, polymorphisms and sulfasalazine as an in vivo probe. *Pharmacogenet. Genomics* 2008;**18**(5):439–448.

246. Azarpira N, Aghdaie MH, Behzad-Behbahanie A, Geramizadeh B, Behzadi S, Malekhoseinie SA, et al. Association between cyclosporine concentration and genetic polymorphisms of CYP3A5 and MDR1 during the early stage after renal transplantation. *Exp. Clin. Transplant.* 2006;**4**(1):416–419.

247. Adkison KK, Vaidya SS, Lee DY, Koo SH, Li L, Mehta AA, et al. The ABCG2 C421A polymorphism does not affect oral nitrofurantoin pharmacokinetics in healthy Chinese male subjects. *Br. J. Clin. Pharmacol.* 2008;**66**(2):233–239.

248. Hahn NM, Marsh S, Fisher W, Langdon R, Zon R, Browning M, et al. Hoosier oncology group randomized phase II study of docetaxel, vinorelbine, and estramustine in combination in hormone-refractory prostate cancer with pharmacogenetic survival analysis. *Clin. Cancer Res.* 2006;**12**(20 Pt. 1):6094–6099.

249. Erdilyi DJ, Kamory E, Csokay B, Andrikovics H, Tordai A, Kiss C, et al. Synergistic interaction of ABCB1 and ABCG2 polymorphisms predicts the prevalence of toxic encephalopathy during anticancer chemotherapy. *Pharmacogenomics J.* 2008; **8**(5):321–327.

250. Morisaki K, Robey RW, Ozvegy-Laczka C, Honjo Y, Polgar O, Steadman K, et al. Single nucleotide polymorphisms modify the transporter activity of ABCG2. *Cancer Chemother. Pharmacol.* 2005;**56**(2):161–172.

251. Mizuarai S, Aozasa N, Kotani H. Single nucleotide polymorphisms result in impaired membrane localization and reduced atpase activity in multidrug transporter ABCG2. *Int. J. Cancer.* 2004;**109**(2):238–246.

252. Kondo C, Suzuki H, Itoda M, Ozawa S, Sawada J, Kobayashi D, et al. Functional analysis of SNPs variants of BCRP/ABCG2. *Pharm. Res.* 2004;**21**(10):1895–1903.

253. Furukawa T, Wakabayashi K, Tamura A, Nakagawa H, Morishima Y, Osawa Y, et al. Major SNP (Q141K) variant of human ABC transporter ABCG2 undergoes lysosomal and proteasomal degradations. *Pharm. Res.* 2009;**26**(2):469–479.

254. Kobayashi D, Ieiri I, Hirota T, Takane H, Maegawa S, Kigawa J, et al. Functional assessment of ABCG2 (BCRP) gene polymorphisms to protein expression in human placenta. *Drug Metab. Dispos.* 2005;**33**(1):94–101.

255. Zamber CP, Lamba JK, Yasuda K, Farnum J, Thummel K, Schuetz JD, et al. Natural allelic variants of breast cancer resistance protein (BCRP) and their relationship to BCRP expression in human intestine. *Pharmacogenetics* 2003;**13**(1):19–28.

256. Takada T, Weiss HM, Kretz O, Gross G, Sugiyama Y. Hepatic transport of PKI166, an epidermal growth factor receptor kinase inhibitor of the pyrrolo-pyrimidine class, and its main metabolite, ACU154. *Drug. Metab. Dispos.* 2004;**32**(11):1272–1278.

257. Lu WJ, Tamai I, Nezu J, Lai ML, Huang JD. Organic anion transporting polypeptide-C mediates arsenic uptake in HEK-293 cells. *J. Biomed. Sci.* 2006;**13**(4):525–533.

258. Lau YY, Okochi H, Huang Y, Benet LZ. Multiple transporters affect the disposition of atorvastatin and its two active hydroxy metabolites: application of in vitro and ex situ systems. *J. Pharmacol. Exp. Ther.* 2006;**316**(2):762–771.

259. Katz DA, Carr R, Grimm DR, Xiong H, Holley-Shanks R, Mueller T et al. Organic anion transporting polypeptide 1B1 activity classified by SLCO1B1 genotype influences atrasentan pharmacokinetics. *Clin. Pharmacol. Ther.* 2006;**79**(3):186–196.

260. Treiber A, Schneiter R, Hausler S, Stieger B. Bosentan is a substrate of human OATP1B1 and OATP1B3: inhibition of hepatic uptake as the common mechanism of its interactions with cyclosporin A, rifampicin, and sildenafil. *Drug. Metab. Dispos.* 2007;**35**(8):1400–1407.

261. van Giersbergen PL, Treiber A, Schneiter R, Dietrich H, Dingemanse J. Inhibitory and inductive effects of rifampin on the pharmacokinetics of bosentan in healthy subjects. *Clin. Pharmacol. Ther.* 2007;**81**(3):414–419.

262. Sandhu P, Lee W, Xu X, Leake BF, Yamazaki M, Stone JA et al. Hepatic uptake of the novel antifungal agent caspofungin. *Drug. Metab. Dispos.* 2005;**33**(5):676–682.

263. Shitara Y, Hirano M, Sato H, Sugiyama Y. Gemfibrozil and its glucuronide inhibit the organic anion transporting polypeptide 2 (OATP2/OATP1B1:SLC21A6)-mediated hepatic uptake and CYP2C8-mediated metabolism of cerivastatin: analysis of the mechanism of the clinically relevant drug-drug interaction between cerivastatin and gemfibrozil. *J. Pharmacol. Exp. Ther.* 2004;**311**(1):228–236.

264. Meier-Abt F, Faulstich H, Hagenbuch B. Identification of phalloidin uptake systems of rat and human liver. *Biochim. Biophys. Acta.* 2004;**1664**(1):64–69.

265. Liu L, Cui Y, Chung AY, Shitara Y, Sugiyama Y, Keppler D et al. Vectorial transport of enalapril by Oatp1a1/Mrp2 and OATP1B1 and OATP1B3/MRP2 in rat and human livers. *J. Pharmacol. Exp. Ther.* 2006;**318**(1):395–402.

266. Oswald S, Konig J, Lutjohann D, Giessmann T, Kroemer HK, Rimmbach C et al. Disposition of ezetimibe is influenced by polymorphisms of the hepatic uptake carrier OATP1B1. *Pharmacogenet. Genomics* 2008;**18**(7):559–568.

267. Nakagomi-Hagihara R, Nakai D, Kawai K, Yoshigae Y, Tokui T, Abe T et al. OATP1B1, OATP1B3, and mrp2 are involved in hepatobiliary transport of olmesartan, a novel angiotensin II blocker. *Drug. Metab. Dispos.* 2006;**34**(5):862–869.

268. Yamada A, Maeda K, Kamiyama E, Sugiyama D, Kondo T, Shiroyanagi Y et al. Multiple human isoforms of drug transporters contribute to the hepatic and renal transport of olmesartan, a selective antagonist of the angiotensin II AT1-receptor. *Drug. Metab. Dispos.* 2007;**35**(12):2166–2176.

269. Fehrenbach T, Cui Y, Faulstich H, Keppler D. Characterization of the transport of the bicyclic peptide phalloidin by human hepatic transport proteins. *Naunyn. Schmiedebergs. Arch. Pharmacol.* 2003;**368**(5):415–420.

270. Hirano M, Maeda K, Shitara Y, Sugiyama Y. Contribution of OATP2 (OATP1B1) and OATP8 (OATP1B3) to the hepatic uptake of pitavastatin in humans. *J. Pharmacol. Exp. Ther.* 2004;**311**(1):139–146.

271. Fujino H, Nakai D, Nakagomi R, Saito M, Tokui T, Kojima J. Metabolic stability and uptake by human hepatocytes of pitavastatin, a new inhibitor of HMG-CoA reductase. *Arzneimittelforschung* 2004;**54**(7):382–388.

272. Nakai D, Nakagomi R, Furuta Y, Tokui T, Abe T, Ikeda T et al. Human liver-specific organic anion transporter, LST-1, mediates uptake of pravastatin by human hepatocytes. *J. Pharmacol. Exp. Ther.* 2001;**297**(3):861–867.

273. Sasaki M, Suzuki H, Ito K, Abe T, Sugiyama Y. Transcellular transport of organic anions across a double-transfected Madin-Darby canine kidney II cell monolayer expressing both human organic anion-transporting polypeptide (OATP2/SLC21A6) and Multidrug resistance-associated protein 2 (MRP2/ABCC2). *J. Biol. Chem.* 2002; **277**(8):6497–6503.

274. Vavricka SR, Van Montfoort J, Ha HR, Meier PJ, Fattinger K. Interactions of rifamycin SV and rifampicin with organic anion uptake systems of human liver. *Hepatology* 2002;**36**(1):164–172.

275. Tirona RG, Leake BF, Wolkoff AW, Kim RB. Human organic anion transporting polypeptide-C (SLC21A6) is a major determinant of rifampin-mediated pregnane X receptor activation. *J. Pharmacol. Exp. Ther.* 2003;**304**(1):223–228.

276. Schneck DW, Birmingham BK, Zalikowski JA, Mitchell PD, Wang Y, Martin PD et al. The effect of gemfibrozil on the pharmacokinetics of rosuvastatin. *Clin. Pharmacol. Ther.* 2004;**75**(5):455–463.

277. Sakamoto S, Kusuhara H, Horie K, Takahashi K, Baba T, Ishizaki J et al. Identification of the transporters involved in the hepatobiliary transport and intestinal efflux of methyl 1-(3,4-dimethoxyphenyl)-3-(3-ethylvaleryl)-4-hydroxy-6,7,8-trimethoxy-2-naphthoat e (S-8921) glucuronide, a pharmacologically active metabolite of S-8921. *Drug. Metab. Dispos.* 2008;**36**(8):1553–1561.

278. Sakamoto K, Mikami H, Kimura J. Involvement of organic anion transporting polypeptides in the toxicity of hydrophilic pravastatin and lipophilic fluvastatin in rat skeletal myofibres. *Br. J. Pharmacol.* 2008;**154**(7):1482–1490.

279. Tsuda-Tsukimoto M, Maeda T, Iwanaga T, Kume T, Tamai I. Characterization of hepatobiliary transport systems of a novel alpha4beta1/alpha4beta7 dual antagonist, TR-14035. *Pharm. Res.* 2006;**23**(11):2646–2656.

280. Nozawa T, Sugiura S, Nakajima M, Goto A, Yokoi T, Nezu J et al. Involvement of organic anion transporting polypeptides in the transport of troglitazone sulfate: implications for understanding troglitazone hepatotoxicity. *Drug. Metab. Dispos.* 2004;**32**(3):291–294.

281. Yamashiro W, Maeda K, Hirouchi M, Adachi Y, Hu Z, Sugiyama Y. Involvement of transporters in the hepatic uptake and biliary excretion of valsartan, a selective antagonist of the angiotensin II AT1-receptor, in humans. *Drug. Metab. Dispos.* 2006;**34**(7):1247–1254.

282. Letschert K, Faulstich H, Keller D, Keppler D. Molecular characterization and inhibition of amanitin uptake into human hepatocytes. *Toxicol. Sci.* 2006;**91**(1):140–149.

283. Konig J, Cui Y, Nies AT, Keppler D. Localization and genomic organization of a new hepatocellular organic anion transporting polypeptide. *J. Biol. Chem.* 2000; **275**(30):23161–23168.

284. Shimizu M, Fuse K, Okudaira K, Nishigaki R, Maeda K, Kusuhara H et al. Contribution of OATP (organic anion-transporting polypeptide) family transporters to the hepatic uptake of fexofenadine in humans. *Drug. Metab. Dispos.* 2005;**33**(10):1477–1481.

285. Baldes C, Koenig P, Neumann D, Lenhof HP, Kohlbacher O, Lehr CM. Development of a fluorescence-based assay for screening of modulators of human organic anion transporter 1B3 (OATP1B3). *Eur. J. Pharm. Biopharm.* 2006;**62**(1):39–43.

286. Fischer WJ, Altheimer S, Cattori V, Meier PJ, Dietrich DR, Hagenbuch B. Organic anion transporting polypeptides expressed in liver and brain mediate uptake of microcystin. *Toxicol. Appl. Pharmacol.* 2005;**203**(3):257–263.

287. Komatsu M, Furukawa T, Ikeda R, Takumi S, Nong Q, Aoyama K et al. Involvement of mitogen-activated protein kinase signaling pathways in microcystin-LR-induced apoptosis after its selective uptake mediated by OATP1B1 and OATP1B3. *Toxicol. Sci.* 2007;**97**(2):407–416.

288. Takeda M, Khamdang S, Narikawa S, Kimura H, Kobayashi Y, Yamamoto T et al. Human organic anion transporters and human organic cation transporters mediate renal antiviral transport. *J. Pharmacol. Exp. Ther.* 2002;**300**(3):918–924.

289. Nies AT, Herrmann E, Brom M, Keppler D. Vectorial transport of the plant alkaloid berberine by double-transfected cells expressing the human organic cation transporter 1 (OCT1, SLC22A1) and the efflux pump MDR1 P-glycoprotein (ABCB1). *Naunyn. Schmiedebergs. Arch. Pharmacol.* 2008;**376**(6):449–461.

290. Tahara H, Kusuhara H, Endou H, Koepsell H, Imaoka T, Fuse E et al. A species difference in the transport activities of H2 receptor antagonists by rat and human renal organic anion and cation transporters. *J. Pharmacol. Exp. Ther.* 2005;**315**(1):337–345.

291. Ming X, Ju W, Wu H, Tidwell RR, Hall JE, Thakker DR. Transport of dicationic drugs pentamidine and furamidine by human organic cation transporters. *Drug. Metab. Dispos.* 2009;**37**(2):424–430.

292. Kang HJ, Lee SS, Lee CH, Shim JC, Shin HJ, Liu KH et al. Neurotoxic pyridinium metabolites of haloperidol are substrates of human organic cation transporters. *Drug. Metab. Dispos.* 2006;**34**(7):1145–1151.

293. Minuesa G, Volk C, Molina-Arcas M, Gorboulev V, Erkizia I, Arndt P et al. Transport of Lamivudine (3TC) and High-Affinity Interaction of Nucleoside Reverse Transcriptase Inhibitors With Human Organic Cation Transporters 1 2, and 3. *J. Pharmacol. Exp. Ther.* 2009.

294. Sato T, Masuda S, Yonezawa A, Tanihara Y, Katsura T, Inui K. Transcellular transport of organic cations in double-transfected MDCK cells expressing human organic cation transporters hOCT1/hMATE1 and hOCT2/hMATE1. *Biochem. Pharmacol.* 2008;**76**(7):894–903.

295. Bourdet DL, Pritchard JB, Thakker DR. Differential substrate and inhibitory activities of ranitidine and famotidine toward human organic cation transporter 1 (hOCT1; SLC22A1), hOCT2 (SLC22A2), and hOCT3 (SLC22A3). *J. Pharmacol. Exp. Ther.* 2005;**315**(3):1288–1297.

296. Busch AE, Karbach U, Miska D, Gorboulev V, Akhoundova A, Volk C et al. Human neurons express the polyspecific cation transporter hOCT2, which translocates monoamine neurotransmitters, amantadine, and memantine. *Mol. Pharmacol.* 1998;**54**(2):342–352.

297. Biermann J, Lang D, Gorboulev V, Koepsell H, Sindic A, Schroter R et al. Characterization of regulatory mechanisms and states of human organic cation transporter 2. *Am. J. Physiol. Cell. Physiol.* 2006;**290**(6):C1521–C1531.

298. Chen Y, Zhang S, Sorani M, Giacomini KM. Transport of paraquat by human organic cation transporters and multidrug and toxic compound extrusion family. *J. Pharmacol. Exp. Ther.* 2007;**322**(2):695–700.

299. Thuerauf N, Fromm MF. The role of the transporter P-glycoprotein for disposition and effects of centrally acting drugs and for the pathogenesis of CNS diseases. *Eur. Arch. Psychiatry Clin. Neurosci.* 2006;**256**(5):281–286.

300. Deeken JF, Figg WD, Bates SE, Sparreboom A. Toward individualized treatment: prediction of anticancer drug disposition and toxicity with pharmacogenetics. *Anticancer. Drugs.* 2007;**18**(2):111–126.

301. Kock K, Grube M, Jedlitschky G, Oevermann L, Siegmund W, Ritter CA et al. Expression of adenosine triphosphate-binding cassette (ABC) drug transporters in peripheral blood cells: relevance for physiology and pharmacotherapy. *Clin. Pharmacokinet.* 2007;**46**(6):449–470.

302. Deng JW, Song IS, Shin HJ, Yeo CW, Cho DY, Shon JH et al. The effect of SLCO1B1*15 on the disposition of pravastatin and pitavastatin is substrate dependent: the contribution of transporting activity changes by SLCO1B1*15. *Pharmacogenet. Genomics.* 2008; **18**(5):424–433.

303. Han JY, Lim HS, Shin ES, Yoo YK, Park YH, Lee JE et al. Influence of the organic anion-transporting polypeptide 1B1 (OATP1B1) polymorphisms on irinotecan-pharmacokinetics and clinical outcome of patients with advanced non-small cell lung cancer. *Lung Cancer* 2008;**59**(1):69–75.

304. He YJ, Zhang W, Chen Y, Guo D, Tu JH, Xu LY et al. Rifampicin alters atorvastatin plasma concentration on the basis of SLCO1B1 521T>C polymorphism. *Clin. Chim. Acta.* 2009;**405**(1–2):49–52.

305. Kalliokoski A, Neuvonen M, Neuvonen PJ, Niemi M. Different effects of SLCO1B1 polymorphism on the pharmacokinetics and pharmacodynamics of repaglinide and nateglinide. *J. Clin. Pharmacol.* 2008;**48**(3):311–321.

306. Kalliokoski A, Neuvonen M, Neuvonen PJ, Niemi M. No significant effect of SLCO1B1 polymorphism on the pharmacokinetics of rosiglitazone and pioglitazone. *Br. J. Clin. Pharmacol.* 2008;**65**(1):78–86.

307. Kajosaari LI, Niemi M, Neuvonen M, Laitila J, Neuvonen PJ, Backman JT. Cyclosporine markedly raises the plasma concentrations of repaglinide. *Clin. Pharmacol. Ther.* 2005; **78**(4):388–399.

308. Niemi M, Kivisto KT, Diczfalusy U, Bodin K, Bertilsson L, Fromm MF et al. Effect of SLCO1B1 polymorphism on induction of CYP3A4 by rifampicin. *Pharmacogenet Genomics.* 2006;**16**(8):565–568.

309. Niemi M, Neuvonen PJ, Hofmann U, Backman JT, Schwab M, Lutjohann D et al. Acute effects of pravastatin on cholesterol synthesis are associated with SLCO1B1 (encoding OATP1B1) haplotype *17. *Pharmacogenet. Genomics.* 2005;**15**(5):303–309.

310. Niemi M, Pasanen MK, Neuvonen PJ. SLCO1B1 polymorphism and sex affect the pharmacokinetics of pravastatin but not fluvastatin. *Clin. Pharmacol. Ther.* 2006; **80**(4):356–366.

311. Suwannakul S, Ieiri I, Kimura M, Kawabata K, Kusuhara H, Hirota T et al. Pharmacokinetic interaction between pravastatin and olmesartan in relation to SLCO1B1 polymorphism. *J. Hum. Genet.* 2008;**53**(10):899–904.

312. Takane H, Miyata M, Burioka N, Kurai J, Fukuoka Y, Suyama H et al. Severe toxicities after irinotecan-based chemotherapy in a patient with lung cancer: a homozygote for the SLCO1B1*15 allele. *Ther. Drug. Monit.* 2007;**29**(5):666–668.

313. Zhang W, He YJ, Gan Z, Fan L, Li Q, Wang A et al. OATP1B1 polymorphism is a major determinant of serum bilirubin level but not associated with rifampicin-mediated bilirubin elevation. *Clin. Exp. Pharmacol. Physiol.* 2007;**34**(12):1240–1244.

314. Tzvetkov MV, Vormfelde SV, Balen D, Meineke I, Schmidt T, Sehrt D et al. The Effects of Genetic Polymorphisms in the Organic Cation Transporters OCT1, OCT2, and OCT3 on the Renal Clearance of Metformin. *Clin. Pharmacol. Ther.* 2009;**86**(3):299–306.

315. Becker ML, Visser LE, van Schaik RH, Hofman A, Uitterlinden AG, Stricker BH. Genetic variation in the organic cation transporter 1 is associated with metformin response in patients with diabetes mellitus. *Pharmacogenomics. J.* 2009;**9**(4):242–247.

316. Bernsdorf A, Giessmann T, Modess C, Wegner D, Igelbrink S, Hecker U et al. Simvastatin does not influence the intestinal P-glycoprotein and MPR2, and the disposition of talinolol after chronic medication in healthy subjects genotyped for the ABCB1, ABCC2 and SLCO1B1 polymorphisms. *Br J Clin Pharmacol* 2006; **61**(4):440–450.

317. Gardner ER, Burger H, van Schaik RH, van Oosterom AT, de Bruijn EA, Guetens G et al. Association of enzyme and transporter genotypes with the pharmacokinetics of imatinib. *Clin. Pharmacol. Ther.* 2006;**80**(2):192–201.

318. Weiss J, Ten Hoevel MM, Burhenne J, Walter-Sack I, Hoffmann MM, Rengelshausen J et al. CYP2C19 genotype is a major factor contributing to the highly variable pharmacokinetics of voriconazole. *J. Clin. Pharmacol.* 2009;**49**(2):196–204.

319. Yamaguchi H, Hishinuma T, Endo N, Tsukamoto H, Kishikawa Y, Sato M et al. Genetic variation in ABCB1 influences paclitaxel pharmacokinetics in Japanese patients with ovarian cancer. *Int. J. Gynecol. Cancer.* 2006;**16**(3):979–985.

320. Naesens M, Kuypers DR, Verbeke K, Vanrenterghem Y. Multidrug resistance protein 2 genetic polymorphisms influence mycophenolic acid exposure in renal allograft recipients. *Transplantation* 2006;**82**(8):1074–1084.

321. Niemi M, Arnold KA, Backman JT, Pasanen MK, Godtel-Armbrust U, Wojnowski L et al. Association of genetic polymorphism in ABCC2 with hepatic multidrug resistance-associated protein 2 expression and pravastatin pharmacokinetics. *Pharmacogenet. Genomics.* 2006;**16**(11):801–808.

322. Jada SR, Lim R, Wong CI, Shu X, Lee SC, Zhou Q et al. Role of UGT1A1*6, UGT1A1*28 and ABCG2 c. 421C > A polymorphisms in irinotecan-induced neutropenia in Asian cancer patients. *Cancer Sci.* 2007;**98**(9):1461–1467.

323. Sparreboom A, Gelderblom H, Marsh S, Ahluwalia R, Obach R, Principe P et al. Diflomotecan pharmacokinetics in relation to ABCG2 421C > A genotype. *Clin. Pharmacol. Ther.* 2004;**76**(1):38–44.

324. Sparreboom A, Loos WJ, Burger H, Sissung TM, Verweij J, Figg WD et al. Effect of ABCG2 genotype on the oral bioavailability of topotecan. *Cancer Biol. Ther.* 2005;**4**(6):650–658.

325. Hedman M, Neuvonen PJ, Neuvonen M, Holmberg C, Antikainen M. Pharmacokinetics and pharmacodynamics of pravastatin in pediatric and adolescent cardiac transplant recipients on a regimen of triple immunosuppression. *Clin. Pharmacol. Ther.* 2004Jan; **75**(1):101–9.

CHAPTER 5

Pharmacogenetics of Drug Targets

ANN K. DALY
Newcastle University, Newcastle upon Tyne, UK

MARIA ARRANZ
King's College London, London, UK

5.1 INTRODUCTION

As described in detail in Chapters 2 and 3, there is a good understanding now of pharmacogenetic polymorphisms affecting drug metabolism, and it is well established that a number of pharmacogenetic polymorphisms are important to the pharmacokinetics of commonly prescribed drugs. There is currently much less understanding of the relationship between polymorphisms that affect drug targets and drug response. For a number of reasons, pharmacogenetic studies on pharmacodynamics have not progressed as rapidly as those concerned with pharmacokinetics. These include poorer understanding of the genes encoding the relevant targets, the difficulties involved in performing studies on functional effects of polymorphisms in some of these genes, and, in many cases, difficulties in quantitating and defining drug response. The availability of improved information on the extent of polymorphism in all genes from projects such as the HapMap has been beneficial for pharmacogenetic studies on drug targets. In addition, detailed *in vitro* studies on the consequences of polymorphisms have now been initiated, especially for important drug targets such as certain adrenergic receptors.

Drug targets include drug receptors, enzymes, and transporters such as those involved in reuptake of serotonin (5-hydroxytryptamine or 5HT) and dopamine. This chapter considers a number of specific pharmacogenetic examples relevant to each of these. Drugs generally target specific receptors or enzymes, but overall response will involve a number of different proteins often as part of a complex pathway. Any component of such a pathway may contribute to pharmacogenetic variability in

Pharmacogenetics and Individualized Therapy, First Edition.
Edited by Anke-Hilse Maitland-van der Zee and Ann K. Daly.

response, but the main emphasis here is on the primary target as overall understanding of pathway effects is currently very limited.

5.2 RECEPTORS

5.2.1 Introduction

At least four different receptor types can be distinguished on the basis of their signal transduction mechanism. These include the ionotropic receptors, metabotropic receptors, and kinase-linked receptors, which are all located on the plasma membrane together with the nuclear receptors, which are intracellular and target gene transcription directly. A more detailed account is given by Rang et al. [1, Chapter 3]. Up to the present, the majority of pharmacogenetic studies on receptors have been concerned with the metabotropic receptors that are G-protein-linked receptors with a characteristic 7 transmembrane domain structure. Pharmacogenetic information on other receptor types such as the ionotropic nicotinic acetylcholine receptor or steroid hormone receptors is still very limited and is not considered further. The receptors that have been well studied pharmacogenetically are summarized in Table 5.1, and each is described in more detail below.

5.2.2 Dopamine

5.2.2.1 Introduction

Dopamine (DA) is a catecholamine neurotransmitter that regulates locomotor functions, cognition, emotion, positive reinforcement, and food intake [2]. Dopamine and serotonin receptors are important targets for drugs used in the treatment of psychotic disorders, given the involvement of both systems in the etiology and

TABLE 5.1 Pharmacogenetic Studies on Receptors as Drug Targets

Receptor (Gene)	Functionally Significant Polymorphisms	Relevance to Drug Response
Dopamine receptor DR_2 (DRD2)	Yes	+ +
Dopamine receptor DR_3 (DRD3)	Yes	+ +
Dopamine receptor DR_4 (DRD4)	Yes	+
Serotonin receptor 5-HTR_{1A} (HTR1A)	Yes	+
Serotonin receptor 5-HTR_{2A} (HTR2A)	Yes	+ +
Serotonin receptor 5-HTR_{2C} (HTR2C)	Yes	+
Adrenergic receptor α_{2B} (ADRA2B)	Yes	+
Adrenergic receptor α_{2C} (ADRA2C)	Yes	+ +
Adrenergic receptor β_1 (ADRB1)	Yes	+ + +
Adrenergic receptor β_2 (ADRB2)	Yes	+ + +
Adrenergic receptor β_3 (ADRB3)	Yes	+

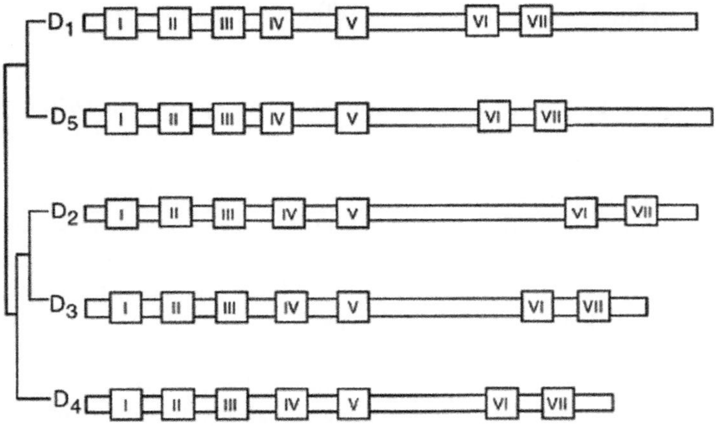

FIGURE 5.1 Dendrogram of the family of dopamine receptors. The D_1 and D_5 receptors are characterized by a short third intracellular loop and long intracellular carboxy termini. The D_2, D_3, and D_4 receptors possess a long third intracellular loop and a short intracellular carboxy termini. Boxes represent transmembrane domains I–VII. (Reproduced from Levant [176] with permission.)

pathological processes of mental disorders. The classical hypothesis of schizophrenia states that the positive symptoms of the disease (hallucinations, delusions, thought disorder) are caused by hyperactivity of dopamine neurotransmission in mesolimbic brain regions. This hypothesis is supported by the observation that all currently available antipsychotic drugs, without exception, bind to dopamine D_2 receptors to varying extents. In addition, the level of D_2 occupancy is directly related to improvement in psychotic symptoms and side effect improvement. A 60% D_2 occupancy level is required to observe antipsychotic activity, but occupancy levels higher than 80% lead to the development of movement disorders or extra-pyramidal side effects caused by dopamine depletion (EPS) [3,4].

There are five subtypes of dopamine receptors (from D_1 to D_5) classified into two subfamilies, the D_1-like (D_1 and D_5) and D_2- like (D_2, D_3 and D_4 receptors) (see Fig. 5.1).

5.2.2.2 Dopamine D_2 Receptors

The D_2-like receptors are G-protein-coupled receptors, with seven transmembrane regions, that inhibit adenylyl cyclase and stimulate K^+ channels [2,5]. The D_2 receptor is abundant in the striatum, olfactory tubercle, and nucleus accumbens, and is also moderately expressed in other brain areas [2]. D_2 receptors are the main target of first-generation antipsychotics such as haloperidol and chlorpromazine; it is believed that blockade of dopamine receptors in the mesolimbic system leads to antipsychotic activity over the positive symptoms of schizophrenia, whereas EPS are a result of the antipsychotic blockade of D_2 receptors in the striatum [2,5,6]. D_2 receptors are also targeted by second-generation antipsychotics (i.e., risperidone, olanzapine, ziprasidone), although to a lesser extent [7]. Interestingly, amisulpride, a newer antipsychotic that displays high mesolimbic affinity for D_2 receptors, retains antipsychotic efficacy but without causing movement disorders [8].

Dopamine D_2 receptors were the first subtype to be cloned, facilitating genetic studies on the coding genes. Two functional polymorphisms in *DRD2*, the gene encoding this receptor, Ser311Cys and −141-C *Ins/Del*, have been associated with response to antipsychotics [9–11]. The −141-C *Del* promoter variant, associated with decreased expression of the D_2 receptor protein [12]; and the 311Cys variant, associated with lower receptor functioning [13], showed poorer responses to antipsychotics, suggesting that the D_2 receptors mediate response to these medications. Some studies have provided evidence relating DRD2 polymorphisms and treatment-induced tardive dyskinesia (TD), a severe and longlasting movement disorder [14]. Although negative reports have been published, two more recent meta-analyses have confirmed these associations and the involvement of D_2 receptors in the development of movement disorders [15,16]. In these meta-analyses, the low expression allele −141-C *Del* was associated with a higher risk of developing TD, probably due to the lower receptor availability facilitating higher levels of occupancy. A *Taq*I polymorphism located 10 kb downstream of the DRD2 gene has also been associated with TD, with the A2 allele conferring a higher risk [15,16]. The same allelic variant has been associated with poorer response to the antipsychotic aripiprazol [17,18]. This polymorphism has now been mapped to ANKK1 [19], a gene adjacent to the DRD2 gene, but its functionality is still unclear.

5.2.2.3 Dopamine D_3 Receptors

The D_3 receptors are most abundant in limbic areas, mainly postsynaptically in nucleus accumbens, and poorly expressed in other brain regions. D_3 receptors inhibit adenylyl cyclase and have an inhibitory role on locomotor activity. This finding is supported by the observation that D_3 agonists inhibit locomotor activity, whereas D_3 antagonists evoke motor activation [2]. D_3 receptors are also involved in cognitive, emotional, and endocrine functions.

Several polymorphisms of potential functional relevance have been described in the promoter (−7685-G/C, −712-G/C, and −205-A/G) and coding region (Ser9Gly, Ala38Thr) of the DRD3 gene, which codes for this receptor. The 9Gly variant, which results in an *N*-terminal amino acid substitution, shows higher dopamine binding affinity than the more common Ser9 allele. The functionality of the other polymorphisms is as yet unknown. The DRD3 Ser9Gly polymorphism has been associated with response to antipsychotic treatment, with the 9Gly variant associated with better improvement of positive psychotic symptoms [20,21]. This polymorphism has also been associated with drug-induced tardive dyskinesia [22]. The 9Gly variant is more frequent in patients presenting TD as a result of antipsychotic treatment. Although discrepant reports for both findings exist, these observations reflect the mediation of dopamine in cognition and motor activities. The higher affinity of the 9Gly allele for dopamine may lead to faster binding of drugs, increasing response and the movement disorders associated with higher receptor occupancy. Additionally, the −205-A/G promoter polymorphism, of yet unknown functionality, has been related to positive symptom improvement in patients treated with the antipsychotic olanzapine [21].

5.2.2.4 Dopamine D_4 Receptors

The D_4 receptors are highly enriched in the prefrontal cortex, where they modulate GABAergic signaling transmission in pyramidal neurons, which may underlie their role in cognition. D_4 receptors are also found in amygdale, hippocampus, and hypothalamus [2,23,24]. The role of D_4 receptors in the dopamine system remains unclear. However, the brain location of these receptors (abundant in limbic but not in striatal areas) and their role in modulating cognition and exploratory behavior made them attractive targets for antipsychotic medication. However, in clinical trials, D_4 antagonists have failed to live up to promise [25,26].

There is less pharmacogenetic evidence relating this receptor gene termed DRD4 with antipsychotic response than for genes encoding other dopamine D_2-like receptors, indicating perhaps a secondary role in mediating antipsychotic activity. The antipsychotic clozapine displays relatively higher affinity for D_4 receptors than for any other dopamine subtype. This led to the hypothesis that these receptors were responsible for the superior efficacy of clozapine over other antipsychotics in treatment of positive and negative symptoms of schizophrenia. Initial reports of an association between a 48-bp polymorphic repeat in DRD4 resulting in size variation in the putative third cytoplasmic loop of the D_4 receptor and clozapine response and other antipsychotics were not universally replicated [27–30], and the association remains unclear. This repeat polymorphism has also been associated with attention deficit and hyperactivity disorder (ADHD) [31]. The DRD4 variant containing 7 repeats of the 48-bp sequence shows lower expression of the receptor protein [32], and is associated with novelty seeking behavior [33] and heroin craving [34]. This allele has been related to a reduced improvement with methylphenidate, a dopamine transporter blocker used for the treatment of ADHD [31,35]. However, it is not clear if these associations are a direct result of the functionality of the polymorphism or of an alternative variant in linkage disequilibrium with the 7 repeat allele. A second functional polymorphism, a −521-C/T change in the promoter region of the gene, influences DRD4 expression with the T allele showing lower levels. Individuals with the −521-C/C genotype show higher novelty seeking behaviour [36], and, not surprisingly, higher risk of heroin addiction [37]. A haplotype combining several polymorphisms in the DRD4 gene, including the 48-bp repeat, was found to be associated with TD [38]. Although the gene is highly polymorphic, no other variant has provided clear associations.

On the whole, pharmacogenetic studies have proved that dopamine receptors are major role players in the mechanism of action of currently available antipsychotic medications. However, it is more difficult to discern the involvement of genetic variants in the peripheral functions modulated by dopamine, where other systems may be major participants.

5.2.3 Serotonin

Serotonin is involved in the regulation of mood states, food intake, anxiety, sleep, reproductory activity, and cognitive function [39–41]. Not surprisingly, serotonin or 5-hydroxytryptamine has been hypothesized to play a significant role in the etiology and treatment of disorders such as anxiety, depression, schizophrenia, and anorexia nervosa, among others. Serotonin response is mediated by serotonin receptors widely distributed pre- and postsynaptically in the central nervous system (CNS) and can also be found in peripheral tissues. There are seven classes of serotonin receptors ($5HT_1$–$5HT_7$) further subdivided into 14 subtypes, according to their structural and functional characteristics; 13 of these subtypes are G-protein-coupled receptors and one ligand-gated ion channel receptor ($5HT_3$). Of these, the $5HT_1$ and $5HT_2$ families have been closely related to antipsychotic and antidepressant mechanisms.

5.2.3.1 $5HT_{1A}$ Receptors

$5HT_{1A}$ receptors are widely distributed in the CNS and highly abundant in cortical and hippocampal pyramidal neurons and induce hyperpolarization and subsequent inhibition of pyramidal neurons [42–44]. $5HT_{1A}$ receptors are located in brain regions associated with cognition and memory functions, and have been hypothesised to mediate in their regulation [42,45,46]. The observation that $5HT_{1A}$ partial agonists show some effectiveness in improving cognition in schizophrenia supports this hypothesis [42].

In comparison to other serotonin receptors, relatively few pharmacogenetic studies have investigated variants in HTR1A, the gene encoding $5HT_{1A}$. Interestingly, three studies on a HTR1A −1019-G/C functional polymorphism have observed an association with treatment response, with the −1019-G allele associated with less improvement in negative symptoms of schizophrenia [47–49]. This same polymorphism has been associated to antidepressant response [50–52] with the −1019-G allele showing poorer response. Only one study reported association of the −1019-C allele with nonresponse [53]. The −1019-G allele reduces inhibition of $5HT_{1A}$ gene expression, which results in a reduction of 5HT transmission, predisposing to depression, anxiety, and other personality traits [47] and providing biological plausibility to these findings. Several other *HTR1A* polymorphisms were found associated with antidepressant response in an Asian population [54], confirming the involvement of this gene in treatment response.

5.2.3.2 $5HT_{2A}$ Receptors

The $5HT_2$ family of receptors comprises the $5HT_{2A}$, $5HT_{2B}$, and $5HT_{2C}$ subtypes, of which $5HT_{2A}$ and $5HT_{2C}$ are strongly targeted by psychotropic medications. The genes encoding the $5HT_{2A}$ and $5HT_{2C}$ receptors, *HTR2A* and *HTR2C*, were among the first 5HT receptor clones isolated, and thus have been extensively studied.

The $5HT_{2A}$ receptors are widely distributed in peripheral and central tissues, being abundant in the cerebral cortex, claustrum, basal ganglia, and peripheral blood vessels [43]. $5HT_{2A}$ receptors are G-protein-coupled and stimulate phospholipase (PLC) activity. The effects of $5HT_{2A}$ receptors are opposite those of $5HT_{1A}$ receptors as they have an excitatory function over pyramidal neurons. $5HT_{2A}$ antagonists have shown a modest improvement in cognition in schizophrenia patients [42]. They mediate vasoconstriction and platelet aggregation, and are involved in depression, anxiety, and eating behavior. LSD activation of brain $5HT_{2A}$ receptors leads to hallucinations and psychotic-like symptoms. Strong binding by atypical antipsychotic drugs was suggested to be the main reason for antipsychotic efficacy without extrapyramidal side effects. However, it has been suggested that low affinity or rapid dissociation from D_2 receptor are the reasons behind clinical efficacy without adverse reactions [55,56]. Antagonism of $5HT_{2A}$ receptors has been suggested to improve the negative symptoms of schizophrenia and to reduce the EPS caused by dopamine binding [7]. There are numerous genetic and pharmacogenetic association studies of HTR2A polymorphisms in relation to mental disorders. In particular, the 102-T/C and −1438-A/G polymorphisms, which have been found in nearly complete linkage disequilibrium in Caucasian populations, have been associated with schizophrenia [57], bipolar disorder [58], Alzheimer's disease [59], and antipsychotic response [60–62]. However, many negative studies have also been published, as would be expected from a gene with moderate effects. In Caucasian populations the −1438-G and 102-C alleles are generally associated with a higher risk for developing mental disorders and to poorer treatment response [61], but in other ethnic groups an opposite effect may be observed [63,64], indicating differences in linkage disequilibrium status among populations. A structural His452Tyr polymorphic change has also been associated with treatment response, with the Tyr452 variant conferring a higher risk of failure in response to clozapine treatment [60]. Functional studies have shown the −1438-G variant, in linkage disequilibrium with the 102-C allele, to be associated with a lower expression of the receptors protein [65,66], and the Tyr452 variant with reduced calcium release and phospholipase activation [67], thus reinforcing $5HT_{2A}$ as a mediator of antipsychotic activity. Two major studies on antidepressant medications have also associated $5HT_{2A}$ with clinical outcome. The STAR*D study investigated a large cohort of depression sufferers treated with citalopram and found a $5HT_{2A}$ polymorphism, rs7997012, associated with response [68]. A more recent European study, GENDEP, investigating patients treated with the antidepressants escitalopram and nortriptyline, found associations between two HTR2A polymorphisms (rs9316233 and rs2224721) and level of response [69]. Not surprisingly, the same study found other variants in genes coding for serotonin signaling pathways associated with response to escitalopram, a selective serotonin reuptake inhibitor (SSRI), and that variants in genes encoding for norepinephine signaling influenced response to nortriptyline, a norepinephrine reuptake inhibitor. Serotonin inhibition of dopamine function has been hypothesized to contribute to the movement disorders associated with antipsychotic treatment. A study provided supporting evidence by associating HTR2A polymorphisms with drug-induced tardive dyskinesia [70]. This association became more evident when the age of the patient was considered [71].

5.2.3.3 $5HT_{2C}$ Receptors

The $5HT_{2C}$ subtype was initially named $5HT_{1C}$, but cloning revealed structural similarities with the $5HT_2$ family and was later renamed $5HT_{2C}$. This subtype is particularly abundant in the choroid plexus, but widely distributed in other brain areas [43]. $5HT_{2C}$ receptors mediate feeding behaviour and appetite [7]. Antagonism of $5HT_{2C}$ receptors protects against EPS and D_2-induced hyperprolactinemia [7].

The role of this receptor in regulating feeding behavior has been confirmed by several studies associating HTR2C genetic variants with antipsychotic-drug-induced weight gain. Pharmacogenetic studies revealed an association of a promoter polymorphism, −759-T/C with weight gain in antipsychotic treated patients [72,73]. The −759-T allele reduces receptor expression and may be the cause of resistance to weight gain [74]. Although some contradictory findings followed, indicating heterogeneity, a meta-analysis has confirmed a modest association of this polymorphism with weight gain [75]. Other polymorphic HTR2C variants have been reported in association with obesity and metabolic syndrome [76]. There is less evidence supporting an involvement of HTR2C variants on the level of antipsychotic response [77] or drug-induced tardive dyskinesia [78,79]. However, a possible role of $5HT_{2C}$ in movement disorders, via inhibition of dopamine neurotransmission, cannot be refuted.

Antipsychotic medication display varied levels of affinity for other serotonergic receptors, namely, $5HT_3$, $5HT_6$, and $5HT_7$ subtypes. However, a few genetic association studies have attempted to investigate a possible involvement in mediating, at least partially, antipsychotic activity [80–82], but no definite reports has been published to date.

Although the role of serotonin receptors and pathways in mediating treatment efficacy may be an indirect result of their regulatory roles on dopaminergic and glutamatergic systems, these pharmacogenetic findings support the hypothesis that serotonin targeting mediates, at least partially, antipsychotic and antidepressant activity.

5.2.4 Adrenergic Receptors

5.2.4.1 Introduction

Adrenergic receptors are G-protein-coupled receptors that bind epinephrine and norepinephrine and mainly use cAMP as second messenger with a role for inositol triphosphate in the case of the α1 receptors only. Structurally, these receptors show considerable homology, with all featuring seven transmembrane domains. They are divided into α1 and β subfamilies which are further divided into α1 and α2 subfamilies; α1, α2 and β each have three subtypes, all encoded by separate genes. The genes encoding these receptors have been relatively well studied, and information is also available on pharmacogenomic aspects. Collectively, the adrenergic receptors play major roles in the cardiovascular and respiratory systems and also contribute to a range of other physiological processes. These major roles mean that they are important drug targets, especially in the case of the β receptors, with both agonists and antagonists that are selective for specific receptors useful for treatment of various diseases. This section considers selected adrenergic receptors from a pharmacogenomic standpoint. There is considerable information available on the extent of polymorphism in each adrenergic receptor with detailed studies on functional significance performed on a number of the more common polymorphisms. The majority of clinically based studies linking drug response to particular genotypes and haplotypes have been on the β1 and β2 receptors, probably because they are the major adrenergic receptors targeted by widely used drugs.

More detailed general information on pharmacological function can be obtained from a variety of sources [1], and there are detailed reviews available on their pharmacogenomic aspects in relation to both cardiovascular medicine and respiratory medicine [83–86]. Other information on clinical relevance is also included in Chapter 6 (on pharmacogenetics of cardiovascular therapy) and Chapter 9 (on pharmacogenetics of asthma and chronic obstructive pulmonary disease).

5.2.4.2 α–Adrenergic Receptors

There are three members of the α1 subfamily: α1A, α1B and α1D, each encoded by separate genes. Although polymorphisms in coding regions of each gene have been described, pharmacogenetic knowledge is limited possibly because these receptors are not important drug targets.

On the other hand, the α2 subfamily, which again includes three separate receptors, α2A, α2B, and α2C, is a major regulator of sympathetic nervous system activity and has roles in regulation of blood pressure, platelet aggregation, and vasoconstriction and vasodilatation, making this group of receptors more important pharmacological targets [84]. In this group of G-protein-linked receptors, agonist binding results in inhibition of adenyl cyclase. The main focus of pharmacogenetic studies has been on the α2B and α2C encoding genes (*ADRA2B* and *ADRA2C*). Both genes have common deletion polymorphisms [87]. In the case of *ADRA2B*, a 9-bp deletion results in the absence of three amino acids located within the third cytoplasmic loop (see Fig. 5.2). This polymorphism is found in a number of ethnic groups but is particularly common in Europeans (frequency ~0.3) with a lower frequency in African-Americans. The variant form of the receptor is associated with decreased phosphorylation by G-protein receptor kinase and with loss of receptor desensitization. *ADRA2C* also shows a common deletion polymorphism that affects the third cytoplasmic loop (Fig. 5.2). In this case, four amino acids are lost and the polymorphism is more common in African-Americans (allele frequency 0.4) compared with Europeans (0.04). As with the *ADRA2B* deletion, this deletion appears to be associated with lower receptor activity with impaired inhibition of adenylcyclase following binding of agonist and poorer agonist-induced stimulation of the enzyme mitogen-activated protein (MAP) kinase. The number of clinical studies in relation to the two α-adrenergic deletion polymorphisms is small, with slightly more data on the clinical significance of the *ADRA2C* polymorphism available. The most potentially interesting observation for *ADRA2C* is not concerned directly with drug response but concerns a study suggesting that homozygous carriers of the *ADRA2C* deletion (of African-American origin) had an increased risk of developing heart failure [88]. This is a biologically plausible observation in that decreased inhibition of norepinephrine release from presynaptic nerve terminals would be expected in those positive for the deletion resulting in increased adrenergic drive. More recent studies in healthy volunteers subject to stress have provided limited support for this hypothesis [89], but attempts to confirm the original observation of the deletion being associated with increased risk of heart failure have not been successful [90]. The limited current use

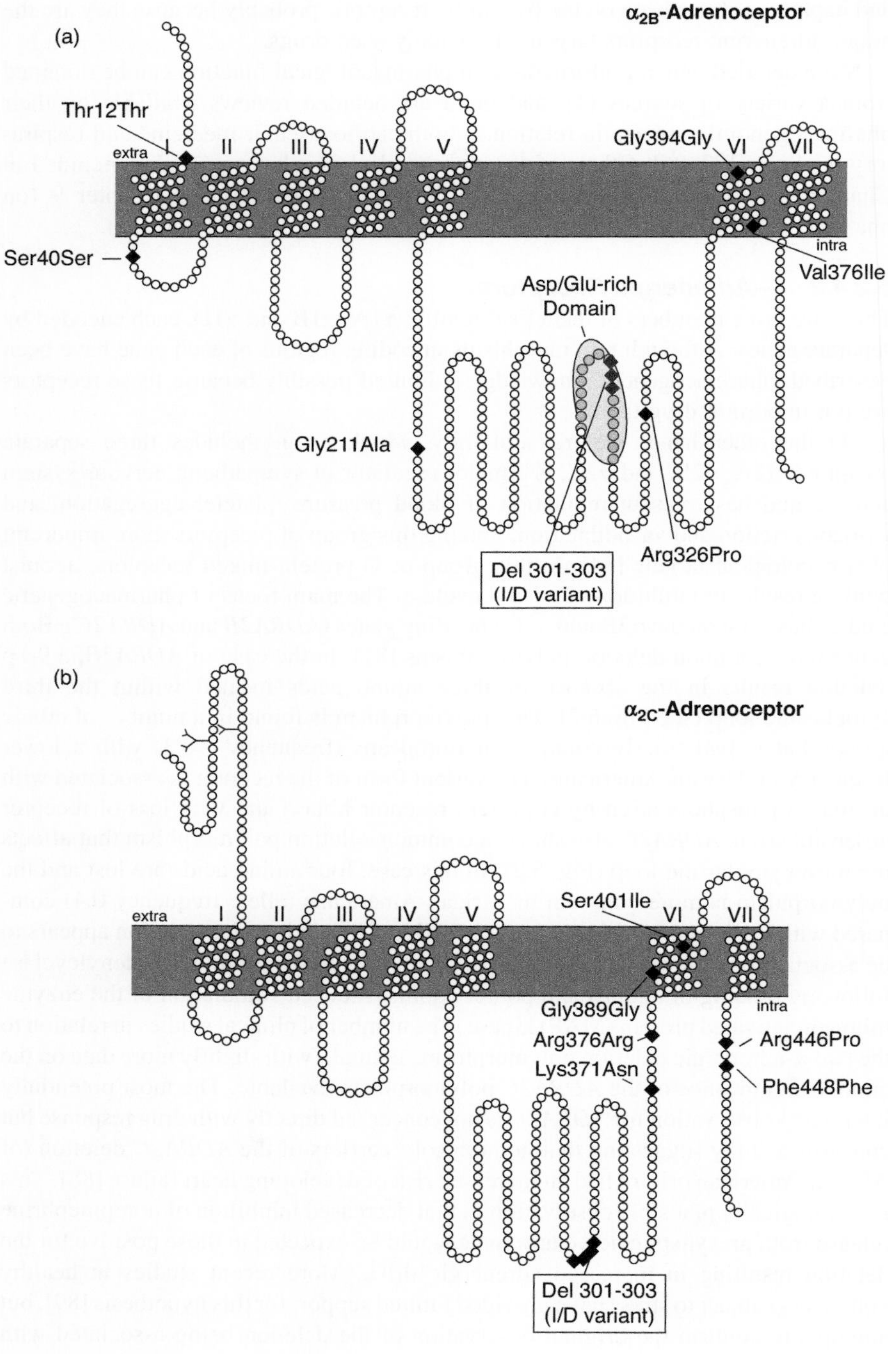
(a)
α2B-Adrenoceptor
Thr12Thr
extra
I
II
III
IV
V
Gly394Gly
VI
VII
Ser40Ser
intra
Val376Ile
Asp/Glu-rich
Domain
Gly211Ala
Arg326Pro
Del 301-303
(I/D variant)
(b)
α2C-Adrenoceptor
extra
I
II
III
IV
V
Ser401Ile
VI
VII
Gly389Gly
intra
Arg376Arg
Arg446Pro
Lys371Asn
Phe448Phe
Del 301-303
(I/D variant)

of drugs targeting α-receptors means that little data on the relevance of the α2 deletion polymorphisms to drug response are available. However, the regulation by α2C receptors of norepinephrine release means that *ADRA2C* genotype may affect response to β-adrenergic antagonists. This has been demonstrated in a study showing that response to metoprolol in heart failure patients is affected by ADRA2C genotype in addition to ADRB1 genotype [91]. This interesting observation needs to be confirmed in larger studies.

5.2.4.3 β1-Adrenergic Receptor (ADRB1 Gene)

β1-adrenergic receptors are the major adrenoreceptor class found in the heart with a key role in regulation of heart rate. They act by stimulating adenyl cyclase, in a mechanism common to all three classes of β-adrenergic receptors. The ADRB1 gene is located on chromosome 10 with a common nonsynonymous polymorphism in codon 398 (Gly389Arg) that has been well studied. Although the Gly variant was the first cDNA clone isolated, the frequency of the Arg variant (~0.70 in Europeans) is higher [92,93]. Another nonsynonymous polymorphism, Ser49Gly, has also been described, but the variant form is relatively uncommon in both Europeans and African-Americans with a frequency of ~ 0.08 [93]. For the Arg389 variant, transfection studies demonstrated slightly higher basal levels of expression compared with the Gly form, but when stimulated with isoproterenol, the Arg variant showed ~3-fold higher levels of activity [92]. In the case of the Ser49Gly polymorphism, the rare Gly variant appears to be more susceptible to agonist-induced downregulation, and this finding may be helpful in chronic heart failure [94,95].

As the Gly389Arg polymorphism is common and clearly functionally significant, it has formed the basis for a large number of clinical studies, particularly on the relationship between genotype and response to β-receptor antagonist treatment. Several studies have shown significant differences in response on the basis of genotype, in studies on hypertension and heart failure. A general conclusion from these studies is that patients homozygous for the Gly489 variant may show a poor response to β-antagonists and might benefit from higher drug doses but, as suggested more recently [83], larger prospective studies are needed to assess the clinical relevance of this concept.

FIGURE 5.2 α2-Adrenergic receptor structure and polymorphisms: (a) Topological model of the α2B-AR. Variants to the coding sequence are indicated by diamonds. The deletion allele of the I/D variant (rs29000568) has been associated with enhanced receptor function. Other variants in the coding sequence include the rare SNPs T12T (rs9333567), S40S (rs35812638), A211G (rs9333568), and R326P (rs45494291), and the more frequent I376V (rs29000569) and G394G (rs2229169). (b) Topological model of the α2C-AR. Glycosylation sites are denoted by y-like structures at the external loop. Variants to the coding sequence are indicated by diamonds. The frequent insertion/deletion variant affects amino acids 321–325 (rs61767072). Rare variants in the coding region include N371K (rs1800037), R376R (rs7435505), G389G (rs7434630), I401S (rs1133450), P446R (rs1133451), and F448F (rs1133453). (Reproduced with permission from Rosskopf and Michel [84].)

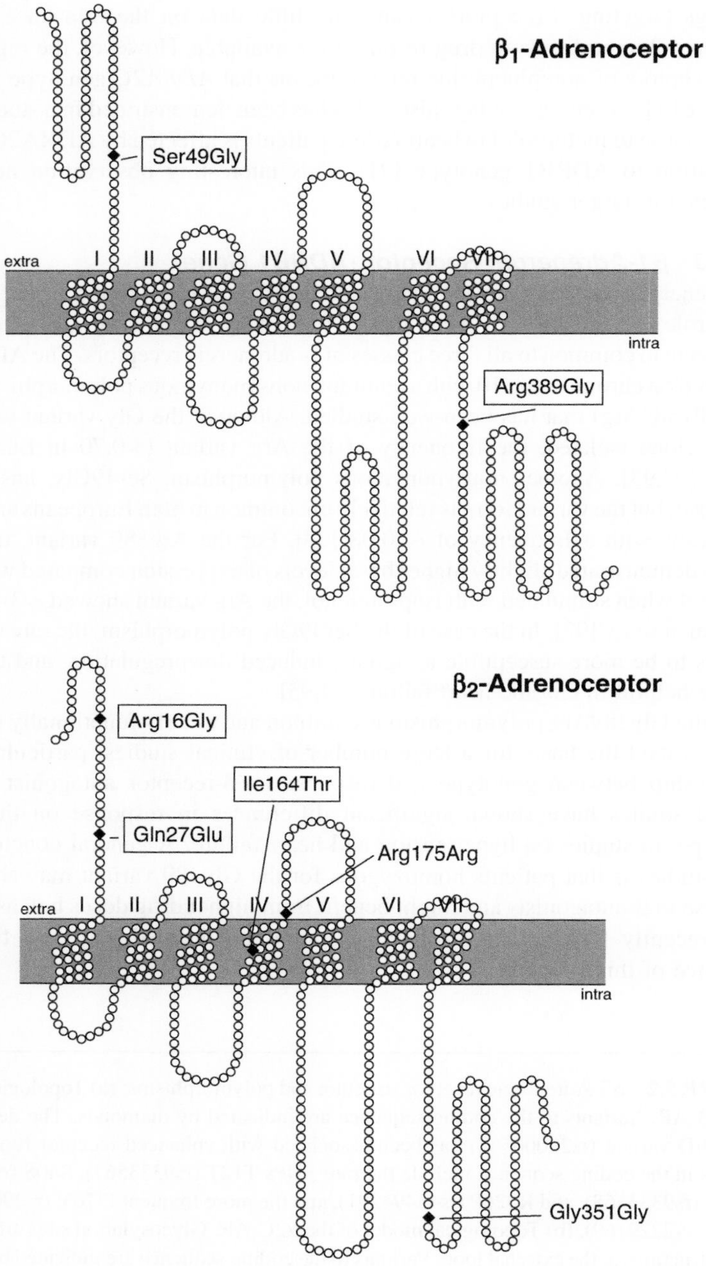
(a)
β1-Adrenoceptor
Ser49Gly
extra
I
II
III
IV
V
VI
VII
intra
Arg389Gly
(b)
β2-Adrenoceptor
Arg16Gly
Ile164Thr
Gln27Glu
Arg175Arg
extra
I
II
III
IV
V
VI
VII
intra
Gly351Gly

5.2.4.4 β2-Adrenergic Receptor (ADRB2 Gene)

The β2-adrenergic receptor is probably the best studied receptor from the pharmacogenetic standpoint, mainly due to its importance as a target for β-agonists in asthma. β2-Adrenergic receptors are classic G-protein-linked receptors that are expressed in smooth muscle. Activation involves elevation of intracellular cAMP. The receptor is encoded by a small intronless gene termed *ADRB2* on chromosome 5. *ADRB2* is unusually polymorphic compared with other adrenergic receptors, especially in the coding sequence, and this has resulted in considerable interest in assessing the relevance of these polymorphisms to drug response and also, to some extent, to disease susceptibility.

There are at least nine polymorphisms in the coding region, with four of these resulting in aminoacid substitutions (nonsynonymous polymorphisms) (see Fig. 5.3). In addition, there is a single nonsynonymous polymorphism in the region encoding the leader peptide and a number of upstream polymorphisms close to the transcription start site. A limited number of haplotypes have been observed, with only four showing frequencies above 5% in any population studied to date, but there is considerable variation between haplotype frequency in different ethnic groups, especially those of European, African, and East Asian origin [96]. For example, among Europeans, three haplotypes are common. Two of these differ mainly at codon 16, with one having a sequence encoding glycine and the second arginine at this position. The Gly encoding form can be further subdivided into two haplotypes, one encoding glutamine at position 27 and the second, which is less common, glutamic acid. These three haplotypes are also common in other ethnic groups, although overall frequencies differ from those seen in Europeans, and there is also a fourth haplotype, which is common in African-Americans [96]. Most clinical studies have focused on the codon 16 polymorphism probably because this SNP is seen at a relatively high population frequency and also because it was the first coding region polymorphism to be identified.

Although the codon 16 polymorphism was identified around 1995, data on its functional significance are quite limited and rather contradictory. Early studies involving transfection of cell cultures with cDNA constructs of defined sequence suggested that the Gly-containing receptor showed enhanced downregulation following agonist binding compared with the Arg-containing form [97]. This downregulation is the main mechanism by which long-term agonist-promoted desensitization of β2-adrenergic receptors occurs [98]. The presence of the codon 27 Glu variant alone had no effect on downregulation, but a double mutant, including

FIGURE 5.3 α-Adrenergic receptor structure and polymorphisms: (a) Topological model of the β1-AR. Glycosylation sites are denoted by y-like structures at the external loop. Variants to the coding sequence are indicated by diamonds. S49G (rs1801252) and G389R (rs1801253) are common variants. (b) Topological model of the β2-AR. Glycosylation sites are denoted by y-like structures at the external loop. Variants to the coding sequence are indicated by diamonds. R16G (rs1042713), Q27E (rs1042714), and I164T (rs1800888) are common nonsynoymous variants. (Reproduced with permission from Rosskopf and Michel [84].)

both Gly at codon 16 and Glu at codon 27 (the more common combination seen *in vivo*), resulted in a downregulation broadly similar to that for receptors, including the Gly variant only [97]. More recently, in a number of separate studies using either cells (lymphocytes and lung cells) of known genotype or genotyped patients receiving β2-adrenergic receptor–agonist treatment for asthma, it was found that the Arg16-containing form of *ADRB2* was associated with increased agonist-induced downregulation and with a poorer response to inhaled short-acting β-agonists [99–102]. The poorer response to β2-adrenergic receptor agonists appears to be specific to short-acting agonists since a large study involving patients undergoing treatment with longer-acting agonists and with an inhaled steroid for asthma failed to show any difference in outcome on the basis of codon 16 genotype [103]. In general, it is now accepted that codon 16 genotype does appear to affect response to short-acting agonists but that this may not be clinically important as current treatments mainly involve use of longer-acting agonists. Further studies would be useful in resolving the question of whether genotyping patients taking β2-adrenergic receptor agonists for polymorphisms in *ADRB2* and personalizing their treatment on this basis is of benefit.

The *ADRB2* genotype may also be relevant to response to β-antagonists. However, since most antagonists tend to have equal affinities for β1 and β2-receptors or preferential interaction with β1 receptors, assessing the contribution of *ADRB2* genotype to response is more difficult. However, a few studies have studied this aspect in patients receiving β-antagonists for treatment of heart failure or hypertension. Most studies, especially larger, more recent ones, have failed to detect any difference in response in relation to genotype for either codon 16 or codon 27 of *ADRB2* [104–106].

5.2.4.5 β3-Adrenergic Receptors

β3-Adrenergic receptors are expressed mainly in adipose tissue, although there is some limited evidence that they may also be expressed in heart tissue (for review, see Ref. 107). There is a common polymorphism at codon 64 (Trp64Arg) at the start of the first intracellular loop. As reviewed by Strosberg [108], this polymorphism varies in frequency between different ethnic groups, and there have been some suggestions that the variant allele might be associated with higher body mass index or susceptibility to type II diabetes. In general, these suggested associations have not been confirmed [107]. Some suggested differences in agonist response between expressed receptors of different codon 64 genotypes [109] was not confirmed in a more detailed study [110]. However, the possibility that noncoding polymorphisms contribute to variability in response to β3-agonists that are in clinical development needs further investigation [110].

5.3 ENZYMES

As well as contributing to drug metabolism, enzymes are important drug targets. Widely used drugs targeting enzymes include the coumarin anticoagulants which inhibit vitamin K epoxide reductase; ACE inhibitors, which target the angiotensin-

TABLE 5.2 Pharmacogenetic Studies on Enzymes as Drug Targets

Enzyme (Gene)	Functionally Significant Polymorphisms	Relevance to Drug Response
Vitamin K epoxide reductase (VKORC1)	Yes	+ + +
HMGCoA reductase (HMGCR)	Yes	+
Cycloxygenase 1 (PTGS1)	Yes	+
Angiotensin-converting enzyme (ACE)	Yes	+ +
Monoamine oxidase (MAOA and MAOB)	Yes	ND
Dihydrofolate reductase (DHFR)	Yes	Possible

converting enzyme; statins, which inhibit HMGCoA reductase, nonsteroidal antiinflammatory drugs (NSAIDs), which inhibit prostaglandin H-synthases I and II; and monoamine oxidase inhibitors. Table 5.2 lists the main enzyme targets whose pharmacogenetics is well studied and will be considered in detail here. In cancer chemotherapy, enzymes expressed in tumor tissue are also an important drug target. Tumor genotype is the key predictor of response to such drugs. This area is outside the scope of the present chapter but is discussed in Chapter 8.

In general, as discussed below, there are clear pharmacogenetic data showing associations between certain genotypes and drug response only for VKOR and HMGCoA reductase. There have also been some studies on PGHS and ACE genotypes in relation to drug response, but, as discussed below, these are generally more limited. Pharmacogenetic studies on other important enzyme targets such as MAO have been concerned mainly with disease susceptibility and are not discussed further.

5.3.1 Vitamin K Epoxide Reductase

Coumarin anticoagulants, including warfarin, acenocoumarol, and phenprocoumon, act by inhibiting the enzyme vitamin K epoxide reductase (VKOR). As shown in Figure 5.4, this enzyme regenerates reduced vitamin K from vitamin K epoxide that is generated during γ carboxylation of coagulation factors [111]. The human enzyme has not been studied extensively but is known to be an integral membrane protein within the endoplasmic reticulum and to have a molecular weight of approx 21,000 daltons [112,113].

Coumarin anticoagulants are among the most widely prescribed drugs worldwide [114]. Unlike most drugs, individualization of coumarin anticoagulant dosing is needed to ensure that adequate anticoagulation is achieved without the patient developing potentially fatal bleeding. Currently, coumarin anticoagulant overdose remains one of the most common reasons for hospital admission due to adverse drug reaction [115] and is also a common cause of adverse drug reaction among inpatients [116].

It is now well established that interindividual variation in the dose of coumarin anticoagulant required to achieve appropriate anticoagulation is due in part to genetic factors affecting both response to the drugs and metabolism by cytochrome P450

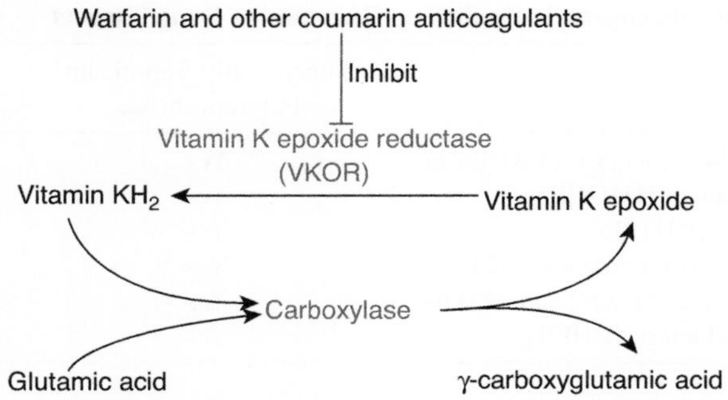

FIGURE 5.4 The vitamin K cycle. The two main enzymes involved are γ-glutamylcarboxylase, which carboxylates glutamate residues on a number of clotting factors in a vitamin K–dependent reaction. Vitamin K epoxide reductase then converts the newly formed vitamin K epoxide back to vitamin K. Warfarin and other coumarin anticoagulants inhibit this reaction, causing lack of vitamin K for the carboxylation reaction.

(see Chapter 2) as well as additional factors such as patient age and body mass index [117]. *VKORC1*, the gene encoding the enzyme vitamin K epoxide reductase in humans, was identified only quite recently [112,118]. It is a small gene located on chromosome 16 with 3 exons. A small proportion of patients treated with coumarin anticoagulants fail to respond at doses within the normal range and are termed *coumarin-resistant*. This lack of response is due mainly to non-synonymous mutations in VKORC1 that appear to affect binding of the anticoagulant to the enzyme. Polymorphisms in coding sequences of VKORC1 are rare but are relatively common in noncoding sequences. A polymorphism at position -1639 ($G \rightarrow A$) is in linkage disequilibrium with a number of other polymorphisms in noncoding sequences [119–121]. The polymorphism has been shown to affect levels of VKORC1 gene expression [120,122], which probably results in interindividual variation in the amount of protein present in hepatocytes. The basis for this is that the A variant is associated with lower transcription than the G found more commonly in European populations [122]. VKOR protein levels appear to be a direct determinant of the required dose of anticoagulant. A clear association between G-1639A genotype and warfarin dose requirement has been reported in a large number of independent studies [120,121,123] and similar associations for the coumarin anticoagulants acenocoumarol and phenprocoumon have also been detected [124,125]. There is ethnic variation in the frequency of the A variant. Although A at position -1639 is less frequent than G in Europeans, it is seen at a higher frequency in East Asians, and as a result, the average dose of coumarin anticoagulant required in East Asian patients is significantly lower than that required in Europeans [126].

It is estimated that approximately 20% of the variability in coumarin anticoagulant dose requirement can be explained by VKORC1 genotype [117]. Anticoagulant dosage is already individualized by measurement of response (coagulation rate measured by prothrombin time), but the possibility that problems with excessive bleeding or lack of response during the initial induction period may be decreased by incorporation of genotyping for VKORC1 and also for CYP2C9, the gene encoding the main metabolizing enzyme (see Chapter 2), is currently under investigation (see also Chapter 6). The potential value of VKORC1 genotyping is also illustrated by the US FDA's recent recommendation that genotyping for common polymorphisms in this gene and CYP2C9 be considered in patients receiving warfarin treatment [127].

5.3.2 HMGCoA Reductase

3-Hydroxy-3-methylglutaryl coenzyme A (HMGCoA) reductase converts 3-hydroxy-3-methylglutaryl coenzyme A to mevalonic acid, which is the rate limiting step in the biosynthesis of cholesterol [128]. It is also the target enzyme for the statins that act to lower plasma cholesterol levels. In view of the large number of patients worldwide now taking statins, the possibility that pharmacogenetic factors, especially those affecting the target, might determine response is of considerable interest. Two polymorphisms in noncoding regions of HMGCR, the gene encoding HMGCoA reductase, are associated with a decreased response to statin treatment and form part of a relatively rare haplotype, including a polymorphism in the 3′-untranslated sequence that may affect RNA stability [129]. The haplotype frequency is approximately 7% in the US population but is more common in African-Americans than in whites [130]. The low haplotype frequency means that up to the present, it has only be possible to study statin response in heterozygotes due to homozygous mutants being extremely rare. The original study reported that this haplotype results in a significantly smaller reduction in both total cholesterol and LDL cholesterol in response to pravastatin treatment, and several more recent studies have attempted to replicate this for both pravastatin and other statins [129–134]. Only two of the five more recent studies have confirmed the original findings [130,134], but there are limitations, with several of the other studies including use of different statins, and failure to provide data on total cholesterol and small sample sizes. The largest more recent study included only white patients with diabetes and did report a significantly smaller decrease in total cholesterol in heterozygotes but no effect on LDL cholesterol [134].

Because of the reported effect on response being relatively small and the low frequency of the SNP, it was suggested in the original report that it is not cost-effective to genotype for polymorphisms in this haplotype as a predictor of statin response [135]. This conclusion seems in line with the findings in the subsequently published studies.

Statins response may be determined by a number of additional pharmacodynamic factors including genotype for other genes that contribute to lipid homeostasis [136] and genes that are independent of the cholesterol pathway [137]. No very clear associations have yet emerged. Some further discussion of this topic can be found in Chapter 6.

5.3.3 Angiotensin-Converting Enzyme (ACE)

Angiotensin-converting enzyme (ACE) catalyzes conversion of the peptide angiotensin I to angiotensin II by removal of two amino acids from the *C* terminus. This reaction is important in regulating blood pressure and maintaining normal electrolyte balance in the body. Because of this, ACE is a important drug target and ACE inhibitors such as enalapril are of value in the treatment of hypertension. ACE is encoded by a large gene of 25 exons located on chromosome 17. A 287-bp deletion/insertion polymorphism in intron 16 has been studied extensively, from the standpoint of both disease susceptibility and drug response (see also Chapter 6). Individuals positive for the deletion have higher plasma levels of ACE activity compared with those positive for the insertion Ref. [138].

The possibility that the insertion/deletion polymorphism genotype might affect response to ACE inhibitors when used for the treatment of cardiovacular disease, including hypertension generally or specifically in diabetics for the prevention of renal and cardiovascular complications, has been the subject of a number of studies [139]. Unfortunately, no clear consensus has emerged from these studies as to whether ACE genotype is a determinant of ACE inhibitor response. The most positive data are from a large study in an Asian population showing that diabetics homozygous for the deletion genotype showed a poorer response to treatment with drugs targeting the renin–angiotensin system, mainly ACE inhibitors in terms of renal endpoint [140]. There is also more limited data from non-Asians in a meta-analysis suggesting that the best response to ACE inhibitor treatment in renal disease prevention is seen in those homozygous for the insertion [141]. It was also suggested on the basis of these findings that treatment with angiotensin 2 inhibitors might be more appropriate for achieving renal protection in those positive for deletion alleles [141]. In separate studies concerned with treatment of cardiovascular disease more generally, no significant association between ACE genotype and outcome of treatment with ACE inhibitors was found [142,143]. The lack of agreement on the relevance of ACE genotype to outcome of treatment with ACE inhibitors may be due to a number of factors, including the possibility that the deletion/insertion polymorphism is not the main SNP determining enzyme levels but simply in linkage disequilibrium with other polymorphisms, including some promoter region polymorphisms. Other complications include the possibility that ACE genotype may also contribute to susceptibility to hypertension and renal disease directly [139].

5.3.4 Other Enzyme Targets

More limited studies on pharmacogenetic relevance have been performed for several other enzyme targets, including prostaglandin H synthase or cycloxygenase, monoamine oxidase, and dihydrofolate reductase; however, up to the present, it is not clear whether genotype for the genes encoding these proteins is relevant to drug response. Cyclooxygenase is the target enzyme for NSAIDs, including aspirin. At least two isoforms, encoded by the genes PGHS1 and PGHS2, occur. Most of the limited pharmacogenetic studies relating to these genes is concerned with studies on aspirin response in relation to its use as an anti-platelet drug. Cyclooxygenase 1, encoded by PGHS1, is expressed in platelets and the target for the antiplatelet effect of aspirin. A more recent large genetic study has indicated that response to aspirin is heritable though this did not include studies on specific genes [144]. Several studies have investigated possible relationships between *PGHS1* genotype and anti-platelet response to aspirin [145,146]. In particular, some evidence for a decreased response associated with an upstream variant allele was reported by Maree and colleagues [146], whereas a separate study found a haplotype including this SNP was associated with greater inhibition of aggregation [145]. Such discrepancies are likely to reflect a number of issues, including small sample size and differences in methods used to determine platelet aggregation, but particularly the complexity of the aggregation pathway, which makes it difficult to study single-gene effects in isolation. There is further coverage of this area in Chapter 6.

Our understanding of the contribution by polymorphism in the gene encoding another important drug target, dihydrofolate reductase, is more limited. Methotrexate, which is widely used in the treatment of cancer and for immunosuppression, is an inhibitor of dihydrofolate reductase. This inhibition results in decreased levels of tetrahydrofolate that will affect *de novo* synthesis of purines and pyrimidines. The folate pathway is complex, with levels of tetrahydrofolate and purine and pyrimidine biosynthesis also subject to regulation by other gene products, including methylene tetrahydrofolate reductase and the reduced folate carrier. Polymorphisms in the genes encoding these proteins may also affect methotrexate response, making it difficult to predict the contribution to variability in response to methotrexate when only the target gene is considered [147]. Only one detailed study on the DHFR gene in relation to methotrexate response has so far been reported. This study on the influence of a range of upstream polymorphisms in *DHFR* on outcome of treatment in acute lymphoblastic leukemia patients, found that poorer event-free survival was associated with a haplotype that the investigators denoted as *1 [148]. The *1 haplotype was also found to be associated with higher DHFR mRNA levels, which would be consistent with poorer inhibition of enzyme activity.

Finally, polymorphisms in the monoamine oxidase genes *MAOA* and *MAOB* have been studied fairly extensively as risk factors for psychiatric disease but also in studies on response to selective serotonin reuptake inhibitors, where monoamine oxidase will be a determinant in levels of 5HT and thus drug response. However, there have been hardly any studies on MAO genotype and response to monoamine oxidase inhibitors, which target monoamine oxidase directly. This probably reflects the fact that monoamine oxidase inhibitors are currently not widely used as antidepressants, mainly because other antidepressant classes are associated with fewer serious side effects.

5.4 TRANSPORTERS

5.4.1 Introduction

Transporters or carrier proteins play an important role in transporting ions and small molecules across cell membranes. This is especially important in the reuptake of a range of neurotransmitters by nerve terminals and receptors that contribute to this process represent an important drug target (for more background, see Chapter 3 in

Rang et al. [1]). The pharmacogenetics of two important neurotransmitter transporters has been well studied, as discussed in detail below.

5.4.2 Serotonin Transporter (5HTT)

The serotonin transporter (5HTT/SERT) mediates 5HT availability in the neurotransmitter pool. After serotonin release in the synapse, the transporter recaptures the neurotransmitter and takes it up to the presynaptic neuron (see Fig. 5.5).

5HTT is a direct target of the selective serotonin reuptake inhibitors (SSRIs) and tricyclic compounds used as antidepressant medications, and may also mediate the toxic effect of cocaine and amphetamines.

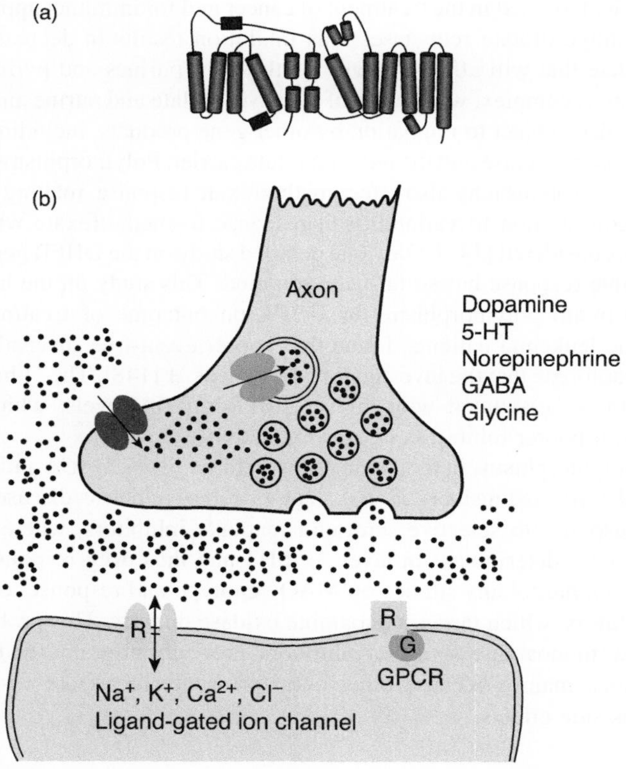

FIGURE 5.5 SLC6 gene family transporter structure: (a) the structure with transmembrane domains shown in red; (b) in the presynaptic nerve terminals of dopamine-, 5HT-, norepinephrine-, glycine-, and GABA-containing synapses, the vesicular transporters [shown in green (e.g., VMAT1 and VMAT2)] sequester neurotransmitters into synaptic vesicles. Released neurotransmitter exerts its effects via receptors such as dopamine receptors, adrenoceptors, and 5HT receptors (light blue, with associated G protein in gray). The plasma membrane transporters encoded by the SLC6 gene family (red) are located in the membrane of the presynaptic neuron (DAT, SERT, NET, GlyT2, GAT1, and GAT2). (Adapted from Gether et al. [177] and reproduced with permission.) (See insert for color representation.)

The 5HTT gene (SLC6A4) spans 31 kb, includes 14 exons [149], and is highly polymorphic, with several polymorphisms of known functional significance. The transcriptional activity of the gene is modulated by a repetitive element upstream of the transcription start site [40]. A common functional polymorphism was described within this region, consisting of a 44-bp insertion or deletion and referred to as *short* (deletion) and *long linked polymorphic region* (LPR) variants. Luciferase reporter gene experiments using human cell lines expressing the 5HTT gene revealed a lower expression of the LPR short variant in comparison with the long variant [150].

A second functional polymorphic repeat with a core sequence of 16/17 bp has been described in intron 2 of the gene, with two common variants of 10 and 12 repeats, and a rarer 9-repeat allele. Transgenic mice including this polymorphism and an associated reporter gene showed higher expression of the 12-repeat variant in comparison to the 10-repeat variant during embryonic development, suggesting a role in brain development and synaptic plasticity [40,41].

Several additional polymorphic single-nucleotide changes and microrepeats have been described [151]. Of particular importance is an A/G single-nucleotide change (rs25331) within the LPR region that alters the functionality of the LPR polymorphism, with the G allele converting the LPR long variant to a low-expression allele (L_G), showing similar levels to those of the LPR short variant, whereas the long variant with the A nucleotide (L_A) retains higher levels of expression [152]. Allele and genotype frequencies of all these polymorphisms show significant geographic variation.

Several studies and meta-analyses have confirmed the association between the 5HTT LPR repeat polymorphism and response to SSRI drugs. The LPR long variant is associated with greater response to antidepressant medications [153,154] although this association is not universally replicated, and geographic differences can be observed. The L variant tends to be more frequent among responders in Caucasian populations, whereas the short variant is the one associated with good response in some Japanese and Korean populations [155]. The association of the L variant with response may reflect the greater availability of the transporter targeted by the drugs. The biological plausibility of the association with the low-expression allele is more complicated to interpret, and require confirmation in further studies, including the function altering rs23551 polymorphism. Surprisingly, a large study conducted in citalopram patients (STAR*D) did not observe any association with response [68], but did find an association with treatment associated side effects [156]. Differences in patient subgroups, population stratification, and heterogeneity may explain this discrepancy. Additional associations have been reported between 5HTT polymorphisms and bipolar disorder [157,158] which may reflect the importance of the transporter in modulating serotonin transmission.

5.4.3 Dopamine Transporter (DAT)

The dopamine transporter (DAT) is a membrane protein that mediates the reuptake of dopamine from the synaptic cleft. The dopamine transporter is the main regulator of dopamine transmission and has been implicated in the aetiology of Parkinson's disease, Tourette's syndrome, bipolar disorder, and substance abuse [159–161]. Disruption of the DAT gene in mouse leads to hyperlocomotion [162], and increased levels of DAT have been observed in brain striatal areas of ADHD patients [31].

The gene encoding the DAT transporters, SLC6A3, is highly polymorphic [163] and contains several common single-nucleotide polymorphisms in the promoter region (−67A/T, −839C/T) as well as two common polymorphic repeats (VNTRs) in the 5′- and 3′-untranslated regions. The polymorphic repeat in the 3′-untranslated region has been widely investigated and exists in two forms, a 9-repeat allele and a 10-repeat allele or a core 40-bp sequence, although rarer alleles occur in different population groups [164]. Messenger RNA levels were higher in the cerebellum, temporal lobe, and lymphocytes of carriers of the 10-repeat allele [165]. Luciferase expression studies using COS7 recombinant cell lines containing this polymorphism agreed with this observation, with vectors containing the 10-repeat showing significantly higher expression levels [166]. However, a study using similar luciferase expression techniques but different cell lines revealed opposite results, with significantly higher expression levels in the vectors containing the 9-repeat allele in comparison with those containing the 10-repeat allele [167]. More recent neuroimaging SPECT studies have revealed higher brain striatal DAT expression in carriers of the 9-repeat allele than in those with the 10-repeat allele [168], thus confirming the latter finding.

The majority of pharmacogenetic investigations report associations of the 3′-polymorphism with response to methylphenidate, a drug used for the treatment of ADHD. This drug blocks the DAT protein, leading to an increased level of synaptic catecholamines and regulating dopamine transmission. The 10 allele repeat of the 3′-VNTR, associated with lower DAT expression, is generally found in higher frequencies in individuals with poorer response to methylphenidate [31,169–172], reflecting the lower availability of the drug target. This polymorphism has also been reported in association with response to antidepressant drugs, but the underlying mechanisms are unclear [173]. These studies confirmed the validity of the DAT transporter as a therapeutic target for the treatment of ADHD, but further investigation on its suitability for the treatment of motor disorders is required.

5.5 CONCLUDING REMARKS

Our knowledge and understanding of the relevance of a variety of polymorphisms in drug targets has increased greatly since 2000 but is still quite limited. It is clear that polymorphisms in VKORC1 affect coumarin anticoagulant response, and there is also increasing evidence that polymorphisms in genes encoding other drug targets such as HMGCoA reductase and ADRB1 affect drug response. However, despite a large number of published studies, our understanding of the relevance of polymorphisms in receptor genes such as those encoding the dopaminergic and serotonergic receptors to drug response is still poor. In addition, there is a need to investigate pharmacogenetic factors affecting response to newly developed drugs. For example, the glutamatergic receptors are targeted by new-generation drugs specific for mGluR2/3 receptors that have shown promising results during clinical trials [174], raising the expectations for improved antipsychotic treatments. Other contemporary examples include drugs such as the newly developed antiplatelet drugs clopidogrel and plasugrel. Though we now understand that not all patients benefit from clopidogrel, due to failure to activate it in CYP2C19 poor metabolizers [175], the possibility that the ability to inhibit platelet activity may be a further source of variability with potentially not all patients showing clear benefit also need to be considered. In general, studies on genetic factors affecting drug response are now beginning to form part of the drug development process, although they still lag behind genetic studies related to drug disposition. Even if studies are not performed during clinical trials, DNA samples from trial participants are increasingly being archived and may provide information on drug response in the future, subject to both ethical and commercial considerations.

REFERENCES

1. Rang HP, Dale MM, Ritter JM, Flower RJ, Henderson G. *Rang and Dale's Pharmacology.* 2011.
2. Missale C, Nash SR, Robinson SW, Jaber M, Caron MG. Dopamine receptors: From structure to function. *Physiol. Rev.* 1998;**78**:189–225.
3. Miyamoto S, Duncan GE, Marx CE, Lieberman JA. Treatments for schizophrenia: A critical review of pharmacology and mechanisms of action of antipsychotic drugs. *Mol. Psychiatry* 2005;**10**:79–104.
4. Jauss M, Krack P, Franz M, Klett R, Bauer R, Gallhofer B, et al. Imaging of dopamine receptors with [123I]iodobenzamide single-photon emission-computed tomography in neuroleptic malignant syndrome. *Mov. Disord.* 1996;**11**:726–728.
5. De KJ. Subtypes and localization of dopamine receptors in human brain. *Neurochem. Int.* 1993;**22**:83–93.
6. Pilowsky LS, Mulligan RS, Acton PD, Ell PJ, Costa DC, Kerwin RW. Limbic selectivity of clozapine. *Lancet* 1997;**350**:490–491.
7. Reynolds GP. Receptor mechanisms in the treatment of schizophrenia. *J. Psychopharmacol.* 2004;**18**:340–345.
8. Natesan S, Reckless GE, Barlow KB, Nobrega JN, Kapur S. Amisulpride the "atypical" atypical antipsychotic–comparison to haloperidol, risperidone and clozapine. *Schizophr. Res.* 2008;**105**:224–235.
9. Himei A, Koh J, Sakai J, Inada Y, Akabame K, Yoneda H. The influence on the schizophrenic symptoms by the DRD2Ser/Cys311 and −141C Ins/Del polymorphisms. *Psychiatry Clin. Neurosci.* 2002;**56**:97–102.
10. Schafer M, Rujescu D, Giegling I, Guntermann A, Erfurth A, Bondy B, et al. Association of short-term response to haloperidol treatment with a polymorphism in the dopamine D (2) receptor gene. *Am. J. Psychiatry* 2001;**158**:802–804.
11. Suzuki A, Kondo T, Mihara K, Yasui-Furukori N, Ishida M, Furukori H, et al. The −141C Ins/Del polymorphism in the dopamine D2 receptor gene promoter region is associated with anxiolytic and antidepressive effects during treatment with dopamine antagonists in schizophrenic patients. *Pharmacogenetics* 2001;**11**:545–550.

12. Arinami T, Gao M, Hamaguchi H, Toru M. A functional polymorphism in the promoter region of the dopamine D2 receptor gene is associated with schizophrenia 1. *Hum. Mol. Genet.* 1997;**6**:577–582.
13. Cravchik A, Sibley DR, Gejman PV. Functional analysis of the human D2 dopamine receptor missense variants. *J. Biol. Chem.* 1996;**271**:26013–26017.
14. Liou YJ, Lai IC, Liao DL, Chen JY, Lin CC, Lin CY, et al. The human dopamine receptor D2 (DRD2) gene is associated with tardive dyskinesia in patients with schizophrenia. *Schizophr. Res.* 2006;**86**:323–325.
15. Zai CC, De LV, Hwang RW, Voineskos A, Muller DJ, Remington G, et al. Meta-analysis of two dopamine D2 receptor gene polymorphisms with tardive dyskinesia in schizophrenia patients. *Mol. Psychiatry* 2007;**12**:794–795.
16. Bakker PR, van Harten PN, van OJ. Antipsychotic-induced tardive dyskinesia and polymorphic variations in COMT, DRD2, CYP1A2 and MnSOD genes: A meta-analysis of pharmacogenetic interactions. *Mol. Psychiatry* 2008;**13**:544–556.
17. Shen YC, Chen SF, Chen CH, Lin CC, Chen SJ, Chen YJ, et al. Effects of DRD2/ANKK1 gene variations and clinical factors on aripiprazole efficacy in schizophrenic patients. *J. Psychiatr. Res.* 2009;**43**:600–606.
18. Kwon JS, Kim E, Kang DH, Choi JS, Yu KS, Jang IJ, et al. Taq1A polymorphism in the dopamine D2 receptor gene as a predictor of clinical response to aripiprazole. *Eur. Neuropsychopharmacol.* 2008;**18**:897–907.
19. Neville MJ, Johnstone EC, Walton RT. Identification and characterization of ANKK1: A novel kinase gene closely linked to DRD2 on chromosome band 11q23.1. *Hum. Mutat.* 2004;**23**:540–545.
20. Reynolds GP, Yao Z, Zhang X, Sun J, Zhang Z. Pharmacogenetics of treatment in first-episode schizophrenia: D3 and 5-HT2C receptor polymorphisms separately associate with positive and negative symptom response. *Eur. Neuropsychopharmacol.* 2005;**15**:143–151.
21. Staddon S, Arranz MJ, Mancama D, Mata I, Kerwin RW. Clinical applications of pharmacogenetics in psychiatry. *Psychopharmacology (Berlin)* 2002;**162**:18–23.
22. Lerer B, Segman RH, Fangerau H, Daly AK, Basile VS, Cavallaro R, et al. Pharmacogenetics of tardive dyskinesia. Combined analysis of 780 patients supports association with dopamine D3 receptor gene Ser9Gly polymorphism. *Neuropsychopharmacology* 2002;**27**:105–119.
23. Wang X, Zhong P, Yan Z. Dopamine D4 receptors modulate GABAergic signaling in pyramidal neurons of prefrontal cortex. *J. Neurosci.* 2002;**22**:9185–9193.
24. Yuen EY, Yan Z. Dopamine D4 receptors regulate AMPA receptor trafficking and glutamatergic transmission in GABAergic interneurons of prefrontal cortex. *J. Neurosci.* 2009;**29**:550–562.
25. Kramer MS, Last B, Getson A, Reines SA. The effects of a selective D4 dopamine receptor antagonist (L-745, 870) in acutely psychotic inpatients with schizophrenia. D4 dopamine antagonist group. *Arch. Gen. Psychiatry* 1997;**54**:567–572.
26. Truffinet P, Tamminga CA, Fabre LF, Meltzer HY, Riviere ME, Papillon-Downey C. Placebo-controlled study of the D4/5-HT2A antagonist fananserin in the treatment of schizophrenia. *Am. J. Psychiatry* 1999;**156**:419–425.
27. Shaikh S, Collier D, Kerwin RW, Pilowsky LS, Gill M, Xu WM, et al. Dopamine D4 receptor subtypes and response to clozapine. *Lancet* 1993;**341**:116.

28. Shaikh S, Kerwin R, Sham P, Sharma T, Collier D. D4 polymorphisms in schizophrenic patients treated with clozapine. *Schizophr. Res.* 1994;**15**:165–166.
29. Kohn Y, Ebstein RP, Heresco-Levy U, Shapira B, Nemanov L, Gritsenko I, et al. Dopamine D4 receptor gene polymorphisms: Relation to ethnicity, no association with schizophrenia and response to clozapine in Israeli subjects. *Eur. Neuropsychopharmacol.* 1997;**7**:39–43.
30. Rao PA, Pickar D, Gejman PV, Ram A, Gershon ES, Gelernter J. Allelic variation in the D4 dopamine receptor (DRD4) gene does not predict response to clozapine. *Arch. Gen. Psychiatry* 1994;**51**:912–917.
31. McGough JJ. Attention-deficit/hyperactivity disorder pharmacogenomics. *Biol. Psychiatry* 2005;**57**:1367–1373.
32. Schoots O, Van Tol HH. The human dopamine D4 receptor repeat sequences modulate expression. *Pharmacogenomics J.* 2003;**3**:343–348.
33. Ebstein RP, Novick O, Umansky R, Priel B, Osher Y, Blaine D, et al. Dopamine D4 receptor (D4DR) exon III polymorphism associated with the human personality trait of novelty seeking 1. *Nat. Genet.* 1996;**12**:78–80.
34. Shao C, Li Y, Jiang K, Zhang D, Xu Y, Lin L, et al. Dopamine D4 receptor polymorphism modulates cue-elicited heroin craving in Chinese. *Psychopharmacology (Berlin)* 2006;**186**:185–190.
35. Cheon KA, Kim BN, Cho SC. Association of 4-repeat allele of the dopamine D4 receptor gene exon III polymorphism and response to methylphenidate treatment in Korean ADHD children. *Neuropsychopharmacology* 2007;**32**:1377–1383.
36. Schinka JA, Letsch EA, Crawford FC. DRD4 and novelty seeking: Results of meta-analyses. *Am. J. Med. Genet.* 2002;**114**:643–648.
37. Szilagyi A, Boor K, Szekely A, Gaszner P, Kalasz H, Sasvari-Szekely M, et al. Combined effect of promoter polymorphisms in the dopamine D4 receptor and the serotonin transporter genes in heroin dependence. *Neuropsychopharmacol. Hung.* 2005;**7**:28–33.
38. Zai CC, Tiwari AK, Basile V, De LV, Muller DJ, King N, et al. Association study of tardive dyskinesia and five DRD4 polymorphisms in schizophrenia patients. *Pharmacogenomics J.* 2009;**9**:168–174.
39. Terry AV, Jr., Buccafusco JJ, Wilson C. Cognitive dysfunction in neuropsychiatric disorders: Selected serotonin receptor subtypes as therapeutic targets. *Behav. Brain Res.* 2008;**195**:30–38.
40. Lesch KP, Gutknecht L. Pharmacogenetics of the serotonin transporter. *Prog. Neuropsychopharmacol. Biol. Psychiatry* 2005;**29**:1062–1073.
41. Lesch KP. Genetic alterations of the murine serotonergic gene pathway: The neurodevelopmental basis of anxiety. *Handbook Exp. Pharmacol.* 2005;**169**:71–112.
42. Roth BL, Hanizavareh SM, Blum AE. Serotonin receptors represent highly favorable molecular targets for cognitive enhancement in schizophrenia and other disorders. *Psychopharmacology (Berlin)* 2004;**174**:17–24.
43. Hannon J, Hoyer D. Molecular biology of 5-HT receptors. *Behav. Brain Res.* 2008;**195**:198–213.
44. Hoyer D, Hannon JP, Martin GR. Molecular, pharmacological and functional diversity of 5-HT receptors. *Pharmacol. Biochem. Behav.* 2002;**71**:533–554.

45. Ogren SO, Eriksson TM, Elvander-Tottie E, D'Addario C, Ekstrom JC, Svenningsson P, et al. The role of 5-HT (1A) receptors in learning and memory. *Behav. Brain Res.* 2008;**195**:54–77.

46. Meltzer HY, Sumiyoshi T. Does stimulation of 5-HT (1A) receptors improve cognition in schizophrenia? *Behav. Brain Res.* 2008;**195**:98–102.

47. Reynolds GP, Arranz B, Templeman LA, Fertuzinhos S, San L. Effect of 5-HT1A receptor gene polymorphism on negative and depressive symptom response to antipsychotic treatment of drug-naive psychotic patients. *Am. J. Psychiatry* 2006;**163**:1826–1829.

48. Wang L, Fang C, Zhang A, Du J, Yu L, Ma J, et al. The –1019 C/G polymorphism of the 5-HT (1)A receptor gene is associated with negative symptom response to risperidone treatment in schizophrenia patients. *J. Psychopharmacol.* 2008;**22**:904–909.

49. Mossner R, Schuhmacher A, Kuhn KU, Cvetanovska G, Rujescu D, Zill P, et al. Functional serotonin 1A receptor variant influences treatment response to atypical antipsychotics in schizophrenia. *Pharmacogenet. Genomics* 2009;**19**:91–94.

50. Lemonde S, Du L, Bakish D, Hrdina P, Albert PR. Association of the C(–1019)G 5-HT1A functional promoter polymorphism with antidepressant response. *Int. J. Neuropsychopharmacol.* 2004;**7**:501–506.

51. Lemonde S, Turecki G, Bakish D, Du L, Hrdina PD, Bown CD, et al. Impaired repression at a 5-hydroxytryptamine 1A receptor gene polymorphism associated with major depression and suicide. *J. Neurosci.* 2003;**23**:8788–8799.

52. Serretti A, Artioli P, Lorenzi C, Pirovano A, Tubazio V, Zanardi R. The C (–1019)G polymorphism of the 5-HT1A gene promoter and antidepressant response in mood disorders: Preliminary findings. *Int. J. Neuropsychopharmacol.* 2004;**7**:453–460.

53. Baune BT, Hohoff C, Roehrs T, Deckert J, Arolt V, Domschke K. Serotonin receptor 1A-1019C/G variant: Impact on antidepressant pharmacoresponse in melancholic depression? *Neurosci. Lett.* 2008;**436**:111–115.

54. Kato M, Fukuda T, Wakeno M, Okugawa G, Takekita Y, Watanabe S, et al. Effect of 5-HT1A gene polymorphisms on antidepressant response in major depressive disorder. *Am. J. Med. Genet. B Neuropsychiatr. Genet.* 2009;**150B**:115–123.

55. Kapur S, Remington G. Dopamine D (2) receptors and their role in atypical antipsychotic action: Still necessary and may even be sufficient. *Biol. Psychiatry* 2001;**50**:873–883.

56. Kapur S, Seeman P. Does fast dissociation from the dopamine d (2) receptor explain the action of atypical antipsychotics? A new hypothesis. *Am. J. Psychiatry* 2001;**158**:360–369.

57. Spurlock G, Heils A, Holmans P, Williams J, D'Souza UM, Cardno A, et al. A family based association study of T102C polymorphism in 5HT2A and schizophrenia plus identification of new polymorphisms in the promoter. *Mol. Psychiatry* 1998;**3**:42–49.

58. Bonnier B, Gorwood P, Hamon M, Sarfati Y, Boni C, Hardy-Bayle MC. Association of 5-HT (2A) receptor gene polymorphism with major affective disorders: The case of a subgroup of bipolar disorder with low suicide risk. *Biol. Psychiatry* 2002;**51**:762–765.

59. Nacmias B, Tedde A, Forleo P, Piacentini S, Guarnieri BM, Bartoli A, et al. Association between 5-HT (2A) receptor polymorphism and psychotic symptoms in Alzheimer's disease. *Biol. Psychiatry* 2001;**50**:472–475.

60. Arranz MJ, Munro J, Owen MJ, Spurlock J, Sham P, Zhao J, et al. Evidence for association between polymorphisms in the promoter and coding regions of the 5-HT2A receptor gene and response to clozapine. *Mol. Psychiatry* 1998;**3**:61–66.

61. Arranz MJ, Munro J, Sham P, Kirov G, Murray RM, Collier DA, et al. Meta-analysis of studies on genetic variation in 5-HT2A receptors and clozapine response. *Schizophr. Res.* 1998;**32**:93–99.

62. Lane HY, Chang YC, Chiu CC, Chen ML, Hsieh MH, Chang WH. Association of risperidone treatment response with a polymorphism in the 5-HT (2A) receptor gene. *Am. J. Psychiatry* 2002;**159**:1593–1595.

63. Benmessaoud D, Hamdani N, Boni C, Ramoz N, Hamon M, Kacha F, et al. Excess of transmission of the G allele of the −1438A/G polymorphism of the 5-HT2A receptor gene in patients with schizophrenia responsive to antipsychotics. *BMC Psychiatry* 2008;**8**:40.

64. Kim B, Choi EY, Kim CY, Song K, Joo YH. Could HTR2A T102C and DRD3 Ser9Gly predict clinical improvement in patients with acutely exacerbated schizophrenia? Results from treatment responses to risperidone in a naturalistic setting. *Hum. Psychopharmacol.* 2008;**23**:61–67.

65. Parsons MJ, D'Souza UM, Arranz MJ, Kerwin RW, Makoff AJ. The −1438A/G polymorphism in the 5-hydroxytryptamine type 2A receptor gene affects promoter activity. *Biol. Psychiatry* 2004;**56**:406–410.

66. Myers RL, Airey DC, Manier DH, Shelton RC, Sanders-Bush E. Polymorphisms in the regulatory region of the human serotonin 5-HT (2A) receptor gene (HTR2A) influence gene expression. *Biol. Psychiatry* 2007;**61**:167–173.

67. Hazelwood LA, Sanders-Bush E. His452Tyr polymorphism in the human 5-HT2A receptor destabilizes the signaling conformation. *Mol. Pharmacol.* 2004;**66**:1293–1300.

68. McMahon FJ, Buervenich S, Charney D, Lipsky R, Rush AJ, Wilson AF, et al. Variation in the gene encoding the serotonin 2A receptor is associated with outcome of antidepressant treatment. *Am. J. Hum. Genet.* 2006;**78**:804–814.

69. Uher R, Huezo-Diaz P, Perroud N, Smith R, Rietschel M, Mors O, et al. Genetic predictors of response to antidepressants in the GENDEP project. *Pharmacogenomics J.* 2009;**9**:225–233.

70. Segman RH, Heresco-Levy U, Finkel B, Goltser T, Shalem R, Schlafman M, et al. Association between the serotonin 2A receptor gene and tardive dyskinesia in chronic schizophrenia. *Mol. Psychiatry* 2001;**6**:225–229.

71. Lerer B, Segman RH, Tan EC, Basile VS, Cavallaro R, Aschauer HN, et al. Combined analysis of 635 patients confirms an age-related association of the serotonin 2A receptor gene with tardive dyskinesia and specificity for the non-orofacial subtype. *Int. J. Neuropsychopharmacol.* 2005;**8**:411–425.

72. Reynolds GP, Zhang ZJ, Zhang XB. Association of antipsychotic drug-induced weight gain with a 5-HT2C receptor gene polymorphism. *Lancet* 2002;**359**:2086–2087.

73. Ryu S, Cho EY, Park T, Oh S, Jang WS, Kim SK, et al. −759 C/T polymorphism of 5-HT2C receptor gene and early phase weight gain associated with antipsychotic drug treatment. *Prog. Neuropsychopharmacol. Biol. Psychiatry* 2007;**31**:673–677.

74. Hill MJ, Reynolds GP. 5-HT2C receptor gene polymorphisms associated with antipsychotic drug action alter promoter activity. *Brain Res.* 2007;**1149**:14–17.

75. De LV, Mueller DJ, de BA, Kennedy JL. Association of the HTR2C gene and antipsychotic induced weight gain: A meta-analysis. *Int. J. Neuropsychopharmacol.* 2007;**10**:697–704.

76. Mulder H, Cohen D, Scheffer H, Gispen-de WC, Arends J, Wilmink FW, et al. HTR2C gene polymorphisms and the metabolic syndrome in patients with schizophrenia: A replication study. *J. Clin. Psychopharmacol.* 2009;**29**:16–20.

77. Sodhi M, Sham P, Makoff A, Collier DA, Arranz MJ, Munro J, et al. Replication and meta-analysis of alleleic association of a 5-HT2C receptor polymorphism with good response to clozapine. *Mol. Psychiatry* 1999;**4**:225–226.

78. Zhang ZJ, Zhang XB, Sha WW, Zhang XB, Reynolds GP. Association of a polymorphism in the promoter region of the serotonin 5-HT2C receptor gene with tardive dyskinesia in patients with schizophrenia 1. *Mol. Psychiatry* 2002;**7**:670–671.

79. Segman RH, Lerer B. Age and the relationship of dopamine D3, serotonin 2C and serotonin 2A receptor genes to abnormal involuntary movements in chronic schizophrenia. *Mol. Psychiatry* 2002;**7**:137–139.

80. Gutierrez B, Arranz MJ, Huezo-Diaz P, Dempster D, Matthiasson P, Travis M, et al. Novel mutations in 5-HT3A and 5-HT3B receptor genes not associated with clozapine response. *Schizophr. Res.* 2002;**58**:93–97.

81. Yu YWY, Tsai SJ, Lin CH, Hsu CP, Ynakg KH, Hong CJ. Serotonin-6 receptor variant (C267T) and clinical response to clozapine. *Neuroreport* 1999;**10**:1231–1233.

82. Wei Z, Wang L, Xuan J, Che R, Du J, Qin S, et al. Association analysis of serotonin receptor 7 gene (HTR7) and risperidone response in Chinese schizophrenia patients. *Prog. Neuropsychopharmacol. Biol. Psychiatry* 2009;**33**:547–551.

83. Brodde OE. Beta-1 and beta-2 adrenoceptor polymorphisms: Functional importance, impact on cardiovascular diseases and drug responses. *Pharmacol. Ther.* 2008;**117**:1–29.

84. Rosskopf D, Michel MC. Pharmacogenomics of G protein-coupled receptor ligands in cardiovascular medicine. *Pharmacol. Rev.* 2008;**60**:513–535.

85. Hawkins GA, Weiss ST, Bleecker ER. Clinical consequences of ADRbeta2 polymorphisms. *Pharmacogenomics* 2008;**9**:349–358.

86. Hall IP, Sayers I. Pharmacogenetics and asthma: False hope or new dawn? *Eur. Respir. J.* 2007;**29**:1239–1245.

87. Small KM, Liggett SB. Identification and functional characterization of alpha (2)-adrenoceptor polymorphisms. *Trends Pharmacol. Sci.* 2001;**22**:471–477.

88. Small KM, Wagoner LE, Levin AM, Kardia SL, Liggett SB. Synergistic polymorphisms of beta1- and alpha2C-adrenergic receptors and the risk of congestive heart failure. *New Engl. J. Med.* 2002;**347**:1135–1142.

89. Kurnik D, Friedman EA, Muszkat M, Sofowora GG, Xie HG, Dupont WD, et al. Genetic variants in the alpha2C-adrenoceptor and G-protein contribute to ethnic differences in cardiovascular stress responses. *Pharmacogenet. Genomics* 2008;**18**:743–750.

90. Canham RM, Das SR, Leonard D, Abdullah SM, Mehta SK, Chung AK, et al. Alpha2cDel322-325 and beta1Arg389 adrenergic polymorphisms are not associated with reduced left ventricular ejection fraction or increased left ventricular volume. *J. Am. Coll. Cardiol.* 2007;**49**:274–276.

91. Lobmeyer MT, Gong Y, Terra SG, Beitelshees AL, Langaee TY, Pauly DF, et al. Synergistic polymorphisms of beta1 and alpha2C-adrenergic receptors and the influence

on left ventricular ejection fraction response to beta-blocker therapy in heart failure. *Pharmacogenet. Genomics* 2007;**17**:277–282.

92. Mason DA, Moore JD, Green SA, Liggett SB. A gain-of-function polymorphism in a G-protein coupling domain of the human beta1-adrenergic receptor. *J. Biol. Chem.* 1999;**274**:12670–12674.
93. Belfer I, Buzas B, Evans C, Hipp H, Phillips G, Taubman J, et al. Haplotype structure of the beta adrenergic receptor genes in US Caucasians and African Americans. *Eur. J. Hum. Genet.* 2005;**13**:341–351.
94. Levin MC, Marullo S, Muntaner O, Andersson B, Magnusson Y. The myocardium-protective Gly-49 variant of the beta 1-adrenergic receptor exhibits constitutive activity and increased desensitization and down-regulation. *J. Biol. Chem.* 2002;**277**:30429–30435.
95. Rathz DA, Brown KM, Kramer LA, Liggett SB. Amino acid 49 polymorphisms of the human beta1-adrenergic receptor affect agonist-promoted trafficking. *J. Cardiovasc. Pharmacol.* 2002;**39**:155–160.
96. Drysdale CM, McGraw DW, Stack CB, Stephens JC, Judson RS, Nandabalan K, et al. Complex promoter and coding region beta 2-adrenergic receptor haplotypes alter receptor expression and predict in vivo responsiveness. *Proc. Natl. Acad. Sci. USA* 2000;**97**:10483–10488.
97. Green SA, Turki J, Innis M, Liggett SB. Amino-terminal polymorphisms of the human beta 2-adrenergic receptor impart distinct agonist-promoted regulatory properties. *Biochemistry* 1994;**33**:9414–9419.
98. Collins S, Caron MG, Lefkowitz RJ. From ligand binding to gene expression: New insights into the regulation of G-protein-coupled receptors. *Trends Biochem. Sci.* 1992;**17**:37–39.
99. Chong LK, Chowdry J, Ghahramani P, Peachell PT. Influence of genetic polymorphisms in the beta2-adrenoceptor on desensitization in human lung mast cells. *Pharmacogenetics* 2000;**10**:153–162.
100. Moore PE, Laporte JD, Abraham JH, Schwartzman IN, Yandava CN, Silverman ES, et al. Polymorphism of the beta (2)-adrenergic receptor gene and desensitization in human airway smooth muscle. *Am. J. Respir. Crit. Care. Med.* 2000;**162**:2117–2124.
101. Taylor DR, Drazen JM, Herbison GP, Yandava CN, Hancox RJ, Town GI. Asthma exacerbations during long term beta agonist use: Influence of beta (2) adrenoceptor polymorphism. *Thorax* 2000;**55**:762–767.
102. Israel E, Chinchilli VM, Ford JG, Boushey HA, Cherniack R, Craig TJ, et al. Use of regularly scheduled albuterol treatment in asthma: Genotype-stratified, randomised, placebo-controlled cross-over trial. *Lancet* 2004;**364**:1505–1512.
103. Bleecker ER, Postma DS, Lawrance RM, Meyers DA, Ambrose HJ, Goldman M. Effect of ADRB2 polymorphisms on response to longacting beta2-agonist therapy: A pharmacogenetic analysis of two randomised studies. *Lancet* 2007;**370**:2118–2125.
104. de Groote P, Helbecque N, Lamblin N, Hermant X, Mc Fadden E, Foucher-Hossein C, et al. Association between beta-1 and beta-2 adrenergic receptor gene polymorphisms and the response to beta-blockade in patients with stable congestive heart failure. *Pharmacogenet. Genomics* 2005;**15**:137–142.
105. Sehnert AJ, Daniels SE, Elashoff M, Wingrove JA, Burrow CR, Horne B, et al. Lack of association between adrenergic receptor genotypes and survival in heart failure patients treated with carvedilol or metoprolol. *J. Am. Coll. Cardiol.* 2008;**52**:644–651.

106. Pacanowski MA, Gong Y, Cooper-Dehoff RM, Schork NJ, Shriver MD, Langaee TY, et al. beta-adrenergic receptor gene polymorphisms and beta-blocker treatment outcomes in hypertension. *Clin. Pharmacol. Ther.* 2008;**84**:715–721.

107. Leineweber K, Buscher R, Bruck H, Brodde OE. Beta-adrenoceptor polymorphisms. *Naunyn. Schmiedebergs Arch. Pharmacol.* 2004;**369**:1–22.

108. Strosberg AD. Association of beta 3-adrenoceptor polymorphism with obesity and diabetes: current status. *Trends Pharmacol. Sci.* 1997;**18**:449–454.

109. Pietri-Rouxel F, St John Manning B, Gros J, Strosberg AD. The biochemical effect of the naturally occurring Trp64-- > Arg mutation on human beta3-adrenoceptor activity. *Eur. J. Biochem.* 1997;**247**:1174–1179.

110. Vrydag W, Alewijnse AE, Michel MC. Do gene polymorphisms alone or in combination affect the function of human beta3-adrenoceptors? *Br. J. Pharmacol.* 2009;**156**:127–134.

111. Stafford DW. The vitamin K cycle. *J. Thromb. Haemost.* 2005;**3**:1873–1878.

112. Li T, Chang CY, Jin DY, Lin PJ, Khvorova A, Stafford DW. Identification of the gene for vitamin K epoxide reductase. *Nature* 2004;**427**:541–544.

113. Tie JK, Nicchitta C, von Heijne G, Stafford DW. Membrane topology mapping of vitamin K epoxide reductase by in vitro translation/cotranslocation. *J. Biol. Chem.* 2005;**280**:16410–16416.

114. Hirsh J, Dalen J, Anderson DR, Poller L, Bussey H, Ansell J, et al. Oral anticoagulants: Mechanism of action, clinical effectiveness, and optimal therapeutic range. *Chest* 2001;**119**:8S–21S.

115. Pirmohamed M, James S, Meakin S, Green C, Scott AK, Walley TJ, et al. Adverse drug reactions as cause of admission to hospital: Prospective analysis of 18 820 patients. *Br. Med. J.* 2004;**329**:15–19.

116. Davies EC, Green CF, Taylor S, Williamson PR, Mottram DR, Pirmohamed M. Adverse drug reactions in hospital in-patients: A prospective analysis of 3695 patient-episodes. *PLoS ONE* 2009;**4**:e4439.

117. Klein TE, Altman RB, Eriksson N, Gage BF, Kimmel SE, Lee MT, et al. Estimation of the warfarin dose with clinical and pharmacogenetic data. *New Engl. J. Med.* 2009;**360**:753–764.

118. Rost S, Fregin A, Ivaskevicius V, Conzelmann E, Hortnagel K, Pelz HJ, et al. Mutations in VKORC1 cause warfarin resistance and multiple coagulation factor deficiency type 2. *Nature* 2004;**427**:537–541.

119. Bodin L, Verstuyft C, Tregouet DA, Robert A, Dubert L, Funck-Brentano C, et al. Cytochrome P4502C9 (CYP2C9) and vitamin K epoxide reductase (VKORC1) genotypes as determinants of acenocoumarol sensitivity. *Blood* 2005;**106**:135–140.

120. Rieder MJ, Reiner AP, Gage BF, Nickerson DA, Eby CS, McLeod HL, et al. Effect of VKORC1 haplotypes on transcriptional regulation and warfarin dose. *New Engl. J. Med.* 2005;**352**:2285–2293.

121. Sconce EA, Khan TI, Wynne HA, Avery P, Monkhouse L, King BP, et al. The impact of CYP2C9 and VKORC1 genetic polymorphism and patient characteristics upon warfarin dose requirements: Proposal for a new dosing regimen. *Blood* 2005;**106**: 2329–2333.

122. Wang D, Chen H, Momary KM, Cavallari LH, Johnson JA, Sadee W. Regulatory polymorphism in vitamin K epoxide reductase complex subunit 1 (VKORC1) affects gene expression and warfarin dose requirement. *Blood* 2008;**112**:1013–1021.

123. D'Andrea G, D'Ambrosio R L, Di Perna P, Chetta M, Santacroce R, Brancaccio V, et al. A polymorphism in VKORC1 gene is associated with an inter-individual variability in the dose-anticoagulant effect of warfarin. *Blood* 2005;**105**:645–649.
124. Schalekamp T, Brasse BP, Roijers JF, Chahid Y, van Geest-Daalderop JH, de Vries-Goldschmeding H, et al. VKORC1 and CYP2C9 genotypes and acenocoumarol anticoagulation status: Interaction between both genotypes affects overanticoagulation. *Clin. Pharmacol. Ther.* 2006;**80**:13–22.
125. Reitsma PH, van der Heijden JF, Groot AP, Rosendaal FR, Buller HR. A C1173T dimorphism in the VKORC1 gene determines coumarin sensitivity and bleeding risk. *PLoS Med* 2005;**2**:e312.
126. Veenstra DL, You JH, Rieder MJ, Farin FM, Wilkerson HW, Blough DK, et al. Association of vitamin K epoxide reductase complex 1 (VKORC1) variants with warfarin dose in a Hong Kong Chinese patient population. *Pharmacogenet. Genomics* 2005;**15**:687–691.
127. Gage BF, Lesko LJ. Pharmacogenetics of warfarin: Regulatory, scientific, and clinical issues. *J. Thromb. Thrombolysis* 2008;**25**:45–51.
128. Goldstein JL, Brown MS. Regulation of the mevalonate pathway. *Nature* 1990;**343**:425–430.
129. Chasman DI, Posada D, Subrahmanyan L, Cook NR, Stanton VP Jr, Ridker PM. Pharmacogenetic study of statin therapy and cholesterol reduction. *JAMA* 2004;**291**:2821–2827.
130. Krauss RM, Mangravite LM, Smith JD, Medina MW, Wang D, Guo X, et al. Variation in the 3-hydroxyl-3-methylglutaryl coenzyme a reductase gene is associated with racial differences in low-density lipoprotein cholesterol response to simvastatin treatment. *Circulation* 2008;**117**:1537–1544.
131. Thompson JF, Man M, Johnson KJ, Wood LS, Lira ME, Lloyd DB, et al. An association study of 43 SNPs in 16 candidate genes with atorvastatin response. *Pharmacogenomics J.* 2005;**5**:352–358.
132. Singer JB, Holdaas H, Jardine AG, Fellstrom B, Os I, Bermann G, et al. Genetic analysis of fluvastatin response and dyslipidemia in renal transplant recipients. *J. Lipid. Res.* 2007;**48**:2072–2078.
133. Polisecki E, Muallem H, Maeda N, Peter I, Robertson M, McMahon AD, et al. Genetic variation at the LDL receptor and HMG-CoA reductase gene loci, lipid levels, statin response, and cardiovascular disease incidence in PROSPER. *Atherosclerosis* 2008;**200**:109–114.
134. Donnelly LA, Doney AS, Dannfald J, Whitley AL, Lang CC, Morris AD, et al. A paucimorphic variant in the HMG-CoA reductase gene is associated with lipid-lowering response to statin treatment in diabetes: A GoDARTS study. *Pharmacogenet. Genomics* 2008;**18**:1021–1026.
135. Chasman DI, Ridker PM. Pharmacogenetics: The outlook for genetic testing in statin therapy. *Nat. Clin. Pract. Cardiovasc. Med.* 2005;**2**:2–3.
136. Kuivenhoven JA, Jukema JW, Zwinderman AH, de Knijff P, McPherson R, Bruschke AV, et al. The role of a common variant of the cholesteryl ester transfer protein gene in the progression of coronary atherosclerosis. The regression growth evaluation statin study group. *New Engl. J. Med.* 1998;**338**:86–93.
137. Wang CY, Liu PY, Liao JK. Pleiotropic effects of statin therapy: Molecular mechanisms and clinical results. *Trends Mol. Med.* 2008;**14**:37–44.

138. Jeunemaitre X. Genetics of the human renin angiotensin system. *J. Mol. Med.* 2008;**86**:637–641.

139. Rudnicki M, Mayer G. Significance of genetic polymorphisms of the renin-angiotensin-aldosterone system in cardiovascular and renal disease. *Pharmacogenomics* 2009;**10**:463–476.

140. So WY, Ma RC, Ozaki R, Tong PC, Ng MC, Ho CS, et al. Angiotensin-converting enzyme (ACE) inhibition in type 2, diabetic patients—interaction with ACE insertion/deletion polymorphism. *Kidney Int.* 2006;**69**:1438–1443.

141. Ruggenenti P, Bettinaglio P, Pinares F, Remuzzi G. Angiotensin converting enzyme insertion/deletion polymorphism and renoprotection in diabetic and nondiabetic nephropathies. *Clin. J. Am. Soc. Nephrol.* 2008;**3**:1511–1525.

142. Harrap SB, Tzourio C, Cambien F, Poirier O, Raoux S, Chalmers J, et al. The ACE gene I/D polymorphism is not associated with the blood pressure and cardiovascular benefits of ACE inhibition. *Hypertension* 2003;**42**:297–303.

143. Arnett DK, Davis BR, Ford CE, Boerwinkle E, Leiendecker-Foster C, Miller MB, et al. Pharmacogenetic association of the angiotensin-converting enzyme insertion/deletion polymorphism on blood pressure and cardiovascular risk in relation to antihypertensive treatment: The genetics of hypertension-associated treatment (GenHAT) study. *Circulation* 2005;**111**:3374–3383.

144. Faraday N, Yanek LR, Mathias R, Herrera-Galeano JE, Vaidya D, Moy TF, et al. Heritability of platelet responsiveness to aspirin in activation pathways directly and indirectly related to cyclooxygenase-1. *Circulation* 2007;**115**:2490–2496.

145. Halushka MK, Walker LP, Halushka PV. Genetic variation in cyclooxygenase 1: Effects on response to aspirin. *Clin. Pharmacol. Ther.* 2003;**73**:122–130.

146. Maree AO, Curtin RJ, Chubb A, Dolan C, Cox D, O'Brien J, et al. Cyclooxygenase-1 haplotype modulates platelet response to aspirin. *J. Thromb. Haemost.* 2005;**3**:2340–2345.

147. Robien K, Boynton A, Ulrich CM. Pharmacogenetics of folate-related drug targets in cancer treatment. *Pharmacogenomics* 2005;**6**:673–689.

148. Dulucq S, St-Onge G, Gagne V, Ansari M, Sinnett D, Labuda D, et al. DNA variants in the dihydrofolate reductase gene and outcome in childhood ALL. *Blood* 2008;**111**:3692–3700.

149. Lesch KP, Heils A, Riederer P. The role of neurotransporters in excitotoxicity, neuronal cell death, and other neurodegenerative processes. *J. Mol. Med.* 1996;**74**:365–378.

150. Lesch KP, Bengel D, Heils A, Sabol SZ, Greenberg BD, Petri S, et al. Association of anxiety-related traits with a polymorphism in the serotonin transporter gene regulatory region. *Science* 1996;**274**:1527–1531.

151. Nakamura M, Ueno S, Sano A, Tanabe H. The human serotonin transporter gene linked polymorphism (5-HTTLPR) shows ten novel allelic variants. *Mol. Psychiatry* 2000;**5**:32–38.

152. Hu X, Oroszi G, Chun J, Smith TL, Goldman D, Schuckit MA. An expanded evaluation of the relationship of four alleles to the level of response to alcohol and the alcoholism risk. *Alcohol Clin. Exp. Res.* 2005;**29**:8–16.

153. Serretti A, Artioli P, Quartesan R. Pharmacogenetics in the treatment of depression: Pharmacodynamic studies. *Pharmacogenet. Genomics* 2005;**15**:61–67.

154. Serretti A, Kato M, De RD, Kinoshita T. Meta-analysis of serotonin transporter gene promoter polymorphism (5-HTTLPR) association with selective serotonin reuptake inhibitor efficacy in depressed patients. *Mol. Psychiatry* 2007;**12**:247–257.

155. Kraft JB, Peters EJ, Slager SL, Jenkins GD, Reinalda MS, McGrath PJ, et al. Analysis of association between the serotonin transporter and antidepressant response in a large clinical sample. *Biol. Psychiatry* 2007;**61**:734–742.

156. Hu XZ, Rush AJ, Charney D, Wilson AF, Sorant AJ, Papanicolaou GJ, et al. Association between a functional serotonin transporter promoter polymorphism and citalopram treatment in adult outpatients with major depression. *Arch. Gen. Psychiatry* 2007;**64**:783–792.

157. Collier DA, Stober G, Li T, Heils A, Catalano M, Di Bella D, et al. A novel functional polymorphism within the promoter of the serotonin transporter gene: Possible role in susceptibility to affective disorders. *Mol. Psychiatry* 1996;**1**:453–460.

158. Gutierrez B, Arranz MJ, Collier DA, Valles V, Guillamat R, Bertranpetit J, et al. Serotonin transporter gene and risk for bipolar affective disorder: An association study in Spanish population. *Biol. Psychiatry* 1998;**43**:843–847.

159. Yoon DY, Rippel CA, Kobets AJ, Morris CM, Lee JE, Williams PN, et al. Dopaminergic polymorphisms in Tourette syndrome: Association with the DAT gene (SLC6A3). *Am. J. Med. Genet. B Neuropsychiatr. Genet.* 2007;**144B**:605–610.

160. McMahon LR, Li JX, Carroll FI, France CP. Some effects of dopamine transporter and receptor ligands on discriminative stimulus, physiologic, and directly observable indices of opioid withdrawal in rhesus monkeys. *Psychopharmacology (Berlin)* 2009;**203**:411–420.

161. Guindalini C, Howard M, Haddley K, Laranjeira R, Collier D, Ammar N, et al. A dopamine transporter gene functional variant associated with cocaine abuse in a Brazilian sample. *Proc. Natl. Acad. Sci. USA* 2006;**103**:4552–4557.

162. Giros B, Jaber M, Jones SR, Wightman RM, Caron MG. Hyperlocomotion and indifference to cocaine and amphetamine in mice lacking the dopamine transporter. *Nature* 1996;**379**:606–612.

163. Greenwood TA, Schork NJ, Eskin E, Kelsoe Jr., Identification of additional variants within the human dopamine transporter gene provides further evidence for an association with bipolar disorder in two independent samples. *Mol. Psychiatry* 2006;**11**: 125–133, 115.

164. Santovito A, Cervella P, Selvaggi A, Caviglia GP, Burgarello C, Sella G, et al. DAT1 VNTR polymorphisms in a European and an African population: Identification of a new allele. *Hum. Biol.* 2008;**80**:191–198.

165. Mill J, Asherson P, Browes C, D'Souza U, Craig I. Expression of the dopamine transporter gene is regulated by the 3' UTR VNTR: Evidence from brain and lymphocytes using quantitative RT-PCR. *Am. J. Med. Genet.* 2002;**114**:975–979.

166. Fuke S, Suo S, Takahashi N, Koike H, Sasagawa N, Ishiura S. The VNTR polymorphism of the human dopamine transporter (DAT1) gene affects gene expression. *Pharmacogenomics J.* 2001;**1**:152–156.

167. Miller GM, Madras BK. Polymorphisms in the 3'-untranslated region of human and monkey dopamine transporter genes affect reporter gene expression. *Mol. Psychiatry* 2002;**7**:44–55.

168. van de Giessen EM, de Win MM, Tanck MW, van den BW, Baas F, Booij J. Striatal dopamine transporter availability associated with polymorphisms in the dopamine transporter gene SLC6A3. *J. Nucl. Med.* 2009;**50**:45–52.

169. Kooij JS, Boonstra AM, Vermeulen SH, Heister AG, Burger H, Buitelaar JK, et al. Response to methylphenidate in adults with ADHD is associated with a polymorphism in SLC6A3 (DAT1). *Am. J. Med. Genet. B Neuropsychiatr. Genet.* 2008;**147B**:201–208.

170. Winsberg BG, Comings DE. Association of the dopamine transporter gene (DAT1) with poor methylphenidate response. *J. Am. Acad. Child Adolesc. Psychiatry* 1999;**38**:1474–1477.

171. Purper-Ouakil D, Wohl M, Orejarena S, Cortese S, Boni C, Asch M, et al. Pharmacogenetics of methylphenidate response in attention deficit/hyperactivity disorder: Association with the dopamine transporter gene (SLC6A3). *Am. J. Med. Genet. B Neuropsychiatr. Genet.* 2008;**147B**:1425–1430.

172. Purper-Ouakil D, Wohl M, Mouren MC, Verpillat P, Ades J, Gorwood P. Meta-analysis of family-based association studies between the dopamine transporter gene and attention deficit hyperactivity disorder. *Psychiatr. Genet.* 2005;**15**:53–59.

173. Kirchheiner J, Nickchen K, Sasse J, Bauer M, Roots I, Brockmoller J. A 40-basepair VNTR polymorphism in the dopamine transporter (DAT1) gene and the rapid response to antidepressant treatment. *Pharmacogenomics J.* 2007;**7**:48–55.

174. Conn PJ, Lindsley CW, Jones CK. Activation of metabotropic glutamate receptors as a novel approach for the treatment of schizophrenia. *Trends Pharmacol. Sci.* 2009;**30**:25–31.

175. Simon T, Verstuyft C, Mary-Krause M, Quteineh L, Drouet E, Meneveau N, et al. Genetic determinants of response to clopidogrel and cardiovascular events. *New Engl. J. Med.* 2009;**360**:363–375.

176. Levant B. The D3 dopamine receptor: Neurobiology and potential clinical relevance. *Pharmacol. Rev.* 1997;**49**:231–252.

177. Gether U, Andersen PH, Larsson OM, Schousboe A. Neurotransmitter transporters: Molecular function of important drug targets. *Trends Pharmacol. Sci.* 2006;**27**:375–383.

PART II

PHARMACOGENETICS: THERAPEUTIC AREAS

CHAPTER 6

Cardiovascular Pharmacogenetics

BAS J. M. PETERS, ANTHONIUS DE BOER, TOM SCHALEKAMP, OLAF H. KLUNGEL, and ANKE-HILSE MAITLAND-VAN DER ZEE

Utrecht University, Utrecht, The Netherlands

6.1 INTRODUCTION

Cardiovascular disease (CVD) covers a wide range of conditions and diseases, including hypertension, hypercholesterolemia, congestive heart failure, cerebrovascular disease, and coronary heart disease (CHD). Especially in developed countries, CVD is one of the leading causes of death because of its high prevalence and high impact on morbidity and mortality [1].

To reduce the risk of CVD, lifestyle adjustments are generally recommended and have been shown to be very effective in reducing CVD risk. These recommendations include physical activity, smoking cessation, low sodium intake, and low-fat diet. However, lifestyle interventions do not always provide satisfactory CVD risk reductions. Moreover, for a variety of reasons, adherence to a healthy lifestyle is a difficult task for many people. Therefore, cardiovascular drugs are abundantly prescribed globally for the treatment of conditions such as hypertension and hyperlipidemia. Although a huge variety of drugs are available for the treatment of CVD, major essential pharmacological groups are considered platelet aggregation inhibitors (PAIs), statins, antihypertensive drugs, and anticoagulants.

There is notable interindividual variation in response to these drugs, which is partially explained by factors such as gender, age, diet, concomitant drug use, and environmental factors. Nevertheless, a large part of this variability remains unknown. Genetic variability may contribute to the explanation of variability in response to these cardiovascular drugs [2].

Since the 1990s, the pharmacogenetics field has enjoyed a tremendous surge in activity due to advances in technology, and many association studies have been published.

Pharmacogenetics and Individualized Therapy, First Edition.
Edited by Anke-Hilse Maitland-van der Zee and Ann K. Daly.

This chapter gives an overview of the state of affairs of the pharmacogenetics of the most commonly prescribed drugs in the management of cardiovascular disease.

6.2 CARDIOVASCULAR DISEASE

The World Health Organization (WHO) estimated that cardiovascular disease accounted for 17.5 million global deaths in 2005. Deaths due to myocardial infarction (MI) and cerebrovascular accident (CVA) represented the majority of these deaths [3,4]. Estimates demonstrate that in 2005, over 80 million people (about 1 in 3 adults) in the United States were suffering from at least one cardiovascular condition or form of CVD [5]. In more detail, these patients accounted for approximately 73.6 million hypertension, 16.8 million CHD (angina pectoris and myocardial infarction), 6.5 million stroke, and 5.7 million heart failure diagnoses [5]. Future prospects are that CVD will continue to cause a great medical and economic burden [3,4].

6.2.1 Pathophysiology

The majority of deaths due to cardiovascular disease are caused by cardiovascular conditions such as hypertension and hypercholesterolemia. The etiology of most cases of hypertension and hypercholesterolemia is poorly understood and are therefore classified as primary hypertension and primary hypercholesterolemia. Both conditions contribute significantly to the development of atherosclerosis, which is characterized by hardening of the arteries, itself enhancing hypertension severity. Atherosclerotic plaques are the result of accumulation of cholesterol-mediated by low-densitylipoproteins (LDL) in the arterial walls, which, in turn, leads to a macrophage-induced inflammatory process. Rupture of an atherosclerotic plaque exposes the lipid core, smooth-muscle cells, macrophages, and collagen to the bloodstream, resulting in adhesion of blood platelets and the activation of the coagulation cascade. Ultimately, a thrombus is formed that can either completely or incompletely occlude an artery, resulting in clinical events such as MI and CVA [6]. Myocardial necrosis may be a consequence of cardiac ischemia. Loss of cardiac function may initiate other CVD such as congestive heart failure, characterized by a poor prognosis.

6.2.2 Clinical Manifestation

Symptoms of a patient suffering from CVD can vary from none to sudden (cardiac) death. Conditions such as hypercholesterolemia, hypertension, and atherosclerosis may elapse unnoticed, because high cholesterol levels, high blood pressure, and atherosclerosis are ravely symptomatic. A MI or CVA generally does not elapse unnoticed. Preceding a MI, some patients experience chest pains known as *angina pectoris*. Specific symptoms of a patient suffering a MI are pain in the chest, arms, left shoulder, jaw, and/or back. A CVA is often characterized by confusion; impaired understanding of speech, impaired speech and/or sight, unilateral weakness; or numbness of the face, arm, and/or leg.

6.3 CARDIOVASCULAR THERAPY

Cardiovascular conditions such as hypertension and hypercholesterolemia do not necessarily require acute medical treatment. Essential lifestyle changes to reduce the risk of CVD include nonpharmacological cornerstone interventions such as smoking cessation, healthy diet, low sodium intake, weight loss, and physical activity [7]. If these interventions do not achieve the desired level of risk reduction, many pharmacological interventions are available.

Besides smoking, the most prevalent CVD risk factors are hypertension and hypercholesterolemia. Heavily depending on the total cardiovascular risk (including factors such as diabetes status, age, gender, smoking status, BMI, cholesterol level), treatment with an antihypertensive drug may be indicated when the blood pressure (BP) is within the high–normal range (130–139/85–89 mmHg) or higher. All subjects with a total plasma cholesterol of >5 mmol/L (190 mg/dL) and LDL cholesterol of >3 mmol/L (115 mg/dL) should be considered for pharmacological intervention with HMG CoA reductase inhibitors (statins), also depending on the total cardiovascular risk. Similar to the treatment of hypertension, lower total cholesterol and LDL cholesterol target levels reduces the risk of CVD even more in patients with other risk factors such as diabetes [8].

Platelet aggregation inhibitors are another class of drugs that reduce the risk of cardiovascular events. By inhibiting platelet aggregation, drugs such as clopidogrel and aspirin prevent formation of a thrombus that could lead to a MI or CVA. CVDs such as atrial fibrillation give rise to high risk of a thromboembolisms and require anticoagulation with warfarin, phenprocoumon, or acenocoumarol.

6.4 GENETIC DETERMINANTS OF RESPONSE TO CARDIOVASCULAR DRUGS

6.4.1 Platelet Aggregation Inhibitors

Pharmacotherapy with PAI such as aspirin and clopidogrel is an important intervention measure in cardiovascular risk management. In high-risk patients, the efficacy in the primary and particularly secondary prevention of cardiovascular death, myocardial infarction, and stroke, is well established [9]. However, some patients suffer a (recurrent) thromboembolic vascular event despite PAI therapy [10]. Results from meta-analyses have shown that patients resistant for aspirin experience a 4-flod greater risk for cardiovascular events [11] whereas patients resistant for clopidogrel have an 8 times greater risk [12]. A variety of tests and clinical outcomes can be used to measure sensitivity to PAI. However, there is little consistency regarding which measure to use to define nonresponse to PAI. Tests to measure platelet function include thromboxane A2 (TXA2) production (measured as urinary or serum 11-dehydro-thromboxane B2 (dTxB2)), optical aggregometry using agonist such as arachidonic acid (AA), adenosine diphosphate (ADP) and collagen, the platelet function analyzer 100, and others [13]. Numerous studies have been conducted to investigate possible underlying genetic mechanisms leading to treatment failure. Most of these studies used one of the platelet function tests as the outcome measure, and fewer studies included clinically relevant outcomes such as MI.

Aspirin irreversibly inhibits the cycloxygenase 1 (COX1) enzyme, ultimately resulting in a decreased amount of TXA2. TXA2 is responsible for activation of platelet aggregation. Therefore, polymorphisms in the *COX1* gene may affect response to aspirin therapy. In 2005, Maree et al. reported an association between a polymorphism in the *COX1* gene and platelet function in response to aspirin [14]. Five common SNPs were genotyped in 144 patients with cardiovascular disease who were treated with aspirin for at least 2 weeks. Aspirin response, determined by serum dTxB2 levels and AA-induced platelet aggregation, was associated with the *A842G* polymorphism. Patients carrying the *–842G* polymorphism were less sensitive to aspirin treatment [14]. Lepantalo et al. included 101 patients undergoing elective percutaneous coronary intervention and reported similar results: 60% of the non-responders carried the *–842G* allele compared to 17% of the responders [15]. Gonzalez-Conejero et al. investigated the *C50T* polymorphism, which was in complete linkage disequilibrium with the *A842G* polymorphism. Only the results of the TXB2 assay were similar to those reported in literature, whereas no drug–gene interaction was shown using the AA-induced platelet aggregation [16]. Other studies report contradictory results, suggesting *–842G* allele carriers to be more sensitive to aspirin [17,18]. The exact mechanism of the possible interaction between aspirin and the *A842G* and *C50T* polymorphisms has not yet been elucidated.

Another gene that has been investigated many times with regard to the pharmacogenetics of both aspirin and clopidogrel is the gene coding for the platelet glycoprotein IIIa subunit, *ITGB3*. It is part of the glycoprotein IIb/IIIa receptor that is present on the activated platelet surface and responsible for platelet aggregation by binding of fibrinogen. Most research focused on the *ITGB3 PlA1/A2* polymorphism, in which the *P1A1* is the wild-type variant [19]. Undas et al. were first to report on the effect of this polymorphism on platelet functioning after patients were exposed to aspirin, showing that subjects carrying the *PlA1/PlA2* genotype were less sensitive to aspirin than homozygous *PlA1* carriers [20]. These findings have been replicated in small studies [21,22], whereas other, larger studies could not find such an association [23–26] or even showed opposite findings [27] corroborating results from earlier *in vitro* studies [28,29]. Similar to findings for clopidogrel response, some articles report (contradicting) associations [30,31] whereas others report no difference between different genotype groups [24,32,33]. The *PlA1/PlA2* polymorphism does not seem to explain a large part of the interindividual variability in response to PAI when considering current evidence.

In addition to the *COX1* and *ITGB3* gene, genetic variabilities in *ITGA2, COX2, P2Y1, P2Y12,* and several other genes have been investigated with respect to modified response to aspirin, but were studied in a very small number of patients, and larger studies did not replicate these results [34,35].

Goodman et al. conducted a meta-analysis on the pharmacogenetics of aspirin to increase statistical power and to take in account the different biochemical and functional methodologies [34]. Combination of studies could not show a pharmacogenetic interaction between aspirin and the polymorphisms that were included (*ITGA2 C807T, COX1 A842G/C50T, P2Y12 H1/H2, P2Y1 A1622G,* and *ITGB3 PlA1/PlA2*). However, after stratification by study population or measurement technique, the *P1A2* allele of the *ITGB3* gene was associated with aspirin resistance; small but significant effects were found in the healthy population (four studies) and in the studies using bleeding time as the outcome measure (only two studies).

Clopidogrel is a prodrug and has to be activated by hepatic cytochrome P450 (CYP) isoenzymes in order to inhibit platelet aggregation. After activation, clopidogrel irreversibly blocks the ADP receptor on platelet cell membranes and thereby activation of the glycoprotein IIb/IIIa pathway. *CYP2C19**2* is a common genetic variant of the *CYP2C19* gene that encodes a deficient version of the enzyme. Hulot et al. showed in 28 healthy subjects that heterozygous carriers of the *CYP2C19**2* allele had decreased platelet responsiveness to clopidogrel [36]. This finding was confirmed in other studies both pharmacokinetically [37,38] and pharmacodynamically [37–40]. In addition, studies on clinical outcomes showed that carriers of loss-of-function alleles of the *CYP2C19* gene have a higher risk of major adverse cardiovascular events when treated with clopidogrel after suffering acute coronary syndromes [38,41,42]. In conclusion, the *CYP2C19**2* polymorphism explains part of the interindividual response to clopidogrel. It is not yet clear what this compelling evidence means for daily practice: (1) should *CYP2C19**2* carriers receive higher dosages that may overcome the loss of effect, or (2) should those patients be treated with an alternative PAI that does not require metabolism by the CYP2C19 enzyme? In case 1, research should provide the evidence that a higher dose for patients carrying the *CYP2C19**2* allele are as effective as the normal dose in wild-type carriers. If so, patients have to be genotyped before starting clopidogrel. However, genotype information is unlikely to be available when starting clopidogrel treatment in the early high-risk phase of a MI. A P2Y12-mediated platelet function test could be a more rapid approach [43]. Moreover, treating patients with the *CYP2C19**2* genotype with an alternative PAI that does not require activation by the CYP2C19 enzyme may be an appropriate solution. Currently, there is no data available that can shed light on these important questions. A prospective study should demonstrate how patients carrying the *CYP2C19**2* allele should be treated.

Other cytochrome P450 system enzymes have also been investigated with regard to the pharmacogenetics of clopidogrel. However, the current status of evidence shows no convincing or conclusive evidence for interactions between clopidogrel and genetic variance in *CYP3A4*, *CYP3A5*, *CYP2C9*, *CYP2B6,* or *CYP1A2* [44].

The active thiol metabolite of clopidgrel binds irreversibly to the P2Y12 receptor. Genetic variability within the genes coding for the P2Y12 receptor and another ADP-dependent P2Y1 receptor present on the platelet surface have been investigated. Unfortunately, research on polymorphisms within the *P2Y12* [24,45–49] and *P2Y1* gene [24,50] have not been able to explain any of the variability in clopidogrel response.

More comprehensive reviews that cover the pharmacogenetics of aspirin [34,35,44,51] and clopidogrel [44,51] can be found elsewhere.

6.4.2 Anticoagulants

Oral anticoagulants of the coumarin type are highly efficacious for the treatment and prevention of thromboembolic diseases [52]. Warfarin is the most common coumarin, but acenocoumarol and phenprocoumon are frequently being used in several European countries [53,54]. Dosing of coumarins is difficult as a consequence of a narrow therapeutic range and large interindividual and intraindividual differences in dose response [55]. Consequently, an overdose will increase the risk of hemorrhage, and an insufficient dose may lead to failure of thromboembolisms prevention. Large intraindividual variability in response to coumarins [56] and strong overanticoagulation [57] are important risk factors for hemorrhages. Patients' characteristics such as weight, diet, disease state, and concomitant use of other medications have been shown to affect the response to coumarins [58]. In addition, genetic variation contributes to the interindividual variation. To date, studies on the pharmacogenetics of coumarins have focused mainly on polymorphisms within the *CYP2C9* and *VKORC1* gene and their modifying effect on mean daily dosage, overanticoagulation, time to stable anticoagulation, and the risk of bleeding.

The *CYP2C9* gene encodes the CYP2C9 enzyme, which is principally responsible for the metabolism of the pharmacologically more effective *S*-enantiomer of coumarins. The most extensively investigated genetic variants are *CYP2C9**2* (*C430T*) and *CYP2C9**3* (*A1075C*), which both encode enzymes with a decreased activity compared to the wild type, *CYP2C9**1*. Sanderson et al. reported in a systematic review and meta-analysis that lower maintenance doses of warfarin are required in subjects carrying either variant allele. They showed that **2* and **3* carriers have an increased risk of bleeding as a result of higher plasma levels of warfarin due to slow metabolism of warfarin by the CYP2C9 enzyme [55,59]. In another meta-analysis of 39 studies with a total of 7907 warfarin users, Lindh et al. found that being carrier of more than one polymorphism resulted in a progressive reduction in warfarin dose requirements, with warfarin dose in patients with the *CYP2C9**3/*3* genotype as 78% less than in patients with the *CYP2C9**1/*1* genotype [60]. For acenocoumarol, the *CYP2C9**2* and *CYP2C9**3* variants have also been associated with low-dose requirements [61–64]. Moreover, the *CYP2C9**3* genotype has been associated with a decreased chance to achieve stable anticoagulation within 6 months, an increased risk for overanticoagulation [65], and an increased risk for major bleeding events [66]. Although research on phenprocoumon is sparse, and although the contribution of CYP2C9 to the metabolism of phenprocoumon is smaller than for warfarin and acenocoumarol [67], the *CYP2C9**2* and *CYP2C9**3* alleles have also been associated with lower dosage requirements, a decreased chance to achieve stability, and an increased risk for overanticoagulation [68] and bleeding [69]. These results could not be replicated in the Rotterdam study [64,66], possibly because of power problems.

Coumarins exert their anticoagulant effects by inhibiting the vitamin K epoxide reductase complex (VKOR), preventing VKOR from converting vitamin K epoxide to reduced vitamin K [70], which is essential for functioning of several clotting factors such as factors II, VII, IX, and X. The target of coumarins is VKORC1, encoded by the homonymous gene *VKORC1*. Being a carrier of the noncoding SNP 1173C>T has been associated with reduced dose needs of warfarin [55], acenocoumarol [71–73], and phenprocoumon [71,72] compared with noncarriers of this SNP. The single 1173C>T SNP proved to be as informative as five haplotype constructs of 10 SNPs in the *VKORC1* gene that have been allocated to low- and high-dose warfarin haplotype groups and that account for almost all the total haplotypes in Caucasian and Asian American populations. [74]. Furthermore, it has been reported that the *VKORC1* and *CYP2C9* genotypes modify each others' effects on over-anticoagulation in users of acenocoumarol [75], with risk highest in patients with both *CYP2C9* and *VKORC1* polymorphisms. However, a more recent study demonstrated that the bleeding risk in users of warfarin was associated with the CYP2C9, but not with the VKORC1 genotype [76].

Inconclusive results for polymorphisms in the *F2* [77–79], *F7* [77,79], and *F10* [77,79] genes—encoding the vitamin K–dependent clotting factors II, VII, and X—suggest a minor influence of these coagulation genes on warfarin dosing. Genetic variability in other downstream genes of coumarin action such as *GGCX*, *EPHX1*, *PROC*, and *APOE* have shown limited effects, if any, on coumarin dosing [80]. The *GGCX* gene encodes γ-glutamylcarboxylase, the enzyme catalyzing the carboxylation of vitamin K–dependent clotting factors, the *PROC* gene encodes the clotting factors Va and VIIIa inactivating protein C; and the *EPHX1* gene encodes microsomal epoxide hydrolase, a subunit of the VKOR complex harboring a vitamin K epoxide binding site. The *APOE* gene has been considered a candidate gene because it encodes the vitamin K liver uptake facilitating ligand apolipoprotein E.

Moreover, a large study that included 183 polymorphisms in 29 candidate genes could not reveal major importance for genes other than *CYP2C19* and *VKORC1* [80]. Similar conclusions were drawn from the results from the only genomewide association study to date, suggesting that it is unlikely that common SNPs with significant effects on warfarin dose are to be discovered outside of the *CYP2C9* and *VKORC1* gene [81].

The abovementioned polymorphisms of CYP2C9 and VKORC1 are common in Caucasian populations, with allele frequencies ranging from 8% to 19% for *CYP2C9*2*, from 4% to 16% for *CYP2C9*3* [82,83] and from 37% to 41% for the VKORC1 1173C>T allele [80,84].

Large studies have been able to explain around 50% of the variability in warfarin dosing with *CYP2C9* and *VKORC1* genotype [84,85], although estimates vary [58]. The next step would be to use this pharmacogenetic knowledge to develop coumarin dosing algorithms that include *CYP2C9* and *VKORC1* genotype information. However, research should first demonstrate that genotype-guided dosing improves safety and efficacy of coumarin therapy in daily practice. Several small randomized studies assessing genotype-guided warfarin have already been conducted. The one study that included both the *CYP2C9* as well as the *VKORC1* genotype in a randomized controlled trial showed genotype-guided warfarin dosing to be moderately favorable [86]. Generally, other studies of genetic testing for warfarin therapy initiation have not been able to demonstrate improvement of safety or efficacy of warfarin therapy [87]. Large randomized clinical trials to evaluate genotype-guided dosing of coumarins are underway and will guide decisions regarding future implications for treatment with coumarins.

More comprehensive overviews of the pharmacogenetics of coumarins can be found elsewhere [55,58].

6.4.3 Antihypertensive Drugs

The most prevalent indication in cardiovascular drug therapy is hypertension. Its high prevalence and the strong association with cardiovascular morbidity have given rise to the question of whom to treat with which drug. In previous decades, the search for markers that can predict response to therapy has experienced a tremendous surge. The major drug classes available for the treatment of hypertension are diuretics, β-blockers, ACE inhibitors, angiotensin 2 type 1 receptor antagonists, and calcium channel blockers (CCBs). In this chapter, the most important genetic variants within the pharmacogenetics of hypertension are highlighted.

6.4.3.1 Diuretics

Diuretics are considered the first-line pharmacological intervention for most patients with hypertension [88]. The long-term beneficial effects of thiazides are thought to result mainly from a reduction of the peripheral vascular resistance.

To date, many pharmacogenetic studies have been published on the pharmacogenetics of diuretics. The best-studied polymorphism is the *Gly460Trp* variant of the α-adducin (*ADD1*) gene. In addition, multiple studies have been conducted on the angiotensin-converting enzyme (*ACE*) *I/D*, angiotensin (*AGT*) *–6A*, angiotensin receptor (*AGTR1*) *A1166C* and G-protein β-3 subunit (*GNB3*) *C825T* polymorphism, and the response to diuretics.

The *ADD1* gene encodes the α subunit of the adducin protein, which is involved in the activation of the renal Na^+/K^+ ATPase. Carriers of the *ADD1 460Trp* allele have a higher activity of the Na^+/K^+ pump in the nephron. The *ADD1 Gly460Trp* polymorphism has been shown to affect renal proximal tubule sodium reabsorption in hypertension with increased reabsorption in patients carrying the *460Trp allele* [89]. Hypothetically, *460Trp allele* carriers could benefit more from therapy as diuretics could trigger less counterregulatory mechanisms. Cusi et al. were first to report on the *ADD1 Gly460Trp* polymorphism and the association with altered response to hydrochlorothiazide in hypertensive patients [90]. They found that heterozygous hypertensive patients experienced a greater fall in mean arterial pressure in response to 2 months' treatment with hydrochlorothiazide than did wild-type homozygous hypertensive patients [90]. Following this study, these results were replicated in two other studies also showing that carriers of the *ADD1 460Trp allele* respond better to hydrochlorothiazide [91,92]. Retrospective large scale studies with up to 36,000 patients [93] could not replicate these findings [93–96] and thereby suggest a minor role for the *ADD1 Gly460Trp* polymorphism in predicting blood pressure response to diuretics.

Furthermore, the *ADD1 460Trp allele* has been associated with a better response to diuretics with regard to clinical outcomes such as stroke or MI [97], a result that was not found in other studies on clinical outcomes [93,98–100]. It would be a myopic judgment to say the *ADD1 Gly460Trp* does not affect the response to diuretics, for several reasons:

1. There is a good rationale for the pharmacogenetic interaction between *ADD1* and use of diuretics.
2. The positive studies all point in the same direction.
3. A closer look at the study designs that were used shows that the three positive studies on blood pressure conducted excellent studies including patients with a newly discovered diagnosis of hypertension and who were never treated before. On the other hand, large observational studies consistently fail to show such association. The association of the *ADD1 Gly460Trp* polymorphism with altered response to diuretics seems genuine, but so far of no clinical importance.

Besides the *ADD1* gene, researchers have taken interest in polymorphisms in genes involved in the rennin–angiotensin system (RAS), namely, the *ACE* gene encoding the ACE, *AGT* encoding angiotensinogen, and *AGTR1* encoding the angiotensin II receptor, type 1. The rationale for the selection of these candidate genes for the pharmacogenetics of diuretics as well as other antihypertensive drugs is obvious as the RAS system is activated by diuretics and regulates water–electrolyte balance and thereby blood volume and blood pressure.

The *D* allele of the *ACE I/D* polymorphism is associated with increased plasma and tissue levels of ACE [101]. Because low plasma renin activity is a predictor of greater BP response to thiazide diuretics [102], it can be hypothesized that *I* allele carriers would respond better to thiazides. Sciarrone et al. indeed reported *I* allele carriers to respond better to hydrochlorothiazide [92]. Schwartz et al. showed similar results for women and opposite results in men [103]. Although the excellent study of Sciarrone et al. confirms the initial hypothesis, the myriad of studies that could not confirm such association [95,104–106] suggest a minor role for the *ACE I/D* polymorphism. Other than the *ACE I/D* polymorphism, Frazier et al. included polymorphisms within the other RAS genes *AGT* and *AGTR1* and showed an association with both genes in African-American women only [105]. These results were not corroborated by the Doetinchem cohort study [95] and were contradicted by Jiang et al. [107]. More studies are needed to elucidate the possible role of these polymorphisms in the response to diuretics.

Furthermore, an association with the *GNB3 C825T* polymorphism has been reported and replicated, both studies showing that subjects carrying the *TT* genotype would benefit more from diuretics in lowering blood pressure [95,108]. The mechanistic pathway of this possible gene–treatment interaction is that the T allele of the *GNB3*

C825T polymorphism has been associated with low plasma renin and an elevated aldosterone renin ratio [109] that could influence the response to diuretics. A study by Schelleman et al. could not corroborate previous findings concerning the association between the *GNB3 C825T* polymorphism and clinical events [98].

6.4.3.2 β-Blockers

The main target of β-blockers is the β1-adrenoreceptor encoded by the *ADRB1* gene, in which the *Arg389Gly* and the *Ser49Gly* polymorphisms are most extensively investigated. The *Arg389* and *Ser49* alleles may enhance response to β-blockers as receptors containing *Arg389* possess a 3–4-fold higher adenylylcyclase activity [110] and *49Gly* polymorphic receptors are more prone to agonist-promoted receptor downregulation [111]. Initially, O'Shaughnessy did not report an association of the ADRB1 polymorphism and altered response to atenolol or bisoprolol [112]. In the years after, four articles were published reporting an association of the *Arg389* allele (in combination with *Ser49* allele [113,114]) with better response to β-blockers, either SBP [114–116], DBP [113,114], or resting MBP [114,115]. This observation could not be confirmed by other studies [117–121]. Nonetheless, the hypothesis should not be rejected as there is a consistency in findings for studies with the β-blocker metoprolol. Moreover, given the similarities in the pharmacology of β-blockers, differences in study design may well explain the inconsistency of results. The positive associations point in the same direction, as expected with regard to the initial hypothesis, and suggest a true pharmacogenetic interaction. Major clinical importance of the *ADRB1 Arg389Gly* and *Ser49Gly* polymorphisms for the pharmacogenetics of β-blockers seems unlikely.

β-Adrenergic receptors are G-protein coupled-receptors. Therefore the *GNB3 C825T* polymorphism possibly modifies the blood pressure response to β blockade. In females only, the carriers of the *CC* genotype has been associated with better blood pressure response to β-blockers [118], a finding that was not confirmed in the Doetinchem study [95].

Finally, the RAS gene *AGT* [*A(-6)G* polymorphism] has been associated with the pharmacogenetics of β-blockers, but the association has been reported only once [122], whereas other studies failed to confirm this association [123,124].

6.4.3.3 ACE Inhibitors

The aforementioned (See Section 6.4.3.1) *ACE* gene—coding for the drug target of ACE inhibitors—has been studied over 20 times. Studies that evaluated blood pressure response to ACE inhibitors according to *ACE I/D* genotype include treatment duration ranging from single doses to several years, small-scale studies as well as larger studies, and studies in both healthy subjects and patients. Carriers of the *D allele*—accompanied by higher ACE levels [101]—could benefit less from ACE inhibitors because of underdosing or could benefit more as a result of a poorer baseline condition. Initially smaller studies reported a more beneficial effect of ACE inhibitors on blood pressure in subjects carrying II. Large studies that have been published more recently [104,125] could not confirm these results. Uncertainty about the expected biological mechanism-based direction of the association together with many studies showing opposite or no association directions of the association suggest that the *ACE I/D* polymorphism is not likely to be a strong modifier of blood pressure response to treatment with ACE inhibitors. Also, stratification of results by study design, study population, or type of ACE inhibitor cannot explain the inconsistency.

Another gene involved in the RAS that has been associated with modified response to ACE inhibitors is the *AGT* gene. Initially, a prospective study in 125 subjects showed that the *T* allele of the *M235T* polymorphism was associated with better blood pressure lowering response to ACE inhibitors compared to homozygous *M* allele carriers [126]. Bis et al. showed similar results for the outcome stroke [127]. Several other studies, both retrospective and prospective, found no such association [95,96,128–131], concluding that there is very little evidence for an interaction between the *AGT M235T* polymorphism and the response to ACE inhibitors.

6.4.3.4 Other Antihypertensive Drugs

Another category of antihypertensives that act on the RAS is the angiotensin II type 1 receptor antagonists. Studies in the SILVHIA trial, which included almost 50 subjects taking irbesartan, reported that the *ACE I/D* [123] and *CYP11B2 C-344T* polymorphism were associated with modified blood pressure response [123,132]. Both genes acting on the RAS, *CYP11B2*—encoding aldosterone synthase—is required for the final steps of aldosterone biosynthesis. Subjects carrying the *ACE II* polymorphism [123] and subjects carrying the *CYP11B2 TT* variant [132] had a more pronounced blood pressure response to irbesartan. The finding of the *CYP11B2 C-344T* polymorphism association could not be replicated (results point in opposite directions) [133]; nor could a prospective study including 206 subjects treated with telmisartan find an association with any of the RAS genes (*AGT, ACE,* and *AGTR1*) polymorphisms [134]. Currently, the role of polymorphisms in genes of the RAS system and the response to angiotensin II antagonists is unknown.

Calcium channel blockers and central α-adrenergic agonists have been insufficiently investigated, and future research should provide more information about the genetic contribution to variability in response.

6.4.3.5 Antihypertensive Drugs and Side Effects

In addition to the impact of genetic variability on the effectiveness of antihypertensive drugs, several studies have investigated the genetic influence on the incidence of certain side effects. A frequent reason for discontinuation of ACE inhibitor therapy is a persistent, dry cough [135]. As a result of ACE inhibition, metabolism of bradykinin by ACE is impaired. Local accumulation of bradykinin in the airways is thought to cause a persistent, dry cough. Variability in RAS genes as well as the gene coding for the bradykinin B2 receptor (BDKRB2) has been proposed to influence the susceptibility to developing a cough due to ACE inhibition. The *T* allele of the *T-58C* promoter polymorphism in the bradykinin B2 receptor gene (*BDKRB2*) results in a higher transcription rate [136] and has been associated with elicitation of the adverse effect coughing [136,137]. All but except one study [138], have been unable to find a relation between the *ACE I/D* polymorphism and cough [136,137,139]. In addition, beneficial effects of ACE inhibition regarding occurrence of diabetes was seen only in hypertensive subjects homozygous for *AGTR1 1166A* and/or carriers of the *ACE I* allele [140].

A complete review of the large amount of literature of the pharmacogenetics of antihypertensives can be found elsewhere [141–144].

6.4.4 Cholesterol Lowering Drugs (Statins)

Statins primarily reduce the risk for coronary artery disease (CAD) by lowering blood cholesterol through inhibition of the HMG-CoA reductase enzyme. Although large clinical trials found a 27% average relative risk reduction of major coronary events [145], there is wide variability in benefits from statin therapy. Many genes involved in the pharmacodynamic pathway of statins have been part of pharmacogenetic research in patients with hypercholesterolemia, with an emphasis on genes involved in the cholesterol pathway, although genes involved with possible pleiotropic effects of statins have been attracting increasing interest. The enormous amount of candidate genes that have been studied in research on the pharmacogenetics of statins proves the potentially significant impact of future findings on treatment with statins. Moreover, it highlights the complexity of the mechanism by which statins exert their beneficial effect.

The HMG-CoA reductase enzyme, which is encoded by the *HMGCR* gene, is responsible for the conversion of HMG-CoA to mevalonic acid, an intermediate in the cholesterol synthesis. The minor alleles of two SNPs, *SNP12* and *SNP29* (rs17238540), jointly uniquely define haplotype 7 of the *HMGCR* gene [146]. The minor alleles for both these SNPs were associated with less pronounced total cholesterol (TC) and low-density lipoprotein (LDL) cholesterol reduction in response to pravastatin treatment (PRINCE study) [146]. A pharmacogenetic study in the ACCESS trial could not replicate these findings [147]. This may be due to a statistical power problem as both a large observational study in diabetics [148] and a prospective study in hypercholesterolemic patients (treatment with simvastatin) [149] reported comparable results for these SNPs. In addition, no association with lipid response was found in the elderly population of the PROSPER trial [150], and no association was found considering clinical outcomes such as MI and CVA [150,151]. Both SNP12 and SNP29 are located in a noncoding region, and further research should determine whether there is a molecular explanation for the results that were found in several studies. Possibly SNP12 and SNP29 explain a small part of the variability in response to statins due to genetics. More recently, Medina et al. discovered a *HMGCR* isoform, encoded by an alternatively spliced transcript whose expression is influenced by SNP rs3846662. The isoform was shown to affect reponse to statins [152].

Cholesterol is transported throughout the body by apolipoproteins. Apolipoprotein E is a major component of very low-density lipoproteins (VLDLs) and ligand for the LDL receptor. Moreover, apolipoprotein E is involved in intestinal cholesterol absorption and reverse cholesterol transport (RCT). Apolipoprotein E is a genetically polymorphic protein defined by three alleles, *ApoE2*, *E3* and *E4*, encoding proteins with increasing affinity for the LDL receptor. Consequently, lipoproteins carrying the E4 isoform are cleared most efficiently from the circulation and cholesterol synthesis, and thus HMG-CoA reductase levels are lower. As a result, *E4* carriers could benefit less from statin therapy. Ordovas et al. reported that carriers of the *E2* genotype experience greatest LDL reduction in response to statin therapy in comparison to *E3* and *E4* carriers [153]. Many similar studies were conducted in attempts to clarify the role of the ApoE polymorphism in the pharmacogenetics of statins. There is a reasonable body of evidence supporting the findings from Ordovas et al [147,154–160], which include some large-scale studies [147,155,156,160]. Nonetheless, studies that could not show similar results have also been reported frequently [146,161–166]. *ApoE2* carriers seem to benefit most from statin therapy regarding lipid profile improvement; however, a sub study of the Scandinavian simvastatin survival study (S4) and the GISSI prevenzione study (both multicenter, double-blind, randomized trials) reported subjects carrying the ApoE4 genotype to have the largest risk reduction of mortality [167,168]. These results were not replicated in an observational study [169].

Besides ApoE, genetic variations in the genes coding for other apolipoproteins have been included in pharmacogenetic research with inconclusive results [170,171].

Lowering the hepatic cholesterol biosynthesis increases the amount of LDL receptors. Some functional mutations in the *LDLR* gene, encoding the low-density lipoprotein receptor, cause familial hypercholesterolemia (FH). Generally small studies have associated these mutations with variable response to statins [172]. More common genetic variations in the LDLR have been suggested to modify the cholesterol lowering response to statins. However, inconsistent results of *LDLR* polymorphisms in the 3′ UTR region (*LDLR C44857T,* and *A44964G*) [146,150,151] and other intronic SNPs (AvaII, PvuII, and HincII) [147,173,174] have been reported. The genetic contribution of genetic variability of the *LDLR* gene should be investigated in detail for the important reason that the LDL receptor plays a pivotal role in the cholesterol housekeeping–working mechanism of statins. In addition, genetic variation within the *LDLR* expression/degradation regulating *SREBF1*, *SCAP,* and *PCSK9* genes have been subject of research without conclusive or consistent results [170,171].

The cholesteryl ester transfer protein (CETP) enzyme plays a central role in transport of cholesterol from peripheral tissues back to the liver, RCT. *Taq1B* is a common polymorphism in the *CETP* gene and is associated with variations in lipid transfer activity and high-density lipoprotein (HDL) levels [175] and may therefore alter response to statins. CETP concentrations are believed to be highest in homozygous B1 carriers and lowest in CETP homozygous B2 carriers. The effect of *Taq1B* on statin therapy was first investigated by Kuivenhoven et al., showing that pravastatin therapy slowed the progression of coronary atherosclerosis in *B1B1* carriers, whereas *B2B2* carriers did not benefit from pravastatin therapy, although higher HDL levels were observed [176]. Very recently, the same research group performed a 10-year follow-up analysis in the same REGRESS cohort, showing similar results; more benefit from statin therapy for *B1B1* carriers on cardiovascular clinical outcomes and all cause mortality despite higher HDL levels observed in B2 carriers [177]. Several other studies investigated the *CETP* polymorphism as well but could not find an association of the *Taq1B* polymorphism with altered efficacy of statins in preventing cardiovascular diseases [178–181] or found the opposite trend [182]. A large meta-analysis including over 13,000 patients found no gene treatment interaction between statins and the *Taq1B* polymorphism of the *CETP* gene [183]. A common pattern of contradictory results is seen for genes encoding lipoprotein lipase (LPL) and hepatic lipase (LIPC), enzymes that transfer lipids between lipoproteins and mediate lipolysis [147,184,185].

The foremost cause of CAD is atherosclerosis, which is characterized by inflammation [186]. In addition to lowering cholesterol, statins have been shown to exert lipid-independent pleiotropic effects, including beneficial effects on the process of inflammation [187]. Therefore not only candidate genes in the lipid lowering pathway, but also genes involved in the atherosclerosis inflammatory pathway, have been designated as candidate genes.

The kinesin-like protein 6 is encoded by KIF6 and is expressed in many tissues and cell types, including vascular cells. The *Trp719Arg* polymorphism in the *KIF6* gene was associated with CVD [188–191] and altered response to statins in three studies [188,192]. These three pharmacogenetic studies included more than 6200 patients exposed to pravastatin 40 mg daily (vs. placebo) [188] or 80 mg atorvastatin (vs. 40 mg pravastatin) daily [192]. The results from the PROVE IT-TIMI 22 trial [192] are consistent with those observed in two other clinical trial populations (CARE and WOSCOPS [188]). Carriers of the *KIF6 719Arg* allele receive significantly greater benefit from (intensive) statin therapy than do noncarriers. Proteins of the kinesin family are involved in intracellular transport, but the exact role of KIF6, the *Trp719Arg* polymorphism, and response to statins are not understood. The differential benefit from statins has been suggested to be distinct from lipid or CRP lowering [192].

The toll-like receptor mediates innate and adaptive immunity. The *Asp299Gly* polymorphism in the *TLR4* gene has been studied in REGRESS and SAS, both including approximately 650 patients. Both studies showed that *Gly* allele carriers treated with statins had a lower risk for cardiovascular events than did noncarriers treated with statins [193,194], suggesting that statins interact with inflammatory factors such as the toll-like receptor through an unknown biological mechanism. Pharmacogenetic research furthermore focused on polymorphisms in other examples of genes that are putatively involved in pleiotropic statin response: *eNOS*, *IL6*, *ITGB3*, and *PAI-1* [170,171].

Statins undergo different metabolizing pathways. Lovastatin, atorvastatin, simvastatin are metabolized mainly by CYP3A4; fluvastatin, by CYP2C9; and pravastatin, pitavastatin, and rosuvastatin are practically not metabolized by CYP enzymes [195]. There is little evidence for polymorphism within genes encoding CYP enzymes to be of much importance to the pharmacogenetics of statins [170,171].

Genes coding for transporters involved in the hepatic uptake and hepatic elimination of statins may also be of great importance for variability in response. Polymorphisms in pharmacokinetic genes encoding the solute carrier organic transporter (SCLO1B1) involved in the hepatic uptake of statins and the adenosine triphosphate (ATB)-binding cassette (ABC) B1 transporter involved in the hepatobiliary excretion of statins may influence the pharmacokinetics of statins and thereby its lipid lowering response. The variant allele of the *SCLO1B1 T521C* polymorphism—a functional SNP causing a Val > Ala aminoacid change—results in impaired hepatic statin uptake and thereby an attenuated pharmacodynamic effect. This has been shown for both the pharmacokinetics and pharmacodynamics of 'statins [196]. The *TT* genotype of the *SCLO1B1 T521C* polymorphism has been associated with greater response to statins in lowering total cholesterol [197,198], although controversy exists [147,199,200]. Variance in the *SCLO1B1* gene is likely to affect the response to statins to some extent.

Many genes encoding members of the ABC transporter family are involved in the pharmacodynamics (*ABCA1*, *ABCG5*, and *ABCG8*) or pharmacokinetics (*ABCB1*, *ABCC2*, *ABCG2*, and *ABCB11*) of statins [171]. Most of these genes have been subject of pharmacogenetic research related to statins, but the most extensively investigated ABC transporter is the ABCB1 transporter. Research has not been able to produce definitive results to show the role—if any—of the contribution of this gene to statin response [171,201,202].

6.4.4.1 Statins and Side Effects

Adverse effects to statin treatment, in particular statin-induced myopathy, have been associated with genetic variability in certain candidate genes [203]. There is convincing evidence regarding the association between the *SLCO1B1 T521C* polymorphism and statin-induced myopathy. The *C* allele is known to cause high plasma levels of statins [196,204,205], and a genomewide scan by the SEARCH collaboration indeed demonstrated a strong association with statin-induced myopathy. In fact, they reported an increased risk for myopathy by 4.5 times for each copy of a *C* allele and an increased risk of 16.9 times for *CC* versus *TT* [206], supporting the hypothesis that statin-induced myopathy is related to plasma levels of statin.

An excellent review published by Mangravite et al. provides a comprehensive overview of most studies conducted on the pharmacogenetics of statins [170,171,207].

6.5 CLINICAL IMPLICATIONS

By addressing the most extensively investigated pharmacogenetic associated genes in cardiovascular drug therapy, it is clear that there is little clinical implication. Although many initial associations of a polymorphism with modified drug response seemed very promising, the reality is that most associations cannot be replicated. Furthermore, most effects that were found are very small. Therefore, implementation of these interactions in clinical practice is still far away. Only for coumarins is there a real opportunity for pharmacogenetics by genotyping the *VKORC1* and *CYP2C9* gene to optimize anticoagulant therapy. Even though the effect of the existing variations in these genes is quite clear, clinical trials should provide evidence for the effectiveness of genotyping regarding prevention of adverse drug events and cost-effectiveness, before genotype guided dosing can become a part of everyday anticoagulant therapy. These studies are currently underway and will possibly advocate for a global implementation of *VKORC1* and *CYP2C9* genotyping into the anticoagulant therapy guidelines. Nevertheless, in August 2007 the FDA updated the warfarin prescribing information and highlighted the opportunity to use genetic tests to improve their initial estimate of warfarin dose.

For the other cardiovascular drugs discussed in this chapter, future research may well elucidate the exact role of genetics in the response to these drugs, but current knowledge is somewhat disappointing after high expectations of personalized medicine in the late 1990s. Nevertheless, for cardiovascular drugs as well, other than coumarins, some real progress has been made. There is a reasonable body of evidence that clopidogrel response partly depends on *CYP2C19* genotype, response to β-blockers is affected by *ADRB1* genotype status, and statin efficacy is highly likely to depend on variation in the *HMGCR* gene, whereas myopathy is related to a polymorphism in the *SLCO1B1*.

6.6 FUTURE DIRECTIONS

Current approaches in pharmacogenetic research do not seem to lead to results that meet our expectations of individualized medicine. Therefore, new approaches are needed to address issues and challenges such as the number of SNPs studied, study power, study design, and application of new statistical methods in (pharmaco)genetic analysis.

Most studies have examined only one polymorphism in a candidate gene associated with modified response to a certain drug. However, drug response is likely to result from complex interactions among various biologic pathways. Hence, future studies should consider a set of candidate genes and/or a genomewide scan (GWS) rather than addressing a single or small number of SNPs. In more recent years, the costs for a GWS have considerably decreased and will be come increasingly available.

Examining multiple SNPs will require sufficient sample size, which many studies to date lack. Moreover, analysis of large numbers of SNPs to identify a combination of SNPs that influence drug efficacy will pose a huge challenge due to statistical problems. Not only should the issue of multiple testing of many SNP be addressed with new tools in statistical analysis; the possible important effects of gene–gene interactions should be considered as will [208]. Although a definitive statistical method for characterising statistical patterns of epistasis in not known yet, conventional statistical methods alone will not provide the appropriate tool for deciphering the complexity of pharmacogenetics.

Finally, to elucidate mechanisms that lie behind the genetic associations, other fields of research, including proteomics and transcriptomics, should be integrated in the field of pharmacogenomics [209].

6.7 CONCLUSION

In conclusion, although pharmacogenetic testing is already part of everyday clinical practice in some areas (chemotherapy, psychiatry), for cardiovascular drugs currently only oral anticoagulant therapy seems to have a real opportunity to benefit from pharmacogenetic testing. Despite the tremendous amount of publications in this field, there is no reason to advocate for genetic testing for any other cardiovascular drugs as yet. Although future research will certainly benefit from emerging genetic technology as high-throughput genomewide scans will be readily available, finding the genetic profile that will predict response to cardiovascular drugs will be a major challenge.

REFERENCES

1. McGovern PG, et al. Trends in acute coronary heart disease mortality, morbidity, and medical care from 1985 through 1997: The Minnesota heart survey. *Circulation*, 2001; **104**(1):19–24.
2. Weinshilboum R. Inheritance and drug response. *New Engl. J. Med.* 2003;**348**(6): 529–537.
3. World Health Organization (available from `http://www.who.int/cardiovascular_diseases/en/`; accessed 7/01/11).
4. Mackay J, Mensah G. *The Atlas of Heart Disease and Stroke*, World Health Organization, 2004.
5. Lloyd-Jones D, et al. Heart disease and stroke statistics—2009 update. A report from the American Heart Association Statistics Committee and Stroke Statistics Subcommittee. *Circulation* 2009;**119**(3):480–486.
6. Yeghiazarians Y, et al. Unstable angina pectoris. *New Engl. J. Med.* 2000;**342** (2):101–114.
7. Lichtenstein AH, et al. Diet and lifestyle recommendations revision 2006: A scientific statement from the American Heart Association Nutrition Committee. *Circulation* 2006; **114**(1):82–96.
8. Graham I, et al. European guidelines on cardiovascular disease prevention in clinical practice: Executive summary. *Atherosclerosis* 2007;**194**(1):1–45.
9. Antithrombotic Trialists' Collaboration. Collaborative meta-analysis of randomised trials of antiplatelet therapy for prevention of death, myocardial infarction, and stroke in high risk patients. *Br. Med. J.* 2002;**324**(7329):71–86.
10. Grotemeyer KH, Scharafinski HW, Husstedt IW. Two-year follow-up of aspirin responder and aspirin non responder. A pilot-study including 180 post-stroke patients. *Thromb. Res.* 1993;**71**(5):397–403.
11. Krasopoulos G, et al. Aspirin "resistance" and risk of cardiovascular morbidity: Systematic review and meta-analysis. *Br. Med. J.* 2008;**336**(7637):195–198.
12. Snoep JD, et al. Clopidogrel nonresponsiveness in patients undergoing percutaneous coronary intervention with stenting: A systematic review and meta-analysis. *Am. Heart J.* 2007;**154**(2):221–231.
13. Michelson AD, Frelinger AL, 3rd, Furman MI. Current options in platelet function testing. *Am. J. Cardiol.* 2006;**98**(10A):4N–10N.
14. Maree AO, et al. Cyclooxygenase-1 haplotype modulates platelet response to aspirin. *J. Thromb. Haemost.* 2005;**3**(10):2340–2345.

15. Lepantalo A, et al. Polymorphisms of COX-1 and GPVI associate with the antiplatelet effect of aspirin in coronary artery disease patients. *Thromb. Haemost.* 2006;**95**(2): 253–259.
16. Gonzalez-Conejero R, et al. Biological assessment of aspirin efficacy on healthy individuals: Heterogeneous response or aspirin failure? *Stroke* 2005;**36**(2):276–280.
17. Halushka MK, Walker LP, Halushka PV. Genetic variation in cyclooxygenase 1: Effects on response to aspirin. *Clin. Pharmacol. Ther.* 2003;**73**(1):122–130.
18. Lim E, et al. Dose-related efficacy of aspirin after coronary surgery in patients With Pl (A2) polymorphism (NCT00262275). *Ann. Thorac. Surg.* 2007;**83**(1):134–138.
19. Nurden AT. Platelet glycoprotein IIIa polymorphism and coronary thrombosis. *Lancet* 1997;**350**(9086):1189–1191.
20. Undas A, et al. Platelet glycoprotein IIIa polymorphism, aspirin, and thrombin generation. *Lancet* 1999;**353**(9157):982–983.
21. Szczeklik A, et al. Relationship between bleeding time, aspirin and the PlA1/A2 polymorphism of platelet glycoprotein IIIa. *Br. J. Haematol.* 2000;**110**(4): 965–967.
22. Undas A, et al. Pl(A2) polymorphism of beta(3) integrins is associated with enhanced thrombin generation and impaired antithrombotic action of aspirin at the site of microvascular injury. *Circulation* 2001;**104**(22):2666–2672.
23. Pamukcu B, Oflaz H, Nisanci Y. The role of platelet glycoprotein IIIa polymorphism in the high prevalence of in vitro aspirin resistance in patients with intracoronary stent restenosis. *Am. Heart J.* 2005;**149**(4):675–680.
24. Lev EI, et al. Genetic polymorphisms of the platelet receptors P2Y(12), P2Y(1) and GP IIIa and response to aspirin and clopidogrel. *Thromb. Res.* 2007;**119**(3):355–360.
25. Jefferson BK, et al. Aspirin resistance and a single gene. *Am. J. Cardiol.* 2005;**95**(6): 805–808.
26. Papp E, et al. Glycoprotein IIIA gene (PlA) polymorphism and aspirin resistance: Is there any correlation? *Ann. Pharmacother.* 2005;**39**(6):1013–1018.
27. Macchi L, et al. Resistance in vitro to low-dose aspirin is associated with platelet PlA1 (GP IIIa) polymorphism but not with C807T(GP Ia/IIa) and C-5T Kozak (GP Ibalpha) polymorphisms. *J. Am. Coll. Cardiol.* 2003;**42**(6):1115–1119.
28. Cooke GE, et al. PlA2 polymorphism and efficacy of aspirin. *Lancet* 1998;**351**(9111): *p.* 1253.
29. Michelson AD, et al. Platelet GP IIIa Pl(A) polymorphisms display different sensitivities to agonists. *Circulation* 2000;**101**(9):1013–1018.
30. Angiolillo DJ, et al. PlA polymorphism and platelet reactivity following clopidogrel loading dose in patients undergoing coronary stent implantation. *Blood Coagul. Fibrinolysis* 2004;**15**(1):89–93.
31. Dropinski J, et al. Anti-thrombotic action of clopidogrel and P1(A1/A2) polymorphism of beta3 integrin in patients with coronary artery disease not being treated with aspirin. *Thromb. Haemost.* 2005;**94**(6):1300–1305.
32. Cooke GE, et al. Effect of platelet antigen polymorphism on platelet inhibition by aspirin, clopidogrel, or their combination. *J. Am. Coll. Cardiol.* 2006;**47**(3):541–546.
33. Papp E, et al. Does glycoprotein IIIa gene (Pl(A)) polymorphism influence clopidogrel resistance? A study in older patients. *Drugs Aging* 2007;**24**(4):345–350.

34. Goodman T, Ferro A, Sharma P. Pharmacogenetics of aspirin resistance: A comprehensive systematic review. *Br. J. Clin. Pharmacol.* 2008;**66**(2):222–232.

35. Goodman T, Sharma P, Ferro A. The genetics of aspirin resistance. *Int. J. Clin. Pract.* 2007;**61**(5):826–834.

36. Hulot JS, et al. Cytochrome P450 2C19 loss-of-function polymorphism is a major determinant of clopidogrel responsiveness in healthy subjects. *Blood* 2006;**108** (7):2244–2247.

37. Brandt JT, et al. Common polymorphisms of CYP2C19 and CYP2C9 affect the pharmacokinetic and pharmacodynamic response to clopidogrel but not prasugrel. *J. Thromb. Haemost.* 2007;**5**(12):2429–2436.

38. Mega JL, et al. Cytochrome P-450 polymorphisms and response to clopidogrel. *N. Engl. J. Med.* 2009;**360**(4):354–362.

39. Frere C, et al. Effect of cytochrome p450 polymorphisms on platelet reactivity after treatment with clopidogrel in acute coronary syndrome. *Am. J. Cardiol.* 2008;**101**(8): 1088–1093.

40. Fontana P, et al. Influence of CYP2C19 and CYP3A4 gene polymorphisms on clopidogrel responsiveness in healthy subjects. *J. Thromb. Haemost.* 2007;**5**(10):2153–2155.

41. Simon T, et al. Genetic determinants of response to clopidogrel and cardiovascular events. *New Engl. J. Med.* 2009;**360**(4):363–375.

42. Collet JP, et al. Cytochrome P450 2C19 polymorphism in young patients treated with clopidogrel after myocardial infarction: A cohort study. *Lancet* 2009;**373**(9660): 309–317.

43. Storey RF, Clopidogrel in acute coronary syndrome: To genotype or not? *Lancet* 2009;**373**(9660):276–278.

44. Feher G, et al. The genetics of antiplatelet drug resistance. *Clin. Genet.* 2009;**75**(1):1–18.

45. Angiolillo DJ, et al. Lack of association between the P2Y12 receptor gene polymorphism and platelet response to clopidogrel in patients with coronary artery disease. *Thromb. Res.* 2005;**116**(6):491–497.

46. Bura A, et al. Role of the P2Y12 gene polymorphism in platelet responsiveness to clopidogrel in healthy subjects. *J. Thromb. Haemost.* 2006;**4**(9):2096–2097.

47. von Beckerath N, et al. P2Y12 gene H2 haplotype is not associated with increased adenosine diphosphate-induced platelet aggregation after initiation of clopidogrel therapy with a high loading dose. *Blood Coagul. Fibrinolysis* 2005;**16**(3):199–204.

48. Cuisset T, et al. Role of the T744C polymorphism of the P2Y12 gene on platelet response to a 600-mg loading dose of clopidogrel in 597 patients with non-ST-segment elevation acute coronary syndrome. *Thromb. Res.* 2007;**120**(6):893–899.

49. Giusti B, et al. Cytochrome P450 2C19 loss-of-function polymorphism, but not CYP3A4 IVS10 + 12G/A and P2Y12 T744C polymorphisms, is associated with response variability to dual antiplatelet treatment in high-risk vascular patients. *Pharmacogenet. Genomics* 2007;**17**(12):1057–1064.

50. Sibbing D, et al. P2Y1 gene A1622G dimorphism is not associated with adenosine diphosphate-induced platelet activation and aggregation after administration of a single high dose of clopidogrel. *J. Thromb. Haemost.* 2006;**4**(4):912–914.

51. Maree AO, Fitzgerald DJ. Variable platelet response to aspirin and clopidogrel in atherothrombotic disease. *Circulation* 2007;**115**(16):2196–2207.

52. Hirsh J, et al. Antithrombotic and thrombolytic therapy: American College of Chest Physicians Evidence-Based Clinical Practice Guidelines (8th ed.). *Chest* 2008;**133** (6 Suppl.):110S–112S.

53. Ansell J, et al. Descriptive analysis of the process and quality of oral anticoagulation management in real-life practice in patients with chronic non-valvular atrial fibrillation: The international study of anticoagulation management (ISAM). *J. Thromb. Thrombolysis* 2007;**23**(2):83–91.

54. Pengo V, et al. Worldwide management of oral anticoagulant therapy: The ISAM study. *J. Thromb. Thrombolysis* 2006;**21**(1):73–77.

55. Wadelius M, Pirmohamed M. Pharmacogenetics of warfarin: Current status and future challenges. *Pharmacogenomics J.* 2007;**7**(2):99–111.

56. Fihn SD, et al. Risk factors for complications of chronic anticoagulation. A multicenter study. Warfarin optimized outpatient follow-up study group. *Ann. Intern. Med.* 1993;**118** (7):511–520.

57. Hylek EM, Singer DE. Risk factors for intracranial hemorrhage in outpatients taking warfarin. *Ann. Intern. Med.* 1994;**120**(11): 897–902.

58. Yin T, Miyata T. Warfarin dose and the pharmacogenomics of CYP2C9 and VKORC1—rationale and perspectives. *Thromb. Res.* 2007;**120**(1):1–10.

59. Sanderson S, Emery J, Higgins J. CYP2C9 gene variants, drug dose, and bleeding risk in warfarin-treated patients: A HuGEnet systematic review and meta-analysis. *Genet. Med.* 2005;**7**(2):97–104.

60. Lindh JD, et al. Influence of CYP2C9 genotype on warfarin dose requirements—a systematic review and meta-analysis. *Eur. J. Clin. Pharmacol.* 2009;**65**(4):365–375.

61. Thijssen HH, Verkooijen IW, Frank HL. The possession of the CYP2C9*3 allele is associated with low dose requirement of acenocoumarol. *Pharmacogenetics* 2000; **10**(8):757–760.

62. Tassies D, et al. Pharmacogenetics of acenocoumarol: Cytochrome P450 CYP2C9 polymorphisms influence dose requirements and stability of anticoagulation. *Haematologica* 2002;**87**(11):1185–1191.

63. Hermida J, et al. Differential effects of 2C9*3 and 2C9*2 variants of cytochrome P-450 CYP2C9 on sensitivity to acenocoumarol. *Blood* 2002;**99**(11):4237–4239.

64. Visser LE, et al. The risk of overanticoagulation in patients with cytochrome P450 CYP2C9*2 or CYP2C9*3 alleles on acenocoumarol or phenprocoumon. *Pharmacogenetics* 2004;**14**(1):27–33.

65. Schalekamp T, et al. Acenocoumarol stabilization is delayed in CYP2C93 carriers. *Clin. Pharmacol. Ther.* 2004;**75**(5):394–402.

66. Visser LE, et al. The risk of bleeding complications in patients with cytochrome P450 CYP2C9*2 or CYP2C9*3 alleles on acenocoumarol or phenprocoumon. *Thromb. Haemost.* 2004;**92**(1):61–66.

67. Ufer M, et al. Genetic polymorphisms of cytochrome P450 2C9 causing reduced phenprocoumon (S)-7-hydroxylation in vitro and in vivo. *Xenobiotica* 2004;**34**(9):847–859.

68. Schalekamp T, et al. Effects of cytochrome P450 2C9 polymorphisms on phenprocoumon anticoagulation status. *Clin. Pharmacol. Ther.* 2004;**76**(5):409–417.

69. Hummers-Pradier E, et al. Determination of bleeding risk using genetic markers in patients taking phenprocoumon. *Eur. J. Clin. Pharmacol.* 2003;**59**(3):213–219.

70. Suttie JW. The biochemical basis of warfarin therapy. *Adv. Exp. Med. Biol.* 1987;**214**:3–16.

71. Bodin L, et al. Cytochrome P450 2C9 (CYP2C9) and vitamin K epoxide reductase (VKORC1) genotypes as determinants of acenocoumarol sensitivity. *Blood* 2005;**106** (1):135–140.

72. Reitsma PH, et al. A C1173T dimorphism in the VKORC1 gene determines coumarin sensitivity and bleeding risk. *PLoS Med.* 2005;**2**(10):e312.

73. Schalekamp T, et al. VKORC1 and CYP2C9 genotypes and acenocoumarol anticoagulation status: Interaction between both genotypes affects overanticoagulation. *Clin. Pharmacol. Ther.* 2006;**80**(1):13–22.

74. Rieder MJ, et al. Effect of VKORC1 haplotypes on transcriptional regulation and warfarin dose. *New Engl. J. Med.* 2005;**352**(22):2285–2293.

75. Schalekamp T, et al. VKORC1 and CYP2C9 genotypes and phenprocoumon anticoagulation status: Interaction between both genotypes affects dose requirement. *Clin. Pharmacol. Ther.* 2007;**81**(2):185–193.

76. Limdi NA, et al. Influence of CYP2C9 and VKORC1 1173C/T genotype on the risk of hemorrhagic complications in African-American and European-American patients on warfarin. *Clin. Pharmacol. Ther.* 2008;**83**(2):312–321.

77. Aquilante CL, et al. Influence of coagulation factor, vitamin K epoxide reductase complex subunit 1, and cytochrome P450 2C9 gene polymorphisms on warfarin dose requirements. *Clin. Pharmacol. Ther.* 2006;**79**(4):291–302.

78. D'Ambrosio RL, et al. Polymorphisms in factor II and factor VII genes modulate oral anticoagulation with warfarin. *Haematologica* 2004;**89**(12):1510–1516.

79. Shikata E, et al. Association of pharmacokinetic (CYP2C9) and pharmacodynamic (factors II, VII, IX, and X; proteins S and C; and gamma-glutamyl carboxylase) gene variants with warfarin sensitivity. *Blood* 2004;**103**(7):2630–2635.

80. Wadelius M, et al. The largest prospective warfarin-treated cohort supports genetic forecasting. *Blood* 2009;**113**(4):784–792.

81. Cooper GM, et al. A genome-wide scan for common genetic variants with a large influence on warfarin maintenance dose. *Blood* 2008;**112**(4):1022–1027.

82. Mizutani T. PM frequencies of major CYPs in Asians and Caucasians. *Drug. Metab. Rev.* 2003;**35**(2–3):99–106.

83. Xie HG, et al. CYP2C9 allelic variants: Ethnic distribution and functional significance. *Adv. Drug Deliv. Rev.* 2002;**54**(10):1257–1270.

84. Gage BF, et al. Use of pharmacogenetic and clinical factors to predict the therapeutic dose of warfarin. *Clin. Pharmacol. Ther.* 2008;**84**(3):326–331.

85. Wadelius M, et al. The largest prospective warfarin-treated cohort supports genetic forecasting. *Blood* 2009;**113**(4):784–792.

86. Anderson JL, et al. Randomized trial of genotype-guided versus standard warfarin dosing in patients initiating oral anticoagulation. *Circulation* 2007;**116**(22):2563–2570.

87. Hynicka LM, Cahoon WD, Jr, Bukaveckas BL. Genetic testing for warfarin therapy initiation. *Ann. Pharmacother.* 2008;**42**(9):1298–1303.

88. Psaty BM, et al. Health outcomes associated with various antihypertensive therapies used as first-line agents: A network meta-analysis. *JAMA* 2003;**289**(19):2534–2544.

89. Manunta P, et al. Adducin polymorphism affects renal proximal tubule reabsorption in hypertension. *Hypertension* 1999;**33**(2):694–697.

90. Cusi D, et al. Polymorphisms of alpha-adducin and salt sensitivity in patients with essential hypertension. *Lancet* 1997;**349**(9062):1353–1357.

91. Glorioso N, et al. The role of alpha-adducin polymorphism in blood pressure and sodium handling regulation may not be excluded by a negative association study. *Hypertension* 1999;**34**(4 Pt 1):649–654.

92. Sciarrone MT, et al. ACE and alpha-adducin polymorphism as markers of individual response to diuretic therapy. *Hypertension* 2003;**41**(3):398–403.

93. Davis BR, et al. Antihypertensive therapy, the alpha-adducin polymorphism, and cardiovascular disease in high-risk hypertensive persons: The genetics of hypertension-associated treatment study. *Pharmacogenomics J.* 2007;**7**(2):112–122.

94. Turner ST, et al. Effects of endothelial nitric oxide synthase, alpha-adducin, and other candidate gene polymorphisms on blood pressure response to hydrochlorothiazide. *Am. J. Hypertens.* 2003;**16**(10):834–839.

95. Schelleman H, et al. Interactions between five candidate genes and antihypertensive drug therapy on blood pressure. *Pharmacogenomics J.* 2006;**6**(1):22–26.

96. Schelleman H, et al. The influence of the alpha-adducin G460W polymorphism and angiotensinogen M235T polymorphism on antihypertensive medication and blood pressure. *Eur. J. Hum. Genet.* 2006;**14**(7):860–866.

97. Psaty BM, et al. Diuretic therapy, the alpha-adducin gene variant, and the risk of myocardial infarction or stroke in persons with treated hypertension. *JAMA* 2002; **287**(13):1680–1689.

98. Schelleman H, et al. Diuretic-gene interaction and the risk of myocardial infarction and stroke. *Pharmacogenomics J.* 2007;**7**(5):346–352.

99. Gerhard T, et al. Alpha-adducin polymorphism associated with increased risk of adverse cardiovascular outcomes: Results from GENEtic Substudy of the INternational VErapamil SR-trandolapril STudy (INVEST-GENES). *Am. Heart J.* 2008;**156**(2):397–404.

100. van Wieren-de Wijer DB, et al. Interaction between the Gly460Trp alpha-adducin gene variant and diuretics on the risk of myocardial infarction. *J. Hypertens.* 2009;**27**(1): 61–68.

101. Rigat B, et al. An insertion/deletion polymorphism in the angiotensin I-converting enzyme gene accounting for half the variance of serum enzyme levels. *J. Clin. Invest.* 1990;**86**(4):1343–1346.

102. Preston RA, et al. Age-race subgroup compared with renin profile as predictors of blood pressure response to antihypertensive therapy. Department of Veterans Affairs cooperative study group on antihypertensive agents. *JAMA* 1998;**280**(13):1168–1172.

103. Schwartz GL, et al. Interacting effects of gender and genotype on blood pressure response to hydrochlorothiazide. *Kidney Int.* 2002;**62**(5):1718–1723.

104. Arnett DK, et al. Pharmacogenetic association of the angiotensin-converting enzyme insertion/deletion polymorphism on blood pressure and cardiovascular risk in relation to antihypertensive treatment: The Genetics of Hypertension-Associated Treatment (GenHAT) study. *Circulation* 2005;**111**(25):3374–3383.

105. Frazier L, et al. Multilocus effects of the renin-angiotensin-aldosterone system genes on blood pressure response to a thiazide diuretic. *Pharmacogenomics J.* 2004;**4**(1):17–23.

106. Schelleman H, et al. Drug-gene interaction between the insertion/deletion polymorphism of the angiotensin-converting enzyme gene and antihypertensive therapy. *Ann. Pharmacother.* 2006;**40**(2):212–218.

107. Jiang X, et al. Effect of renin-angiotensin-aldosterone system gene polymorphisms on blood pressure response to antihypertensive treatment. *Chin. Med. J. (Engl.)* 2007;**120**(9): 782–786.

108. Turner ST, et al. C825T polymorphism of the G protein beta(3)-subunit and antihypertensive response to a thiazide diuretic. *Hypertension* 2001;**37**(2 Pt. 2):739–743.

109. Schunkert H, et al. Association between a polymorphism in the G protein beta3 subunit gene and lower renin and elevated diastolic blood pressure levels. *Hypertension* 1998; **32**(3):510–513.

110. Mason DA, et al. A gain-of-function polymorphism in a G-protein coupling domain of the human beta1-adrenergic receptor. *J. Biol. Chem.* 1999;**274**(18):12670–12674.

111. Rathz DA, et al. Amino acid 49 polymorphisms of the human beta1-adrenergic receptor affect agonist-promoted trafficking. *J. Cardiovasc. Pharmacol.* 2002;**39**(2):155–160.

112. O'Shaughnessy KM, et al. The gain-of-function G389R variant of the beta1-adrenoceptor does not influence blood pressure or heart rate response to beta-blockade in hypertensive subjects. *Clin. Sci. (London)* 2000;**99**(3):233–238.

113. Johnson JA, et al. Beta 1-adrenergic receptor polymorphisms and antihypertensive response to metoprolol. *Clin. Pharmacol. Ther.* 2003;**74**(1):44–52.

114. Liu J, et al. beta1-adrenergic receptor polymorphisms influence the response to metoprolol monotherapy in patients with essential hypertension. *Clin. Pharmacol. Ther.* 2006;**80**(1):23–32.

115. Liu J, et al. Gly389Arg polymorphism of beta1-adrenergic receptor is associated with the cardiovascular response to metoprolol. *Clin. Pharmacol. Ther.* 2003;**74**(4):372–379.

116. Sofowora GG, et al. A common beta1-adrenergic receptor polymorphism (Arg389Gly) affects blood pressure response to beta-blockade. *Clin. Pharmacol. Ther.* 2003;**73**(4): 366–371.

117. Zateyshchikov DA, et al. Association of CYP2D6 and ADRB1 genes with hypotensive and antichronotropic action of betaxolol in patients with arterial hypertension. *Fundam. Clin. Pharmacol.* 2007;**21**(4):437–443.

118. Filigheddu F, et al. Genetic polymorphisms of the beta-adrenergic system: Association with essential hypertension and response to beta-blockade. *Pharmacogenomics J.* 2004; **4**(3):154–160.

119. Karlsson J, et al. Beta1-adrenergic receptor gene polymorphisms and response to beta1-adrenergic receptor blockade in patients with essential hypertension. *Clin. Cardiol.* 2004;**27**(6):347–350.

120. Lemaitre RN, et al. beta1- and beta2-adrenergic receptor gene variation, beta-blocker use and risk of myocardial infarction and stroke. *Am. J. Hypertens.* 2008;**21**(3):290–296.

121. Pacanowski MA, et al. beta-adrenergic receptor gene polymorphisms and beta-blocker treatment outcomes in hypertension. *Clin. Pharmacol. Ther.* 2008;**84**(6):715–721.

122. Kurland L, et al. Angiotensinogen gene polymorphisms: Relationship to blood pressure response to antihypertensive treatment. Results from the Swedish Irbesartan left ventricular hypertrophy investigation vs atenolol (SILVHIA) trial. *Am. J. Hypertens.* 2004; **17**(1):8–13.

123. Kurland L, et al. Angiotensin converting enzyme gene polymorphism predicts blood pressure response to angiotensin II receptor type 1 antagonist treatment in hypertensive patients. *J. Hypertens.* 2001;**19**(10):1783–1787.
124. Dudley C, et al. Prediction of patient responses to antihypertensive drugs using genetic polymorphisms: Investigation of renin-angiotensin system genes. *J. Hypertens.* 1996; **14**(2):259–262.
125. Harrap SB, et al. The ACE gene I/D polymorphism is not associated with the blood pressure and cardiovascular benefits of ACE inhibition. *Hypertension* 2003;**42**(3): 297–303.
126. Hingorani AD, et al. Renin-angiotensin system gene polymorphisms influence blood pressure and the response to angiotensin converting enzyme inhibition. *J. Hypertens.* 1995;**13**(12 Pt. 2):1602–1609.
127. Bis JC, et al. Angiotensinogen Met235Thr polymorphism, angiotensin-converting enzyme inhibitor therapy, and the risk of nonfatal stroke or myocardial infarction in hypertensive patients. *Am. J. Hypertens.* 2003;**16**(12):1011–1017.
128. Mondorf UF, et al. Contribution of angiotensin I converting enzyme gene polymorphism and angiotensinogen gene polymorphism to blood pressure regulation in essential hypertension. *Am. J. Hypertens.* 1998;**11**(2):174–183.
129. Schelleman H, et al. Angiotensinogen M235T polymorphism and the risk of myocardial infarction and stroke among hypertensive patients on ACE-inhibitors or beta-blockers. *Eur. J. Hum. Genet.* 2007;**15**(4):478–484.
130. Su X, et al. Association between angiotensinogen, angiotensin II receptor genes, and blood pressure response to an angiotensin-converting enzyme inhibitor. *Circulation* 2007;**115**(6):725–732.
131. Yu H, et al. T1198C polymorphism of the angiotensinogen gene and antihypertensive response to angiotensin-converting enzyme inhibitors. *Hypertens. Res.* 2005;**28**(12): 981–986.
132. Kurland L, et al. Aldosterone synthase (CYP11B2) -344 C/T polymorphism is related to antihypertensive response: Result from the Swedish Irbesartan left ventricular hypertrophy investigation versus atenolol (SILVHIA) trial. *Am. J. Hypertens.* 2002;**15**(5): 389–393.
133. Ortlepp JR, et al. Variants of the CYP11B2 gene predict response to therapy with candesartan. *Eur. J. Pharmacol.* 2002;**445**(1–2):151–152.
134. Redon J, et al. Renin-angiotensin system gene polymorphisms: Relationship with blood pressure and microalbuminuria in telmisartan-treated hypertensive patients. *Pharmacogenomics J.* 2005;**5**(1):14–20.
135. Fuller RW, Choudry NB. Increased cough reflex associated with angiotensin converting enzyme inhibitor cough. *Br. Med. J. (Clin. Res. Ed.)* 1987;**295**(6605):1025–1026.
136. Mukae S, et al. Bradykinin B(2) receptor gene polymorphism is associated with angiotensin-converting enzyme inhibitor-related cough. *Hypertension* 2000;**36**(1): 127–131.
137. Mukae S, et al. Association of polymorphisms of the renin-angiotensin system and bradykinin B2 receptor with ACE-inhibitor-related cough. *J. Hum. Hypertens.* 2002; **16**(12):857–863.
138. Lee YJ, Tsai JC. Angiotensin-converting enzyme gene insertion/deletion, not bradykinin B2 receptor -58T/C gene polymorphism, associated with angiotensin-converting enzyme

inhibitor-related cough in Chinese female patients with non-insulin-dependent diabetes mellitus. *Metabolism* 2001;**50**(11):1346–1350.

139. Zee RY, et al. Three candidate genes and angiotensin-converting enzyme inhibitor-related cough: A pharmacogenetic analysis. *Hypertension* 1998;**31**(4):925–928.

140. Bozkurt O, et al. Genetic variation in the renin-angiotensin system modifies the beneficial effects of ACE inhibitors on the risk of diabetes mellitus among hypertensives. *J. Hum. Hypertens.* 2008;**22**(11):774–780.

141. Arnett DK, Claas SA, Glasser SP. Pharmacogenetics of antihypertensive treatment. *Vascul. Pharmacol.* 2006;**44**(2):107–118.

142. Shin J, Johnson JA. Pharmacogenetics of beta-blockers. *Pharmacotherapy* 2007;**27**(6): 874–887.

143. Mellen PB, Herrington DM. Pharmacogenomics of blood pressure response to antihypertensive treatment. *J. Hypertens.* 2005;**23**(7):1311–1325.

144. Schelleman H, et al. Drug-gene interactions between genetic polymorphisms and antihypertensive therapy. *Drugs* 2004;**64**(16):1801–1816.

145. Cheung BM, et al. Meta-analysis of large randomized controlled trials to evaluate the impact of statins on cardiovascular outcomes. *Br. J. Clin. Pharmacol.* 2004;**57** (5):640–651.

146. Chasman DI, et al. Pharmacogenetic study of statin therapy and cholesterol reduction. JAMA 2004;**291**(23):2821–2827.

147. Thompson JF, et al. An association study of 43 SNPs in 16 candidate genes with atorvastatin response. *Pharmacogenomics J.* 2005;**5**(6):352–358.

148. Donnelly LA, et al. A paucimorphic variant in the HMG-CoA reductase gene is associated with lipid-lowering response to statin treatment in diabetes: A GoDARTS study. *Pharmacogenet. Genomics* 2008;**18**(12):1021–1026.

149. Krauss RM, et al. Variation in the 3-hydroxyl-3-methylglutaryl coenzyme a reductase gene is associated with racial differences in low-density lipoprotein cholesterol response to simvastatin treatment. *Circulation* 2008;**117**(12):1537–1544.

150. Polisecki E, et al. Genetic variation at the LDL receptor and HMG-CoA reductase gene loci, lipid levels, statin response, and cardiovascular disease incidence in PROSPER. *Atherosclerosis* 2008;**200**(1):109–114.

151. Hindorff LA, et al. Common genetic variation in six lipid-related and statin-related genes, statin use and risk of incident nonfatal myocardial infarction and stroke. *Pharmacogenet. Genomics* 2008;**18**(8):677–682.

152. Medina MW, et al. Alternative splicing of 3-hydroxy-3-methylglutaryl coenzyme A reductase is associated with plasma low-density lipoprotein cholesterol response to simvastatin. *Circulation* 2008;**118**(4):355–362.

153. Ordovas JM, et al. Effect of apolipoprotein E and A-IV phenotypes on the low density lipoprotein response to HMG CoA reductase inhibitor therapy. *Atherosclerosis* 1995; **113**(2):157–166.

154. Ye P, Shang Y, Ding X. The influence of apolipoprotein B and E gene polymorphisms on the response to simvastatin therapy in patients with hyperlipidemia. *Chin. Med. Sci. J.* 2003;**18**(1):9–13.

155. Pedro-Botet J, et al. Apolipoprotein E genotype affects plasma lipid response to atorvastatin in a gender specific manner. *Atherosclerosis* 2001;**158**(1):183–193.

156. Ballantyne CM, et al. Apolipoprotein E genotypes and response of plasma lipids and progression-regression of coronary atherosclerosis to lipid-lowering drug therapy. *J. Am. Coll. Cardiol.* 2000;**36**(5):1572–1578.

157. Nestel P, et al. A comparative study of the efficacy of simvastatin and gemfibrozil in combined hyperlipoproteinemia: Prediction of response by baseline lipids, apo E genotype, lipoprotein(a) and insulin. *Atherosclerosis* 1997;**129**(2):231–239.

158. Takane H, et al. Pharmacogenetic determinants of variability in lipid-lowering response to pravastatin therapy. *J. Hum. Genet.* 2006;**51**(9):822–826.

159. Ojala JP, et al. Effect of apolipoprotein E polymorphism and XbaI polymorphism of apolipoprotein B on response to lovastatin treatment in familial and non-familial hypercholesterolaemia. *J. Intern. Med.* 1991;**230**(5):397–405.

160. Donnelly LA, et al. Apolipoprotein E genotypes are associated with lipid-lowering responses to statin treatment in diabetes: A Go-DARTS study. *Pharmacogenet. Genomics* 2008;**18**(4):279–287.

161. Pena R, et al. Effect of apoE genotype on the hypolipidaemic response to pravastatin in an outpatient setting. *J. Intern. Med.* 2002;**251**(6):518–525.

162. Sanllehy C, et al. Lack of interaction of apolipoprotein E phenotype with the lipoprotein response to lovastatin or gemfibrozil in patients with primary hypercholesterolemia. *Metabolism* 1998;**47**(5):560–565.

163. Tavintharan S, et al. Apolipoprotein E genotype affects the response to lipid-lowering therapy in Chinese patients with type 2 diabetes mellitus. *Diab. Obes. Metab.* 2007;**9**(1):81–86.

164. Zuccaro P, et al. Tolerability of statins is not linked to CYP450 polymorphisms, but reduced CYP2D6 metabolism improves cholesteraemic response to simvastatin and fluvastatin. *Pharmacol. Res.* 2007;**55**(4):310–317.

165. Maitland-van der Zee AH, et al. Apolipoprotein-E polymorphism and response to pravastatin in men with coronary artery disease (REGRESS). *Acta Cardiol.* 2006; **61**(3):327–331.

166. Fiegenbaum M, et al. Pharmacogenetic study of apolipoprotein E, cholesteryl ester transfer protein and hepatic lipase genes and simvastatin therapy in Brazilian subjects. *Clin. Chim. Acta.* 2005;**362**(1–2):182–188.

167. Gerdes LU, et al. The apolipoprotein epsilon4 allele determines prognosis and the effect on prognosis of simvastatin in survivors of myocardial infarction: A substudy of the Scandinavian simvastatin survival study. *Circulation* 2000;**101**(12):1366–1371.

168. Chiodini BD, et al. Apolipoprotein E polymorphisms influence effect of pravastatin on survival after myocardial infarction in a Mediterranean population: The GISSI-prevenzione study. *Eur. Heart J.* 2007;**28**(16):1977–1983.

169. Maitland-van der Zee AH, et al. The effectiveness of hydroxy-methylglutaryl coenzyme A reductase inhibitors (statins) in the elderly is not influenced by apolipoprotein E genotype. *Pharmacogenetics* 2002;**12**(8):647–653.

170. Mangravite LM, Krauss RM. Pharmacogenomics of statin response. *Curr. Opin. Lipidol.* 2007;**18**(4):409–414.

171. Mangravite LM, Thorn CF, Krauss RM. Clinical implications of pharmacogenomics of statin treatment. *Pharmacogenomics J.* 2006;**6**(6):360–374.

172. Choumerianou DM, Dedoussis GV. Familial hypercholesterolemia and response to statin therapy according to LDLR genetic background. *Clin. Chem. Lab. Med.* 2005;**43**(8): 793–801.

173. Lahoz C, et al. Baseline levels of low-density lipoprotein cholesterol and lipoprotein (a) and the AvaII polymorphism of the low-density lipoprotein receptor gene influence the response of low-density lipoprotein cholesterol to pravastatin treatment. *Metabolism* 2005;**54**(6):741–747.

174. Salazar LA, et al. Lipid-lowering response of the HMG-CoA reductase inhibitor fluvastatin is influenced by polymorphisms in the low-density lipoprotein receptor gene in Brazilian patients with primary hypercholesterolemia. *J. Clin. Lab. Anal.* 2000;**14**(3):125–131.

175. Hannuksela ML, et al. Relation of polymorphisms in the cholesteryl ester transfer protein gene to transfer protein activity and plasma lipoprotein levels in alcohol drinkers. *Atherosclerosis* 1994;**110**(1):35–44.

176. Kuivenhoven JA, et al. The role of a common variant of the cholesteryl ester transfer protein gene in the progression of coronary atherosclerosis. The regression growth evaluation statin study group. *New Engl. J. Med.* 1998;**338**(2):86–93.

177. Regieli JJ, et al. CETP genotype predicts increased mortality in statin-treated men with proven cardiovascular disease: An adverse pharmacogenetic interaction. *Eur. Heart J.* 2008;**29**(22):2792–2799.

178. de Grooth GJ, et al. The cholesteryl ester transfer protein (CETP) TaqIB polymorphism in the cholesterol and recurrent events study: No interaction with the response to pravastatin therapy and no effects on cardiovascular outcome: A prospective analysis of the CETP TaqIB polymorphism on cardiovascular outcome and interaction with cholesterol-lowering therapy. *J. Am. Coll. Cardiol.* 2004;**43**(5):854–857.

179. Freeman DJ, et al. A polymorphism of the cholesteryl ester transfer protein gene predicts cardiovascular events in non-smokers in the west of scotland coronary prevention study. *Eur. Heart J.* 2003;**24**(20):1833–1842.

180. Klerkx AH, et al. Cholesteryl ester transfer protein concentration is associated with progression of atherosclerosis and response to pravastatin in men with coronary artery disease (REGRESS). *Eur. J. Clin. Invest.* 2004;**34**(1):21–28.

181. Marschang P, et al. Plasma cholesteryl ester transfer protein concentrations predict cardiovascular events in patients with coronary artery disease treated with pravastatin. *J. Intern. Med.* 2006;**260**(2):151–159.

182. Carlquist JF, et al. The cholesteryl ester transfer protein Taq1B gene polymorphism predicts clinical benefit of statin therapy in patients with significant coronary artery disease. *Am. Heart J.* 2003;**146**(6):1007–1014.

183. Boekholdt SM, et al. Cholesteryl ester transfer protein TaqIB variant, high-density lipoprotein cholesterol levels, cardiovascular risk, and efficacy of pravastatin treatment: Individual patient meta-analysis of 13, 677 subjects. Circulation 2005;**111**(3):278–287.

184. Sing K, et al. Lipoprotein lipase gene mutations, plasma lipid levels, progression/regression of coronary atherosclerosis, response to therapy, and future clinical events. Lipoproteins and coronary atherosclerosis study. *Atherosclerosis* 1999;**144**(2):435–442.

185. Lahoz C, et al. The -514C/T polymorphism of the hepatic lipase gene significantly modulates the HDL-cholesterol response to statin treatment. *Atherosclerosis* 2005; **182**(1):129–134.

186. Hansson GK, Inflammation, atherosclerosis, and coronary artery disease. *New Engl. J. Med.* 2005;**352**(16):1685–1695.

187. Jain MK, Ridker PM. Anti-inflammatory effects of statins: Clinical evidence and basic mechanisms. *Nat. Rev. Drug. Discov.* 2005;**4**(12):977–987.

188. Iakoubova OA, et al. Association of the Trp719Arg polymorphism in kinesin-like protein 6 with myocardial infarction and coronary heart disease in 2 prospective trials: The CARE and WOSCOPS trials. *J. Am. Coll. Cardiol.* 2008;**51**(4):435–443.

189. Bare LA, et al. Five common gene variants identify elevated genetic risk for coronary heart disease. *Genet. Med.* 2007;**9**(10):682–689.

190. Shiffman D, et al. A kinesin family member 6 variant is associated with coronary heart disease in the women's health study. *J. Am. Coll. Cardiol.* 2008;**51**(4):444–448.

191. Shiffman D, et al. Association of gene variants with incident myocardial infarction in the cardiovascular health study. *Arterioscler. Thromb. Vascul. Biol.* 2008;**28**(1): 173–179.

192. Iakoubova OA, et al. Polymorphism in KIF6 gene and benefit from statins after acute coronary syndromes: Results from the PROVE IT-TIMI 22 study. *J. Am. Coll. Cardiol.* 2008;**51**(4):449–455.

193. Boekholdt SM, et al. Variants of toll-like receptor 4 modify the efficacy of statin therapy and the risk of cardiovascular events. *Circulation* 2003;**107**(19):2416–2421.

194. Holloway JW, Yang IA, Ye S. Variation in the toll-like receptor 4 gene and susceptibility to myocardial infarction. *Pharmacogenet. Genomics* 2005;**15**(1):15–21.

195. Shitara Y, Sugiyama Y, Pharmacokinetic and pharmacodynamic alterations of 3-hydroxy-3-methylglutaryl coenzyme A (HMG-CoA) reductase inhibitors: Drug-drug interactions and interindividual differences in transporter and metabolic enzyme functions. *Pharmacol. Ther.* 2006;**112**(1):71–105.

196. Konig J, et al. Pharmacogenomics of human OATP transporters. *Naunyn. Schmiedebergs Arch. Pharmacol.* 2006;**372**(6):432–443.

197. Tachibana-Iimori R, et al. Effect of genetic polymorphism of OATP-C (SLCO1B1) on lipid-lowering response to HMG-CoA reductase inhibitors. *Drug Metab. Pharmacokinet.* 2004;**19**(5):375–380.

198. Zhang W, et al. SLCO1B1 521T-->C functional genetic polymorphism and lipid-lowering efficacy of multiple-dose pravastatin in Chinese coronary heart disease patients. *Br. J. Clin. Pharmacol.* 2007;**64**(3):346–352.

199. Igel M, et al. Impact of the SLCO1B1 polymorphism on the pharmacokinetics and lipid-lowering efficacy of multiple-dose pravastatin. *Clin. Pharmacol. Ther.* 2006;**79**(5): 419–426.

200. Niemi M, et al. Acute effects of pravastatin on cholesterol synthesis are associated with SLCO1B1 (encoding OATP1B1) haplotype *17. *Pharmacogenet. Genomics* 2005;**15**(5): 303–309.

201. Kajinami K, et al. Polymorphisms in the multidrug resistance-1 (MDR1) gene influence the response to atorvastatin treatment in a gender-specific manner. *Am. J. Cardiol.* 2004;**93**(8):1046–1050.

202. Fiegenbaum M, et al. The role of common variants of ABCB1, CYP3A4, and CYP3A5 genes in lipid-lowering efficacy and safety of simvastatin treatment. *Clin. Pharmacol. Ther.* 2005;**78**(5):551–558.

203. Vladutiu GD, Genetic predisposition to statin myopathy. *Curr. Opin. Rheumatol.* 2008; **20**(6):648–655.

204. Niemi M, et al. High plasma pravastatin concentrations are associated with single nucleotide polymorphisms and haplotypes of organic anion transporting polypeptide-C (OATP-C, SLCO1B1). *Pharmacogenetics* 2004;**14**(7):429–440.

205. Pasanen MK, et al. SLCO1B1 polymorphism markedly affects the pharmacokinetics of simvastatin acid. *Pharmacogenet. Genomics* 2006;**16**(12):873–879.

206. Link E, et al. SLCO1B1 variants and statin-induced myopathy—a genomewide study. *New Engl. J. Med.* 2008;**359**(8):789–799.

207. Mangravite LM, et al. Pharmacogenomics of statin response. *Curr. Opin. Mol. Ther.* 2008;**10**(6):555–561.

208. McKinney BA, et al. Machine learning for detecting gene-gene interactions: A review. *Appl. Bioinform.* 2006;**5**(2):77–88.

209. Evans WE, Relling MV. Moving towards individualized medicine with pharmacogenomics. *Nature* 2004;**429**(6990):464–468.

CHAPTER 7

Pharmacogenetics in Psychiatry

EVANGELIA M. TSAPAKIS, SARAH CURRAN, RUTH I. OHLSEN, NORA S. VYAS, and KATHERINE J. AITCHISON

King's College London, London, UK

ANN K. DALY

Newcastle University, Newcastle upon Tyne, UK

7.1 INTRODUCTION

Interindividual variation in response to medication and in adverse drug reactions (ADRs) is well known in psychiatry [1]. At present, most prescribing relies on the clinician's best judgment but for the most commonly prescribed medications (antipsychotics, antidepressants, and mood stabilizers), in 40–60% of cases, the first medication prescribed at a given dose either does not work or cannot be tolerated [2]. As with any pharmacologically active agent, the overall clinical effect is determined by a complex interplay of many factors, including age, gender, ethnicity, body mass and composition, liver function, other medications, dietary and other substances, and psychological and social factors in addition to pharmacogenetic factors.

Pharmacogenetic studies in psychiatry have to date identified polymorphisms in metabolic enzymes and drug targets, including receptors that have been associated with clinical outcome and ADRs [3–6] (see Chapters 2 and 5 for detailed description). Some centers are now beginning to used the identification of such polymorphisms as a clinical tool for individualized prescribing.

This chapter considers pharmacogenetic aspects of both drug response and susceptibility to ADRs in treatment with antipsychotic drugs, antidepressants, and mood stabilizers.

Pharmacogenetics and Individualized Therapy, First Edition.
Edited by Anke-Hilse Maitland-van der Zee and Ann K. Daly.

7.2 PHARMACOGENETICS OF ANTIPSYCHOTIC TREATMENT

7.2.1 Response

Polymorphisms in genes encoding drug metabolizing enzymes (DMEs), receptors, and transporters may all affect response to antipsychotics (APs) (i.e., antipsychotic medications). CYP2D6 plays a significant role in the metabolism of several APs, including perphenazine, thioridazine, zuclopenthixol, haloperidol, risperidone, and aripiprazole [7]. However, although numerous studies show significant relationships between CYP2D6 genotype and drug levels (see Chapter 2), definitive information in relation to the effect of genotype on drug response is only just emerging [8].

Other commonly used APs included olanzapine and clozapine, for which CYP1A2 plays a significant metabolic role [9]. In the case of the latter, although it exhibits large interindividual variations in bioavailability, steady-state plasma concentrations, and clearance, there is a narrow therapeutic index [10]. A preliminary study suggested that *CYP1A2* polymorphisms may be associated with response to clozapine [11].

Since almost all APs are dopamine receptor antagonists, many drug response studies have focused on genes that code for dopaminergic receptors, such as the dopaminergic D_2, D_3, and D_4 receptors (*DRD2*, *DRD3*, and *DRD4*, respectively). In addition, other relevant targets have been studied, such as the serotonergic $5HT_{2A}$ (*HTR2A*), $5HT_{2C}$ (*HTR2C*), and $5HT_6$ (*HTR6*) receptors, the histaminergic H_1 and H_2 receptors (*HRH1* and *HRH2*), the muscarinic cholinergic receptors, neurotransmitter transporters, and other intracellular signalling molecules.

Several studies have found associations between variants in *DRD2* and response or ADRs to typical APs [12–16]. Associations have also been found with response to clozapine, olanzapine, and risperidone [17–22]. In particular, the deletion (*Del*) allele of the −141-C*Ins/Del* polymorphism, which has been associated with reduced *DRD2* expression *in vitro* [23], has been associated with reduced response to AP treatment [15,16]. This polymorphism has, however, been associated with increased D_2 receptor density in the striatum *in vivo* [24], which may possibly represent a compensatory mechanism in the striatolimbic pathway.

An association between a *DRD3* Ser9Gly polymorphism and improvement in positive symptomatology after AP treatment has been reported, especially in the case of typical APs [25–29]. *In vitro* studies indicate that the Gly variant is associated with higher dopamine binding affinity [30]. The Gly variant has in general been associated with good response in Caucasians but poor response in Chinese, which may relate to the different genetic backgrounds in the different ethnic groups.

An elevation of D_4 receptors in the brain of patients with schizophrenia, combined with the observation that D_4 receptors were more strongly targeted by clozapine than D_2 receptors, led to the hypothesis that D_4 receptors mediate the AP efficacy of clozapine [31,32]. Several studies on the association of a 16-amino acid repeat polymorphism in exon 3 of *DRD4* have been conducted, with conflicting findings. Three studies have suggested that this polymorphism is associated with response to clozapine and risperidone [33–35], while others have been negative in regard to such associations [36–39].

A number of reports have found associations between a silent *HTR2A* polymorphism, the 102-T/C substitution and response to clozapine and risperidone [40–45]. This polymorphism is in high linkage disequilibrium (LD) with the −1438G > A promoter polymorphism in Caucasians, and its G allele may be associated with reduced promoter activity [45]. The −1438G allele tends to be associated with poorer response, suggesting that a lower expression of the $5HT_{2A}$ protein may reduce the serotonin–dopamine regulation exerted by $5HT_{2A}$ antagonists. Another functional variant in *HTR2A* resulting in a His452Tyr change has been associated with response to clozapine response [46,47], and although not replicated [48–52], a meta-analysis seemed to indicate an association of the Tyr variant with worse response [42].

Genetic variants in the promoter (−759T > C and −995G > A) and coding region (Cys23Ser) of the *HTR2C* have also been associated with response to clozapine, with specifically improvement in negative symptoms [28,53,54].

Studies of the $5HT_5$ [55] and $5HT_6$ receptor genes has indicated a minor contribution to response to clozapine [56] or risperidone [22], but replication is required [57].

The $5HT_{1A}$ receptor is hypothetically involved in negative, cognitive, and depressive symptomatology. The presynaptic autoreceptor function leads to its ability to influence efficacy by regulating other serotonin and dopamine receptors. A 2006 study provides support for this theory by reporting an association between the $5HT_{1A}$ −1019C > G polymorphism and improvement in negative symptoms [58].

In addition to receptor variants, polymorphisms in the serotonin transporter gene (*5HTT*) may also influence AP response. The VNTR in the promoter of the *5HTT*, which is usually denoted as the 5HTTLPR promoter polymorphism, seems to contribute to clozapine response [54,59], although this was not replicated in all studies [60,61].

There are many lines of evidence implicating a role for the glutamatergic system in psychosis, and response to antipsychotics in relation to genotype for these receptors has also been considered. Metabotropic glutamate receptor type 3 (*GRM3*) genotypes were associated with negative symptom improvement after treatment in a small sample of Caucasian patients [62], and Chiu et al. [63] found an association between *NMDAR1* receptor subunit 2b variants and the effect of clozapine during treatment of Chinese patients with schizophrenia, replicating the earlier report by Hong et al. [64]. In a Brazilian study, T/T homozygosity of the functional 825C > T polymorphism of *GNB3* (β subunit of a G protein involved in signal transduction of G-protein-coupled receptors) has been reported to be associated with nonresponse to clozapine [65].

7.2.2 Adverse Drug Reactions

A number of different ADRs are associated with AP use, including tardive dyskinesia, weight gain, agranulocytosis, hyperprolactinemia, and neuroleptic malignant syndrome (NMS). As discussed below, there is pharmacogenetic data available on each of these reactions. It is important to stress that NMS and agranulocytosis are rare events during AP treatment; therefore, it is difficult to gather sufficiently large samples for detection of moderate genetic effects.

7.2.2.1 Tardive Dyskinesia

Tardive dyskinesia (TD), an ADR more commonly associated with typical AP medication, is an involuntary movement disorder manifesting typically in the orofacial area, but frequently extending to the limbs and the trunk. Vulnerability to involuntary movements, including TD over a lifetime trajectory of schizophrenia, approaches 100%, with the annual incidence of TD estimated at approximately 5% in patients treated with typical APs [66,67].

Both genetic and nongenetic factors are currently thought to play a role in the etiopathogenesis of TD. Genetic variability in DMEs, neurotransmitters, and oxidative stress pathway genes have all been associated with the development of TD, although mostly with inconsistent results [68]. Impaired activity of the CYP2D6 enzyme was associated with TD as early as 1995 [69]. A meta-analysis of 12 studies on the impact of CYP2D6 variants on TD risk in various ethnicities concluded that *CYP2D6* PM status might predispose to TD in patients with schizophrenia treated with antipsychotics drugs [70], and a case of a CYP2D6 PM who exhibited tardive dyskinesia on risperidone, accompanied by unexpectedly high risperidone levels, was reported by Bork et al. [71], with a study in Chinese patients with schizophrenia, concluding that the *CYP2D6**10* reduced-activity allele might be associated with TD [72]. Interestingly, there is also evidence of increasing risk of TD with increased *CYP2D6* activity. In a study of German patients, *CYP2D6* genotype was as good a predictor of adverse events as plasma haloperidol concentrations [73]. *CYP1A2* variants also appear to constitute genetic risk factors for the development of drug-induced TD, as suggested by positive association findings [74,75]. The evidence overall appears to support the involvement of *CYP1A2* and *CYP2D6* variants in AP-induced movement ADRs, including TD despite several negative reports, such as one from Plesnicar et al. [76].

Polymorphisms in *DRD3* receptor genes were first reported to contribute to drug-induced TD by Steen and colleagues [77] and by Segman et al. [78]. In both studies, individuals with one or two copies of the Gly allele of the *DRD3* Ser9Gly polymorphism were more likely to develop TD with AP treatment. Several subsequent studies failed to replicate this finding [79,80], but a meta-analysis in a large sample of 780 patients of different ethnic backgrounds treated with typical APs [81] and further reports of association [82–84] have confirmed the *DRD3* Ser9Gly association with TD. The Gly variant is reportedly associated with significantly higher dopamine activity, which, in turn, could explain the association with movement disorders [85]. However, the modest odds ratios seen also suggest further contribution of other genes in the development of this severe side effect.

An association between *DRD2* polymorphisms and TD has been reported by two studies [86], but no evidence was found by others [87–94]. Interestingly, two meta-analyses also confirmed the association [95,96].

There is also a reported association between *DRD4* polymorphisms and drug-induced TD [92], increasing the evidence supporting the involvement of dopamine receptors in susceptibility to TD. The contribution of 10 polymorphic sites in six candidate dopaminergic and serotonergic genes to the development of TD was examined in a small Jewish sample, with only the dopamine transporter gene 3′VNTR polymorphism, the serotonin transporter-linked polymorphic region (*5HTTLPR*), and the tryptophan hydroxylase intron 7 polymorphism yielding trends toward a positive association [97].

Serotonin inhibition of dopamine function may also contribute to the pathological events related to movement disorders. Initial reports of association between $5HT_{2A}$ polymorphisms and TD [91,98,99] were not replicated in independent studies [100–102]. The association was later confirmed in a combined analysis controlling for patient age [103], an important factor in the development of TD. Serotonin $5HT_{2C}$ promoter polymorphisms were also reportedly associated with TD [104].

Oxidative stress caused by the increased formation of reactive-oxygen species induced by AP treatment may result in neuronal degeneration and TD. A possible synergistic effect of *DRD3* Ser9Gly and manganese superoxide dismutase genes (*SOD2*) influencing mitochondrial free-radical scavenging on susceptibility to TD has been reported [105], but a study investigating increased activity of plasma MnSOD in TD failed to link this to the *SOD2* Ala9Val polymorphism [104]. Further evidence supporting the oxidative stress hypothesis was provided by studies investigating NAD(P)H quinone oxidoreductase (NQO1) and nitric oxide synthases (NOS1 and NOS3). *NQO1* polymorphisms were found to be associated with TD in Korean patients [106], but not in Taiwanese patients [107]. Although no evidence could be found of a relationship between *NOS1* genetic variants and TD [108,109], positive associations with *NOS3* polymorphisms [110] support a possible role of oxidative stress and neuronal damage in the development of TD.

More recently, a genomewide association study from Japan identified eight GABAergic pathway genes involved in TD [111], but this finding needs additional confirmation.

7.2.2.2 Weight Gain

Side effects such as weight gain can be a serious impediment to successful pharmacotherapy, and a genetic component has been suggested to contribute to this side effect [112,113]. Serotonin and histamine receptors have important roles in controlling eating behavior and are hence obvious candidate genes for study in this area. The adrenergic system is thought to play an important role in regulating energy balance via stimulation of thermogenesis and lipid mobilization in adipose tissue. Genetic variation in these receptors could alter lipolytic activity and contribute to weight alterations during AP treatment. Among APs, clozapine appears to have the greatest weight gain liability, with some patients gaining as much as 50 kg over a 1-year treatment period [114]. Ten genetic polymorphisms across nine candidate genes, namely, the *HTR2C*, *HTR2A*, the H_1 and H_2, the *CYP1A2*, the β3-and α1-adrenergic receptor genes (*ADRB3* and *ADRA1A* respectively), and the tumor necrosis factor α gene (*TNF*α), involved in both central hypothalamic weight regulation and peripheral thermogenic pathways, were investigated in one study [115]; only four of these genes (*ADRB3*, *ADRA1A*, *TNFα*, and *HTR2C*) demonstrated a modest, nonsignificant trend toward a positive association with clozapine-induced weight gain. More recent work has demonstrated a significant association between the −1291C>G polymorphism of the adrenergic α2A-receptor gene and antipsychotic-antipsychotic medication-induced weight gain (clozapine and olanzapine) in Caucasians, and pending further studies, also in African-Americans [116].

Among the genes and their variants known to be associated with AP-induced weight gain is the promoter polymorphism −759C>T, which is thought to alter *HTR2C* gene expression [28,117]. This polymorphism has been shown to be associated with weight gain due to typical antipsychotics, clozapine, and risperidone, with several studies showing a protective effect against weight gain of the −759T variant [117–120], although not all studies agree with this [121–124].

Furthermore, a −2548A>G variant of the leptin gene, a hormone that also plays a role in the regulation of food intake, was found to be associated with weight gain after 9 months of weight gain, but not in the short term in first episode English patients [120]. This finding was replicated in Korean patients with schizophrenia receiving olanzapine treatment [125]. Another study found that changes in body mass index (BMI) from baseline increased significantly in persons with olanzapine plasma levels >20.6 ng/mL for subjects carrying at least one G allele at the −1548G>A polymorphism of the leptin gene and the Gln223Arg polymorphism of the leptin receptor, and concluded that genetic variability in the leptin gene and leptin receptor may predispose some individuals to excessive weight gain from increased exposure to olanzapine [126]. Mueller and Kennedy [127] also found an association between the leptin gene, leptin receptor genes, and *GNB3* and antipsychotic-medication-induced (AMI) weight gain. More recently, another leptin gene variant, rs4731426, was found to be moderately associated with median weight gain and significantly associated with extreme weight gain in an Indian population of patients taking olanzapine [128]. Musil et al. [129] reported three polymorphisms in the synaptosomal-associated protein of 25 kDa (SNAP25 gene) that were positively associated with either AP-induced weight gain or elevated baseline triglyceride levels.

The G variant of a −1291C>G promoter polymorphism in *ADRA2A* was significantly associated with weight gain on clozapine and olanzapine in two separate studies in Chinese and Korean patients, respectively [130,131], and more recently in a study on Europeans [116]. Variants of the β3-adrenergic receptor do not appear to contribute to clozapine-induced weight gain [132].

A study of 11 olanzapine-treated Caucasian patients found an association between *CYP2D6* PM alleles (**3* and **4*) and increased BMI [133], although the mechanism for this is unclear. A more recent study found no significant correlation between olanzapine concentration and weight gain [134], although dose response and weight change (as well as prolactin) were significantly correlated.

A genomewide linkage study of obesity in patients undergoing treatment with typical APs identified suggestive linkage at 12q24 [135]. The gene coding for promelanin-concentrating hormone (*PMCH*), involved in the control of food intake and energy regulation, is located near this region and is a potential candidate gene for drug-induced weight gain. This hypothesis was later tested in patients with schizophrenia receiving APs and in controls by the same researchers, who suggested that the common allele of *PMCH* may be associated with a greater BMI in olanzapine-treated patients with schizophrenia [136].

A physiogenomic study of the genes associated with olanzapine- and risperidone-induced weight gain showed some between drug variations, indicating that the mechanisms of weight gain for these drugs are different—specifically, that risperidone-induced weight gain appears to be associated with SNPs in the leptin receptor, neuropeptide Y, and paroxonase 1, all of which play significant roles in appetite regulation [137]. Another candidate gene that has been suggested as implicated in risperidone-induced weight gain is brain-derived neurotrophic factor (BDNF), which is involved in the regulation of body weight fluctuation and metabolism in both animals and humans. Variants in the *BDNF* gene, specifically the BDNF Val66Met polymorphism [138], appear to be associated with risperidone-induced weight gain. Further associations between BDNF and risperidone include a positive correlation between clinical response to risperidone and increased levels of serum BDNF [139].

7.2.2.3 Agranulocytosis

Although infrequent (0.7–3% of treated patients [140–142]), clozapine-induced agranulocytosis is a potentially lethal side effect, due to its clinical implications. Immune-mediated toxicity, is one of the likely causes of neutropenia. It has been shown to be associated with a dominant gene within the major histocompatibility complex region marked by heatshock protein 70-1 and 70-2 variants, and several reports of associations with the major histocompatibility complex (MHC) seem to confirm this hypothesis [143–145]. Thus, HLA loci may serve as clinically relevant genetic markers to identify patients prone to this severe idiosyncratic drug reaction.

Alternatively, it has been suggested that defective oxidative mechanisms may be the cause of agranulocytosis, and that oxidative mitochondrial stress in neutrophils of clozapine-treated patients probably contributes to it [146]. Myeloperoxidases (MPOs) and NADPH oxidases participate in the oxidative mechanism of neutrophils, and polymorphisms in the genes coding for MPO and for a subunit of NADPH oxidase (NOX1) were found to be related to clozapine-induced agranulocytosis [142]. However, a preliminary study failed to replicate the MPO association [147]. Furthermore, variants of the oxidative gene *NQO1*, which is involved in the detoxification of drugs, were associated with clozapine-induced agranulocytosis [141]. Another more recent candidate for exploration is the gene encoding the cytokine TNFα, whose release is stimulated by AP treatment. Polymorphisms in this gene are found at higher frequencies in patients presenting with agranulocytosis [148].

7.2.2.4 Hyperprolactinaemia

Earlier, AP-induced hyperprolactinaemia was shown to be associated with the *DRD2* Taq1A polymorphism [149], and more recently, a significant association between *DRD2* −141C and hyperprolactinaemia was shown, consistent with *in vitro* work; this association was strengthened by controlling for *CYP2D6* genotypic category, and by haplotype analysis [150]. Moreover, CYP2D6 seems to be an independent contributor to the pituitary pharmacodynamic tissue sensitivity to perphenazine after accounting for the A1 allele of the *Taq*1A polymorphism *3′* of *DRD2*. At a given AP dose, individuals with the A1 allele were shown to achieve a higher occupancy of D_2 receptors by APs, consistent with increased prolactin elevation in the A1/A1 genotype group [151]. These findings provide a basis for further studies of the endogenous substrates and interactions of CYP2D6 and the rational selection of candidate genes for the investigation of AP-induced hyperprolactinaemia.

7.2.2.5 Neuroleptic Malignant Syndrome

Severe dysfunction of the dopaminergic system is thought to be the main pathophysiological mechanism for neuroleptic malignant syndrome (NMS). Its incidence ranges between 0.3% and 2% [152]. Two reports by the same investigators have suggested association between a *DRD2 Taq*IA polymorphism and NMS [153,154], but this association was not confirmed independently [155]. This polymorphism is now known to lie inside a novel kinase gene, *ANKK1* [156], and further research in this area is warranted. Additional support for the involvement of the D_2 receptor was provided by the finding of association between the functional −141-C Ins/Del with NMS, with patients possessing the Del allele showing higher incidence of NMS [157]. The −141-DelC allele was initially reported to be associated with a lower expression of the D_2 receptor protein *in vitro* [23] and higher D_2 density in the striatum *in vivo* [24], whereas the *Taq*I *A1* allele has been related to lower D_2 densities [157]. A single-photon emission-computed tomography study by Jauss et al. [158] has shown that D_2 receptors were completely occupied in patients with acute NMS. This could result either from lower D_2 density or from increased occupancy of D_2 receptors by dopamine in a state of acute psychosis. The *in vivo* observation of higher D_2 density in patients with the −141-DelC allele [24] could support the latter hypothesis.

7.3 PHARMACOGENETICS OF ANTIDEPRESSANT TREATMENT

Pharmacotherapy in depression results in effective treatment for the majority of patients, but over 50% do not respond sufficiently to the initial treatment, and it can take up to 6 weeks before the results of such treatment can be evaluated. It would, therefore, be highly desirable to identify nonresponders prior to initiating therapy such that exposure to long periods of trial and error is avoided. The impact of a test identifying these patients on healthcare costs would, undoubtedly, be enormous. There is a considerable literature on genes affecting the outcome of antidepressant treatment [159]. These include those relevant to drug metabolism, those encoding neurotransmitter transporters, metabolic enzymes, and receptors; and those belonging to a number of miscellaneous categories. This section considers all classes of antidepressants, including selective serotonin reuptake inhibitors (SSRIs), tricyclic antidepressants (TCAs), and monoamine oxidase inhibitors (MAOIs).

7.3.1 Genes Relevant to Drug Metabolism

Most interest has focused on *CYP2D6* (see Chapter 2 for more details on this gene). CYP2D6 poor metabolizers may show increased concentrations of metabolized drugs at conventional doses [160]. At the other extreme, ultrarapid metabolizers may not reach therapeutic concentrations at customary doses, and it has been hypothesised that they would therefore require an increased dose to achieve therapeutic response [161]. For example, with nortriptyline, *CYP2D6* PMs require only 50% of the average effective antidepressant dose, but UMs may require up to 230% of this dose for an effective response [161].

Genetic polymorphism of *CYP2D6* has been a major focus for pharmacogenetic studies in depression, and dosage recommendations in relationship to *CYP2D6* genotypes have been suggested [162]. CYP2D6 plays a significant role in the metabolism of many antidepressants, thus making *CYP2D6* polymorphisms potentially important in determining drug concentrations and clinical outcome.

The CYP2C19 gene is also involved in the metabolism of several antidepressants. The magnitude of the influence of CYP2C19 activity on the pharmacokinetics and clinical effects of such antidepressants is, as with any other drug metabolising enzyme, dependent on the relative contribution of this CYP and the metabolic steps involved, compared with other CYPs (particularly CYP2D6) and other relevant drug metabolizing enzymes (DMEs). Following a single oral dose of moclobemide, a monoamine oxidase inhibitor (MAOI), a 3-fold higher area under the curve (AUC), has been observed in CYP2C19 PM compared with EM subjects [163], and CYP2C19 is extensively inhibited by omeprazole in CYP2C19 EMs but not in PMs [163,164]. The plasma concentration of moclobemide has not been associated with therapeutic efficacy. Instead, there appears to be an association between plasma concentration and side effects such as dizziness, nausea, and insomnia [165], whereby an increased risk of side effects might be expected in CYP2C19 PMs. Amitriptyline, a TCA, is demethylated to nortriptyline by CYP2C19. *CYP2C19* genotype affects the metabolic ratio (MR) of amitriptyline to nortriptyline, as well as the AUC of both [166–168]. However, although a preliminary report found a relationship between *CYP2C19* genotype and response to a variety of TCAs [169], the effect on response was not replicated in a study on amitriptyline alone [170]. CYP2C19 can also affect the risk of ADRs; one study found that a combination of high CYP2C19 activity and low CYP2D6 activity conferred the highest risk of ADRs, since CYP2C19 produces the active metabolite nortriptyline, whereas CYP2D6 metabolizes nortriptyline into the inactive metabolite 4-hydroxynortriptyline [170]. Furthermore, the steady-state plasma concentration of clomipramine has been shown to be affected by the *CYP2C19* genotype [171]. Although it is considered pharmacologically active, the plasma concentration of the metabolite desmethylclomipramine has been reported to be inversely correlated to the clinical effect [172], thus suggesting that CYP2C19 status might influence therapeutic outcome.

The SSRI sertraline is demethylated by CYP2C19 to an almost inactive metabolite, and the areas under the curve (AUCs) of sertraline and desmethylsertraline have been shown to be 41% higher and 35% lower, respectively, in PMs compared with

EMs when sertraline is given as a single oral dose [173]. Although it appears that several P450s are involved in the demethylation of sertraline *in vitro*, CYP2C19 represents the most important enzyme [174–176]. In addition, the dose – response relationship in sertraline treatment may not be straightforward, as evidenced from a lack of improved therapeutic effect when increasing the dose in nonresponders [177]. The SSRI citalopram is metabolized by CYP2C19 into a demethylated metabolite with lower plasma concentration and potency in terms of efficacy than citalopram [178]. CYP2C19 preferentially metabolises the *S*-enantiomer of citalopram (escitalopram), which is considered to mediate the antidepressant effect, and the AUCs of citalopram and *S*-citalopram have been shown to be significantly higher in PMs as compared with EMs [179,180]. Rudberg et al. [181] analyzed therapeutic drug monitoring data and found a lower geometric mean escitalopram serum concentration in patients homozygous for the *CYP2C19*17* ultrarapid allele compared to wild-type (*CYP2C19*1/*1*) patients [181]. A similar analysis was conducted in the prospective study GENDEP, finding an association between *CYP2C19* genotype, including the *CYP2C19*17* allele, and steady-state escitalopram concentration-to-dose ratio and an effect of *CYP2D6* genotype [6]. An increased dose from 10 to 20 mg appears to increase the response rates in severely depressed compared with moderately depressed patients [182], and a relationship between CYPs and ADRs to escitalopram is emerging [8].

There are many different explanations for the lack of correlation between antidepressant dose and/or plasma concentration, which can be well predicted by cytochrome P450 genotype, and clinical response. This includes the complexity of the depression phenotype, which may include various subtypes, as exemplified by the phenomenon that moclobemide (MAOI) non-responders may be treated with sertraline (SSRI) [183]. P450 genotype-adjusted drug dosage may, of course, be only one route for improvement of drug treatment in depression [184], with other means of improving therapeutic outcome also important.

7.3.2 The 5HT Transporter Gene

There is evidence that the influence of life stress in the etiology of depression is moderated by polymorphism in the 5HTT gene [185]. Moreover, since the 5HT transporter (5HTT) is a primary target for many antidepressants, especially the SSRIs, the effect of *5HTT* variants, particularly the *5HTTLPR* (see Chapter 5 for more information on *5HTT* variants) on clinical response to these drugs has been studied, commencing with the Italian studies on clinical response to fluvoxamine and paroxetine [186,187], which showed that the presence of at least one long (l) allele was significantly associated with greater improvement in Hamilton depression rating scale (HDRS) scores. An association between the *5HTTLPR* and response to SSRIs was replicated in Spanish Caucasians, elderly Americans, and Taiwanese [3]. Rausch et al. [188] also reported an association between the *5HTTLPR* l/l genotype and improved response to fluoxetine and a placebo-controlled study confirmed a significant increase in response to sertraline in elderly depressed patients homozygous for the l allele compared with patients carrying one or two copies of the s variant.

No significant difference was observed in the placebo group [189]. A positive trend toward an association between the *5HTTLPR* l/l genotype and response to treatment with TCAs in a group of Caucasian mainly unipolar depressed patients has also been reported [190]. On the other hand, several studies have suggested an association in the opposite direction, not only in East Asian but also in American patients treated with SSRIs [191]. In the East Asian studies, the different results may be due to differential frequency of the l and s alleles (and other length variants) compared to Caucasians as well as different sequence variation in this region. Ito et al. [192] found no association between *5HTTLPR* genotype and response to fluvoxamine after 6 weeks of treatment in 66 patients with major depressive disorder, and these negative findings were later replicated [193]. However, on meta-analysis, there was overall a positive association between l/l or l/s genotypes and better response to SSRIs [3]. Kim et al. [194] have also found a significant association between specific SSRI response and the intron 2VNTR 12/12 genotype in the 5HTT, and in a later study an interaction between the *5HTTLPR* and the intron 2 VNTR in antidepressant response [195]. Moreover, significant associations between the *5HTTLPR* and *SLC6A4* intron 2 genotypes with both remission and response following initial and second switch therapy were found in a 2009 study from Scotland [196]. In the GENDEP study, an association between the *5HTTLPR* and response to escitalopram in men, and also between the functional intron 1 SNP (rs2020933) and response to both escitalopram and nortriptyline has been found [197]. Moreover, in the same study, baseline stressful life events were shown to predict a significantly better response to escitalopram [5], but had no effect on response to nortriptyline, with variation in the *5HTTLPR* and STin4 (an intron 4 short tandem repeat polymorphism in *SLC6A4* not previously studied) significantly modifying these effects [5]. Stressful life events were a specific predictor of reduction in the cognitive symptom dimension on escitalopram but not nortriptyline [198,199]. More complex analytical approaches, including gene–environment interactions, may therefore be required to tease out pharmacogenetic associations.

7.3.3 Genes Relevant to Neurotransmitter Metabolism Pathways

As tryptophan hydroxylase, encoded by the *TPH1* gene, is the rate limiting enzyme in serotonin biosynthesis, a role for TPH in the pathophysiology of mental disorders has long been suspected. In a Finnish sample, the intron 7 A779C polymorphism was associated with suicidality and alcoholism [200]. This polymorphism is in strong linkage disequilibrium with another in intron 7 (A218C), located in a potential transcription factor binding site, which may hence influence gene expression. Associations between the A218C *TPH1* variant and response to both fluvoxamine and paroxetine have been reported in Italians, but not replicated in Asian samples [159].

Although TPH1 may be associated with the regulation of peripheral tryptophan levels and therefore availability of tryptophan to the brain [201], the more recently studied candidate is the centrally expressed *TPH2* locus [202]. In a Germany study, the polymorphisms rs10897346 and Pro312Pro in the *TPH2* gene were suggested to play an important role in TPH2 expression and antidepressant drug response [203]. Peters et al. [204] and Uher et al. [205] included *TPH2* in their studies of antidepressant response, and the latter were negative for both SNPs in both *TPH1* and *TPH2*. SNPs in *TPH1* and *TPH2* were also negative for association with increasing suicidal ideation in GENDEP [206].

Monoamine oxidase A (MAOA) is also a good candidate for an effect on antidepressant response, as it is involved in degradation of monoamines, and it may also influence the mechanism of action of SSRIs through interaction with the 5HT transporter. Mueller et al. [207] investigated the possible correlation between a *MAOA* VNTR (see Chapter 5 for more details on this polymorphism) and the antidepressant response to moclobemide, with negative results. On studying the *MAOA* VNTR polymorphism together with the *TPH1* A218C in Japanese patients with depression, Yoshida et al. [208] did not find any association with fluvoxamine treatment. This negative finding was replicated in a sample of inpatients with major depression and bipolar disorder treated with fluvoxamine or paroxetine [209] and also by Peters et al. [204] in the study described above. The VNTR is, however, to be studied in GENDEP.

For the catechol-*O*-methyltransferase gene (*COMT*), two pharmacogenetic studies revealed similar effects of the Val158Met variant, which is associated with altered COMT enzyme activity on antidepressant treatment, indicating that the Val (high activity) allele was associated with better response to mirtazapine [210], citalopram [211], and milnacipram [212]. This finding was not replicated for response to paroxetine [210,211].

7.3.4 Neurotransmitter Receptor Genes

Other possible candidate genes for pharmacogenetic studies are those coding for receptors, especially those in the serotonin and noradrenaline systems. The postsynaptic $5HT_{2A}$ receptor is thought to influence the efficacy of serotonergic antidepressants. The C-containing variants of the T102C *HTR2A* polymorphism have been associated with response to treatment with SSRIs, TCAs, and electroconvulsive therapy (ECT) [213]. One previous study found suggestive evidence that *HTR2A* was associated with a delayed and sustained pattern of treatment outcome on fluoxetine in a small sample [209], and an earlier study of 443 depressed inpatients detected a marginally significant association between *HTR2A* variants and outcome [208]. Furthermore, a Korean study investigating the relationship between the −1438A/G polymorphism in *HTR2A* and response to citalopram in major depressive disorder (MDD) showed that the G allele of the −1438A/G polymorphism in *HTR2A* was associated with MDD, and that patients homozygous for the −1438G allele had a better response to treatment with citalopram than did patients with the other −1438A/G genotypes [214]. A more recent Japanese study found that the −1438G/G genotype of *HTR2A* was significantly associated with a good response to fluvoxamine, and significantly so with severe nausea in paroxetine-treated MDD patients [215]. In total, 68 candidate genes were genotyped, with 768 single-nucleotide polymorphism markers chosen to detect common genetic variation in 1953 prospectively assessed patients with MDD who were treated with citalopram in the sequenced treatment alternatives for depression (STAR*D) study, and a significant association between treatment outcome and a SNP in *HTR2A* was detected [216]. Participants who were homozygous for the A allele in rs7997012 had an 18% reduction in absolute risk of having no response to treatment, compared with those homozygous for the other allele, while the A allele was over 6 times more frequent in white than in black participants, and treatment was less effective among black participants. The authors, therefore, suggested that the A allele may contribute to racial differences in outcomes of antidepressant treatment [216]. In the GENDEP study, another SNP (rs9316233) in the same intron in *HTR2A* was associated with response to escitalopram, and a haplotypic association comprising four markers was also found [205]. A second study utilizing a second wave of genotype results from STAR*D tested the association between treatment response and 768 markers genotyped in the full set of 1816 eligible patients from this cohort [217]. In addition to the previously identified marker in the *HTR2A* gene, a new marker (rs1954787) in the *GRIK4* gene, which codes for the kainic acid–type glutamate receptor KA1, was observed, suggesting that the glutamate system may play an important role in modulating response to SSRIs [217]. Furthermore, in a 2009 study from Scotland, the *HTR2A* 1354T/C polymorphism was shown to be associated with remission and response following paroxetine therapy [196].

Lemonde et al. [218] found an association between the G allele of the functional −1019G/C variant in the 5HT1A receptor gene (*HTR1A*) and response to various antidepressants in 118 unipolar subjects. These results were replicated by Serretti et al. [219] when investigating fluvoxamine response in a sample of 262 mood disorder patients; the *HTR1A* −1019G allele appeared to be associated with the antidepressant response in bipolar subjects only. Similar findings were reported later, in a naturalistic design study [220]. Nevertheless, studies by Arias et al. [221] and Baune et al. [222] revealed findings in the opposite direction, but the significance of these findings could be seen only after considering *HTR1A* genetic variation together with *5HTTLPR* genetic variants. In the Asian population, three studies reported significant results with better response for G/G compared to C allele carriers [223–225]. A different Gly272Asp polymorphism was explored in Japanese depressive outpatients treated with fluvoxamine [226]. Asp-allele carriers showed a more marked reduction in depressive symptomatology compared to Gly/Gly homozygotes. This finding was not confirmed by subsequent studies [224–227], although this polymorphism was found to be in strong LD with −1019C/G [224]. A significant association of treatment response with two other SNPs, rs10042486 in the promoter region and rs1364043 in the downstream region, has also been reported [225], with the minor allele homozygous combination −1019G–rs10042486C–rs1364043T (all in strong LD) robustly associated with a better response and fast remission. In GENDEP, the corrected p value for SNPs in *HTR1A* in the escitalopram-treated subjects was 0.05, with a higher p value for the combined value or the nortriptyline-treated subjects [205].

A significant association between *HTR3A* 178C/T T homozygotes and better response to SSRIs has been reported, although no association of this SNP with side effects including nausea could be observed in the same study [215]. Two other studies also found no association between the *HTR3A* 195C/T or 178C/T SNPs with gastrointestinal symptoms induced by SSRIs [228,229], but the former found a significant association of the *HTR3B* 129Tyr/Ser (rs1176744) polymorphism with nausea induced by paroxetine.

The serotonergic and dopaminergic systems are interconnected in the brain, with serotonergic projections believed to inhibit dopamine function in the midbrain [230]. SSRIs were shown to enhance dopamine function in the nucleus accumbens through increased expression of postsynaptic D_2 receptors, and Klimke et al. [231] suggested an association between changes in the dopaminergic system and treatment response in major depression. However, a study testing two functional polymorphisms, the *DRD2* 311C/S and the exon three VNTR polymorphism of *DRD4* failed to find any evidence of association with efficacy of SSRIs [232].

7.3.5 Miscellaneous Candidate Genes Affecting Antidepressant Response

Abnormal signal transduction pathways are possibly involved in the response to treatment with antidepressants. A functional polymorphism in *GNB3*, the gene encoding the $\beta 3$ G protein subunit, 825C/T (rs5443) in exon 10, is associated with alternative splicing to a protein truncated by 41 amino acids (GNB-s), which is associated with enhanced signal transduction [233] and an increased risk of major depression. A number of studies have also reported an association between the TT genotype at this SNP and good response to a variety of antidepressants [234–238]. Contradictory findings have, however, been reported [239], and a more recent meta-analysis was negative [240]. Interestingly, more recent analysis of the GENDEP data aiming to elucidate the reason underlying these apparent discrepancies found that the TT genotype was significantly associated with better response to nortriptyline, and these effects were specific to improvements in somatic symptoms. In addition, the same genotype predicted fewer incidents of treatment-emergent insomnia and greater weight gain on the same drug [241].

More recent data suggest that antidepressants increase the synthesis and signaling of brain-derived neurotrophic factor (BDNF), and BDNF signaling appears to be involved in behavioral effects induced by antidepressants [242]. BDNF secretion and intercellular trafficking are regulated by a functional polymorphism in the *BDNF* gene, resulting in a Val $\rightarrow$ Met substitution at codon 66 [243]. Several studies have investigated the effect of this polymorphism or other *BDNF* SNPs [244–246] on antidepressant response with discrepant findings possibly contributing to differentail allelic frequencies in different ethnic groups. In GENDEP, associations between haplotypes of markers in *BDNF* and its receptor (*NTRK2*) and treatment-emergent suicidal ideation were found, with an interactive effect between these two genes [4]. The association with *NTRK2* has been replicated by GWAS analysis [247].

Other candidate genes potentially playing a role in the antidepressant response include an intronic Ins/Del polymorphism in the angiotensin-converting enzyme gene (*ACE*). This polymorphism has a dramatic impact on substance P levels and may affect activity of antidepressants. Indeed, the D allele, which determines higher ACE plasma levels [248] (see also Chapter 5), was associated with higher substance P levels [249] and a faster response to treatment with antidepressants [250], especially among women [251], although negative results were also reported [252].

Some genes coding for components of the hypothalamic–pituitary–adrenal axis have been explored as modulators of antidepressant response. The corticotrophin-releasing hormone receptor 1 gene (*CRHR1*) is a promising candidate as CRHR1 antagonists have consistently demonstrated antidepressant properties in experimental animals and humans [253,254]. Research on *CRHR1* pharmacogenetics is at a very early stage; however, two studies identified associations with three SNP haplotypes to antidepressant response [255,256]. The influence of SNPs within the gene encoding the hsp90 cochaperone *FKBP5* [a part of the mature glucocorticoid receptor (GR) heterocomplex] was also investigated by four studies with inconsistent results [257–260].

7.4 PHARMACOGENETICS OF LITHIUM TREATMENT

Lithium response has long been thought to have a genetic component, and disturbances of the serotonergic system have been repeatedly implicated in the mechanism of action of lithium. No association between response to lithium prophylaxis and the 102T/C or the 1421C/T *HTR2A* polymorphisms was found in an Italian sample, but the same group reported a positive association between presence of the l allele of the 5HTTLPR polymorphism and good response to lithium [261,262], in contrast with an earlier Sardinian study reporting the l/l genotype to be associated with the nonresponder phenotype [263]. In a study from Poland, the 102T/C *HTR2A* and the 68G/C *HTR2C* polymorphisms were not associated with degree of prophylactic lithium response [264], and the same group replicated the positive association between presence of the l allele of the 5HTTLPR polymorphism and good response to lithium treatment [265]. Furthermore, a significant association between *TPH* and prophylactic efficacy of lithium has also been reported [266].

Lithium, at therapeutic doses, inhibits inositol polyphosphate 1-phosphatase, which is involved in recycling inositol phosphatases to inositol [267], and a higher frequency of a phospholipase C $\gamma 1$ gene (*PLCG1*) repeat was shown to be positively associated with lithium response in the treatment of bipolar disorder [268]. In addition, Lovlie et al. [269] reported a *PLCG1* 8 repeat to be more frequent among lithium responders than normal controls, and Steen et al. [270] suggested that the 973A/C polymorphism in the inositol polyphosphate 1-phosphatase gene was an indication of positive lithium response. Other genes involved in the intracellular transduction system or hormonal control have been investigated, including corticotrophin releasing hormone (*CRH*) or proenkephalin (*PENK*) [271]; some polyglutamine coding loci [272], with negative results; three polymorphic sites localized in exons 9, 26, and 31 of the *PLCG1* gene [273]; and six markers on chromosome 18 [274,275].

Washizuka et al. [276] reported an association between the mitochondrial DNA (mtDNA) 10398 polymorphism and response to maintenance lithium treatment in a small Japanese sample of patients with bipolar disorder [275]. Another study from Japan has more recently investigated the association of a breakpoint cluster region (*BCR*) gene polymorphism and response to lithium [276]. *BCR* is one of the two genes in the bcr-abl complex, which is associated with the Philadelphia chromosome.

The allele frequency of Ser796 of the Asn796Ser was significantly higher in nonresponders than in responders [276].

Glycogen synthase kinase 3β (*GSK3β*) gene codes for an enzyme that is a target for the action of lithium [277]. The −50T/C SNP, within the effective promoter region of *GSK3β*, was shown to be possibly involved in the response to lithium [278]. More recently, several polymorphisms in the genes encoding the transcription factors,—cAMP response element binding 1 (*CREB1*), *CREB2*, and *CREB3*,—have been investigated in relation to lithium response in bipolar patients. The *CREB1* 1H and 7H polymorphisms were shown to be positively associated with bipolar disorder and/or lithium response [279].

7.5 CONCLUSIONS

In summary, there has been considerable recent progress in the field of pharmacogenetics in psychiatry. Valuable samples have been collected through collaborative effort, and positive findings are emerging. This review has focused on antipsychotics and antidepressants; however, in other areas, such as ADHD and addictions [280], significant progress is also being made. Atomoxetine is metabolised by *CYP2D6* and used in the treatment of ADHD. Trzepacz et al. [281] reported that *CYP2D6*-poor metabolisers had a lower mean dose and a greater increase in heart rate, with a trend for increased discontinuation rate; further work in this area is warranted.

Indeed, we suggest that further resources should be directed to achieving the maximum potential in this field, including utilization of existing collections that have not yet been fully explored, in order to enhance the clinical care and quality of life of those with mental illnesses. Given that the World Health Organisation has predicted that by 2030, depression will be the most significant health condition in terms of global burden of disease, the known association between depression and other conditions including addictions and physical health disorders [282], and the contribution that pharmacogenetics/genomics may make not only to more cost-effective healthcare but also to elucidating molecular mechanisms of disease, it is in the best interests of society to support such work.

REFERENCES

1. Aitchison KJ, Gill M. Pharmacogenetics in the postgenomic era. In Plomin R, DeFries JC, Craig I, McGuffin P, eds.: *Behavioral Genetics in the Postgenomic Era.* Washington DC: APA Books, 2002.
2. Trivedi MH, Rush AJ, Wisniewski SR, Nierenberg AA, Warden D, Ritz L, Norquist G, Howland RH, Lebowitz B, McGrath PJ, Shores-Wilson K, Biggs MM, Balasubramani GK, Fava M. Evaluation of outcomes with citalopram for depression using measurement-based care in STAR*D: Implications for clinical practice. *Am. J. Psychiatry* 2006;**163**(1): 28–40.

3. Serretti A, Kato M, De RD, Kinoshita T. Meta-analysis of serotonin transporter gene promoter polymorphism (5-HTTLPR) association with selective serotonin reuptake inhibitor efficacy in depressed patients. *Mol. Psychiatry* 2007;**12**(3): 247–257.
4. Perroud N, Aitchison KJ, Uher R, Smith R, Huezo-Diaz P, Marusic A, Maier W, Mors O, Placentino A, Henigsberg N, Rietschel M, Hauser J, Souery D, Kapelski P, et al. Genetic predictors of increase in suicidal ideation during antidepressant treatment in the GENDEP project. *Neuropsychopharmacology* 2009;**34**:2517–2528.
5. Keers R, Uher R, Huezo-Diaz P, Smith R, Jaffee S, Rietschel M, Henigsberg N, Kozel D, Mors O, Maier W, Zobel A, Hauser J, Souery D, Placentino A, Larsen ER, et al. Interaction between serotonin transporter gene variants and life events predicts response to antidepressants in the GENDEP project. *Pharmacogenomics J.* 2011;**11**:138–145.
6. Huezo-Diaz P, Perroud N, Spencer EP, Smith R, Sim S, Virding S, Uher R, Gunasinghe C, Gray J, Campbell D, Hauser J, Maier W, Marusic A, Rietschel M, et al. Effect of CYP2C19 genotype on steady state escitalopram level in GENDEP. *J. Psychopharmacol.* 2011, epub Sept 17.
7. Dahl ML, Bertilsson L. Genetically variable metabolism of antidepressants and neuroleptic drugs in man. *Pharmacogenetics* 1993;**3**(2):61–70.
8. Keers R, Ingelman-Sundberg M, Hauser J, Maier W, Rietschel M, Mors O, McGuffin P, Farmer AE, Craig IW, Aitchison KJ.CYP2D6 and CYP2C19 genotype predicts antidepressant dose in the GENDEP project. Poster and oral presentation to the 2010 ECNP Young Scientists Workshop, Nice.
9. Aitchison KJ, Jann MW, Zhao JH, Sakai T, Zaher H, Wolff K, Collier DA, Kerwin RW, Gonzalez FJ. Clozapine pharmacokinetics and pharmacodynamics studied with CYP1A2-null mice. *J. Psychopharmacol.* 2000;**14**(4):353–359.
10. Murray M. Role of CYP pharmacogenetics and drug-drug interactions in the efficacy and safety of atypical and other antipsychotic agents. *J. Pharm. Pharmacol.* 2006;**58**(7): 871–885.
11. Basu A, Tsapakis E, Aitchison K. Pharmacogenetics and psychiatry. *Curr. Psychiatry. Rep.* 2004;**6**(2):134–142.
12. Dahmen N, Muller MJ, Germeyer S, Rujescu D, Anghelescu I, Hiemke C, Wetzel H. Genetic polymorphisms of the dopamine D2 and D3 receptor and neuroleptic drug effects in schizophrenic patients. *Schizophr. Res.* 2001;**49**(1–2):223–225.
13. Schafer M, Rujescu D, Giegling I, Guntermann A, Erfurth A, Bondy B, Moller HJ. Association of short-term response to haloperidol treatment with a polymorphism in the dopamine D(2) receptor gene. *Am. J. Psychiatry* 2001;**158**(5):802–804.
14. Suzuki A, Kondo T, Mihara K, Yasui-Furukori N, Ishida M, Furukori H, Kaneko S, Inoue Y, Otani K. The −141C Ins/Del polymorphism in the dopamine D2 receptor gene promoter region is associated with anxiolytic and antidepressive effects during treatment with dopamine antagonists in schizophrenic patients. *Pharmacogenetics* 2001;**11**(6): 545–550.
15. Himei A, Koh J, Sakai J, Inada Y, Akabame K, Yoneda H. The influence on the schizophrenic symptoms by the DRD2Ser/Cys311 and −141C Ins/Del polymorphisms. *Psychiatry Clin. Neurosci.* 2002;**56**(1):97–102.
16. Wu S, Xing Q, Gao R, Li X, Gu N, Feng G, He L. Response to chlorpromazine treatment may be associated with polymorphisms of the DRD2 gene in Chinese schizophrenic patients. *Neurosci. Lett.* 2005;**376**(1):1–4.

17. Ikeda M, Yamanouchi Y, Kinoshita Y, Kitajima T, Yoshimura R, Hashimoto S, O'Donovan MC, Nakamura J, Ozaki N, Iwata N. Variants of dopamine and serotonin candidate genes as predictors of response to risperidone treatment in first-episode schizophrenia. *Pharmacogenomics* 2008;**9**(10):1437–1443.

18. Lencz T, Robinson DG, Xu K, Ekholm J, Sevy S, Gunduz-Bruce H, Woerner MG, Kane JM, Goldman D, Malhotra AK. DRD2 promoter region variation as a predictor of sustained response to antipsychotic medication in first-episode schizophrenia patients. *Am. J. Psychiatry* 2006;**163**(3):529–531.

19. Hwang R, Shinkai T, De Luca V, Muller DJ, Ni X, Macciardi F, Potkin S, Lieberman JA, Meltzer HY, Kennedy JL. Association study of 12 polymorphisms spanning the dopamine D(2) receptor gene and clozapine treatment response in two treatment refractory/intolerant populations. Psychopharmacology (Berlin) 2005;**181**(1):179–187.

20. Hwang R, Shinkai T, Deluca V, Macciardi F, Potkin S, Meltzer HY, Kennedy JL. Dopamine D2 receptor gene variants and quantitative measures of positive and negative symptom response following clozapine treatment. *Eur. Neuropsychopharmacol.* 2006; **16**(4):248–259.

21. Yamanouchi Y, Iwata N, Suzuki T, Kitajima T, Ikeda M, Ozaki N. Effect of DRD2, 5-HT2A, and COMT genes on antipsychotic response to risperidone. *Pharmacogenomics J.* 2003;**3**(6):356–361.

22. Lane HY, Lee CC, Chang YC, Lu CT, Huang CH, Chang WH. Effects of dopamine D2 receptor Ser311Cys polymorphism and clinical factors on risperidone efficacy for positive and negative symptoms and social function. *Int. J. Neuropsychopharmacol.* 2004;**7**(4):461–470.

23. Arinami T, Gao M, Hamaguchi H, Toru M. A functional polymorphism in the promoter region of the dopamine D2 receptor gene is associated with schizophrenia 1. *Hum. Mol. Genet.* 1997;**6**(4):577–582.

24. Jonsson EG, Nothen MM, Grunhage F, Farde L, Nakashima Y, Propping P, Sedvall GC. Polymorphisms in the dopamine D2 receptor gene and their relationships to striatal dopamine receptor density of healthy volunteers. *Mol. Psychiatry* 1999;**4**(3): 290–296.

25. Staddon S, Arranz MJ, Mancama D, Mata I, Kerwin RW. Clinical applications of pharmacogenetics in psychiatry. *Psychopharmacology* (Berlin) 2002;**162**(1):18–23.

26. Scharfetter J, Chaudhry HR, Hornik K, Fuchs K, Sieghart W, Kasper S, Aschauer HN. Dopamine D3 receptor gene polymorphism and response to clozapine in schizophrenic Pakistani patients. *Eur. Neuropsychopharmacol.* 1999;**10**(1):17–20.

27. Szekeres G, Keri S, Juhasz A, Rimanoczy A, Szendi I, Czimmer C, Janka Z. Role of dopamine D3 receptor (DRD3) and dopamine transporter (DAT) polymorphism in cognitive dysfunctions and therapeutic response to atypical antipsychotics in patients with schizophrenia. *Am. J. Med. Genet. B Neuropsychiatr. Genet.* 2004;**124B**(1):1–5.

28. Reynolds GP, Yao Z, Zhang X, Sun J, Zhang Z. Pharmacogenetics of treatment in first-episode schizophrenia: D3 and 5-HT2C receptor polymorphisms separately associate with positive and negative symptom response. *Eur. Neuropsychopharmacol.* 2005; **15**(2):143–151.

29. Lane HY, Hsu SK, Liu YC, Chang YC, Huang CH, Chang WH. Dopamine D3 receptor Ser9Gly polymorphism and risperidone response. *J. Clin. Psychopharmacol.* 2005; **25**(1):6–11.

30. Lundstrom K, Turpin MP. Proposed schizophrenia-related gene polymorphism: Expression of the Ser9Gly mutant human dopamine D3 receptor with the Semliki Forest virus system. *Biochem. Biophys. Res. Commun.* 1996;**225**(3):1068–1072.

31. Van Tol HH, Bunzow JR, Guan HC, Sunahara RK, Seeman P, Niznik HB, Civelli O. Cloning of the gene for a human dopamine D4 receptor with high affinity for the antipsychotic clozapine. *Nature* 1991;**350**(6319):610–614.

32. Kapur S, Remington G. Atypical antipsychotics: New directions and new challenges in the treatment of schizophrenia. *Annu. Rev. Med.* 2001;**52**:503–517.

33. Zhao AL, Zhao JP, Zhang YH, Tang BS, Liu ZN, Cheng JD. Distribution of genotype and allele frequencies of dopamine D4 receptor gene 48 bp variable number tandem repeat polymorphism in Chinese Han population in Hunan (Engl. transl.). *Zhonghua Yi Xue Yi Chuan Xue Za Zhi* 2005;**22**(4):470–472.

34. Cohen BM, Ennulat DJ, Centorrino F, Matthysse S, Konieczna H, Chu HM, Cherkerzian S. Polymorphisms of the dopamine D4 receptor and response to antipsychotic drugs. *Psychopharmacology (Berlin)* 1999;**141**(1):6–10.

35. Hwu HG, Hong CJ, Lee YL, Lee PC, Lee SF. Dopamine D4 receptor gene polymorphisms and neuroleptic response in schizophrenia. *Biol. Psychiatry* 1998;**44**(6):483–487.

36. Shaikh S, Collier D, Kerwin RW, Pilowsky LS, Gill M, Xu WM, Thornton A. Dopamine D4 receptor subtypes and response to clozapine. *Lancet* 1993;**341**(8837):116.

37. Rietschel M, Naber D, Oberlander H, Holzbach R, Fimmers R, Eggermann K, Moller HJ, Propping P, Nothen MM. Efficacy and side-effects of clozapine: Testing for association with allelic variation in the dopamine D4 receptor gene. *Neuropsychopharmacology* 1996;**15**(5):491–496.

38. Kaiser R, Konneker M, Henneken M, Dettling M, Muller-Oerlinghausen B, Roots I, Brockmoller J. Dopamine D4 receptor 48-bp repeat polymorphism: No association with response to antipsychotic treatment, but association with catatonic schizophrenia. *Mol. Psychiatry* 2000;**5**(4):418–424.

39. Zalsman G, Frisch A, Lev-Ran S, Martin A, Michaelovsky E, Bensason D, Gothelf D, Nahshoni E, Tyano S, Weizman A. DRD4 exon III polymorphism and response to risperidone in Israeli adolescents with schizophrenia: A pilot pharmacogenetic study. *Eur. Neuropsychopharmacol.* 2003;**13**(3):183–185.

40. Lane HY, Chang YC, Chiu CC, Chen ML, Hsieh MH, Chang WH. Association of risperidone treatment response with a polymorphism in the 5-HT(2A) receptor gene. *Am. J. Psychiatry* 2002;**159**(9):1593–1595.

41. Arranz M, Collier D, Sodhi M, Ball D, Roberts G, Price J, Sham P, Kerwin R. Association between clozapine response and allelic variation in 5-HT2A receptor gene. *Lancet* 1995;**346**(8970):281–282.

42. Arranz MJ, Munro J, Sham P, Kirov G, Murray RM, Collier DA, Kerwin RW. Meta-analysis of studies on genetic variation in 5-HT2A receptors and clozapine response. *Schizophr. Res.* 1998;**32**:93–99.

43. Joober R, Benkelfat C, Brisebois K, Toulouse A, Turecki G, Lal S, Bloom D, Labelle A, Lalonde P, Fortin D, Alda M, Palmour R, Rouleau GA. T102C polymorphism in the 5-HT2A gene and schizophrenia: Relation to phenotype and drug response variability. *J. Psychiatry Neurosci.* 1999;**24**(2):141–146.

44. Yu YW, Tsai SJ, Yang KH, Lin CH, Chen MC, Hong CJ. Evidence for an association between polymorphism in the serotonin-2A receptor variant (102T/C) and increment of

N100 amplitude in schizophrenics treated with clozapine. *Neuropsychobiology* 2001; **43**(2):79–82.

45. Parsons MJ, D'Souza UM, Arranz MJ, Kerwin RW, Makoff AJ. The −1438A/G polymorphism in the 5-hydroxytryptamine type 2A receptor gene affects promoter activity. *Biol. Psychiatry* 2004;**56**(6):406–410.
46. Arranz MJ, Collier DA, Munro J, Sham P, Kirov G, Sodhi M, Roberts G, Price J, Kerwin RW. Analysis of a structural polymorphism in the 5-HT2A receptor and clinical response to clozapine. *Neurosci. Lett.* 1996;**217**(2–3):177–178.
47. Masellis M, Basile V, Meltzer HY, Lieberman JA, Sevy S, Macciardi FM, Cola P, Howard A, Badri F, Nothen MM, Kalow W, Kennedy JL. Serotonin subtype 2 receptor genes and clinical response to clozapine in schizophrenia patients. *Neuropsychopharmacology* 1998;**19**(2):123–132.
48. Nothen MM, Rietschel M, Erdmann J, Oberlander H, Moller HJ, Nober D, Propping P. Genetic variation of the 5-HT2A receptor and response to clozapine. *Lancet* 1995;**346** (8979):908–909.
49. Masellis M, Paterson AD, Badri F, Lieberman JA, Meltzer HY, Cavazzoni P, Kennedy JL. Genetic variation of 5-HT2A receptor and response to clozapine. *Lancet* 1995; **346**(8982):1108.
50. Malhotra AK, Goldman D, Buchanan R, Breier A, Pickar D. 5-HT 2a receptor T102C polymorphism and schizophrenia. *Lancet* 1996;**347**(9018):1830–1831.
51. Jonsson E, Nothen MM, Bunzel R, Propping P, Sedvall G. 5-HT 2a receptor T102C polymorphism and schizophrenia. *Lancet* 1996;**347**(9018):1831.
52. Lin CH, Tsai SJ, Yu YW, Song HL, Tu PC, Sim CB, Hsu CP, Yang KH, Hong CJ. No evidence for association of serotonin-2A receptor variant (102T/C) with schizophrenia or clozapine response in a Chinese population. *Neuroreport* 1999;**10**(1):57–60.
53. Sodhi MS, Arranz MJ, Curtis D, Ball DM, Sham P, Roberts GW, Price J, Collier DA, Kerwin RW. Association between clozapine response and allelic variation in the 5-HT2C receptor gene. *Neuroreport* 1995;**7**(1):169–172.
54. Arranz MJ, Munro J, Birkett J, Bolonna A, Mancama D, Sodhi M, Lesch KP, Meyer JF, Sham P, Collier DA, Murray RM, Kerwin RW. Pharmacogenetic prediction of clozapine response. *Lancet* 2000;**355**(9215):1615–1616.
55. Birkett JT, Arranz MJ, Munro J, Osbourn S, Kerwin RW, Collier DA. Association analysis of the 5-HT5A gene in depression, psychosis and antipsychotic response. *Neuroreport* 2000;**11**(9):2017–2020.
56. Yu YW, Tsai SJ, Lin CH, Hsu CP, Yang KH, Hong CJ. Serotonin-6 receptor variant (C267T) and clinical response to clozapine. *Neuroreport* 1999;**10**(6):1231–1233.
57. Masellis M, Basile VS, Meltzer HY, Lieberman JA, Sevy S, Goldman DA, Hamblin MW, Macciardi FM, Kennedy JL. Lack of association between the T-- >C 267 serotonin 5-HT6 receptor gene (HTR6) polymorphism and prediction of response to clozapine in schizophrenia. *Schizophr. Res.* 2001;**47**(1):49–58.
58. Reynolds GP, Arranz B, Templeman LA, Fertuzinhos S, San L. Effect of 5-HT1A receptor gene polymorphism on negative and depressive symptom response to antipsychotic treatment of drug-naive psychotic patients. *Am. J. Psychiatry* 2006; **163**(10):1826–1829.
59. Arranz MJ, Bolonna AA, Munro J, Curtis CJ, Collier DA, Kerwin RW. The serotonin transporter and clozapine response. *Mol. Psychiatry* 2000;**5**(2):124–125.

60. Tsai SJ, Hong CJ, Yu YW, Lin CH, Song HL, Lai HC, Yang KH. Association study of a functional serotonin transporter gene polymorphism with schizophrenia, psychopathology and clozapine response. *Schizophr. Res.* 2000;**44**(3):177–181.

61. Kaiser R, Tremblay PB, Schmider J, Henneken M, Dettling M, Muller-Oerlinghausen B, Uebelhack R, Roots I, Brockmoller J. Serotonin transporter polymorphisms: No association with response to antipsychotic treatment, but associations with the schizoparanoid and residual subtypes of schizophrenia. *Mol. Psychiatry* 2001;**6**(2):179–185.

62. Bishop JR, Ellingrod VL, Moline J, Miller D. Association between the polymorphic GRM3 gene and negative symptom improvement during olanzapine treatment. *Schizophr. Res.* 2005;**77**(2–3):253–260.

63. Chiu HJ, Wang YC, Liou YJ, Lai IC, Chen JY. Association analysis of the genetic variants of the N-methyl D-aspartate receptor subunit 2b (NR2b) and treatment-refractory schizophrenia in the Chinese. *Neuropsychobiology* 2003;**47**(4):178–181.

64. Hong CJ, Yu YW, Lin CH, Cheng CY, Tsai SJ. Association analysis for NMDA receptor subunit 2B (GRIN2B) genetic variants and psychopathology and clozapine response in schizophrenia. *Psychiatr. Genet.* 2001;**11**(4):219–222.

65. Kohlrausch FB, Salatino-Oliveira A, Gama CS, Lobato MI, Belmonte-de-Abreu P, Hutz MH. G-protein gene 825C > T polymorphism is associated with response to clozapine in Brazilian schizophrenics. *Pharmacogenomics* 2008;**9**(10):1429–1436.

66. Quinn J, Meagher D, Murphy P, Kinsella A, Mullaney J, Waddington JL. Vulnerability to involuntary movements over a lifetime trajectory of schizophrenia approaches 100%, in association with executive (frontal) dysfunction. *Schizophr. Res.* 2001;**49**:79–87.

67. Tarsy D, Baldessarini RJ. Epidemiology of tardive dyskinesia: Is risk declining with modern antipsychotics? *Mov. Disord.* 2006;**21**(5):589–598.

68. Thelma B, Srivastava V, Tiwari AK. Genetic underpinnings of tardive dyskinesia: Passing the baton to pharmacogenetics. *Pharmacogenomics* 2008;**9**(9):1285–1306.

69. Arthur H, Dahl ML, Siwers B, Sjoqvist F. Polymorphic drug metabolism in schizophrenic patients with tardive dyskinesia. *J. Clin. Psychopharmacol.* 1995;**15**(3):211–216.

70. Patsopoulos NA, Ntzani EE, Zintzaras E, Ioannidis JP. CYP2D6 polymorphisms and the risk of tardive dyskinesia in schizophrenia: A meta-analysis. *Pharmacogenet. Genomics* 2005;**15**(3):151–158.

71. Bork JA, Rogers T, Wedlund PJ, de Leon J. A pilot study on risperidone metabolism: The role of cytochromes P450 2D6 and 3A. *J. Clin. Psychiatry* 1999;**60**:469–476.

72. Fu Y, Fan CH, Deng HH, Hu SH, Lv DP, Li LH, Wang JJ, Lu XQ. Association of CYP2D6 and CYP1A2 gene polymorphism with tardive dyskinesia in Chinese schizophrenic patients. *Acta Pharmacol. Sin.* 2006;**27**(3):328–332.

73. Brockmoller J, Kirchheiner J, Schmider J, Walter S, Sachse C, Muller-Oerlinghausen B, Roots I. The impact of the CYP2D6 polymorphism on haloperidol pharmacokinetics and on the outcome of haloperidol treatment. *Clin. Pharmacol. Ther.* 2002;**72**(4): 438–452.

74. Basile VS, Ozdemir V, Masellis M, Walker ML, Meltzer HY, Lieberman JA, Potkin SG, Alva G, Kalow W, Macciardi FM, Kennedy JL. A functional polymorphism of the cytochrome P450 1A2 (CYP1A2) gene: Association with tardive dyskinesia in schizophrenia. *Mol. Psychiatry* 2000;**5**(4):410–417.

75. Tiwari AK, Deshpande SN, Rao AR, Bhatia T, Mukit SR, Shriharsh V, Lerer B, Nimagaonkar VL, Thelma BK. Genetic susceptibility to tardive dyskinesia in chronic

schizophrenia subjects: I. Association of CYP1A2 gene polymorphism. *Pharmacogenomics J.* 2005;**5**(1):60–69.

76. Plesnicar BK, Zalar B, Breskvar K, Dolzan V. The influence of the CYP2D6 polymorphism on psychopathological and extrapyramidal symptoms in the patients on long-term antipsychotic treatment. *J. Psychopharmacol.* 2006;**20**(6):829–833.
77. Steen VM, Lovlie R, MacEwan T, McCreadie RG. Dopamine D3-receptor gene variant and susceptibility to tardive dyskinesia in schizophrenic patients. *Mol. Psychiatry* 1997; **2**(2):139–145.
78. Segman R, Neeman T, Heresco-Levy U, Finkel B, Karagichev L, Schlafman M, Dorevitch A, Yakir A, Lerner A, Shelevoy A, Lerer B. Genotypic association between the dopamine D3 receptor and tardive dyskinesia in chronic schizophrenia. *Mol. Psychiatry* 1999;**4**(3):247–253.
79. Lovlie R, Daly AK, Blennerhassett R, Ferrier N, Steen VM. Homozygosity for the Gly-9 variant of the dopamine D3 receptor and risk for tardive dyskinesia in schizophrenic patients. *Int. J. Neuropsychopharmacol.* 2000;**3**(1):61–65.
80. Rietschel M, Krauss H, Muller DJ, Schulze TG, Knapp M, Marwinski K, Maroldt AO, Paus S, Grunhage F, Propping P, Maier W, Held T, Nothen MM. Dopamine D3 receptor variant and tardive dyskinesia. *Eur. Arch. Psychiatry Clin. Neurosci.* 2000;**250**(1):31–35.
81. Lerer B, Segman RH, Fangerau H, Daly AK, Basile VS, Cavallaro R, Aschauer HN, McCreadie RG, Ohlraun S, Ferrier N, Masellis M, Verga M, et al. Pharmacogenetics of tardive dyskinesia: Combined analysis of 780 patients supports association with dopamine D3 receptor gene Ser9Gly polymorphism. *Neuropsychopharmacology* 2002; **27**(1):105–119.
82. Liao DL, Yeh YC, Chen HM, Chen H, Hong CJ, Tsai SJ. Association between the Ser9Gly polymorphism of the dopamine D3 receptor gene and tardive dyskinesia in Chinese schizophrenic patients. *Neuropsychobiology* 2001;**44**(2):95–98.
83. Woo SI, Kim JW, Rha E, Han SH, Hahn KH, Park CS, Sohn JW. Association of the Ser9Gly polymorphism in the dopamine D3 receptor gene with tardive dyskinesia in Korean schizophrenics. *Psychiatry Clin. Neurosci.* 2002;**56**(4):469–474.
84. de Leon J, Susce MT, Pan RM, Koch WH, Wedlund PJ. Polymorphic variations in GSTM1, GSTT1, PgP, CYP2D6, CYP3A5, and dopamine D2 and D3 receptors and their association with tardive dyskinesia in severe mental illness. *J. Clin. Psychopharmacol.* 2005;**25**(5):448–456.
85. Bakker PR, van Harten PN, van Os J. Antipsychotic-induced tardive dyskinesia and the Ser9Gly polymorphism in the DRD3 gene: A meta analysis. *Schizophr. Res.* 2006; **83**(2–3):185–192.
86. Liou YJ, Lai IC, Liao DL, Chen JY, Lin CC, Lin CY, Chen CM, Bai YM, Chen TT, Wang YC. The human dopamine receptor D2 (DRD2) gene is associated with tardive dyskinesia in patients with schizophrenia. *Schizophr. Res.* 2006;**86**(1–3):323–325.
87. Mihara K, Kondo T, Suzuki A, Yasui N, Ono S, Otani K, Kaneko S. No relationship between −141C Ins/Del polymorphism in the promoter region of dopamine D2 receptor and extrapyramidal adverse effects of selective dopamine D2 antagonists in schizophrenic patients: A preliminary study. *Psychiatry Res.* 2001;**101**(1):33–38.
88. Hori H, Ohmori O, Shinkai T, Kojima H, Nakamura J. Association between three functional polymorphisms of dopamine D2 receptor gene and tardive dyskinesia in schizophrenia. *Am. J. Med. Genet.* 2001;**105**(8):774–778.

89. Kaiser R, Tremblay PB, Klufmoller F, Roots I, Brockmoller J. Relationship between adverse effects of antipsychotic treatment and dopamine D(2) receptor polymorphisms in patients with schizophrenia. *Mol. Psychiatry* 2002;**7**(7):695–705.

90. Chong SA, Tan EC, Tan CH, Mythily, Chan YH. Polymorphisms of dopamine receptors and tardive dyskinesia among Chinese patients with schizophrenia. *Am. J. Med. Genet. B Neuropsychiatr. Genet.* 2003;**116**(1):51–54.

91. Lattuada E, Cavallaro R, Serretti A, Lorenzi C, Smeraldi E. Tardive dyskinesia and DRD2, DRD3, DRD4, 5-HT2A variants in schizophrenia: An association study with repeated assessment. *Int. J. Neuropsychopharmacol.* 2004;**7**(4):489–493.

92. Srivastava V, Varma PG, Prasad S, Semwal P, Nimgaonkar VL, Lerer B, Deshpande SN, Bk T. Genetic susceptibility to tardive dyskinesia among schizophrenia subjects: IV. Role of dopaminergic pathway gene polymorphisms. *Pharmacogenet. Genomics* 2006;**16**(2): 111–117.

93. Wu SN, Gao R, Xing QH, Li HF, Shen YF, Gu NF, Feng GY, He L. Association of DRD2 polymorphisms and chlorpromazine-induced extrapyramidal syndrome in Chinese schizophrenic patients. *Acta Pharmacol. Sin.* 2006;**27**(8):966–970.

94. Dolzan V, Plesnicar BK, Serretti A, Mandelli L, Zalar B, Koprivsek J, Breskvar K. Polymorphisms in dopamine receptor DRD1 and DRD2 genes and psychopathological and extrapyramidal symptoms in patients on long-term antipsychotic treatment. *Am. J. Med. Genet. B Neuropsychiatr. Genet.* 2007;**144B**(6):809–815.

95. Zai CC, Hwang RW, De Luca V, Muller DJ, King N, Zai GC, Remington G, Meltzer HY, Lieberman JA, Potkin SG, Kennedy JL. Association study of tardive dyskinesia and twelve DRD2 polymorphisms in schizophrenia patients. *Int. J. Neuropsychopharmacol.* 2007;**10**(5):639–651.

96. Bakker PR, van Harten PN, van Os J. Antipsychotic-induced tardive dyskinesia and polymorphic variations in COMT, DRD2, CYP1A2 and MnSOD genes: A meta-analysis of pharmacogenetic interactions. *Mol. Psychiatry* 2008;**13**(5):544–556.

97. Segman RH, Goltser T, Heresco-Levy U, Finkel B, Shalem R, Schlafman M, Yakir A, Greenberg D, Strous R, Lerner A, Shelevoy A, Lerer B. Association of dopaminergic and serotonergic genes with tardive dyskinesia in patients with chronic schizophrenia. *Pharmacogenomics J.* 2003;**3**(5):277–283.

98. Segman RH, Heresco-Levy U, Finkel B, Goltser T, Shalem R, Schlafman M, Dorevitch A, Yakir A, Greenberg D, Lerner A, Lerer B. Association between the serotonin 2A receptor gene and tardive dyskinesia in chronic schizophrenia. *Mol. Psychiatry* 2001;**6**(2):225–229.

99. Tan EC, Chong SA, Mahendran R, Dong F, Tan CH. Susceptibility to neuroleptic-induced tardive dyskinesia and the T102C polymorphism in the serotonin type 2A receptor. *Biol. Psychiatry* 2001;**50**(2):144–147.

100. Basile VS, Ozdemir V, Masellis M, Meltzer HY, Lieberman JA, Potkin SG, Macciardi FM, Petronis A, Kennedy JL. Lack of association between serotonin-2A receptor gene (HTR2A) polymorphisms and tardive dyskinesia in schizophrenia. *Mol. Psychiatry* 2001;**6**(2):230–234.

101. Herken H, Erdal ME, Boke O, Savas HA. Tardive dyskinesia is not associated with the polymorphisms of 5-HT2A receptor gene, serotonin transporter gene and catechol-o-methyltransferase gene. *Eur. Psychiatry* 2003;**18**(2):77–81.

102. Deshpande SN, Varma PG, Semwal P, Rao AR, Bhatia T, Nimgaonkar VL, Lerer B, Thelma BK. II. Serotonin receptor gene polymorphisms and their association with tardive

dyskinesia among schizophrenia patients from North India. *Psychiatr. Genet.* 2005; **15**(3):157–158.

103. Lerer B, Segman RH, Tan EC, Basile VS, Cavallaro R, Aschauer HN, Strous R, Chong SA, Heresco-Levy U, Verga M, Scharfetter J, Meltzer HY, Kennedy JL, Macciardi F. Combined analysis of 635 patients confirms an age-related association of the serotonin 2A receptor gene with tardive dyskinesia and specificity for the non-orofacial subtype. *Int. J. Neuropsychopharmacol.* 2005;**8**(3):411–425.

104. Zhang ZJ, Zhang XB, Sha WW, Reynolds GP. Association of a polymorphism in the promoter region of the serotonin 5-HT2C receptor gene with tardive dyskinesia in patients with schizophrenia. *Mol. Psychiatry* 2002;**7**(7):670–671.

105. Zhang ZJ, Zhang XB, Hou G, Yao H, Reynolds GP. Interaction between polymorphisms of the dopamine D3 receptor and manganese superoxide dismutase genes in susceptibility to tardive dyskinesia. *Psychiatr. Genet.* 2003;**13**(3):187–192.

106. Pae CU, Yu HS, Kim JJ, Lee CU, Lee SJ, Jun TY, Lee C, Paik IH. Quinone oxidoreductase (NQO1) gene polymorphism (609C/T) may be associated with tardive dyskinesia, but not with the development of schizophrenia. *Int. J. Neuropsychopharmacol.* 2004;**7**(4):495–500.

107. Liou YJ, Wang YC, Lin CC, Bai YM, Lai IC, Liao DL, Chen JY. Association analysis of NAD(P)Hratioquinone oxidoreductase (NQO1) Pro187Ser genetic polymorphism and tardive dyskinesia in patients with schizophrenia in Taiwan. *Int. J. Neuropsychopharmacol.* 2005;**8**(3):483–486.

108. Shinkai T, Ohmori O, Matsumoto C, Hori H, Kennedy JL, Nakamura J. Genetic association analysis of neuronal nitric oxide synthase gene polymorphism with tardive dyskinesia. *Neuromol. Med.* 2004;**5**(2):163–170.

109. Wang YC, Liou YJ, Liao DL, Bai YM, Lin CC, Yu SC, Chen JY. Association analysis of a neural nitric oxide synthase gene polymorphism and antipsychotics-induced tardive dyskinesia in Chinese schizophrenic patients. *J. Neural. Transm.* 2004;**111**(5):623–629.

110. Liou YJ, Lai IC, Lin MW, Bai YM, Lin CC, Liao DL, Chen JY, Lin CY, Wang YC. Haplotype analysis of endothelial nitric oxide synthase (NOS3) genetic variants and tardive dyskinesia in patients with schizophrenia. *Pharmacogenet. Genomics* 2006; **16**(3):151–157.

111. Inada T, Koga M, Ishiguro H, Horiuchi Y, Syu A, Yoshio T, Takahashi N, Ozaki N, Arinami T. Pathway-based association analysis of genome-wide screening data suggest that genes associated with the [gamma]-aminobutyric acid receptor signaling pathway are involved in neuroleptic-induced, treatment-resistant tardive dyskinesia. *Pharmacogenet. Genomics* 2008;**18**(4):317–323.

112. Theisen FM, Gebhardt S, Haberhausen M, Heinzel-Gutenbrunner M, Wehmeier PM, Krieg JC, Kuhnau W, Schmidtke J, Remschmidt H, Hebebrand J. Clozapine-induced weight gain: A study in monozygotic twins and same-sex sib pairs. *Psychiatr. Genet.* 2005;**15**(4):285–289.

113. Wehmeier PM, Gebhardt S, Schmidtke J, Remschmidt H, Hebebrand J, Theisen FM. Clozapine: Weight gain in a pair of monozygotic twins concordant for schizophrenia and mild mental retardation. *Psychiatry Res.* 2005;**133**(2–3):273–276.

114. Allison DB, Mentore JL, Heo M, Chandler LP, Cappelleri JC, Infante MC, Weiden PJ. Antipsychotic-induced weight gain: A comprehensive research synthesis. *Am. J. Psychiatry* 1999;**156**(11):1686–1696.

115. Basile VS, Masellis M, McIntyre RS, Meltzer HY, Lieberman JA, Kennedy JL. Genetic dissection of atypical antipsychotic-induced weight gain: Novel preliminary data on the pharmacogenetic puzzle. *J. Clin. Psychiatry* 2001;**62** (Suppl 23): 45–66.

116. Sickert L, Muller DJ, Tiwari AK, Shaikh S, Zai C, De Souza R, De Luca V, Meltzer HY, Lieberman JA, Kennedy JL. Association of the alpha2A adrenergic receptor −1291C/G polymorphism and antipsychotic-induced weight gain in European-Americans. *Pharmacogenomics* 2009;**10**(7):1169–1176.

117. Reynolds GP, Zhang Z, Zhang X. Polymorphism of the promoter region of the serotonin 5-HT(2C) receptor gene and clozapine-induced weight gain. *Am. J. Psychiatry* 2003; **160**(4):677–679.

118. Ellingrod VL, Perry PJ, Ringold JC, Lund BC, Bever-Stille K, Fleming F, Holman TL, Miller D. Weight gain associated with the −759C/T polymorphism of the 5-HT2C receptor and olanzapine. *Am. J. Med. Genet. B Neuropsychiatr. Genet.* 2005; **134B**(1):76–78.

119. Miller DD, Ellingrod VL, Holman TL, Buckley PF, Arndt S. Clozapine-induced weight gain associated with the 5-HT2C receptor −759C/T polymorphism. *Am. J. Med. Genet. B Neuropsychiatr. Genet.* 2005;**133B**(1):97–100.

120. Templeman LA, Reynolds GP, Arranz B, San L. Polymorphisms of the 5-HT2C receptor and leptin genes are associated with antipsychotic drug-induced weight gain in Caucasian subjects with a first-episode psychosis. *Pharmacogenet. Genomics* 2005;**15**(4):195–200.

121. Hong CJ, Lin CH, Yu YW, Yang KH, Tsai SJ. Genetic variants of the serotonin system and weight change during clozapine treatment. *Pharmacogenetics* 2001; **11**(3):265–268.

122. Tsai SJ, Hong CJ, Yu YW, Lin CH. −759C/T genetic variation of 5-HT(2C) receptor and clozapine-induced weight gain. *Lancet* 2002;**360**(9347):1790.

123. Theisen FM, Hinney A, Bromel T, Heinzel-Gutenbrunner M, Martin M, Krieg JC, Remschmidt H, Hebebrand J. Lack of association between the −759C/T polymorphism of the 5-HT2C receptor gene and clozapine-induced weight gain among German schizophrenic individuals. *Psychiatr. Genet.* 2004;**14**(3):139–142.

124. Park YM, Cho JH, Kang SG, Choi JE, Lee SH, Kim L, Lee HJ. Lack of association between the −759C/T polymorphism of the 5-HT2C receptor gene and olanzapine-induced weight gain among Korean schizophrenic patients. *J. Clin. Pharm. Ther.* 2008;**33** (1):55–60.

125. Kang SG, Lee HJ, Park YM, Choi JE, Han C, Kim YK, Kim SH, Lee MS, Joe SH, Jung IK, Kim L. Possible association between the −2548A/G polymorphism of the leptin gene and olanzapine-induced weight gain. *Prog. Neuropsychopharmacol. Biol. Psychiatry* 2008;**32**(1):160–163.

126. Ellingrod VL, Bishop JR, Moline J, Lin YC, Miller DD. Leptin and leptin receptor gene polymorphisms and increases in body mass index (BMI) from olanzapine treatment in persons with schizophrenia. *Psychopharmacol Bull* 2007;**40**(1):57–62.

127. Mueller DJ, Kennedy JL. Genetics of antipsychotic treatment emergent weight gain in schizophrenia. *Pharmacogenomics* 2006;**7**(6):863–887.

128. Srivastava V, Deshpande SN, Nimgaonkar VL, Lerer B, Thelma B. Genetic correlates of olanzapine-induced weight gain in schizophrenia subjects from north India: Role of metabolic pathway genes. *Pharmacogenomics* 2008;**9**(8):1055–1068.

129. Musil R, Spellmann I, Riedel M, Dehning S, Douhet A, Maino K, Zill P, Muller N, Moller HJ, Bondy B. SNAP-25 gene polymorphisms and weight gain in schizophrenic patients. *J. Psychiatr. Res.* 2008;**42**(12):963–970.

130. Wang YC, Bai YM, Chen JY, Lin CC, Lai IC, Liou YJ. Polymorphism of the adrenergic receptor alpha 2a −1291C > G genetic variation and clozapine-induced weight gain. *J. Neural. Transm.* 2005;**112**(11):1463–1468.

131. Park YM, Chung YC, Lee SH, Lee KJ, Kim H, Byun YC, Lim SW, Paik JW, Lee HJ. Weight gain associated with the alpha2a-adrenergic receptor −1, 291 C/G polymorphism and olanzapine treatment. *Am. J. Med. Genet. B Neuropsychiatr. Genet.* 2006; **141B**(4):394–397.

132. Tsai SJ, Yu YW, Lin CH, Wang YC, Chen JY, Hong CJ. Association study of adrenergic beta3 receptor (Trp64Arg) and G-protein beta3 subunit gene (C825T) polymorphisms and weight change during clozapine treatment. *Neuropsychobiology* 2004;**50** (1):37–40.

133. Ellingrod VL, Miller D, Schultz SK, Wehring H, Arndt S. CYP2D6 polymorphisms and atypical antipsychotic weight gain. *Psychiatr. Genet.* 2002;**12**(1):55–58.

134. Citrome L, Stauffer VL, Chen L, Kinon BJ, Kurtz DL, Jacobson JG, Bergstrom RF. Olanzapine plasma concentrations after treatment with 10 20, and 40 mg/d in patients with schizophrenia: An analysis of correlations with efficacy, weight gain, and prolactin concentration. *J. Clin. Psychopharmacol.* 2009;**29**(3):278–283.

135. Chagnon YC, Merette C, Bouchard RH, Emond C, Roy MA, Maziade M. A genome wide linkage study of obesity as secondary effect of antipsychotics in multigenerational families of eastern Quebec affected by psychoses. *Mol. Psychiatry* 2004;**9**(12):1067–1074.

136. Chagnon YC, Bureau A, Gendron D, Bouchard RH, Merette C, Roy MA, Maziade M. Possible association of the pro-melanin-concentrating hormone gene with a greater body mass index as a side effect of the antipsychotic olanzapine. *Am. J. Med. Genet. B Neuropsychiatr. Genet.* 2007;**144B**(8):1063–1069.

137. Ruano G, Goethe JW, Caley C, Woolley S, Holford TR, Kocherla M, Windemuth A, de Leon J. Physiogenomic comparison of weight profiles of olanzapine- and risperidone-treated patients. *Mol. Psychiatry* 2007;**12**(5):474–482.

138. Lane HY, Liu YC, Huang CL, Chang YC, Wu PL, Lu CT, Chang WH. Risperidone-related weight gain: Genetic and nongenetic predictors. *J. Clin. Psychopharmacol.* 2006;**26**(2):128–134.

139. Lee BH, Kim YK. Increased plasma brain-derived neurotropic factor, not nerve growth factor-beta, in schizophrenia patients with better response to risperidone treatment. *Neuropsychobiology* 2009;**59**(1):51–58.

140. Munro J, O'Sullivan D, Andrews C, Arana A, Mortimer A, Kerwin R. Active monitoring of 12, 760 clozapine recipients in the UK and Ireland. Beyond pharmacovigilance. *Br. J. Psychiatry* 1999;**175**:576–580.

141. Ostrousky O, Meged S, Loewenthal R, Valevski A, Weizman A, Carp H, Gazit E. NQO2 gene is associated with clozapine-induced agranulocytosis. *Tissue Antigens* 2003; **62**(6):483–491.

142. Mosyagin I, Dettling M, Roots I, Mueller-Oerlinghausen B, Cascorbi I. Impact of myeloperoxidase and NADPH-oxidase polymorphisms in drug-induced agranulocytosis. *J. Clin. Psychopharmacol.* 2004;**24**(6):613–617.

143. Amar A, Segman RH, Shtrussberg S, Sherman L, Safirman C, Lerer B, Brautbar C. An association between clozapine-induced agranulocytosis in schizophrenics and HLA-DQB1*0201. *Int. J. Neuropsychopharmacol.* 1998;**1**(1):41–44.

144. Valevski A, Klein T, Gazit E, Meged S, Stein D, Elizur A, Narinsky ER, Kutzuk D, Weizman A. HLA-B38 and clozapine-induced agranulocytosis in Israeli Jewish schizophrenic patients. *Eur. J. Immunogenet.* 1998;**25**(1):11–13.

145. Meged S, Stein D, Sitrota P, Melamed Y, Elizur A, Shmuelian I, Gazit E. Human leukocyte antigen typing, response to neuroleptics, and clozapine-induced agranulocytosis in jewish Israeli schizophrenic patients. *Int. Clin. Psychopharmacol.* 1999; **14**(5):305–312.

146. Fehsel K, Loeffler S, Krieger K, Henning U, Agelink M, Kolb-Bachofen V, Klimke A. Clozapine induces oxidative stress and proapoptotic gene expression in neutrophils of schizophrenic patients. *J. Clin. Psychopharmacol.* 2005;**25**(5):419–426.

147. Dettling M, Sachse C, Muller-Oerlinghausen B, Roots I, Brockmoller J, Rolfs A, Cascorbi I. Clozapine-induced agranulocytosis and hereditary polymorphisms of clozapine metabolizing enzymes: No association with myeloperoxidase and cytochrome P4502D6. *Pharmacopsychiatry* 2000;**33**(6):218–220.

148. Turbay D, Lieberman J, Alper CA, Delgado JC, Corzo D, Yunis JJ, Yunis EJ. Tumor necrosis factor constellation polymorphism and clozapine-induced agranulocytosis in two different ethnic groups. *Blood* 1997;**89**(11):4167–4174.

149. Mihara K, Kondo T, Suzuki A, Yasui N, Nagashima U, Ono S, Otani K, Kaneko S. Prolactin response to nemonapride, a selective antagonist for D2 like dopamine receptors, in schizophrenic patients in relation to Taq1A polymorphism of DRD2 gene. *Psychopharmacology* (Berlin) 2000;**149**(3):246–250.

150. Aitchison K, Pereira J, Purcell S. An association study of DRD2 and CYP2D6 and hyperprolactinaemia. *Proc. Int. Congress Schizophrenia Research*, Colorado Springs, 2003.

151. Aklillu E, Kalow W, Endrenyi L, Harper P, Miura J, Ozdemir V. CYP2D6 and DRD2 genes differentially impact pharmacodynamic sensitivity and time course of prolactin response to perphenazine. *Pharmacogenet. Genomics* 2007;**17**(11):989–993.

152. Ananth J, Parameswaran S, Gunatilake S, Burgoyne K, Sidhom T. Neuroleptic malignant syndrome and atypical antipsychotic drugs. *J. Clin. Psychiatry* 2004;**65**(4):464–470.

153. Suzuki A, Kondo T, Otani K, Mihara K, Yasui-Furukori N, Sano A, Koshiro K, Kaneko S. Association of the TaqI A polymorphism of the dopamine D(2) receptor gene with predisposition to neuroleptic malignant syndrome. *Am. J. Psychiatry* 2001;**158**(10): 1714–1716.

154. Mihara K, Kondo T, Suzuki A, Yasui-Furukori N, Ono S, Sano A, Koshiro K, Otani K, Kaneko S. Relationship between functional dopamine D2 and D3 receptors gene polymorphisms and neuroleptic malignant syndrome. *Am. J. Med. Genet. B Neuropsychiatr. Genet.* 2003;**117B**(1):57–60.

155. Kishida I, Kawanishi C, Furuno T, Matsumura T, Hasegawa H, Sugiyama N, Suzuki K, Yamada Y, Kosaka K. Lack of association in Japanese patients between neuroleptic malignant syndrome and the TaqI A polymorphism of the dopamine D2 receptor gene. *Psychiatr. Genet.* 2003;**13**(1):55–57.

156. Casey DE. Implications of the CATIE trial on treatment: Extrapyramidal symptoms. *CNS Spectrums* 2006;**11**(7 Suppl. 7):25–31.

157. Kishida I, Kawanishi C, Furuno T, Kato D, Ishigami T, Kosaka K. Association in Japanese patients between neuroleptic malignant syndrome and functional polymorphisms of the dopamine D(2) receptor gene. *Mol. Psychiatry* 2004;**9**(3):293–298.

158. Jauss M, Krack P, Franz M, Klett R, Bauer R, Gallhofer B, Dorndorf W. Imaging of dopamine receptors with [123I]iodobenzamide single-photon emission-computed tomography in neuroleptic malignant syndrome. *Mov. Disord.* 1996;**11**(6):726–728.

159. Gupta B, Keers R, Uher R, McGuffin P, Aitchison KJ. Pharmacogenetics of antidepressant response. In Pariante CM, Nesse R, Nutt D, Wolpert L, eds.: *Depression: Translational Approaches to Understanding and Treating*. Oxford, UK: Oxford Univ. Press, 2009. pp. 299–314.

160. Brosen K. Drug-metabolizing enzymes and therapeutic drug monitoring in psychiatry. *Ther. Drug Monit.* 1996;**18**(4):393–396.

161. Bertilsson L, Dahl ML, Sjoqvist F, Aberg-Wistedt A, Humble M, Johansson I, Lundqvist E, Ingelman-Sundberg M. Molecular basis for rational megaprescribing in ultrarapid hydroxylators of debrisoquine. *Lancet* 1993;**341**(8836):63.

162. Thuerauf N, Lunkenheimer J. The impact of the CYP2D6-polymorphism on dose recommendations for current antidepressants. *Eur. Arch. Psychiatry Clin. Neurosci.* 2006;**256**(5):287–293.

163. Yu KS, Yim DS, Cho JY, Park SS, Park JY, Lee KH, Jang IJ, Yi SY, Bae KS, Shin SG. Effect of omeprazole on the pharmacokinetics of moclobemide according to the genetic polymorphism of CYP2C19. *Clin. Pharmacol. Ther.* 2001;**69**(4):266–273.

164. Cho JY, Yu KS, Jang IJ, Yang BH, Shin SG, Yim DS. Omeprazole hydroxylation is inhibited by a single dose of moclobemide in homozygotic EM genotype for CYP2C19. *Br. J. Clin. Pharmacol.* 2002;**53**(4):393–397.

165. Bonnet U. Moclobemide: Therapeutic use and clinical studies. *CNS Drug Rev.* 2003; **9**(1):97–140.

166. Jiang ZP, Shu Y, Chen XP, Huang SL, Zhu RH, Wang W, He N, Zhou HH. The role of CYP2C19 in amitriptyline N-demethylation in Chinese subjects. *Eur. J. Clin. Pharmacol.* 2002;**58**(2):109–113.

167. Shimoda K, Someya T, Yokono A, Morita S, Hirokane G, Takahashi S, Okawa M. The impact of CYP2C19 and CYP2D6 genotypes on metabolism of amitriptyline in Japanese psychiatric patients. *J. Clin. Psychopharmacol.* 2002;**22**(4):371–378.

168. van der Weide J, van Baalen-Benedek EH, Kootstra-Ros JE. Metabolic ratios of psychotropics as indication of cytochrome P450 2D6/2C19 genotype. *Ther. Drug Monit.* 2005;**27**(4):478–483.

169. Tandon K, Huezo-Diaz P, Kinirons M, Gustafsson L, Gill M, McGuffin P, Kerwin RW, Craig I, Aitchison KJ.The pharmacogenetics of response to tricyclic antidepressants in relation to CYP2D6 genotype and phenotype and CYP2C19 genotype. Oral presentation by KJ Aitchison at 2005 Cold Spring Harbor Pharmacogenomics Conf.

170. Steimer W, Zopf K, von Amelunxen S, Pfeiffer H, Bachofer J, Popp J, Messner B, Kissling W, Leucht S. Amitriptyline or not, that is the question: Pharmacogenetic testing of CYP2D6 and CYP2C19 identifies patients with low or high risk for side effects in amitriptyline therapy. *Clin. Chem.* 2005;**51**(2):376–385.

171. Yokono A, Morita S, Someya T, Hirokane G, Okawa M, Shimoda K. The effect of CYP2C19 and CYP2D6 genotypes on the metabolism of clomipramine in Japanese psychiatric patients. *J. Clin. Psychopharmacol.* 2001;**21**(6):549–555.

172. Noguchi T, Shimoda K, Takahashi S. Clinical significance of plasma levels of clomipramine, its hydroxylated and desmethylated metabolites: Prediction of clinical outcome in mood disorders using discriminant analysis of therapeutic drug monitoring data. *J. Affect. Disord.* 1993;**29**(4):267–279.

173. Wang JH, Liu ZQ, Wang W, Chen XP, Shu Y, He N, Zhou HH. Pharmacokinetics of sertraline in relation to genetic polymorphism of CYP2C19. *Clin. Pharmacol. Ther.* 2001;**70**(1):42–47.

174. Kobayashi K, Ishizuka T, Shimada N, Yoshimura Y, Kamijima K, Chiba K. Sertraline N-demethylation is catalyzed by multiple isoforms of human cytochrome P-450 *in vitro*. *Drug Metab. Dispos.* 1999;**27**(7):763–766.

175. Xu ZH, Wang W, Zhao XJ, Huang SL, Zhu B, He N, Shu Y, Liu ZQ, Zhou HH. Evidence for involvement of polymorphic CYP2C19 and 2C9 in the N-demethylation of sertraline in human liver microsomes. *Br. J. Clin. Pharmacol.* 1999;**48**(3):416–423.

176. Obach RS, Cox LM, Tremaine LM. Sertraline is metabolized by multiple cytochrome P450 enzymes, monoamine oxidases, and glucuronyl transferases in human: An *in vitro* study. *Drug Metab. Dispos.* 2005;**33**(2):262–270.

177. Schweizer E, Rynn M, Mandos LA, Demartinis N, Garcia-Espana F, Rickels K. The antidepressant effect of sertraline is not enhanced by dose titration: Results from an outpatient clinical trial. *Int. Clin. Psychopharmacol.* 2001;**16**(3):137–143.

178. Hyttel J. Citalopram—pharmacological profile of a specific serotonin uptake inhibitor with antidepressant activity. *Prog. Neuropsychopharmacol. Biol. Psychiatry* 1982;**6**(3): 277–295.

179. Herrlin K, Yasui-Furukori N, Tybring G, Widen J, Gustafsson LL, Bertilsson L. Metabolism of citalopram enantiomers in CYP2C19/CYP2D6 phenotyped panels of healthy Swedes. *Br. J. Clin. Pharmacol.* 2003;**56**(4):415–421.

180. Yu BN, Chen GL, He N, Ouyang DS, Chen XP, Liu ZQ, Zhou HH. Pharmacokinetics of citalopram in relation to genetic polymorphism of CYP2C19. *Drug Metab. Dispos.* 2003;**31**(10):1255–1259.

181. Rudberg, I, Mohebi, B, Hermann, M, Refsum, H, Molden, E. Impact of the ultrarapid CYP2C19*17 allele on serum concentration of escitalopram in psychiatric patients. *Clin. Pharmacol. Ther.* 2008;**83**:322–327.

182. Bech P, Andersen HF, Wade A. Effective dose of escitalopram in moderate versus severe DSM-IV major depression. *Pharmacopsychiatry* 2006;**39**(4):128–134.

183. George T, Theodoros MT, Chiu E, Krapivensky N, Hokin A, Tiller JW. An open study of sertraline in patients with major depression who failed to respond to moclobemide. *Austral. NZ J. Psychiatry* 1999;**33**(6):889–895.

184. Kootstra-Ros JE, Van Weelden MJ, Hinrichs JW, De Smet PA, van der Weide J. Therapeutic drug monitoring of antidepressants and cytochrome p450 genotyping in general practice. *J. Clin. Pharmacol.* 2006;**46**(11):1320–1327.

185. Caspi A, Sugden K, Moffitt TE, Taylor A, Craig IW, Harrington H, et al. Influence of life stress on depression: Moderation by a polymorphism in the 5-HTT gene. *Science* 2003;**301**:386–389.

186. Smeraldi E, Zanardi R, Benedetti F, Di Bella D, Perez J, Catalano M. Polymorphism within the promoter of the serotonin transporter gene and antidepressant efficacy of fluvoxamine. *Mol. Psychiatry* 1998;**3**(6):508–511.

187. Zanardi R, Benedetti F, Di Bella D, Catalano M, Smeraldi E. Efficacy of paroxetine in depression is influenced by a functional polymorphism within the promoter of the serotonin transporter gene. *J. Clin. Psychopharmacol.* 2000;**20**(1):105–107.

188. Rausch JL, Johnson ME, Fei YJ, Li JQ, Shendarkar N, Hobby HM, Ganapathy V, Leibach FH. Initial conditions of serotonin transporter kinetics and genotype: Influence on SSRI treatment trial outcome. *Biol. Psychiatry* 2002;**51**(9):723–732.

189. Durham LK, Webb SM, Milos PM, Clary CM, Seymour AB. The serotonin transporter polymorphism, 5-HTTLPR, is associated with a faster response time to sertraline in an elderly population with major depressive disorder. *Psychopharmacology* (Berlin) 2004;**174**(4):525–529.

190. Tsapakis E, Checkley S, Kerwin RW, Aitchison KJ. Association between the serotonin transporter linked polymorphic region gene and response to tricyclic antidepressants. *Eur. Neuropsychopharmacol.* 2005;**15**:S26–S27.

191. Serretti A, Lilli R, Smeraldi E. Pharmacogenetics in affective disorders. *Eur. J. Pharmacol.* 2002;**438**(3):117–128.

192. Ito K, Yoshida K, Sato K, Takahashi H, Kamata M, Higuchi H, Shimizu T, Itoh K, Inoue K, Tezuka T, Suzuki T, Ohkubo T, Sugawara K, Otani K. A variable number of tandem repeats in the serotonin transporter gene does not affect the antidepressant response to fluvoxamine. *Psychiatry Res.* 2002;**111**(2–3):235–239.

193. Yoshida K, Ito K, Sato K, Takahashi H, Kamata M, Higuchi H, Shimizu T, Itoh K, Inoue K, Tezuka T, Suzuki T, Ohkubo T, Sugawara K, Otani K. Influence of the serotonin transporter gene-linked polymorphic region on the antidepressant response to fluvoxamine in Japanese depressed patients. *Prog. Neuropsychopharmacol. Biol. Psychiatry* 2002;**26**(2):383–386.

194. Kim DK, Lim SW, Lee S, Sohn SE, Kim S, Hahn CG, Carroll BJ. Serotonin transporter gene polymorphism and antidepressant response. *Neuroreport* 2000; **11**(1):215–219.

195. Kim H, Lim SW, Kim S, Kim JW, Chang YH, Carroll BJ, Kim DK. Monoamine transporter gene polymorphisms and antidepressant response in koreans with late-life depression. *JAMA* 2006;**296**(13):1609–1618.

196. Wilkie MJ, Smith G, Day RK, Matthews K, Smith D, Blackwood D, Reid IC, Wolf CR. Polymorphisms in the SLC6A4 and HTR2A genes influence treatment outcome following antidepressant therapy. *Pharmacogenomics J.* 2009;**9**(1):61–70.

197. Huezo-Diaz P, Uher R, Smith R, Rietschel M, Henigsberg N, Marusic A, Mors O, Maier W, Hauser J, Souery D, Placentino A, Zobel A, Larsen ER, Czerski PM, et al. Moderation of antidepressant response by the serotonin transporter gene. *Br. J. Psychiatry* 2009;**195**:30–38.

198. Uher R, Maier W, Hauser J, Marusic A, Schmael C, Mors O, Henigsberg N, Souery D, Placentino A, Rietschel M, Zobel A, Dmitrzak-Weglarz M, Petrovic A, et al. Differential efficacy of escitalopram and nortriptyline on dimensional measures of depression. *Br. J. Psychiatry* 2009;**194**:252–259.

199. Keers R, Uher R, Gupta B, Rietschel M, Schulze T, Hauser J, Skibinska M, Henigsberg N, Kalember P, Maier W, Zobel A, Mors O, Kristensen AS, Kozel O, et al. Stressful life events, cognitive symptoms of depression and response to antidepressants in GENDEP. *J. Affect. Disord.* 2010;**127**:337–342

200. Rotondo A, Schuebel K, Bergen A, Aragon R, Virkkunen M, Linnoila M, Goldman D, Nielsen D. Identification of four variants in the tryptophan hydroxylase promoter and association to behavior. *Mol. Psychiatry* 1999;**4**(4):360–368.

201. Porter RJ, Mulder RT, Joyce PR, Miller AL, Kennedy M. Tryptophan hydroxylase gene (TPH1) and peripheral tryptophan levels in depression. *J. Affect. Disord.* 2008; **109**(1–2):209–212.

202. Austin MC and O'Donnell SM. Regional distriubtion and cellular expression of tryptophan hydroxylase messenger RNA in postmortem human brainstem and pineal gland. *J. Neureochem.* 1999;**72**:2065–2073.

203. Tzvetkov MV, Brockmoller J, Roots I, Kirchheiner J. Common genetic variations in human brain-specific tryptophan hydroxylase-2 and response to antidepressant treatment. *Pharmacogenet. Genomics* 2008;**18**(6):495–506.

204. Peters EJ, Slager SL, McGrath PJ, Knowles JA, Hamilton SP. Investigation of serotonin-related genes in antidepressant response. *Mol. Psychiatry* 2004;**9**(9):879–89.

205. Uher R, Huezo-Diaz P, Perroud N, Smith R, Rietchel M, Mors O, Hauser J, Maier W, Kozel D, Henigsberg N, Barreto M, Placentino A, Dernovsek MZ, Schulze TG, et al. Genetic predictors of response to antidepressants in the GENDEP project. *Pharmacogenomics J.* 2009;**9**:225–233.

206. Perroud N, Aitchison KJ, Uher R, Smith R, Huezo-Diaz P, Marusic A, Maier W, Mors O, Placentino A, Henigsberg N, Rietschel M, Hauser J, Souery D, Kapelski P, et al. Genetic predictors of increase in suicidal ideation during antidepressant treatment in the GENDEP project. *Neuropsychopharmacology* 2009;**34**:2517–2528.

207. Mueller DJ, Schulze TG, Macciardi F, Ohlraun S, Gross MM, Scherk H, Neidt H, Syagailo YV, Grassle M, Nothen MM, Maier W, Lesch KP, Rietschel M. Moclobemide response in depressed patients: Association study with a functional polymorphism in the monoamine oxidase A promoter. *Pharmacopsychiatry* 2002;**35**(4):157–158.

208. Yoshida K, Naito S, Takahashi H, Sato K, Ito K, Kamata M, Higuchi H, Shimizu T, Itoh K, Inoue K, Tezuka T, Suzuki T, Ohkubo T, Sugawara K, Otani K. Monoamine oxidase: A gene polymorphism, tryptophan hydroxylase gene polymorphism and antidepressant response to fluvoxamine in Japanese patients with major depressive disorder. *Prog. Neuropsychopharmacol. Biol. Psychiatry* 2002;**26**(7–8):1279–1283.

209. Cusin C, Serretti A, Zanardi R, Lattuada E, Rossini D, Lilli R, Lorenzi C, Smeraldi E. Influence of monoamine oxidase A and serotonin receptor 2A polymorphisms in SSRI antidepressant activity. *Int. J. Neuropsychopharmacol.* 2002;**5**(1):27–35.

210. Szegedi A, Rujescu D, Tadic A, Muller MJ, Kohnen R, Stassen HH, Dahmen N. The catechol-O-methyltransferase Val108/158Met polymorphism affects short-term treatment response to mirtazapine, but not to paroxetine in major depression. *Pharmacogenomics J.* 2005;**5**(1):49–53.

211. Arias B, Serretti A, Lorenzi C, Gasto C, Catalan R, Fananas L. Analysis of COMT gene (Val 158 Met polymorphism) in the clinical response to SSRIs in depressive patients of European origin. *J. Affect. Disord.* 2006;**90**(2–3):251–256.

212. Yoshida K, Higuchi H, Takahashi H, Kamata M, Sato K, Inoue K, Suzuki T, Itoh K, Ozaki N. Influence of the tyrosine hydroxylase val81met polymorphism and catechol-O-methyltransferase val158met polymorphism on the antidepressant effect of milnacipran. *Hum. Psychopharmacol.* 2008;**23**(2):121–128.

213. Minov C, Baghai TC, Schule C, Zwanzger P, Schwarz MJ, Zill P, Rupprecht R, Bondy B. Serotonin-2A-receptor and -transporter polymorphisms: Lack of association in patients with major depression. *Neurosci. Lett.* 2001;**303**(2):119–122.

214. Choi MJ, Kang RH, Ham BJ, Jeong HY, Lee MS. Serotonin receptor 2A gene polymorphism (−1438A/G) and short-term treatment response to citalopram. *Neuropsychobiology* 2005;**52**(3):155–162.

215. Kato M, Fukuda T, Wakeno M, Fukuda K, Okugawa G, Ikenaga Y, Yamashita M, Takekita Y, Nobuhara K, Azuma J, Kinoshita T. Effects of the serotonin type 2A, 3A and 3B receptor and the serotonin transporter genes on paroxetine and fluvoxamine efficacy and adverse drug reactions in depressed Japanese patients. *Neuropsychobiology* 2006;**53** (4):186–195.

216. McMahon FJ, Buervenich S, Charney D, Lipsky R, Rush AJ, Wilson AF, Sorant AJ, Papanicolaou GJ, Laje G, Fava M, Trivedi MH, Wisniewski SR, Manji H. Variation in the gene encoding the serotonin 2A receptor is associated with outcome of antidepressant treatment. *Am. J. Hum. Genet.* 2006;**78**(5):804–814.

217. Paddock S, Laje G, Charney D, Rush AJ, Wilson AF, Sorant AJ, Lipsky R, Wisniewski SR, Manji H, McMahon FJ. Association of GRIK4 with outcome of antidepressant treatment in the STAR*D cohort. *Am. J. Psychiatry* 2007;**164**(8):1181–1188.

218. Lemonde S, Du L, Bakish D, Hrdina P, Albert PR. Association of the C(−1019)G 5-HT1A functional promoter polymorphism with antidepressant response. *Int. J. Neuropsychopharmacol.* 2004;**7**(4):501–506.

219. Serretti A, Artioli P, Lorenzi C, Pirovano A, Tubazio V, Zanardi R. The C(−1019)G polymorphism of the 5-HT1A gene promoter and antidepressant response in mood disorders: Preliminary findings. *Int. J. Neuropsychopharmacol.* 2004;**7**:453–460.

220. Parsey RV, Olvet DM, Oquendo MA, Huang YY, Ogden RT, Mann JJ. Higher 5-HT1A receptor binding potential during a major depressive episode predicts poor treatment response: Preliminary data from a naturalistic study. *Neuropsychopharmacology* 2006; **31**(8):1745–1749.

221. Arias B, Catalan R, Gasto C, Gutierrez B, Fananas L. Evidence for a combined genetic effect of the 5-HT(1A) receptor and serotonin transporter genes in the clinical outcome of major depressive patients treated with citalopram. *J. Psychopharmacol.* 2005;**19**(2):166–172.

222. Baune BT, Hohoff C, Roehrs T, Deckert J, Arolt V, Domschke K. Serotonin receptor 1A-1019C/G variant: Impact on antidepressant pharmacoresponse in melancholic depression? *Neurosci. Lett.* 2008;**436**(2):111–115.

223. Hong CJ, Chen TJ, Yu YW, Tsai SJ. Response to fluoxetine and serotonin 1A receptor (C-1019G) polymorphism in Taiwan Chinese major depressive disorder. *Pharmacogenomics J.* 2006;**6**(1):27–33.

224. Yu YW, Tsai SJ, Liou YJ, Hong CJ, Chen TJ. Association study of two serotonin 1A receptor gene polymorphisms and fluoxetine treatment response in Chinese major depressive disorders. *Eur. Neuropsychopharmacol.* 2006;**16**(7):498–503.

225. Kato M, Fukuda T, Wakeno M, Okugawa G, Takekita Y, Serretti A, Azuma J, Kinoshita T. 5-HT1A gene polymorphisms contributed to antidepressant response in major depression (in Japanese). *Nihon Shinkei Seishin Yakurigaku Zasshi* 2009;**29**(1):23–31.

226. Suzuki Y, Sawamura K, Someya T. The effects of a 5-hydroxytryptamine 1A receptor gene polymorphism on the clinical response to fluvoxamine in depressed patients. *Pharmacogenomics J.* 2004;**4**(4):283–286.

227. Levin GM, Bowles TM, Ehret MJ, Langaee T, Tan JY, Johnson JA, Millard WJ. Assessment of human serotonin 1A receptor polymorphisms and SSRI responsiveness. *Mol. Diagn. Ther.* 2007;**11**(3):155–160.

228. Sugai T, Suzuki Y, Sawamura K, Fukui N, Inoue Y, Someya T. The effect of 5-hydroxytryptamine 3A and 3B receptor genes on nausea induced by paroxetine. *Pharmacogenomics J.* 2006;**6**(5):351–356.

229. Suzuki Y, Sawamura K, Someya T. Polymorphisms in the 5-hydroxytryptamine 2A receptor and CytochromeP4502D6 genes synergistically predict fluvoxamine-induced side effects in japanese depressed patients. *Neuropsychopharmacology* 2006;**31**(4): 825–831.

230. Kapur S, Remington G. Serotonin-dopamine interaction and its relevance to schizophrenia. *Am. J. Psychiatry* 1996;**153**(4):466–476.

231. Klimke A, Larisch R, Janz A, Vosberg H, Muller-Gartner HW, Gaebel W. Dopamine D2 receptor binding before and after treatment of major depression measured by [123I] IBZM SPECT. *Psychiatry Res.* 1999;**90**(2):91–101.

232. Serretti A, Zanardi R, Cusin C, Rossini D, Lilli R, Lorenzi C, Lattuada E, Smeraldi E. No association between dopamine D(2) and D(4) receptor gene variants and antidepressant activity of two selective serotonin reuptake inhibitors. *Psychiatry Res.* 2001;**104**(3): 195–203.

233. Siffert W, Rosskopf D, Siffert G, Busch S, Moritz A, Erbel R, Sharma AM, Ritz E, Wichmann HE, Jakobs KH, Horsthemke B. Association of a human G-protein beta3 subunit variant with hypertension. *Nat. Genet.* 1998;**18**(1):45–48.

234. Zill P, Baghai TC, Zwanzger P, Schule C, Minov C, Riedel M, Neumeier K, Rupprecht R, Bondy B. Evidence for an association between a G-protein beta3-gene variant with depression and response to antidepressant treatment. *Neuroreport* 2000;**11**(9): 1893–1897.

235. Joyce PR, Mulder RT, Luty SE, McKenzie JM, Miller AL, Rogers GR, Kennedy MA. Age-dependent antidepressant pharmacogenomics: Polymorphisms of the serotonin transporter and G protein beta3 subunit as predictors of response to fluoxetine and nortriptyline. *Int. J. Neuropsychopharmacol.* 2003;**6**(4):339–346.

236. Lee HJ, Cha JH, Ham BJ, Han CS, Kim YK, Lee SH, Ryu SH, Kang RH, Choi MJ, Lee MS. Association between a G-protein beta 3 subunit gene polymorphism and the symptomatology and treatment responses of major depressive disorders. *Pharmacogenomics J.* 2004;**4**(1):29–33.

237. Serretti A, Lorenzi C, Cusin C, Zanardi R, Lattuada E, Rossini D, Lilli R, Pirovano A, Catalano M, Smeraldi E. SSRIs antidepressant activity is influenced by G beta 3 variants. *Eur. Neuropsychopharmacol.* 2003;**13**(2):117–122.

238. Wilkie MJ, Smith D, Reid IC, Day RK, Matthews K, Wolf CR, Blackwood D, Smith G. A splice site polymorphism in the G-protein beta subunit influences antidepressant efficacy in depression. *Pharmacogenet. Genomics* 2007;**17**(3):207–215.

239. Kang RH, Hahn SW, Choi MJ, Lee MS. Relationship between G-protein beta-3 subunit C825T polymorphism and mirtazapine responses in Korean patients with major depression. *Neuropsychobiology* 2007;**56**(1):1–5.

240. Kato M, Serretti A. Review and meta-analysis of antidepressant pharmacogenetic findings in major depressive disorder. *Mol. Psychiatry* 2010;**15**:473–500.

241. Keers R, Bonvicini C, Scassellati C, Uher R, Placentino A, Giovannini C, Rietschel M, Henigsberg N, Kozel D, Mors O, Maier W, Hauser J, Souery D, et al. Variation in *GNB3* predicts response and adverse reactions to antidepressants. *J. Psychopharmaco.* (in press).

242. Duman RS. Role of neurotrophic factors in the etiology and treatment of mood disorders. *Neuromol. Med.* 2004;**5**(1):11–25.

243. Egan MF, Weinberger DR, Lu B. Schizophrenia, III: Brain-derived neurotropic factor and genetic risk. *Am. J. Psychiatry* 2003;**160**(7):1242.

244. Yoshida K, Higuchi H, Kamata M, Takahashi H, Inoue K, Suzuki T, Itoh K, Ozaki N. The G196A polymorphism of the brain-derived neurotrophic factor gene and the antidepressant effect of milnacipran and fluvoxamine. *J. Psychopharmacol.* 2007;**21**(6):650–656.

245. Gratacos M, Soria V, Urretavizcaya M, Gonzalez JR, Crespo JM, Bayes M, de Cid R, Menchon JM, Vallejo J, Estivill X. A brain-derived neurotrophic factor (BDNF) haplotype is associated with antidepressant treatment outcome in mood disorders. *Pharmacogenomics J.* 2008;**8**(2):101–112.

246. Kang RH, Chang HS, Wong ML, Choi MJ, Park JY, Lee HY, Jung IK, Joe SH, Kim L, Kim SH, Kim YK, Han CS, Ham BJ, Lee HJ, Ko YH, Lee MS, Lee MS. Brain-derived neurotrophic factor gene polymorphisms and mirtazapine responses in Koreans with major depression. *J. Psychopharmacol.* 2010;**24**:1755–1763.

247. Perroud N, Uher R, Ng MY, Guipponi M, Hauser J, Henigsberg N, Maier W, Mors O, Pacentino A, Rietschel M, Souery D, Kozel D, Lathrop M, Farmer A, Breen G, et al. Genome-wide association study of increasing suicidal ideation during antidepressant treatment in the GENDEP project. *Pharmacogenomics J.* 2010; epub Sept 28.

248. Rigat B, Hubert C, Alhenc-Gelas F, Cambien F, Corvol P, Soubrier F. An insertion/deletion polymorphism in the angiotensin I-converting enzyme gene accounting for half the variance of serum enzyme levels. *J. Clin. Invest.* 1990;**86**(4):1343–1346.

249. Arinami T, Li L, Mitsushio H, Itokawa M, Hamaguchi H, Toru M. An insertion/deletion polymorphism in the angiotensin converting enzyme gene is associated with both brain substance P contents and affective disorders. *Biol. Psychiatry* 1996;**40**(11):1122–1127.

250. Baghai TC, Schule C, Zwanzger P, Minov C, Schwarz MJ, de Jonge S, Rupprecht R, Bondy B. Possible influence of the insertion/deletion polymorphism in the angiotensin I-converting enzyme gene on therapeutic outcome in affective disorders. *Mol. Psychiatry* 2001;**6**(3):258–259.

251. Baghai TC, Schule C, Zill P, Deiml T, Eser D, Zwanzger P, Ella R, Rupprecht R, Bondy B. The angiotensin I converting enzyme insertion/deletion polymorphism influences therapeutic outcome in major depressed women, but not in men. *Neurosci. Lett.* 2004; **363**(1):38–42.

252. Hong CJ, Wang YC, Tsai SJ. Association study of angiotensin I-converting enzyme polymorphism and symptomatology and antidepressant response in major depressive disorders. *J. Neural. Transm.* 2002;**109**(9):1209–1214.

253. Seymour PA, Schmidt AW, Schulz DW. The pharmacology of CP-154,526, a non-peptide antagonist of the CRH1 receptor: A review. *CNS Drug Rev.* 2003;**9**(1):57–96.

254. Overstreet DH, Keeney A, Hogg S. Antidepressant effects of citalopram and CRF receptor antagonist CP-154,526 in a rat model of depression. *Eur. J. Pharmacol.* 2004;**492**(2–3):195–201.

255. Licinio J, O'Kirwan F, Irizarry K, Merriman B, Thakur S, Jepson R, Lake S, Tantisira KG, Weiss ST, Wong ML. Association of a corticotropin-releasing hormone receptor 1

haplotype and antidepressant treatment response in Mexican-Americans. *Mol. Psychiatry* 2004;**9**(12):1075–1082.

256. Liu Z, Zhu F, Wang G, Xiao Z, Tang J, Liu W, Wang H, Liu H, Wang X, Wu Y, Cao Z, Li W. Association study of corticotropin-releasing hormone receptor1 gene polymorphisms and antidepressant response in major depressive disorders. *Neurosci. Lett.* 2007; **414**(2):155–158.
257. Binder EB, Salyakina D, Lichtner P, Wochnik GM, Ising M, Putz B, Papiol S, Seaman S, Lucae S, Kohli MA, Nickel T, Kunzel HE, Fuchs B, Majer M, Pfennig A, et al. Polymorphisms in FKBP5 are associated with increased recurrence of depressive episodes and rapid response to antidepressant treatment. *Nat. Genet.* 2004;**36**(12): 1319–1325.
258. Tsai SJ, Hong CJ, Chen TJ, Yu YW. Lack of supporting evidence for a genetic association of the FKBP5 polymorphism and response to antidepressant treatment. *Am. J. Med. Genet. B Neuropsychiatr. Genet.* 2007;**144B**(8):1097–1098.
259. Papiol S, Arias B, Gasto C, Gutierrez B, Catalan R, Fananas L. Genetic variability at HPA axis in major depression and clinical response to antidepressant treatment. *J. Affect. Disord.* 2007;**104**(1–3):83–90.
260. Lekman M, Laje G, Charney D, Rush AJ, Wilson AF, Sorant AJ, Lipsky R, Wisniewski SR, Manji H, McMahon FJ, Paddock S. The FKBP5-gene in depression and treatment response—an association study in the sequenced treatment alternatives to relieve depression (STAR*D) cohort. *Biol. Psychiatry* 2008;**63**(12):1103–1110.
261. Serretti A, Lilli R, Mandelli L, Lorenzi C, Smeraldi E. Serotonin transporter gene associated with lithium prophylaxis in mood disorders. *Pharmacogenomics J.* 2001; **1**(1):71–77.
262. Serretti A, Malitas PN, Mandelli L, Lorenzi C, Ploia C, Alevizos B, Nikolaou C, Boufidou F, Christodoulou GN, Smeraldi E. Further evidence for a possible association between serotonin transporter gene and lithium prophylaxis in mood disorders. *Pharmacogenomics J.* 2004;**4**(4):267–273.
263. Del Zompo M, Ardau R, Palmas MA, Bocchetta A, Reina A, Piccardi MP. Lithium response: Association study with two candidate genes. *Mol. Psychiatry* 1999;**4**:S66–S67.
264. Dmitrzak-Weglarz M, Rybakowski JK, Suwalska A, Slopien A, Czerski PM, Leszczynska-Rodziewicz A, Hauser J. Association studies of 5-HT2A and 5-HT2C serotonin receptor gene polymorphisms with prophylactic lithium response in bipolar patients. *Pharmacol Rep* 2005;**57**(6):761–765.
265. Rybakowski JK, Suwalska A, Czerski PM, Dmitrzak-Weglarz M, Leszczynska-Rodziewicz A, Hauser J. Prophylactic effect of lithium in bipolar affective illness may be related to serotonin transporter genotype. *Pharmacol. Rep.* 2005;**57**(1):124–127.
266. Serretti A, Lilli R, Lorenzi C, Gasperini M, Smeraldi E. Tryptophan hydroxylase gene and response to lithium prophylaxis in mood disorders. *J. Psychiatr. Res.* 1999;**33**(5):371–377.
267. Manji HK, Moore GJ, Chen G. Lithium at 50: Have the neuroprotective effects of this unique cation been overlooked? *Biol. Psychiatry* 1999;**46**(7):929–940.
268. Turecki G, Grof P, Cavazzoni P, Duffy A, Grof E, Ahrens B, Berghofer A, Muller-Oerlinghausen B, Dvorakova M, Libigerova E, Vojtechovsky M, Zvolsky P, et al. Evidence for a role of phospholipase C-gamma1 in the pathogenesis of bipolar disorder. *Mol. Psychiatry* 1998;**3**(6):534–538.

269. Lovlie R, Berle JO, Stordal E, Steen VM. The phospholipase C-gamma1 gene (PLCG1) and lithium-responsive bipolar disorder: Re-examination of an intronic dinucleotide repeat polymorphism. *Psychiatr. Genet.* 2001;**11**(1):41–43.

270. Steen VM, Lovlie R, Osher Y, Belmaker RH, Berle JO, Gulbrandsen AK. The polymorphic inositol polyphosphate 1-phosphatase gene as a candidate for pharmacogenetic prediction of lithium-responsive manic-depressive illness. *Pharmacogenetics* 1998;**8**(3):259–268.

271. Alda M, Turecki G, Grof P, Cavazzoni P, Duffy A, Grof E, Ahrens B, Berghofer A, Muller-Oerlinghausen B, Dvorakova M, Libigerova E, Vojtechovsky M, et al. Association and linkage studies of CRH and PENK genes in bipolar disorder: A collaborative IGSLI study. *Am. J. Med. Genet.* 2000;**96**(2):178–181.

272. Turecki G, Alda M, Grof P, Joober R, Lafreniere R, Cavazzoni P, Duffy A, Grof E, Ahrens B, Berghofer A, Muller-Oerlinghausen B, Dvorakova M, Libigerova E, et al. Polyglutamine coding genes in bipolar disorder: Lack of association with selected candidate loci. *J. Affect. Disord.* 2000;**58**(1):63–68.

273. Ftouhi-Paquin N, Alda M, Grof P, Chretien N, Rouleau G, Turecki G. Identification of three polymorphisms in the translated region of PLC-gamma1 and their investigation in lithium responsive bipolar disorder. *Am. J. Med. Genet.* 2001;**105**(3):301–305.

274. Turecki G, Alda M, Grof P, Martin R, Cavazzoni PA, Duffy A, Maciel P, Rouleau GA. No association between chromosome-18 markers and lithium-responsive affective disorders. *Psychiatry Res.* 1996;**63**(1):17–23.

275. Washizuka S, Ikeda A, Kato N, Kato T. Possible relationship between mitochondrial DNA polymorphisms and lithium response in bipolar disorder. *Int. J. Neuropsychopharmacol.* 2003;**6**(4):421–424.

276. Masui T, Hashimoto R, Kusumi I, Suzuki K, Tanaka T, Nakagawa S, Suzuki T, Iwata N, Ozaki N, Kato T, Takeda M, Kunugi H, Koyama T. A possible association between missense polymorphism of the breakpoint cluster region gene and lithium prophylaxis in bipolar disorder. *Prog. Neuropsychopharmacol. Biol. Psychiatry* 2008;**32**(1):204–208.

277. Jope RS, Bijur GN. Mood stabilizers, glycogen synthase kinase-3beta and cell survival. *Mol. Psychiatry* 2002;**7** (Suppl 1): S35–S45.

278. Benedetti F, Serretti A, Pontiggia A, Bernasconi A, Lorenzi C, Colombo C, Smeraldi E. Long-term response to lithium salts in bipolar illness is influenced by the glycogen synthase kinase 3-beta −50T/C SNP. *Neurosci. Lett.* 2005;**376**(1):51–55.

279. Mamdani F, Alda M, Grof P, Young LT, Rouleau G, Turecki G. Lithium response and genetic variation in the CREB family of genes. *Am. J. Med. Genet. B Neuropsychiatr. Genet.* 2008;**147B**(4):500–504.

280. Wolff K, Tsapakis EM, Pariante CM, Holt D, Winstock AR, Kerwin RW, Forsling ML, Aitchison KJ. Pharmacogenetic studies of change in cortisol on ecstasy (MDMA) consumption. *J. Psychopharmacol.* 2011, epub Oct 3.

281. Trzepacz PT, Williams DW, Feldman PD, Wrishko RE, Witcher JW, Buitelaar JK. CYP2D6 metabolizer status and atomoxetine dosing in children and adolescents with ADHD. *Eur Neuropsychopharmacol.* 2008;**18**(2):79–86.

282. Korszun A, Owen M, Craddock N, Jones L, Jones I, Gray J, Williamson R, McGuffin P. Medical disorders in people with recurrent depression Br. *J. Psychiatry* 2008;**192**:351–355.

CHAPTER 8

Pharmacogenetics in Cancer

SHARON MARSH
University of Alberta, Edmonton, Alberta, Canada

8.1 INTRODUCTION

For many cancer types there are multiple possible treatment options. Selection of the most appropriate therapy would benefit from guidelines to allow for successful therapy to be initiated at the earliest possible stage. Failed treatment or unacceptable toxicity leading to a change of medication or dose can significantly reduce the optimal therapeutic window. Pharmacogenomics can be a useful tool in the selection of appropriate therapy based on individual variability in chemotherapy pathway genes [1].

Many technologies are now marketed for pharmacogenomics in either the research or clinical setting [2–4], and more recently the US FDA has approved genetic tests and altered package label inserts for chemotherapy medications on the basis of pharmacogenomics studies (Table 8.1). Although still in its infancy, the translation of pharmacogenomics into oncology clinical practice is now underway.

Oncology offers its own set of challenges for pharmacogenomics research. In addition to the typical genetic variability seen in the germline genome (single–nucleotide polymorphisms (SNPs), tandem repeats (VNTRs), insertions/deletions (INDELS), etc), the tumor genome can often be quite distinct [5]. Studies have shown a good concordance between the presence of polymorphisms in paired tumor and germline samples [6–8]; however, this does not take into account other sources of variability affecting the tumor genome, including somatic mutations, microsatellite instability, loss of heterozygosity, gross chromosomal rearrangements (e.g., translocations), amplification or deletion, and epigenetic factors such as methylation. Markers for toxicity (in particular markers in pharmacokinetic genes) are more likely to be linked to germline DNA variation. However, tumor markers in pharmacodynamic genes may be more relevant for outcome prediction [9].

Pharmacogenetics and Individualized Therapy, First Edition.
Edited by Anke-Hilse Maitland-van der Zee and Ann K. Daly.

TABLE 8.1 Approved FDA Tests for Personalised Cancer Treatment

Drug	Biomarker	Test Status (US FDA)	Test Type
Cetuximab	EGFR expression	Required	Immunohistochemistry
Trastuzumab	ERBB2 over-expression	Required	Immunohistochemistry or fluorescence in situ hybridization (FISH)
Azathioprine	TPMT variants	Recommended	Genotype
Irinotecan	UGT1A1 variants	Recommended	Genotype
Tamoxifen	CYP2D6 variants	Pending	Genotype

[a]Approved at time of publication of this volume.

8.2 PERSONALIZED THERAPY

The use of monocolonal antibodies for targeted therapy in oncology is gaining momentum. In these situations the target would typically be screened for in advance of therapy selection, as the therapies will work only if the target is present. In some cases, for example, trastuzumab, the target needs to be over expressed for the therapy to have a significant effect on outcome.

8.2.1 Cetuximab

Cetuximab is a monoclonal antibody that specifically targets the epidermal growth factor receptor (EGFR) [10]. It is approved for therapy in EGFR-expressing metastatic colorectal cancer that has failed to respond to previous irinotecan-based therapy [11]. EGFR expression is typically determined using immunohistochemistry (Table 8.1).

8.2.2 Trastuzumab

Overexpression of ERBB2 (Her 2/neu) occurs in approximately 30% of breast cancer cases and is consistently associated with reduced survival [12–14]. Trastuzumab (Herceptin) is a monoclonal antibody, which was developed as a targeted therapy for breast cancer patients overexpressing the gene product Her2/neu through amplification or overexpression of the gene ERBB2 [15,16]. Trastuzumab was approved for use in 1998 [12–14] and represents one of the earliest FDA approved treatments involving screening markers for personalized therapy selection (Table 8.1).

8.2.2.1 ERBB2

Amplification of ERBB2 can be identified clinically using fluorescence *in situ* hybridization (FISH), and overexpression is assessed by immunohistochemistry [13,17]. Further assessment of serum Her2/neu levels may improve patient selection [18]. Early-stage or metastatic breast cancer patients with ERBB2 amplification/overexpression are selected for trastuzumab therapy and also receive standard chemotherapy. In addition, trastuzumab monotherapy is used in patients with ERBB2 overexpressing metastatic breast cancer who have previously received chemotherapy. There is overwhelming evidence to support the use of trastuzumab in ERBB2 amplified/overexpressed breast cancer [13]. In a large study of early-stage breast cancer patients with amplified/overexpressed ERBB2 (combined trial data consisting of 3351 patients), patients had significantly improved overall survival and disease-free survival after 4 years of treatment (paclitaxel with trastuzumab) compared to paclitaxel alone [19]. This and other studies have demonstrated the effectiveness of trastuzumab therapy [13].

Despite the success of trastuzumab, overall or progression-free survival is still not 100% in patients overexpressing ERBB2, according to immunohistochemistry or FISH data [20]. An analysis of four trastuzumab trials in metastatic breast cancer suggests that measuring serum levels of the extracellular domain of the Her2 protein using enzyme-linked immunoadsorbent (ELISA) may also be an important diagnostic tool [21]. In addition, there are factors beyond ERBB2 overexpression that can also influence response to trastuzumab. For example, germline ERBB2 polymorphisms and acquired mutations in tumor ERBB2 could impact gene expression or activity [22]. Additional therapeutic strategies may also help to overcome trastuzumab resistance in some patients [20].

8.3 PHARMACOGENOMIC MARKERS

There is a growing list of examples of genetic tests approved by the US FDA that could impact response to cancer therapy (Table 8.1). Currently (as of 2011) these tests are not required prior to therapy, but recommendations for screening can be found in the package inserts for the relevant medications.

8.3.1 6-Mercaptopurine

6-Mercaptopurine is a commonly used oral medication for childhood acute lymphocytic leukemia (ALL). Typically patients receive the therapy daily for 2–3 years. 6-Mercaptopurine exerts its activity by incorporating thioguanine nucleotides into DNA. 6-Mercaptopurine is also methylated to form methylmercaptopurine via thiopurine methyltransferase (TPMT) and oxidized to thioruic acid by xanthine oxidase (XDH). Underexpression of TPMT leads to increased accumulation of thioguanine nucleotides. This can cause intolerance to mercaptopurine and lead to severe, life-threatening hematopoietic toxicities [23,24]. In addition to variation in the TPMT gene, polymorphisms in other members of the 6-mercaptopurine pathway can also play a role. The gene encoding inosine triphosphate pyrophospatase (ITPA) has been associated with toxicity [25]. ITPA deficiency leads to a lack of inosine monophosphate (IMP) [26]. The lack of IMP leads to an accumulation of the metabolite 6-thio-ITP following 6-mercaptopurine therapy, potentially leading to toxicity [27].

8.3.1.1 Thiopurine Methyltransferase (TPMT)

Activity of TPMT is reduced in patients carrying single nucleotide polymorphisms (SNPs) in the coding region of the gene. Approximately 10% of patients have an intermediate enzyme activity, and 0.3% are deficient for TPMT activity [28]. Patients with intermediate TPMT activity have a greater incidence of thiopurine toxicity, whereas TPMT–deficient patients have severe or fatal toxicity from 6-mercaptopurine therapy. Reduction of starting dose is essential in patients with reduced 6-mercaptopurine activity to avoid toxicity [29].

Several genetic variants in the TPMT gene have been associated with low TPMT enzyme activity [24]. Three of these variants (TPMT*2, TPMT*3A, and TPMT*3C) account for up to 95% of low TPMT activity phenotypes [24]. Patients heterozygous for these alleles have intermediate TPMT levels and tolerate approximately 65% of the standard mercaptopurine dose [30]. Patients homozygous for the variant TPMT alleles are at high risk for severe, potentially life-threatening toxicity, requiring significant reductions in drug doses (1/10–1/15th of the standard dose). Reducing dose in TPMT–deficient individuals does not affect outcome. Patients receiving dose reduction because of the presence of variant TPMT alleles have similar or superior survival compared to patients homozygous for the wild-type TPMT allele [30].

The TPMT*2 variant leads to an amino acid substitution (A80P), causing a cleft in the protein. TPMT*3A is a combination of two variants leading to amino acid substitutions (A154T and Y240C). A154T is in the cosubstrate binding site, and the Y240C allele causes the loss of protein side-chain contacts. The combination of A154T and Y240C in TPMT*3A causes a distorted protein structure [31]. TPMT*3C contains the Y240C substitution but not the A154T variant.

In Caucasian populations, TPMT*3A is the most common allele, with a frequency of 3.2–5.7%. TPMT*2 and TPMT*3C alleles are present in 0.2–0.8% of Caucasians. Significant variation in TPMT allele frequencies is seen among different world populations. TPMT*3A is the only variation found in Southwest Asians (1%), whereas TPMT*3 is the predominant allele in African populations (5.4–7.6%) [24]. Although the commonly studied variants TPMT*2, *3A, and *3C are convincingly associated with azathioprine toxicity, other variants are prevalent in non-Caucasian populations. For example, in sub-Saharan African populations, TPMT*8 accounts for the majority of nonfunctional alleles [32], but this would not be routinely screened for as it is uncommon in other populations.

In 118 children with ALL, TPMT genotype correlated with TPMT activity only before the initiation of 6-mercaptopurine treatment [33]. Consequently, prescreening patients prior to therapy is the most appropriate way to determine the likelihood of hematological toxicity. Although currently not a requirement for prescribing 6-mercaptopurine, pretreatment knowledge of a patient's TPMT genotype status is recommended by the US FDA (Table 8.1) and is often screened in major centers for dose optimization in order to prospectively reduce the likelihood of toxicity in children with ALL [34].

8.3.1.2 TPMT Copy Number

Gain of chromosomes can occur in leukemia cells. Gain of chromosome 6 (containing the TPMT gene) was shown in a study of 147 children with ALL. There was no bias for the chromosome 6 (maternal or paternal chromosome) that was amplified. In patients where a chromosome 6 containing a variant TPMT allele was amplified, leading to multiple copies of the variant allele, a significant decrease in TPMT activity was seen [35]. Currently, there are no tests for screening the tumor genome prior to 6-mercaptopurine dosing. However, screening germline DNA alone will miss the increase in variant allele copy number and lead to underestimation of TPMT activity, meaning that the starting 6-mercaptopurine dose would not be appropriately reduced.

8.3.1.3 ITPA

The gene for inosine triphosphate pyrophospatase (ITPA) has been associated with 6-mercaptopurine toxicity. A coding variant, ITPA 94C > A, is predicted to cause ITPA deficiency [26] and is present at a frequency of 1–19% in different populations. In Caucasians the minor allele frequency is approximately 7%.

Studies revealed TPMT genotype to be more important than ITPA P32T in childhood ALL patients for predicting toxicity only in patients not prestratified for 6-mercaptopurine dosing on the basis of the TPMT genotype. However, in childhood ALL patients whose 6-mercaptopurine dose was regulated on the basis of the TPMT genotype, the ITPA P32T allele was significantly associated with the incidence of febrile neutropenia [25]. In other words, the ITPA P32T polymorphism identified patients still likely to suffer 6-mercaptopurine–induced toxicity even after selection for the common toxicity-related TPMT polymorphisms.

If ITPA is validated as a marker for toxicity from mercaptopurine, variants will need to be screened in conjunction with TPMT polymorphisms and TPMT gene amplification to better determine the likelihood of toxicity prior to therapy selection [36]. This would be particularly relevant in populations where the frequency of TPMT variants is low, as these populations tend to have a correspondingly high frequency of ITPA P32T. For example, Asian patients, who have a low incidence of the common TPMT variants, may be more susceptible to toxicity from mercaptopurine on the basis of the ITPA P32T allele, whereas Hispanic patients have low ITPA P32T frequency but have some of the highest common TPMT allele frequencies, suggesting that TPMT is of greater importance for predicting 6-mercaptopurine toxicity in these populations [36].

8.3.2 5-Fluorouracil (5FU)

5-Fluorouracil (5FU) was developed as a chemotherapy drug in the 1950s [37] following the discovery that uracil is preferentially taken up by cancer cells. It is still one of most commonly used treatments (in combination with irinotecan or oxaliplatin) for colorectal cancer. However, some patients experience potentially life-threatening toxicities from 5FU treatment, including severe gastrointestinal toxicities and neutropenia [38]. 5FU is inactivated via metabolism by dihydropyrimidine dehydrogenase, and its main target of action is to block the conversion of dUMP to dTMP by forming a stable ternary complex with the metabolite FdUMP, thymidylate synthase, and a methyl cofactor.

8.3.2.1 Dihydropyrimidine Dehydrogenase (DPYD)

Dihydropyrimidine dehydrogenase (DPD) is encoded for by the gene DPYD [39] and is responsible for the degradation of over 80% of all 5-fluorouracil. As the starting dose typically accounts for this level of degradation, individuals with decreased DPD activity have a greater than 4-fold risk of life-threatening toxicity from standard doses of 5FU [40].

Over 30 polymorphisms in the gene encoding DPD (DPYD) have been described to date [41–43]. The most frequently studied DPYD polymorphism, DPYD∗2A, is a G → A transition located in an intron/exon splice junction. This results in exon 14 being skipped and absent from the DPD protein [41]. Patients heterozygous for this polymorphism have low DPD activity and typically experience severe, life-threatening toxicity from 5FU therapy [40,41]. Although commonly screened for in patients who have experienced 5FU toxicity, the incidence of DPYD∗2A in the general population is very low (< 1%) [44]. In addition, a prospective study of 683 cancer patients treated with 5FU identified that the sensitivity of DPYD∗2A predicting 5FU toxicity was low (5.5% for overall toxicity) [45]. Consequently, it has become apparent DPYD∗2A is not the sole cause of 5FU toxicity, or the only variant responsible for DPD deficiency.

Although it is a marker for toxicity, DPYD∗2A is too rare to justify screening for it alone in every patient prior to the selection of 5FU at this time. Other more frequently occurring DPYD polymorphisms may also have an impact on 5FU toxicity. For example, there is an association between DPYD∗5 and moderate to severe 5FU toxicity in gastro intestinal (GI) and colon cancer patients [46].

Variability in the frequencies of DPYD polymorphisms is seen between different world populations [44,47], as well as differences in haplotype structure for the commonly studied polymorphisms [44]. The relative contribution of the multiple polymorphisms in DPYD remains to be assessed, and it is likely that a combination of polymorphisms or a functional haplotype for DPYD would need to be screened in patients to predict the incidence of 5FU toxicity. Finally, other genes in the degradation pathway, specifically UPB1 and DPYS, could also play a role in the predisposition of patients to toxicity from 5FU therapy [48–50]. These genes have, to date, not been comprehensively assessed in a pharmacogenomics context.

8.3.2.2 DPYD Methylation

Epigenetic silencing of transcription via aberrant methylation in tumor cells can lead to reduced or absent gene expression. The methylation status of pharmacogenomically relevant genes in tumors could influence drug response [51]. It has been shown that various CpG loci (methylation sites) around the transcription start site of DPYD are abnormally methylated in cells with low expression of the DPD enzyme. Reversal of this methylation decreased sensitivity to 5FU in cultured cells [52], suggesting methylation status as a possible pharmacogenomic marker. A positive association between DPD deficiency and DPYD promoter hypermethylation was also seen, suggesting the possibility of using methylation of the DPYD promoter as an alternative mechanism for DPD deficiency in cancer patients [53]. As with many potential markers, however, a contradictory study showed that DPD RNA expression did not differ between DPYD methylated and unmethylated tumors [54,55]. It is possible that the effect of DPYD promoter methylation on DPD activity can be tissue-specific, and more work needs to be done to clarify the use of DPYD methylation as a marker for DPD deficiency and 5FU toxicity.

8.3.2.3 Thymidylate Synthase (TYMS)

Thymidylate synthase (TYMS), along with the cofactor 5,10-methylenetetrahydrofolate, catalyzes the conversion of dUMP to dTMP. This is the sole *de novo* source of thymidine in the cell. The 5FU metabolite, FdUMP, inhibits this conversion, leading to a depletion of thymidine in the cell and consequently inhibiting DNA synthesis. Overexpression of TYMS, leading to an excess of TYMS protein, has been linked to resistance to 5FU [56,57]. To date, three common polymorphisms in the TYMS gene have been identified [58].

The most commonly studied TYMS variant is a 28-bp polymorphic repeat in the promoter enhancer region of the 5′ untranslated region (5′UTR). This polymorphism consists of varying numbers of repeats (2, 3, 4, 5 and 9 copies have been identified so far) and is typically denoted TSER [59–61]. Studies have suggested that an increased number of repeats increases TYMS RNA and protein expression [58,59,62,63]. The frequency of the TYMS TSER alleles among different ethnic groups shows an interesting pattern. Caucasian and African populations have similar frequencies of the TSER∗3 (3 repeats) allele (49–54%) [60,64,65]; however, Asian populations have significantly higher frequency of TSER∗3 (62–95%) [61,64,66]. TSER∗2 (2 repeats) makes up the majority of the other alleles. The TSER∗4 (4 repeats) alleles are found mainly in African populations at low frequency (1–7%) [60,65]; TSER∗5 (5 repeats) has been identified in Chinese populations ($\leq 4\%$) [61] and TSER∗9 (9 repeats) alleles have been identified only in a population from Ghana (1%), although many African populations remain unstudied for this polymorphism [60]. The effect on expression of the 4, 5, and 9 repeats remains unknown.

The clinical impact of the TYMS TSER polymorphism has been assessed in multiple studies [58]. Associations with outcome to 5FU therapy have been identified. In 117 patients receiving 5FU adjuvant therapy compared to 104 patients receiving surgery alone, no significant benefit of chemotherapy on survival was observed for homozygous TSER∗3 patients. Improved survival was seen in patients receiving 5FU compared with surgery alone for patients with at least one TSER∗2 allele [67]. In a pivotal study the TYMS TSER was also linked to tumor downstaging in 65 rectal cancer patients treated preoperatively with 5FU and radiation [68]. Patients with at least one TSER∗2 allele had a significantly increased frequency of tumor downstaging compared to patients homozygous for TSER∗3 [68]. This and similar studies led to the development of a genotype-guided clinical cancer trial [69].

Rectal cancer patients with at least one TSER∗2 allele were treated with standard therapy (radiation and 5FU), and patients homozygous for TSER∗3 received the standard therapy in combination with irinotecan [68]. Preliminary data were promising for both treatment strategies based on genotype [69], suggesting that treating rectal cancer patients with respect to genotype might improve response.

Not all studies show associations with TSER and 5FU outcome. For example, in a study of 135 Japanese colorectal cancer patients there was no association between TSER genotype and efficacy of oral 5FU chemotherapy [70]. In addition, even in studies with positive correlations, not all patients with the TSER∗2 allele respond to 5FU, and not all patients with TSER∗3 alleles fail 5FU therapy. Some of these discrepancies may be explained by the presence of a SNP located within the TYMS TSER [71]. This is an unusual variant in that the SNP lies in the 12th nucleotide of the second repeat of the TSER∗3 allele (often denoted TSER∗3G > A), and is consequently seen only in patients with at least one TSER∗3 allele. Subsequently a further polymorphism in the TSER∗2 allele has also been described, however, the function is currently unknown [72,73]. The TSER∗3G > C polymorphism disrupts a USF1 transcription factor binding site [71], leading to significantly higher RNA expression [63]. Consequently, it is possible that this SNP will allow TSER∗3 carriers to be further stratified into categories of high and low TYMS expression. Clinical data on the significance of this SNP are conflicting. In 89 metastatic colorectal cancer patients receiving 5FU, patients without any TSER∗3G alleles had improved overall response [74]; however, in 129 colorectal cancer patients treated with 5FU the TSER∗3G > C SNP did not improve prognosis beyond that associated with the TSER polymorphism [75].

The third commonly studied polymorphism in the TYMS gene is a 6-bp deletion located in the 3′-untranslated region, 447 bp downstream from the stop codon (commonly denoted TYMSdel) [76] and is significantly associated with red blood cell folate levels and homocysteine concentrations [77]. This deletion causes the expression of approximately 3-fold less TYMS RNA than patients homozygous for the presence of the 6 bp [78]. It is possible that the deletion allele exerts its effect by altering TYMS RNA stability in the cell. The deletion allele is found in 27–29% of Caucasians [76,78]. Once again, clinical data are conflicting. Two studies of patients receiving 5FU therapy have found positive associations with outcome and the deletion allele [75,79], reinforcing the theory that the deletion leads to reduced TYMS expression. However, a study of patients receiving capecitabine (an oral 5FU prodrug) and raltitrexed found a significant association between the deletion allele and poor response to therapy [80].

Assessing the combination of the three common TYMS polymorphisms using haplotype analysis may be more informative than assessing each variant individually. A significantly higher risk for tumor recurrence was seen in colorectal cancer patients who had received 5Fu containing therapy who were also TSER∗3, or TSER∗3G and did not have the TYMSdel allele [81]. Although there is compelling evidence to suggest the involvement of TYMS polymorphisms, in particular the TSER, with response to 5FU therapy, more studies are required to clarify the extent of the relationship between polymorphism(s) and outcome.

8.3.2.4 *TYMS in Tumor Cells*

Along with TYMS polymorphisms identified in germline DNA, TYMS expression in the tumor genome also needs to be taken into account. TYMS amplification has been shown *in vitro* and *in vivo* to influence resistance to 5FU [82,83]. *TYMS* gene amplification was seen in the tumor cells of 23% of 31 patients treated with 5FU, whereas no amplification was observed in metastases of patients who had not been treated with 5FU. Patients with metastases containing TYMS amplification had a significantly worse median survival than those without amplification [82]. Conversely, loss of the TYMS-containing region of chromosome 18p is common in colorectal cancer [84]. A study of TYMS gene copy number in 52 untreated colorectal tumor samples has shown that 27% of the tumors had a deletion of TYMS, which would be predicted to be a beneficial deletion for patients receiving 5FU [85].

Clearly, the absence of TYMS in the tumor, or the presence of multiple gene copies, will affect response to 5FU irrespective of germline polymorphisms, whereas the presence of germline polymorphisms could enhance the deleterious effect of TYMS amplification in the tumor. Consequently, a comprehensive profile of TYMS in both tumor and germline DNA from each patient is ultimately needed to better predict response to 5FU therapy.

8.3.3 Irinotecan

Irinotecan is typically used in combination with 5-fluorouracil or oxaliplatin for colorectal cancer and other solid tumors. The active form of irinotecan, SN38, is inactivated through glucuronidation by a member of the UDP-glucuronosyltransferase family, UGT1A1. The UGT1A1 enzyme is responsible for hepatic bilirubin glucuronidation and is the main UGT1A enzyme involved in the glucuronidation of SN38. Underexpression of UGT1A1 leads to excess SN38 in the cell, causing severe, life-threatening diarrhea and/or neutropenia [86].

8.3.3.1 *UGT1A1*

Expression of UGT1A1 is altered by a polymorphism in the TATA box of the gene promoter [87]. This polymorphism is a dinucleotide TA repeat, $(TA)_nTAA$, and the number of repeats ranges from 5 to 8 copies. $(TA)_6TAA$ represents the most common allele (considered wild-type for UGT1A1 expression), and $(TA)_7TAA$ (UGT1A1∗28) is the most common variant allele (leading to reduced UGT1A1 expression) [88]. UGT1A1∗28 is present at a frequency of between 15% (Asians) and 30% (Caucasians) of the general population [88]. Reduced UGT1A1 expression is linked to an increased risk of severe toxicity (diarrhea and neutropenia) from irinotecan [89]. Several studies have shown a link between UGT1A1∗28 and irinotecan toxicity [86]. In a definitive prospective study of 66 patients with advanced disease treated with irinotecan, patients homozygous for UGT1A1∗28 had a significantly higher risk of toxicity (grade IV neutropenia) compared to heterozygous or homozygous wild-type patients [89]. Based on the wealth of information showing a link between UGT1A1∗28 and irinotecan toxicity, the US FDA approved a genotype test for UGT1A1∗28 [90,91] and included toxicity and dosing warnings relating to the UGT1A1*28 allele in the irinotecan package insert [91] (Table 8.1).

One of the current problems with altering package inserts to reflect pharmacogenomics data is that there is often little or no information available to suggest what the appropriate starting dose would be for patients carrying the variant alleles. In addition, for UGT1A1 and irinotecan, work conducted subsequent to the package insert change suggests that the relationship between UGT1A1*28 and irinotecan toxicity may be dependent on the irinotecan regimen used. At low doses (50–180 mg/m^2) the relationship between UGT1A1*28 genotype and toxicity was not clinically significant, whereas at moderate to high doses (200–350 mg/m^2) the risk of severe hematological toxicity in patients homozygous for UGT1A1*28 was 27.8 times higher than for patients heterozygous or homozygous for wild-type UGT1A1 [92]. Consequently, further amendments to the irinotecan package insert may be required in the future.

In addition to dosing criteria, in populations with a low frequency of UGT1A1*28, for example, Asian populations [93], other genetic variants within UGT1A1 may also play a role in irinotecan toxicity [86,89,94,95]. For example, an intron 1 polymorphism, UGT1A1*6 (G71R), which is rarely seen in Caucasians but found in Asians at approximately 10% frequency is associated with altered irinotecan pharmacokinetics and toxicity from irinotecan therapy [94,95].

8.3.3.2 UGT1A1 Methylation

Variation in expression of UGT1A1 could also be linked to methylation status of the gene promoter in tumor cells. A study of cancer cell lines has shown UGT1A1 expression to be increased in cell lines with UGT1A1 promoter hypomethylation, and decreased in cell lines with UGT1A1 promoter hypermethylation. Direct methylation of the UGT1A1 promoter in cell lines resulted in the complete repression of transcriptional activity. Loss of UGT1A1 methylation was also associated with an increase in UGT1A1 protein levels and with an enhanced inactivation of SN38 in a cancer cell line [96]. Although this study has not yet been validated *in vivo*, it represents an important mechanism of control of UGT1A1 expression, and is another indicator that the tumor genome can provide important markers for treatment response.

8.3.3.3 Other Genes Implicated in Irinotecan Toxicity

Several studies have suggested that polymorphisms in other metabolism and transport genes may also play a role in irinotecan pharmacokinetics and toxicity [86,97–99]. Genetic variants in other members of the UGT1A gene family, specifically UGT1A7 and UGT1A9, are associated with irinotecan toxicities [100,101]. In addition, a haplotype in the multidrug transporter ABCC2 predicts toxicity in patients without UGT1A1*28 [99], and variants in the transporter ABCC1 impact the variability in SN38 pharmacokinetics [102].

Pharmacodynamic irinotecan genes have not been well characterized, but one study suggests that neutropenia from irinotecan is associated with topoisomerase I (TOP1) genetic variants [97].

8.3.4 Tamoxifen

Tamoxifen is used for the advanced and adjuvant treatment of breast cancer and has been the mainstay of breast cancer therapy for over 20 years [103]. Acquired resistance is a major problem, and side effects from tamoxifen include hot flushes, thromboembolic events, secondary endometrial cancer, endometrial polyps, irregular menses, and ovarian cysts [103]. Tamoxifen is catalyzed into the active form 4-hydroxytamoxifen (4-OH TAM) by the metabolizing enzyme CYP2D6. In addition CYP2D6 also converts the metabolite *N*-desmethyltamoxifen to 4-hydroxy-*N*-desmethyltamoxifen (endoxifen) [104].

8.3.4.1 CYP2D6

The CYP2D6 gene is responsible for the metabolism of a wide range of medications and has consequently been well characterized in the field of pharmacogenomics (see Chapter 3). There are multiple functional polymorphisms, ranging from SNPs to whole-gene amplification or deletion [105]. These polymorphisms have a range of effects that correspond to poor, intermediate, extensive, and ultrarapid metabolism. The wild-type (normal) CYP2D6 gene corresponds to the extensive metabolism classification [106]. Variations in CYP2D6, particularly those leading to a lack of or reduced CYP2D6 function (poor or intermediate metabolism), have been associated with tamoxifen outcome in breast cancer patients.

In 80 breast cancer patients CYP2D6∗4 (loss of CYP2D6 function) carriers had significantly lower endoxifen levels than did patients with wild-type CYP2D6 [107]. In 223 estrogen-receptor-positive patients receiving tamoxifen, patients homozygous for CYP2D6∗4 experienced significantly poorer survival than patients with at least one wild-type CYP2D6 allele [108]. CYP2D6∗4 is present at a frequency of approximately 21% Caucasian populations; however, it is less common in other populations where other CYP2D6 polymorphisms may play a more important role [106]. For example, a reduced-function variant, CYP2D6∗10, has been identified in Asian breast cancer patients to be associated with tamoxifen response [109,110].

In October 2006 an advisory committee for the US FDA recommended an update to the tamoxifen package insert to include CYP2D6 pharmacogenomic information [111]. The US FDA has also approved an AmpliChip CYP450 test through Roche that screens multiple CYP2D6 variants (33 alleles, including ∗4 and ∗10) [112].

8.3.4.2 Other Genes Implicated in Tamoxifen Outcome

The CYP2D6 gene is not the only marker for outcome to tamoxifen therapy. Metabolites of tamoxifen are conjugated via SULT1A1 leading to excretion by sulfurylation, and are also subjected to glucurondation, via UGT2B15 [113].

Studies have revealed a correlation between SULT1A1∗2 (R213H) and decreased 4-OH TAM sulfation and survival in breast cancer patients [114,115]. In addition, a nonsynonymous polymorphism in UGT2B15 (UGT2B15∗2; D85Y) was assessed in 165 tamoxifen-receiving breast cancer patients. When present in patients with SULT1A1∗2 alleles, patients carrying at least one UGT2B15∗2 allele had significantly reduced 5-year survival rates [114].

8.3.5 Taxanes

For some oncology treatments there are no clear DNA-based markers for pharmacogenomic therapy selection. For example, for the taxanes, paclitaxel and docetaxel, commonly used in the treatment of several solid tumors, there are limited data on putative pharmacogenomic markers despite being assessed in multiple studies [116–120]. To date (as of 2011) no putative association has been validated in subsequent studies [116–120].

One marker that shows early promise is CYP1B1∗3 [121]. This was shown to be significantly associated with progression-free survival in breast cancer patients receiving very high-dose combination chemotherapy (including paclitaxel) [122]. In addition, a further study in prostate cancer found an association between CYP1B1∗3 and survival in patients treated with docetaxel [123]. This finding was not reproduced in a large ovarian cancer study [118], however, it is possible that the effect is tumor-site-dependent.

8.3.5.1 Expression

For treatments where conclusive DNA markers cannot be identified, other sources of biomarkers may be more useful. Expression profiles, of either individual genes or panels of genes, can provide a method of predicting tumor response.

For taxanes, overexpression of class III β–tubulin (the target for taxanes) has been shown *in vitro* and *in vivo* to predict response to ovarian tumors following taxane treatment [124]. DNA variants in β–tubulin have yet to be validated as a predictor of taxane response [116]; consequently, measuring expression would be an alternative solution.

Some studies have identified panels of genes that can be used to predict taxane response in breast cancer, for example, the commercially available oncotype Dx panel [125–127]. This is a 21-gene panel consisting of 5 reference genes (ACTB, GAPDH, GUS, RPLPO, and TFRC) and 16 cancer-related genes (AURKA, BAG1, BCL2, BIRC5, CCNB1, CD68, CTSL2, ERBB2, ESR1, GRB7, GSTM1, MKI67, MMP11, MYBL2, PGR, and SCUBE2) [127].

8.4 CONCLUSIONS

With the exception of EGFR and ERBB2, where identification of the marker is required for the relevant therapy to be administered, one of the major problems with integrating pharmacogenomics into clinical practice is how to interpret the data. For example, there is presently no indication of how to select the appropriate irinotecan dose according to the UGT1A1∗28 status of the patient. Consequently, in the near future studies including genotype-directed clinical trials will be essential to elucidate the role of pharmacogenomics in individualizing therapy. In addition, for chemotherapeutics where there are no known validated markers, studies involving gene/SNP detection strategies will be essential to identify new potential markers [128,129].

Another factor to take into account is the variability in allele frequencies, and also variability in the relevant functional allele between different populations. A more global approach to pharmacogenomics is required to ensure that marker selection is relevant to all countries [130,131].

Despite these challenges, pharmacogenomics has made significant progress since 2000, and for many chemotherapeutics it should be possible to screen for clinically relevant biomarkers to aid therapy selection in the not too distant future.

REFERENCES

1. Evans WE, McLeod HL. Pharmacogenomics—drug disposition, drug targets, and side effects. *New Engl. J. Med.* 2003;**348**:538–49.
2. Freimuth RR, Ameyaw M-M, Pritchard SC, et al. High-throughput genotyping methods for pharmacogenomic studies. *Curr. Pharmacogenomics* 2004;**2**:21–33.
3. Syvanen AC. Toward genome-wide SNP genotyping. *Nat, Genet.* 2005;**37S**:S5–S10.
4. Kim S, Misra A. SNP genotyping: Technologies and biomedical applications. *Annu. Rev. Biomed. Eng.* 2007;**9**:289–320.
5. Marsh S. Pharmacogenomics. *Ann. Oncol.* 2007;**18** (Suppl. 9): 24–28.
6. Marsh S, Mallon MA, Goodfellow P, et al. Concordance of pharmacogenetic markers in germline and colorectal tumor DNA. *Pharmacogenomics* 2005;**6**:873–877.
7. Marsh S. Concordance between tumor and germline DNA. In Innocenti F, ed.: *Genomics and Pharmacogenomics in Anticancer Drug Development and Clinical Response*. Ed.; Totowa, NJ: Humana Press, 2008, pp. 91–101.
8. McWhinney SR, Mcleod HL. Using germline genotype in cancer pharmacogenetic studies. *Pharmacogenomics* 2009;**10**:489–493.
9. Hoskins JM, Mcleod HL. The move from pharmacokinetics to pharmacodynamics. *Curr. Pharmacogenomics* 2006;**4**:39–46.
10. Labianca R, La Verde N, Garassino MC. Development and clinical indications of cetuximab. *Int. J. Biol. Markers* 2007;**22**:S40–S46.
11. Wong SF. Cetuximab: An epidermal growth factor receptor monoclonal antibody for the treatment of colorectal cancer. *Clin. Ther.* 2005;**27**:684–694.
12. Plosker GL, Keam SJ. Spotlight on Trastuzumab in the management of HER2-positive metastatic and early-stage breast cancer. *BioDrugs* 2006;**20**:259–262.
13. Plosker GL, Keam SJ. Trastuzumab: A review of its use in the management of HER2-positive metastatic and early-stage breast cancer. *Drugs* 2006;**66**: 449–475.
14. Ross JS, Slodkowska EA, Symmans WF, et al. The HER-2 receptor and breast cancer: Ten years of targeted anti-HER-2 therapy and personalized medicine. *Oncologist* 2009;**14**:320–368.
15. Bange J, Zwick E, Ullrich A. Molecular targets for breast cancer therapy and prevention. *Nat. Med.* 2001;**7**:548–552.
16. Engel RH, Kaklamani VG. HER2-positive breast cancer: Current and future treatment strategies. *Drugs* 2007;**67**:1329–1341.

17. Kim MA, Jung EJ, Lee HS, et al. Evaluation of HER-2 gene status in gastric carcinoma using immunohistochemistry, fluorescence in situ hybridization, and real-time quantitative polymerase chain reaction. *Hum. Pathol.* 2007;**38**:1386–1393.
18. Carney WP. Hidden HER-2/neu-positive breast cancer: How to maximize detection. *IDrugs* 2009;**12**:238–242.
19. Romond EH, Perez EA, Bryant J, et al. Trastuzumab plus adjuvant chemotherapy for operable HER2-positive breast cancer. *New Engl. J. Med.* 2005;**353**:1673–1684.
20. Nahta R, Esteva FJ. Trastuzumab: Triumphs and tribulations. *Oncogene* 2007;**26**: 3637–3643.
21. Lennon S, Barton C, Banken L, et al. Utility of serum HER2 extracellular domain assessment in clinical decision making: Pooled analysis of four trials of trastuzumab in metastatic breast cancer. *J. Clin. Oncol.* 2009;**27**:1685–1693.
22. Ameyaw MM, Tayeb M, Thornton N, et al. Ethnic variation in the HER-2 codon 655 genetic polymorphism previously associated with breast cancer. *J. Hum. Genet.* 2002;**47**:172–175.
23. McLeod HL, Relling MV, Liu Q, et al. Polymorphic thiopurine methyltransferase in erythrocytes is indicative of activity in leukemic blasts from children with acute lymphoblastic leukemia. *Blood* 1995;**85**:1897–1902.
24. McLeod HL, Siva C. The thiopurine S-methyltransferase gene locus—implications for clinical pharmacogenomics. *Pharmacogenomics* 2002;**3**:89–98.
25. Stocco G, Cheok MH, Crews KR, et al. Genetic polymorphism of inosine triphosphate pyrophosphatase is a determinant of mercaptopurine metabolism and toxicity during treatment for acute lymphoblastic leukemia. *Clin. Pharmacol. Ther.* 2009;**85**:164–172.
26. Cao H, Hegele RA. DNA polymorphisms in ITPA including basis of inosine triphosphatase deficiency. *J, Hum. Genet.* 2002;**47**:620–622.
27. Marinaki AM, Ansari A, Duley JA, et al. Adverse drug reactions to azathioprine therapy are associated with polymorphism in the gene encoding inosine triphosphate pyrophosphatase (ITPase). *Pharmacogenetics* 2004;**14**:181–187.
28. McLeod HL, Lin JS, Scott EP, et al. Thiopurine methyltransferase activity in American white subjects and black subjects. *Clin. Pharmacol. Ther.* 1994;**55**:15–20.
29. Relling MV, Hancock ML, Boyett JM, et al. Prognostic importance of 6-mercaptopurine dose intensity in acute lymphoblastic leukemia. *Blood* 1999;**93**:2817–2823.
30. Relling MV, Hancock ML, Rivera GK, et al. Mercaptopurine therapy intolerance and heterozygosity at the thiopurine S-methyltransferase gene locus. *J. Natl. Cancer Inst.* 1999;**91**:2001–2008.
31. Rutherford K, Daggett V. Four human thiopurine S-methyltransferase alleles severely affect protein structure and dynamics. *J. Mol. Biol.* 2008;**379**:803–814.
32. Oliveira E, Quental S, Alves S, et al. Do the distribution patterns of polymorphisms at the thiopurine S-methyltransferase locus in sub-Saharan populations need revision? Hints from Cabinda and Mozambique. *Eur. J. Clin. Pharmacol.* 2007;**63**:703–706.
33. Fakhoury M, Andreu-Gallien J, Mahr A, et al. Should TPMT genotype and activity be used to monitor 6-mercaptopurine treatment in children with acute lymphoblastic leukaemia? *J. Clin. Pharm. Ther.* 2007;**32**:633–639.
34. Sahasranaman S, Howard D, Roy S. Clinical pharmacology and pharmacogenetics of thiopurines. *Eur. J. Clin. Pharmacol.* 2008;**64**:753–767.

35. Cheng Q, Yang W, Raimondi SC, et al. Karyotypic abnormalities create discordance of germline genotype and cancer cell phenotypes. *Nat. Genet.* 2005;**37**:878–882.

36. Marsh S, Van Booven DJ. The increasing complexity of mercaptopurine pharmacogenomics. *Clin. Pharmacol. Ther.* 2009;**85**:139–141.

37. Heidelberger C, Chaudhuri NK, Danneberg P, et al. Fluorinated pyrimidines, a new class of tumour-inhibitory compounds. *Nature* 1957;**179**:663–666.

38. Marsh S. Pharmacogenetics of colorectal cancer. *Expert Opin. Pharmacother.* 2005;**6**:2607–2616.

39. McLeod HL, Collie-Duguid ES, Vreken P. et al. Nomenclature for human DPYD alleles. *Pharmacogenetics* 1998;**8**:455–459.

40. Van Kuilenburg AB, Meinsma R, Zoetekouw L, et al. High prevalence of the IVS14 + 1G > A mutation in the dihydropyrimidine dehydrogenase gene of patients with severe 5-fluorouracil-associated toxicity. *Pharmacogenetics* 2002;**12**:555–558.

41. Wei X, Elizondo G, Sapone A, et al. Characterization of the human dihydropyrimidine dehydrogenase gene. *Genomics* 1998;**51**:391–400.

42. Ezzeldin H, Johnson MR, Okamoto Y, et al. Denaturing high performance liquid chromatography analysis of the DPYD gene in patients with lethal 5-fluorouracil toxicity. *Clin. Cancer Res.* 2003;**9**:3021–3028.

43. Seck K, Riemer S, Kates R, et al. Analysis of the DPYD gene implicated in 5–fluorouracil catabolism in a cohort of Caucasian individuals. *Clin. Cancer Res.* 2005;**11**:5886–5892.

44. Ahluwalia R, Freimuth R, McLeod HL, et al. Use of pyrosequencing to detect clinically relevant polymorphisms in dihydropyrimidine dehydrogenase. *Clin. Chem.* 2003;**49**: 1661–1664.

45. Schwab M, Zanger UM, Marx C, et al. Role of genetic and nongenetic factors for fluorouracil treatment-related severe toxicity: A prospective clinical trial by the German 5-FU toxicity study group. *J. Clin. Oncol.* 2008;**26**:2131–2138.

46. Zhang H, Li YM, Jin X. DPYD*5 gene mutation contributes to the reduced DPYD enzyme activity and chemotherapeutic toxicity of 5-FU: Results from genotyping study on 75 gastric carcinoma and colon carcinoma patients. *Med. Oncol.* 2007;**24**:251–258.

47. Maekawa K, Saeki M, Saito Y, et al. Genetic variations and haplotype structures of the DPYD gene encoding dihydropyrimidine dehydrogenase in Japanese and their ethnic differences. *J. Hum. Genet.* 2007;**52**:804–819.

48. Thomas HR, Ezzeldin HH, Guarcello V, et al. Genetic regulation of dihydropyrimidinase and its possible implication in altered uracil catabolism. *Pharmacogenet. Genomics* 2007;**17**:973–987.

49. Thomas HR, Ezzeldin HH, Guarcello V, et al. Genetic regulation of beta-ureidopropionase and its possible implication in altered uracil catabolism. *Pharmacogenet. Genomics.* 2008;**18**:25–35.

50. van Kuilenburg AB, Meinsma R, Zonnenberg BA, et al. Dihydropyrimidinase deficiency and severe 5-fluorouracil toxicity. *Clin. Cancer Res.* 2003;**9**:4363–4367.

51. Stebbing J, Bower M, Syed N, et al. Epigenetics: An emerging technology in the diagnosis and treatment of cancer. *Pharmacogenomics* 2006;**7**:747–757.

52. Noguchi T, Tanimoto K, Shimokuni T, et al. Aberrant methylation of DPYD promoter, DPYD expression, and cellular sensitivity to 5-fluorouracil in cancer cells. *Clin. Cancer Res.* 2004;**10**:7100–7107.

53. Ezzeldin HH, Lee AM, Mattison LK, et al. Methylation of the DPYD promoter: An alternative mechanism for dihydropyrimidine dehydrogenase deficiency in cancer patients. *Clin. Cancer Res.* 2005;**11**:8699–8705.
54. Yu J, Freimuth RR, Culverhouse R, et al. DNA methylotype analysis in colorectal cancer. *Oncol. Rep.* 2008;**20**:921–927.
55. Yu J, McLeod HL, Ezzeldin HH, et al. Methylation of the DPYD promoter and dihydropyrimidine dehydrogenase deficiency. *Clin. Cancer Res.* 2006;**12**:3864.
56. Johnston PG, Lenz HJ, Leichman CG, et al. Thymidylate synthase gene and protein expression correlate and are associated with response to 5-fluorouracil in human colorectal and gastric tumors. *Cancer Res.* 1995;**55**:1407–1412.
57. Leichman CG, Lenz HJ, Leichman L, et al. Quantitation of intratumoral thymidylate synthase expression predicts for disseminated colorectal cancer response and resistance to protracted-infusion fluorouracil and weekly leucovorin. *J. Clin. Oncol.* 1997;**15**: 3223–3229.
58. Marsh S. Thymidylate synthase pharmacogenetics. Invest. *New Drugs* 2005;**23**:533–537.
59. Horie N, Aiba H, Oguro K, et al. Functional analysis and DNA polymorphism of the tandemly repeated sequences in the 5′-terminal regulatory region of the human gene for thymidylate synthase. *Cell Struct. Funct.* 1995;**20**:191–197.
60. Marsh S, Ameyaw MM, Githang'a J. et al. Novel thymidylate synthase enhancer region alleles in African populations. *Hum. Mutat.* 2000;**16**:528.
61. Luo HR, Lu XM, Yao YG, et al. Length polymorphism of thymidylate synthase regulatory region in Chinese populations and evolution of the novel alleles. *Biochem. Genet.* 2002;**40**:41–51.
62. Kawakami K, Omura K, Kanehira E, et al. Polymorphic tandem repeats in the thymidylate synthase gene is associated with its protein expression in human gastrointestinal cancers. *Anticancer Res.* 1999;**19**:3249–3252.
63. Morganti M, Ciantelli M, Giglioni B, et al. Relationships between promoter polymorphisms in the thymidylate synthase gene and mRNA levels in colorectal cancers. *Eur. J. Cancer* 2005;**41**:2176–2183.
64. Marsh S, Collie-Duguid ES, Li T, et al. Ethnic variation in the thymidylate synthase enhancer region polymorphism among Caucasian and Asian populations. *Genomics* 1999;**58**:310–312.
65. Marsh S, McLeod HL. Thymidylate synthase pharmacogenetics in colorectal cancer. *Clin. Colorectal Cancer* 2001;**1**: *175-178;* discussion pp. 9–81.
66. Horie N, Takeishi K. Functional structure of the promoter region of the human thymidylate synthase gene and nuclear factors that regulate the expression of the gene. *Nucleic Acids Symp. Ser.* 1995;**34**:77–78.
67. Iacopetta B, Grieu F, Joseph D, et al. A polymorphism in the enhancer region of the thymidylate synthase promoter influences the survival of colorectal cancer patients treated with 5-fluorouracil. *Br. J. Cancer* 2001;**85**:827–830.
68. Villafranca E, Okruzhnov Y, Dominguez MA, et al. Polymorphisms of the repeated sequences in the enhancer region of the thymidylate synthase gene promoter may predict downstaging after preoperative chemoradiation in rectal cancer. *J. Clin. Oncol.* 2001;**19**:1779–1786.
69. McLeod HL, Tan B, Malyapa R, et al. Genotype-guided neoadjuvant therapy for rectal cancer. *Proc. Am. Soc. Clin. Oncol.* 2005;**23**:197.

70. Tsuji T, Hidaka S, Sawai T, et al. Polymorphism in the thymidylate synthase promoter enhancer region is not an efficacious marker for tumor sensitivity to 5-fluorouracil-based oral adjuvant chemotherapy in colorectal cancer. *Clin. Cancer Res.* 2003;**9**: 3700–3704.

71. Mandola MV, Stoehlmacher J, Muller-Weeks S, et al. A novel single nucleotide polymorphism within the 5′ tandem repeat polymorphism of the thymidylate synthase gene abolishes USF-1 binding and alters transcriptional activity. *Cancer Res.* 2003;**63**: 2898–2904.

72. Gusella M, Bolzonella C, Crepaldi G, et al. A novel G/C single-nucleotide polymorphism in the double 28-bp repeat thymidylate synthase allele. *Pharmacogenomics J.* 2006;**6**: 421–424.

73. Lincz LF, Scorgie FE, Garg MB, et al. Identification of a novel single nucleotide polymorphism in the first tandem repeat sequence of the thymidylate synthase 2R allele. *Int. J. Cancer* 2007;**120**:1930–1934.

74. Marcuello E, Altes A, del Rio E, et al. Single nucleotide polymorphism in the 5' tandem repeat sequences of thymidylate synthase gene predicts for response to fluorouracil-based chemotherapy in advanced colorectal cancer patients. *Int. J. Cancer* 2004;**112**: 733–737.

75. Dotor E, Cuatrecases M, Martinez-Iniesta M, et al. Tumor thymidylate synthase 1494del6 genotype as a prognostic factor in colorectal cancer patients receiving fluorouracil-based adjuvant treatment. *J. Clin. Oncol.* 2006;**24**:1603–1611.

76. Ulrich CM, Bigler J, Velicer CM, et al. Searching expressed sequence tag databases: Discovery and confirmation of a common polymorphism in the thymidylate synthase gene. *Cancer Epidemiol. Biomarkers Prev.* 2000;**9**:1381–1385.

77. Kealey C, Brown KS, Woodside JV, et al. A common insertion/deletion polymorphism of the thymidylate synthase (TYMS) gene is a determinant of red blood cell folate and homocysteine concentrations. *Hum. Genet.* 2005;**116**:347–353.

78. Lenz H-J, Zhang W, Zahedy S, et al. A 6 base-pair deletion in the 3 UTR of the thymidylate synthase (TS) gene predicts TS mRNA expression in colorectal tumors. A possible candidate gene for colorectal cancer risk [abstract]. *Proc. Am. Assoc. Cancer Res.* 2002;**43**:660.

79. Ruzzo A, Graziano F, Loupakis F, et al. Pharmacogenetic profiling in patients with advanced colorectal cancer treated with first-line FOLFIRI chemotherapy. *Pharmacogenomics J.* 2008;**8**:278–288.

80. Salgado J, Zabalegui N, Gil C, et al. Polymorphisms in the thymidylate synthase and dihydropyrimidine dehydrogenase genes predict response and toxicity to capecitabine-raltitrexed in colorectal cancer. *Oncol. Rep.* 2007;**17**:325–328.

81. Lurje G, Zhang W, Yang D, et al. Thymidylate synthase haplotype is associated with tumor recurrence in stage II and stage III colon cancer. *Pharmacogenet. Genomics* 2008;**18**:161–168.

82. Wang TL, Diaz LA, Jr., Romans K, et al. Digital karyotyping identifies thymidylate synthase amplification as a mechanism of resistance to 5-fluorouracil in metastatic colorectal cancer patients. *Proc. Natl. Acad. Sci. USA* 2004;**101**:3089–3094.

83. Rooney PH, Stevenson DA, Marsh S, et al. Comparative genomic hybridization analysis of chromosomal alterations induced by the development of resistance to thymidylate synthase inhibitors. *Cancer Res.* 1998;**58**:5042–5045.

84. Rooney PH, Murray GI, Stevenson DA, et al. Comparative genomic hybridization and chromosomal instability in solid tumours. *Br. J. Cancer* 1999;**80**:862–873.

85. Yu J, Miller R, Zhang W, et al. Copy-number analysis of topoisomerase and thymidylate synthase genes in frozen and FFPE DNAs of colorectal cancers. *Pharmacogenomics* 2008;**9**:1459–1466.

86. Marsh S, McLeod HL. Pharmacogenetics of irinotecan toxicity. *Pharmacogenomics* 2004;**5**:835–843.

87. Bosma PJ, Chowdhury JR, Bakker C, et al. The genetic basis of the reduced expression of bilirubin UDP-glucuronosyltransferase 1 in Gilbert's syndrome. *New Engl. J. Med.* 1995;**333**:1171–1175.

88. Beutler E, Gelbart T, Demina A. Racial variability in the UDP-glucuronosyltransferase 1 (UGT1A1) promoter: A balanced polymorphism for regulation of bilirubin metabolism? *Proc. Natl. Acad. Sci. USA* 1998;**95**:8170–8174.

89. Innocenti F, Undevia SD, Iyer L, et al. Genetic variants in the UDP-glucuronosyltransferase 1A1 gene predict the risk of severe neutropenia of irinotecan. *J. Clin. Oncol.* 2004;**22**:1382–1388.

90. FDA clears third wave pharmacogenetic test. *Pharmacogenomics* 2005;**6**:671–672.

91. Ratain MJ. From bedside to bench to bedside to clinical practice: An odyssey with irinotecan. *Clin. Cancer Res.* 2006;**12**:1658–1660.

92. Hoskins JM, Goldberg RM, Qu P, et al. UGT1A1*28 genotype and irinotecan-induced neutropenia: Dose matters. *J. Natl. Cancer Inst.* 2007;**99**:1290–1295.

93. Premawardhena A, Fisher CA, Liu YT, et al. The global distribution of length polymorphisms of the promoters of the glucuronosyltransferase 1 gene (UGT1A1): Hematologic and evolutionary implications. *Blood Cells Mol. Dis.* 2003;**31**:98–101.

94. Han JY, Lim HS, Shin ES, et al. Comprehensive analysis of UGT1A polymorphisms predictive for pharmacokinetics and treatment outcome in patients with non-small-cell lung cancer treated with irinotecan and cisplatin. *J. Clin. Oncol.* 2006;**24**:2237–2244.

95. Sai K, Saeki M, Saito Y, et al. UGT1A1 haplotypes associated with reduced glucuronidation and increased serum bilirubin in irinotecan-administered Japanese patients with cancer. *Clin. Pharmacol. Ther.* 2004;**75**:501–515.

96. Gagnon JF, Bernard O, Villeneuve L, et al. Irinotecan inactivation is modulated by epigenetic silencing of UGT1A1 in colon cancer. *Clin. Cancer Res.* 2006;**12**: 1850–1858.

97. Hoskins JM, Marcuello E, Altes A, et al. Irinotecan pharmacogenetics: Influence of pharmacodynamic genes. *Clin. Cancer Res.* 2008;**14**:1788–1796.

98. Mathijssen RH, Marsh S, Karlsson MO, et al. Irinotecan pathway genotype analysis to predict pharmacokinetics. *Clin. Cancer Res.* 2003;**9**:3246–3253.

99. de Jong FA, Scott-Horton TJ, Kroetz DL, et al. Irinotecan-induced diarrhea: functional significance of the polymorphic ABCC2 transporter protein. *Clin. Pharmacol. Ther.* 2007;**81**:42–49.

100. Carlini LE, Meropol NJ, Bever J, et al. UGT1A7 and UGT1A9 polymorphisms predict response and toxicity in colorectal cancer patients treated with capecitabine/irinotecan. *Clin. Cancer Res.* 2005;**11**:1226–1236.

101. Cecchin E, Innocenti F, D'Andrea M, et al. Predictive role of the UGT1A1, UGT1A7, and UGT1A9 genetic variants and their haplotypes on the outcome of metastatic

colorectal cancer patients treated with fluorouracil, leucovorin, and irinotecan. *J. Clin. Oncol.* 2009;**27**:2457–2465.

102. Innocenti F, Kroetz DL, Schuetz E, et al. Comprehensive pharmacogenetic analysis of irinotecan neutropenia and pharmacokinetics. *J. Clin. Oncol.* 2009;**27**:2604–2614.

103. Osborne CK. Tamoxifen in the treatment of breast cancer. *New Engl. J. Med.* 1998;**339**:1609–1618.

104. Desta Z, Ward BA, Soukhova NV, et al. Comprehensive evaluation of tamoxifen sequential biotransformation by the human cytochrome P450 system in vitro: Prominent roles for CYP3A and CYP2D6. *J. Pharmacol. Exp. Ther.* 2004;**310**: 1062–1075.

105. Ingelman-Sundberg M. Genetic polymorphisms of cytochrome P450 2D6 (CYP2D6): Clinical consequences, evolutionary aspects and functional diversity. *Pharmacogenomics J.* 2005;**5**:6–13.

106. Beverage JN, Sissung TM, Sion AM, et al. *CYP2D6 polymorphisms and the impact on tamoxifen therapy. J. Pharm. Sci.* 2007;**96**:2224–2231.

107. Jin Y, Desta Z, Stearns V, et al. CYP2D6 genotype, antidepressant use, and tamoxifen metabolism during adjuvant breast cancer treatment. *J. Natl. Cancer Inst.* 2005;**97**: 30–39.

108. Goetz MP, Rae JM, Suman VJ, et al. Pharmacogenetics of tamoxifen biotransformation is associated with clinical outcomes of efficacy and hot flashes. *J. Clin. Oncol.* 2005;**23**: 9312–9318.

109. Xu Y, Sun Y, Yao L, et al. Association between CYP2D6 *10 genotype and survival of breast cancer patients receiving tamoxifen treatment. *Ann. Oncol.* 2008;**19**: 1423–1429.

110. Kiyotani K, Mushiroda T, Sasa M, et al. Impact of CYP2D6*10 on recurrence-free survival in breast cancer patients receiving adjuvant tamoxifen therapy. *Cancer Sci.* 2008;**99**:995–999.

111. Reynolds S. SPORE study provides new guidelines for tamoxifen use., *NCI Cancer Bull.* 2006;**3**:1–2.

112. Rebsamen MC, Desmeules J, Daali Y, et al. The AmpliChip CYP450 test: Cytochrome P450 2D6 genotype assessment and phenotype prediction. *Pharmacogenomics J.* 2009;**9**:34–41.

113. Nishiyama T, Ogura K, Nakano H, et al. Reverse geometrical selectivity in glucuronidation and sulfation of cis- and trans-4-hydroxytamoxifens by human liver UDP-glucuronosyltransferases and sulfotransferases. *Biochem. Pharmacol.* 2002;**63**: 1817–1830.

114. Nowell SA, Ahn J, Rae JM, et al. Association of genetic variation in tamoxifen-metabolizing enzymes with overall survival and recurrence of disease in breast cancer patients. *Breast Cancer Res. Treat.* 2005;**91**:249–258.

115. Nowell S, Sweeney C, Winters M, et al. Association between sulfotransferase 1A1 genotype and survival of breast cancer patients receiving tamoxifen therapy. *J. Natl. Cancer Inst.* 2002;**94**:1635–1640.

116. Marsh S. Taxane pharmacogenetics. *Personal. Med.* 2006;**3**:33–43.

117. Marsh S, King CR, McLeod HL, et al. ABCB1 2677G>T/A genotype and paclitaxel pharmacogenetics in ovarian cancer. *Clin. Cancer Res.* 2006;**12**: *4127* (author reply p. 4129).

118. Marsh S, Paul J, King CR, et al. Pharmacogenetic assessment of toxicity and outcome after platinum plus taxane chemotherapy in ovarian cancer: The Scottish randomised trial in ovarian cancer. *J. Clin. Oncol.* 2007;**25**:4528–4535.

119. Marsh S, McLeod HL. Pharmacogenetics and oncology treatment for breast cancer. *Expert Opin. Pharmacother.* 2007;**8**:119–127.

120. Green H. Pharmacogenomics of importance for paclitaxel chemotherapy. *Pharmacogenomics* 2008;**9**:671–674.

121. Sissung TM, Price DK, Sparreboom A, et al. Pharmacogenetics and regulation of human cytochrome P450 1B1: Implications in hormone-mediated tumor metabolism and a novel target for therapeutic intervention. *Mol. Cancer Res.* 2006;**4**:135–150.

122. Marsh S, Somlo G, Li X, et al. Pharmacogenetic analysis of paclitaxel transport and metabolism genes in breast cancer. *Pharmacogenomics J.* 2007;**7**:362–365.

123. Sissung TM, Danesi R, Price DK, et al. Association of the CYP1B1*3 allele with survival in patients with prostate cancer receiving docetaxel. *Mol. Cancer Ther.* 2008;**7**:19–26.

124. Aoki D, Oda Y, Hattori S, et al. Overexpression of class III beta-tubulin predicts good response to taxane-based chemotherapy in ovarian clear cell adenocarcinoma. *Clin. Cancer Res.* 2009;**15**:1473–1480.

125. Chang JC, Makris A, Gutierrez MC, et al. Gene expression patterns in formalin-fixed, paraffin-embedded core biopsies predict docetaxel chemosensitivity in breast cancer patients. *Breast Cancer Res. Treat.* 2008;**108**:233–240.

126. Gianni L, Zambetti M, Clark K, et al. Gene expression profiles in paraffin-embedded core biopsy tissue predict response to chemotherapy in women with locally advanced breast cancer. *J. Clin. Oncol.* 2005;**23**:7265–7277.

127. Kaklamani VG, Gradishar WJ. Gene expression in breast cancer. *Curr. Treat. Options Oncol.* 2006;**7**:123–128.

128. Shukla SJ, Dolan ME. Use of CEPH and non-CEPH lymphoblast cell lines in pharmacogenetic studies. *Pharmacogenomics* 2005;**6**:303–310.

129. Watters JW, Kraja A, Meucci MA, et al. Genome-wide discovery of loci influencing chemotherapy cytotoxicity. *Proc. Natl. Acad. Sci. USA* 2004;**101**:11809–11814.

130. Engen RM, Marsh S, Van Booven DJ, et al. Ethnic differences in pharmacogenetically relevant genes. *Curr. Drug Targets* 2006;**7**:1641–1648.

131. Marsh S, Van Booven DJ, McLeod HL. Global pharmacogenetics: Giving the genome to the masses. *Pharmacogenomics* 2006;**7**:625–631.

CHAPTER 9

Pharmacogenetics of Asthma and COPD

ELLEN S. KOSTER, JAN A. M. RAAIJMAKERS, and
ANKE-HILSE MAITLAND-VAN DER ZEE
Utrecht University, Utrecht, The Netherlands

GERARD H. KOPPELMAN
University Medical Center Groningen, Groningen, The Netherlands

9.1 INTRODUCTION

Asthma and chronic obstructive pulmonary disease (COPD) are chronic airway diseases that are among the most common chronic disorders in the world. Because of their high prevalence and chronicity, they induce a great economic and social burden [1,2]. In the United States, asthma is the most common reason for paediatric hospital admission [3] and COPD is the fourth leading cause of chronic morbidity and mortality [2].

Although the etiology of asthma is still not fully clear, there are effective treatments for asthma. Treatment is based on regular use of inhaled corticosteroids (ICSs) in combination with $\beta 2$-agonists and leukotriene antagonists to prevent asthma exacerbations, retain proper lung function, and modulate inflammatory responses. Exacerbations are treated with oral steroids [4–8]. For COPD patients, treatment is based on use of both short- and long-acting bronchodilating agents ($\beta 2$-agonists and anticholinergics). ICSs are recommended for patients with frequent exacerbations and in some (severe) cases antibiotics are prescribed [2,9].

Response to pharmacotherapy can be highly variable among individual patients. Currently available drugs are effective in most asthmatic patients, whereas treatment response in COPD is variable. There remains a group of patients who are not adequately controlled on existing treatments [10]. Suboptimal effects in asthma and COPD therapy can hamper a person's wellbeing; many of these patients have

Pharmacogenetics and Individualized Therapy, First Edition.
Edited by Anke-Hilse Maitland-van der Zee and Ann K. Daly.

recurrent exacerbations, increased bronchial obstruction, and chronically impaired lung function. The quality of life of these patients is negatively affected by disease. Furthermore, these patients contribute disproportionately to healthcare costs through increased medical care and medication consumption. Therefore, further research and the development of new and more effective therapies for those who cannot be treated effectively with current available therapeutics is needed.

It is not fully clear what factors determine interindividual variations in responsiveness to drugs. Environmental factors, the genetic background, and the involvement of inflammatory cells contribute to the development of several clinical phenotypes of asthma and COPD, ranging from seasonal allergies to difficult to treat late-onset asthma. To which extend inter-individual variability in treatment response is genetic is not certain. Variability in individual treatment response may be due to many factors, such as severity and type of disease, compliance, comorbidity, comedication (drug–drug interactions), environmental exposures, and age. However, calculations of repeatability of treatment response among individuals suggest that a substantial fraction of the variance could be genetic. A study of response to antiasthma drugs showed that up to 60–80% of the variance in treatment response may be due to differences among individuals [4]. Several genetic variants have been discovered in genes that are involved in action or metabolism of antiasthma drugs and are associated with altered therapeutic responses [10].

Pharmacogenetics, with personalized prescription as the ultimate goal, could help to administer therapies to asthma and COPD patients to those least likely to experience adverse effects and to whom can benefit the most. Genes involved in the different drug pathways can play a role in treatment response. Several asthma and COPD pharmacogenetic studies (discussed in this chapter) have been described to assess the relationship between variation in these genes and response to treatment.

9.2 ASTHMA AND COPD

Asthma and COPD present distinct features; however, patients may present with overlapping clinical symptoms, which makes it difficult to distinguish the two diseases. Both are characterized by two components: airflow obstruction (in COPD chronic obstruction and in asthma recurrent episodes of obstruction) and inflammation of the airways. Both result from gene–environment interactions, and both are characterized by mucus secretion, bronchoconstriction, and exacerbations [11].

Although there are similarities, it is the differences between the diseases that define their natural history and clinical presentations (Table 9.1). The first clear difference between the two diseases is that in COPD both the airways and parenchyma are affected, while in asthma only the airways are affected. In COPD, emphysema (irreversible destruction of the lung parenchyma) is present, but not in asthma. Another important difference is the nature of inflammation; in asthma inflammation is characterized by increased numbers of eosinophils, $CD4^+$ lymphocytes and mast cells, while in COPD inflammation is primarily neutrophilic with

TABLE 9.1 Differences between Asthma and COPD

Characteristics	Asthma	COPD
Anatomic site	Airways	Airways and parenchyma
Nature of inflammation	Eosinophilic	Neutrophilic
Treatment response to ICS	Reduction of inflammation	Mostly nonresponsive
Cause of inflammation	Allergens	Particles and gasses
Progression of disease	Chronic	Chronic and progressive
Age of onset	Usually childhood	(Late) adult life
Atopy	Common feature	Not prominent feature
Lung function	Normal	Airflow limitation
Reversibility of airway obstruction	Mostly reversible	Mostly irreversible

increased numbers of neutrophils, $CD8^+$ lymphocytes and macrophages [11,12]. This could also affect response to pharmacotherapy. In contrast to asthma patients, where ICS therapy reduces airway inflammation, treatment of COPD patients with ICS remains questionable, because of the low benefit (inflammation is mostly nonresponsive to steroid therapy) and potential drug toxicity [13,14].

Chronic airway inflammation in COPD patients is an amplification of the normal inflammatory response in the airways after exposure to chronic irritants such as tobacco smoke or chemical irritants. Airway inflammation is then further amplified by oxidative stress and proteinases in the lung. Tobacco smoke and airway pollution are the main causes of COPD [2], while in asthma inhaled allergens (such as house dust mite) are important environmental factors in the pathogenesis. The natural histories of both diseases also differ, COPD is a chronic progressive disease characterized by not fully reversible airflow limitation. Asthma is a chronic, but not progressive, disease characterized by reversible airflow limitation [11]. However, in a subgroup, asthma results in ongoing, irreversible airflow obstruction and increased lung function decline over time.

Besides the different disease characteristics, there are also differences in the clinical features of asthma and COPD (Table 9.1). One of these features is the age of onset; asthma usually begins in childhood, and COPD becomes clinically apparent in adult life. A history of atopic disorders is common in asthma, while in COPD this is not a prominent feature. Furthermore, lung function in asthma is still normal in patients with mild disease, while in COPD airflow obstruction is a hallmark and becomes progressively greater as the disease advances. If reversibility of airflow limitation is found, asthma is likely to be the diagnosis. If the airflow limitation is irreversible, the diagnosis is most likely COPD [11].

9.2.1 Asthma

Allergic asthma is a multifactorial polygenic inflammatory disease of the airways, which is characterized physiologically by recurrent airway obstruction that resolves spontaneously or as a result of treatment [15,16]. According to the global initiative for asthma (GINA) [1,17], asthma is defined as:

> A chronic inflammatory disorder of the airways in which many cells and cellular elements play a role. The chronic inflammation is associated with airway hyperresponsiveness that leads to recurrent episodes of wheezing, breathlessness, chest tightness and coughing, particularly at night or in the early morning. These episodes are usually associated with widespread, but variable, airflow obstruction within the lung that is often reversible either spontaneously or with treatment.

Asthma is a very complex disease that has many clinical phenotypes in both adults and children. Bronchial asthma exists at all ages, but for many patients the disease begins in infancy [18]. Both genetic factors (atopy) and environmental factors contribute to its inception and evolution [15].

9.2.2 COPD

In the Global Initiative for *Chronic Obstructive Lung Disease* (GOLD) guidelines [2,19], COPD is defined as:

> A preventable and treatable disease with some significant extrapulmonary effects that may contribute to the severity in individual patients. Its pulmonary component is characterized by airflow limitation that is not fully reversible. The airflow limitation is usually progressive and associated with an abnormal inflammatory response of the lung to noxious particles or gases.

The chronic airflow limitation in COPD patients is caused by a combination of small airway disease and emphysema. The most common cause of COPD is cigarette smoking, although COPD may also be caused by exposure to other particles and gasses [2,19].

9.3 ASTHMA AND COPD TREATMENT

The treatment strategy for both asthma and COPD consist of two steps: treatment with bronchodilating agents for symptomatic relief and treatment with antiinflammatory drugs to modulate the inflammatory response. However, in COPD treatment it is still questionable whether ICS should be prescribed for every patient [13,20].

9.3.1 Asthma Treatment

Asthma therapy is induced to reduce clinical symptoms such as wheeze and cough, to reduce the number of acute exacerbations and minimize sleep disturbances [6]. Currently, there are three main drug classes for asthma available: (both short- and long-acting) $\beta2$-agonists, inhaled corticosteroids, and leukotriene inhibitors [4,6–8,21]. The main form of long-term treatment of asthmatic patients is the use of ICS to retain proper lung function and modulate inflammatory responses combined with as-needed use of short-acting $\beta2$-agonists for symptomatic treatment [5,6]. ICSs are the most effective agents available for control of airway inflammation and improvement of lung function. However, the potential side effects of ICS when used on a long-term basis and in escalating doses have led to the use of adjunctive therapies. Treatment with long-acting $\beta 2$-agonists and leukotriene antagonists has been shown to help control asthma symptoms while sometimes reducing ICS use [22].

9.3.2 COPD Treatment

The treatment regime for COPD includes smoking cessation, pulmonary rehabilitation, treatment of exacerbations, and, where necessary, oxygen therapy. Pharmacotherapy in COPD patients is used to prevent and control symptoms, reduce the frequency and severity of exacerbations, improve health status, and improve exercise tolerance. Pharmacotherapy has been shown to reduce the rate of lung function decline (measured by FEV1) in COPD patients, thus slowing disease progression [23]. The main form of long-term management involves the use of inhaled bronchodilators (long-acting $\beta 2$-agonists and anticholinergics) and the use of inhaled corticosteroids (in moderate to severe COPD) [9].

9.3.3 Treatment Response in Asthma and COPD

Polymorphisms in the genes encoding relevant drug targets may contribute significantly to the variability in drug response. In this chapter we will discuss mainly asthma pharmacogenetic studies, as these are investigated in greater depth in the literature than is COPD.

9.4 STUDIES OF ASTHMA AND COPD PHARMACOGENETICS

Currently, most studies focused on the pharmacogenetic effects of the $\beta 2$-adrenergic receptor, because most other pharmacogenetic effects are likely to be of smaller magnitude or less common. Many studies have been performed to study associations between genetic variation and altered treatment response. However, not all studies address clinically relevant outcomes. Outcomes that are used in asthma or COPD pharmacogenetic studies are change in FEV1 (forced expiratory volume at 1 s), change in PEF (peak expiratory flow), PC20 measurement (airway responsiveness for metacholine), asthma control (mostly questionnaire-based, including number of exacerbations, nighttime awakenings, and short-acting $\beta 2$-agonist use), gene and protein expression levels, gene transcription activity, and dexamethasone suppression testing. In this chapter we will focus on studies with clinically relevant endpoints defined as treatment response measured by improvement in lung function or asthma control.

9.4.1 $\beta 2$-Agonists

Short-acting inhaled $\beta 2$-agonists (SABAs) are used for the treatment of acute asthma exacerbations and for quick relief of symptoms in asthma and COPD patients.

Long-acting β2-agonists (LABAs) are used as maintenance symptomatic treatment in both asthma and COPD [5,6].

β2-Agonists reduce the bronchoconstriction by activating the β2-receptors in the lung, which leads to smooth-muscle relaxation, decreased hyperreactivity, improved mucociliary clearance, and reduced airway obstruction [10]. The β2-adrenergic receptors are expressed on a variety of lung cells, including epithelial cells, smooth muscle cells, vascular endothelium, and immune cells [24]. When a β2-agonist binds to the receptor, the receptor evokes a number of signals. Briefly, binding of β2-agonists to the β2-adrenergic receptor results in the activation of adenylcyclase via stimulatory G proteins. This results in an increase in cAMP and activation of protein kinase A (PKA). PKA phosphorylates target proteins, decreases intracellular calcium levels, and leads to smooth-muscle relaxation. When the β2-adrenergic receptor is activated by the β2-agonist, a complex process of desensitization occurs. This process functions to attenuate the effects of β2-agonists and is mediated by both short-term (uncoupling of the receptor) and long-term (downregulation of receptor expression) mechanisms. Although many genes are likely to be involved in the response to β2-agonists, most β2-agonist pharmacogenetic studies focus on polymorphisms in the drug target, the β2-adrenergic receptor, itself. Several studies have shown an association between β2-adrenergic receptor gene (ADRB2) polymorphisms and altered response to β2-agonists. As shown in Table 9.2, findings of these studies vary.

The ADRB2 gene is located on chromosome 5q31–32. The structure of the β2-adrenergic receptor is the same as that of other G-protein-coupled receptors. Nine single base substitutions have been identified in the ADRB2 coding region (see also Chapter 6). Five of these are synonymous and unlikely to be functionally important. Of the remaining four non-synonymous polymorphisms, three (an arginine substitution for cystine at codon 16 (A $\rightarrow$ G change at basepair 46), glutamine substitution for glutamic acid at codon 27 (C $\rightarrow$ G change at basepair 79), and a threonine substitution for isoleucine at codon 164 (C $\rightarrow$ T change at basepair 491) have functional effects. One rare polymorphism (valine substitution for methionine at codon 34) seems to have no influence on receptor function [24].

The polymorphisms at codon 16 (allele frequency approximately 40%) and 27 (allele frequency approximately 45%) are quite common [24–28] and have been shown to be functionally important *in vitro* with respect to receptor binding affinity [29]. The polymorphisms at loci 34 and 164 are infrequent and found only in heterozygous state; the polymorphism at codon 34 is very rare (allele frequency $< 1\%$) and the polymorphism at codon 164 is also uncommon (allele frequency $< 5\%$) [24,26–28].

Several studies showed that the previously mentioned nonsynonymous polymorphisms are associated with decreased response to β2-agonist treatment. Most pharmacogenetic studies with respect to β2-agonists focused on short-acting β2-agonists. Patients who are homozygous for arginine at position 16 showed improved lung function and therapeutic response after treatment with short-acting β2-agonists when compared to patients homozygous for glycine at position 16 [30,31]. Subsequent pharmacogenetic studies found opposite results (improved treatment response for homozygous glycine carriers) or no association [32–36].

TABLE 9.2 Pharmacogenetic Studies Performed on β2-Agonists

Gene	Variant	Population	Outcome	Association	Reference
ADRB2	Gly16Arg	2225 asthmatics	Treatment response (severe exacerbations) to LABA (formoterol or salmeterol)	Gly16Arg genotype had no effect on treatment response across all treatment groups	25
ADRB2	Gly16Arg	405 asthmatics	Treatment response was closely similar for all genotypes	—	25
ADRB2	Gly16Arg and Gln27Glu	209 children with reduced FEV1	Treatment response (change in FEV1) to SABA (albuterol)	Homozygous Arg16 carriers showed increased response compared to homozygous Gly19 carriers Haplotypes of Arg16Gln27 showed the highest response; Haplotypes with Arg16 also showed better treatment response	30
ADRB2	Gly16Arg and Gln27Glu	269 children	Treatment response (change in FEV1) to SABA (albuterol)	Homozygous Arg16 carriers showed increased response compared to homozygous Gly16 carriers	31
ADRB2	Gly16Arg	149 asthmatics	Treatment response (PEF) to LABA (salmeterol)	Homozygous Arg16 carriers showed reduced response compared to Gly16 carriers	32
ADRB2	Gly16Arg and Gln27Glu	22 severe asthmatics	Treatment response (change in FEV1) to LABA (formoterol)	Homozygous Gly16 and Glu27 carriers showed increased response	33
ADRB2	Gly16Arg and Gln27Glu	190 asthmatics	Treatment response (PEF) to SABA (albuterol)	Homozygous Arg16 carriers who used albuterol regularly showed a decline in PEF compared to as-needed users; Gly16 carriers showed no such decline	34

(continued)

TABLE 9.2 *(Continued)*

Gene	Variant	Population	Outcome	Association	Reference
ADRB2	Haplotypes	560 asthmatics and 625 controls	Treatment response (FEV1/FVC ratio) to SABA (albuterol)	No association between ADRB2 haplotypes and response; one SNP was associated with albuterol response in African-Americans	35
ADRB2	Haplotypes	121 asthmatics	Treatment response (change in FEV1) to SABA (albuterol)	Treatment response was associated with haplotype pairs, but not with single SNPs; haplotypes associated with better response *in vivo* were also associated with increased ADRB2 protein expression in vitro	36
ADRB2	Gly16Arg	78 mild asthmatics	Treatment response (PEF) to SABA (albuterol)	Homozygous Arg16 carriers showed reduced response compared to homozygous Gly16 carriers	37
ADRB2	Gly16Arg	183 asthmatics	Treatment response (PEF) to LABA (salmeterol)	Treatment response did not vary between ADRB2 genotypes	39
ADRB2	Gly16Arg and Gln27Glu	104 COPD patients	Treatment response (change in FEV1) to LABA (salmeterol)	No association between ADRB2 genotype and treatment response	40
ADRB2	Haplotypes: Gly16Glu27	107 COPD patients	Treatment response (change in FEV1 and PEF) to SABA (salbutamol)	Haplotypes may affect severity of obstructive impairment, but no association with immediate bronchodilator response	41
ADRB2	Gly16Arg and Gln27Glu	246 COPD patients	Treatment response (change in FEV1) to SABA (salbutamol)	Arg16 allele and and Arg16Gln27 haplotype were associated with decreased response	42

Notation: SABA—short-acting β-agonist; LABA—long-acting β-agonist; FEV1—forced expiratory volume in 1 s; PEF = peak expiratory flow.

At codon 27, patients homozygous for glutamine showed reduced treatment response compared to patients homozygous for glutamic acid [30,33,36]. The polymorphisms at codons 16 and 27 are in partial linkage disequilibrium in Western populations [31,33]. In addition to retrospective studies that suggest reduced treatment response after short-acting β2-agonist treatment in patients homozygous for argininine at position 16, the BARGE study [37], a large prospective clinical trial, investigated genotype-dependent differences in short-acting β2-agonist treatment response. This study confirmed that patients who were homozygous for arginine at position 16 did not benefit from treatment and suggested that patients with this genotype should discontinue β2-agonist therapy and use as-needed anticholinergics instead. However, a large multiethnic asthma case–control study showed no clear association between ADRB2 haplotypes and treatment response [35].

Studies on long-acting β2-agonists are consistent with studies on short-acting β2-agonists; they also demonstrate a reduced treatment response in arginine carriers at position 16 [32,38]. In contrast to this and earlier described studies on short acting β2-agonist treatment response, a study by Bleecker et al. showed no pharmacogenetic effect of ADRB2 variation on long-acting β2-agonist therapeutic response (severe asthma exacerbations and secondary endpoints such as lung function, use of as-needed medication, and nights with interrupted sleep) in asthma [25]. Another study that analyzed the effect of ADRB2 genotype on salmeterol response (determined by lung function, use of as-needed medication, and asthma symptoms) confirmed these results [39].

Few studies have focused on therapeutic responses to β2-agonist treatment in COPD patients. Its results are conflicting; some studies could not demonstrate an association between ADRB2 genotype and effect on lung function or immediate bronchodilator response of treatment with β2-agonists in COPD patients [40,41], while in another study, patients with an arginine allele at codon 16 showed reduced response to treatment with β2-agonists [42].

There are also polymorphisms discovered within the promoter region of the ADRB2 gene, which may have the potential to alter ADRB2 gene expression and therefore change the level of receptor expression at the cell surface [43]. Promoter region ADRB2 haplotypes alter receptor expression and can therefore influence therapeutic efficacy [36].

Only a few studies have been performed to assess the effect of polymorphisms in other genes in the β-agonist pathway on treatment response. However, because asthma is a complex disorder and response phenotypes to inhaled β2-agonists are also complex, it is plausible that genes other than the ADRB2 may also play a role in treatment response [44]. Tantisira et. al. [45] showed that a polymorphism in the AC9 gene (adenylylcyclase 9), which plays a role in the β-agonist pathway, is associated with a different treatment response to β2-agonist use under conditions of cortico-steroid exposure. Furthermore, polymorphisms in the arginase 1 gene (ARG1), which is involved in the regulation of airway function by regulating the production of nitric oxide [46], were associated with bronchodilator response [47].

Research has highlighted associations between polymorphisms in genes involved in the β-agonist pathway. The β2-receptor is the most studied target in this pathway and has genetic polymorphisms that are of functional importance. Particularly the two common polymorphisms at codons 16 and 27 in the β2-receptor are important in β2-agonist response in asthmatics, because they have shown functional effects and are quite common. In contrast to asthma patients, ADRB2 gene polymorphisms are not well studied in COPD patients. So far, it seems unclear whether polymorphisms in the ADRB2 gene influence treatment response in COPD. More studies are needed in this area. Future research should also focus on other genes involved in the β-agonist pathway that may influence drug response. Furthermore, the study of haplotypes and multiple genes instead of single polymorphisms will contribute to a better prediction of treatment response in individuals using β2-agonists.

9.4.2 Corticosteroids

Inhaled corticosteroids are the basis of the maintenance therapy for asthma and are used to reduce clinical symptoms and to improve lung function [5,6]. Oral corticosteroids may be prescribed when inhaled corticosteroids fail to control symptoms. The most important effect of corticosteroids is to switch off a variety of inflammatory genes (encoding cytokines, inflammatory enzymes, receptors, and proteins) that have been activated during the inflammation process [48,49]. Furthermore, they induce gene transcription, resulting in secretion of antiinflammatory proteins. Corticosteroids may also interact with recognition sites of activated inflammatory genes to inhibit transcription. Corticosteroids also have effects on signal transduction pathways through increased transcription of inhibitors of these pathways or repression of critical enzymes [48–50].

Corticosteroids bind to the cytoplasmic glucocorticoid receptors (GRs) in the cytoplasm. GRs are bound to chaperone proteins which protect the receptor. The human GR is encoded by a single gene, of which several variants are known as a result of alternative transcript splicing and alternative translation. GRα binds corticosteroids, and the GRβ variant binds to DNA but cannot be activated by corticosteroids. When corticosteroids have bound to GRs, changes in structure of the receptor result in dissociation of the chaperone proteins and exposition of nuclear localisation signals on the GR. This results in transport of the activated GR–corticosteroid complex into the nucleus, where it binds to DNA of corticosteroid responsive genes known as *glucocorticoid response elements* (GREs) leading to changes in gene transcriptions [48,49]. Between 10 and 100 genes are assumed to be directly regulated by the glucocorticoid receptor, and many other genes are indirectly regulated through an interaction between the glucocorticoid receptor and transcription factors and coactivators. Corticosteroids have complex effects on multiple signal transduction pathways. The major effect of corticosteroids is to inhibit the synthesis of inflammatory cells and proteins by suppressing the genes that encode them. Besides switching off inflammatory genes, corticosteroids switch on genes that have antiinflammatory effects [48,49].

Corticotrophin releasing hormone (CRH) and related hormones regulate the release of glucocorticoids via the hypothalamic pituitary adrenal (HPA) axis. The HPA axis sets the level of circulating glucocorticoid in the (human) body. CRH regulates adrenocorticotropin (ACTH) secretion, which stimulates adrenal glucocorticoid secretion. Corticotropin releasing hormone receptor type 1 (CRHR1) and the homologous receptor type 2 (CRHR2) are the two receptors that mediate biological activity in this pathway. CRHR1, a major regulator of glucocorticoid synthesis, has been implicated in the pathogenesis of asthma. Absence of CRH results in a decreased production of endogenous glucocorticoids and an increase in allergen-induced airway inflammation and lung dysfunction [10]. Defects in CRHR1 could cause a similar increase because of insufficient glucocorticoid production, resulting in an increased response to exogenous glucocorticoids.

A considerable number of pharmacogenetic studies have been performed to study differences in treatment response after corticosteroid use (Table 9.3). Most studies focused on polymorphisms that alter the glucocorticoid receptor itself and the CRHR1 gene, which is involved in the CRF pathway. The human glucocorticoid receptor (NR3C1) gene is located on chromosome 5q31, and several polymorphisms have been described [51–54].

Several studies showed associations between GR polymorphisms and altered corticosteroid response, although results are not always consistent [53]. A three-point haplotype within intron B is associated with enhanced sensitivity to corticosteroids [55]. In contrast, an aminoacid substitution (isoleucine for valine) at codon 729 impairs the function of the GR and is likely a cause of cortisol resistance [56]. Furthermore, an aminoacid substitution at position 641 (valine for aspartic acid) results in lower binding affinity of the GR receptor and therefore imparts glucocorticoid resistance [57]. There is also evidence that the BclI polymorphism is associated with response to corticosteroids [58].

Variation in the CRHR1 gene is associated with enhanced response to therapy. CRHR1 plays a very important role in steroid biology. It exerts antiinflammatory effects through the mediation of ACTH release, which regulates endogenous cortisol levels, which underlie antiinflammatory effects and furthermore direct proinflammatory effects through mast cell degranulation. Polymorphisms in this gene might therefore affect airway inflammation and treatment effects of corticosteroids. Indeed, multiple polymorphisms in the CRHR1 gene have been shown to be associated with treatment response. Individuals homozygous for the variant gene (a haplotype called GAT) manifested an enhanced lung function (FEV1) response to corticosteroids compared to wild-type carriers [59,60]. However, results are not consistent with another study finding no association between CRHR1 variants and treatment response (FEV1) [61].

Other genes may also be relevant in corticosteroid pharmacogenetics. Variation in the TBX21 gene, which influences T lymphocyte development and has been implicated in asthma pathogenesis, is associated with improved response to corticosteroid therapy in asthmatic children [62]. Furthermore, variation in FCER2, the low-affinity IgE receptor gene, is also associated with response to steroid treatment [63].

The glucocorticoid receptor is part of a multiprotein complex that may be involved in the glucocorticoid resistance phenotype. Focus in future studies should be on these genes coding for proteins in the entire complex. Genes involved in the CRH pathway are candidates for pharmacogenetic studies, especially CRHR1 and CRHR2, which are major regulators of the pathway.

TABLE 9.3 Pharmacogenetic Studies Performed on Corticosteroids

Gene	Variant	Population	Outcome	Association	Reference
NR3C1	R477H, G679S	12 patients with primary cortisol resistance	Transactivating capacity, ligand binding capacity	Both variant NR3C1 genotypes caused impaired receptor function	52
NR3C1	S651F, T504S, 2314insA	DNA from 88 allergic patients and cell lines from 73 different individuals	mRNA and protein expression levels, transcriptional activity and inhibition of NFkB transactivation	S651F and 2314insA NR3C1 variant were associated with altered protein and mRNA expression levels, reduced transcriptional activity, and reduction of NFkB transactivation and were suggested to influence glucocorticosteroid response	54
NR3C1	Three-point haplotype within intron B	40 psoriasis patients and 76 controls	Dexamethasone suppression	NR3C1 haplotype within intron B was associated with enhanced sensitivity to glucocorticoids	55
NR3C1	Ile729Val	DNA from patient with primary cortisol resistance, mother and 2 healthy controls	Dexamathasone binding affinity	NR3C1 variant was associated with impaired receptor function	56
NR3C1	Val641Asp	DNA from 3 patients with familial glucocorticoid resistance	Dexamathasone binding affinity	NR3C1 variant was associated with impaired receptor function	57
NR3C1	BclI, N363S, ER22/23EK	119 IBD patients	Treatment response to glucocorticoids (corticosteroid withdrawal without need for steroids for at least 1 year)	NR3C1 variant genotype was associated with better response to corticosteroid treatment	58

MDR1	C3435T, G2677T	119 IBD patients	Treatment response to glucocorticoids (corticosteroid withdrawal without need for steroids for at least 1 year)	No association was found between variant MDR1 genotypes and response to corticosteroid treatment	58
CRHR1	rs242941 and haplotypes	470 asthmatics, 311 asthmatic children and 336 asthmatics	Treatment response to ICS (change in FEV1)	CRHR1 variant genotypes were associated with an enhanced response to corticosteroid treatment	59
CRHR1	rs1876828, rs242939, rs242941	470 asthmatics, 311 asthmatic children and 336 asthmatics	Treatment response to ICS (change in FEV1)	CRHR1 variant genotypes were associated with an enhanced response to corticosteroid treatment	60
CRHR1	rs1876828, rs242939, rs242941	281 asthmatics	Treatment response to ICS (change in FEV1)	CRHR1 polymorphisms were not associated with immediate or long-term improvement in lung function	61
TBX21	His33Glu	701 asthmatics	Treatment response to budesonide (improvement in PC20)	TBX21 Glu33 carriers showed improvement in airway responsiveness after budesonide use	62

Notation: FEV1—forced expiratory volume in 1 s; PC20—provocative concentration of metacholine causing a 20% fall in FEV1.

9.4.3 Leukotriene Antagonists

Leukotriene antagonists are used in the treatment of asthma to inhibit bronchoconstriction by interfering with the synthesis or action of the leukotrienes, lipid mediators that take part in the inflammatory response. Leukotrienes are important mediators in the pathophysiology of asthma; they are responsible for a variety of effects such as activation of inflammatory cells, increased mucus release, increased smooth-muscle cell contractility, and increased vascular endothelial cell permeability. Leukotrienes are products of the 5-lipoxygenase pathway of arachidonic acid metabolism [64]. They act by binding to specific receptors located on structural and inflammatory cells. Leukotrienes are synthesized from arachidonic acid via the action of 5-lipoxygenase (5LO) and 5-lipoxygenase activating protein (FLAP). Arachidonic acid is converted to 5-hydroperoxyeicosatetraenoic acid and subsequently to leukotriene A4 (LTA4) by a catalytic complex consisting of 5LO and FLAP. LTA4 is unstable and transformed to leukotriene B4 (LTB4), which is involved in eosinophil and neutrophil chemotaxis. In the presence of leukotriene C4 (LTC4) synthase, LTA4 is converted to LTC4. LTC4 is cleaved to form the active entity, leukotriene D4 (LTD4). Out of LTD4, leukotriene E4 (LTE4) is formed. LTC4, LTD4, and LTE4 are all known as *cysteinyl leukotrienes*, because they all contain a cysteine group. Leukotrienes act by binding to specific receptors. LTB4 binds to the leukotriene B4 receptor, and the cysteinyl leukotrienes bind to two receptors: cysteinyl leukotriene receptor 1 (CYSLT1) and 2 (CYSLT2). Stimulation of the CYSLT1 receptors leads to smooth-muscle contraction and stimulation of CYSLT2 leads to smooth muscle contraction and chemotaxis. There are two main pharmacological treatment strategies developed to inhibit leukotriene activity: (1) inhibition of 5-lipoxygenase, which results in a decreased leukotriene synthesis, and (2) antagonists to the CYSLT2 receptor to prevent cysteinyl leukotrienes from binding and inhibit activity [65].

Several studies showed that variation in genes in the leukotriene pathway can alter response to leukotriene antagonists, and polymorphisms have been identified in various genes in the pathway (Table 9.4). The most frequently studied genes are ALOX5 and LTC4S.

5-Lipoxygenase is coded by the ALOX5 gene that has a tandem repeat polymorphism within the transcription factor binding region of its promoter. A decreased treatment response to leukotriene inhibitors is seen in carriers of other than the 5-tandem-repeat allele in the ALOX5 promotor region [66–69]. However, a study by Lima et. al. [70] showed an increased response to leukotriene inhibitors in carriers of the mutant allele. These data suggest that the ALOX5 tandem repeat polymorphism may be an interesting pharmacogenetic locus. Polymorphisms in the LTC4S gene are also associated with treatment response. Several studies showed that the LTC4S A-444C polymorphism is associated with an improved response to treatment [70–73].

Besides polymorphisms in the ALOX5 and LTC4S genes, there are polymorphisms in other genes in the leukotriene pathway described that can influence treatment response. Polymorphisms in the multidrug resistance protein 1 (MRP1)

TABLE 9.4 Pharmacogenetic Studies Performed on Leukotriene Antagonists

Gene	Variant	Population	Phenotype	Outcome	Reference
ALOX5	Number of tandem Sp1 repeats	221 asthmatics	Treatment response to ABT761 (change in FEV1)	Variant ALOX5 genotypes were associated with decreased response to treatment	66
ALOX5	Number of tandem Sp1 repeats	61 asthmatics	Treatment response to montelukast (exacerbation rate, SABA use, change in FEV1)	5/5 and 5/4 ALOX5 genotypes were associated with improved treatment response	67
ALOX5	rs4987105, rs4986832	174 asthmatics	Treatment response to montelukast (change in PEF and FEV1)	Variant ALOX5 genotypes were associated with improved treatment response	68
ALOX5	Number of tandem Sp1 repeats, rs2115819, haplotypes	252 asthmatics	Treatment response to montelukast (exacerbation rate and change in FEV1)	Variant ALOX5 tandem repeat genotypes were associated with reduced risk of exacerbations; SNP rs2115819 was associated with increased FEV1; Haplotypes were associated with risk for exacerbations	70
CYSLT2	rs91227, rs192278	174 asthmatics	Treatment response to montelukast (change in PEF and FEV1)	Variant CYSLT2 genotypes were associated with improved treatment response	68
LTC4S	A444C polymorphism (rs730012)	252 asthmatics	Treatment response to montelukast (exacerbation rate and change in FEV1)	Variant LTC4S genotype was associated with reduced risk for exacerbations	70

(continued)

TABLE 9.4 (*Continued*)

Gene	Variant	Population	Phenotype	Outcome	Reference
LTC4S	A444C polymorphism	59 asthmatics	Treatment response to montelukast (asthma symptoms, SABA use, change in PEF)	Variant LTC4S genotype was associated with improved response to montelukast	71
LTC4S	A444C polymorphism	23 asthmatics	Treatment response to zafirlukast (change in FEV1, FVC and PEF)	Variant LTC4S genotypes were associated with increased treatment response	72
LTC4S	A444C polymorphism	50 asthmatics	Treatment response to pranlukast (change in FEV1)	Variant LTC4S genotypes were associated with increased treatment response	73
LTA4H	rs2660845	252 asthmatics	Treatment response to montelukast (exacerbation rate and change in FEV1)	Variant LTA4H genotype was associated with increased risk for exacerbations	70
MRP1	rs119774	252 asthmatics	Treatment response to montelukast (exacerbation rate and change in FEV1)	Variant MRP1 genotype was associated with increased response to treatment	70
IL13	–1512A/C, –1112C/T, +2044G/A and haplotypes	374 asthmatics and 242 controls	Treatment response to montelukast (change in FEV1)	Variant IL13 genotype and IL13 haplotypes were associated with improved response to treatment	74

Notation: FEV1—forced expiratory volume in 1 s; PEF—peak expiratory factor.

are associated with treatment response [70]. As discussed in Chapter 5, the MRP1 gene is highly polymorphic and a mutation in the last transmembrane part influences LTC4 transport and could therefore alter response to leukotriene inhibitors. Furthermore, CYSLT2 could be a plausible candidate gene in leukotriene inhibitor pharmacogenetic studies. CYSLT2 variants may enhance response to leukotriene inhibitors [68]. Pharmacogenetic associations are also found for LTA4H genes [70].

Genes other than those involved in the leukotriene pathway may also influence treatment response to leukotriene inhibitors. Several studies have shown associations for IL13 polymorphisms and polymorphisms in the TBXA2R gene (a negative regulator of LTC4) [74,75].

9.4.4 Anticholinergics

Cholinergic nerves are the major bronchoconstriction neural mechanism in the airways. They originate in the brainstem and pass down the vagus nerve to relay in local ganglia situated in the airway walls. From these ganglia, fibers connect to airway smooth muscle cells and submucosal glands. Stimulation of the vagus nerve results in acetylcholine release, which activates muscarinic receptors leading to bronchoconstriction and mucus secretion in the airways [76]. Anticholinergic drugs act by blocking muscarinic receptors and are known to be effective in the treatment of acute exacerbations in asthma and bronchodilation in COPD.

The muscarinic receptors are G-protein-coupled receptors like the $\beta 2$-receptor, with seven transmembrane spanning proteins. Anticholinergic therapy is directed toward muscarinic receptors within the lung. Three out of the five known muscarinic receptors—M1, M2, and—M3 are expressed in the lung [77]. M1 receptors in the airways are localized mainly to parasympathetic ganglia, and their stimulation acts to facilitate cholinergic neurotransmission. M2 receptors can be found on smooth-muscle cells within the airways. Acute stimulation of these receptors results in inhibition of adenylate cyclase activation via coupling to an inhibitory G protein, and this results in a decrease of the degree of cAMP-induced airway smooth-muscle relaxation. M3 receptors are found on airway smooth muscle and mucus glands; they mediate smooth-muscle contraction and mucus hypersecretion [78]. Polymorphic variations within the muscarinic M2 and M3 receptors could alter treatment response to anticholinergic agents used in asthma and COPD therapy.

The muscarinic M2 and M3 receptors were screened for genetic variation [79]. Two polymorphisms were found in the coding region of the M2 receptor that did not result in aminoacid substitutions. Another polymorphism was found in the untranslated region of this gene. In this study, no polymorphisms were found in the screened DNA samples for M3 receptor gene. Another study also showed variability in the M2 receptor gene [80]. But hitherto none of the detected polymorphisms in previous studies of pharmacogenetics on anticholinergic drugs have been shown to be clinically or functionally relevant. Therefore, it is unlikely that variation in the M2 and M3 receptor contributes to interindividual variation in response to anticholinergic drugs.

9.5 CHALLENGES IN ASTHMA AND COPD PHARMACOGENETICS

A considerable number of studies on asthma and COPD pharmacogenetics are retrospective assessment of clinical trials. In these trials the effect of genetic variation on treatment response is determined by measuring, for example, changes in lung function or differences in number of severe exacerbations between carriers of a polymorphism and wild-type carriers after (a few weeks) of $\beta 2$-agonist or corticosteroid use. These trials are limited in their ability to identify adverse drug effects and long-term treatment effects, due to their relatively small size and short duration. Therefore, well-designed case–control or cohort studies might be a better approach. The first step in developing better pharmacogenetic research strategies for case–control or cohort studies requires correct diagnosis of patients and an accurate definition of different disease phenotypes.

Correct diagnosis is a problem, especially in pediatric asthma patients below the age of 5 years, because they are not able to perform a lung function test and symptoms are often transient [5].

Furthermore, asthma and COPD are both very heterogeneous diseases with recurrent episodes of respiratory symptoms. This makes it difficult to distinguish different disease phenotypes and to define true endpoints. Asthma or COPD control (used as an endpoint for response to treatment) is defined as surrogate endpoints determined by a variety of clinical parameters, such as lung function measurement (FEV1, FVC, PEF), clinical symptoms (number of severe exacerbations, awakenings at night), and rescue medication use (SABA). This hampers the definition of responders and nonresponders to treatment. This is really a major challenge in asthma and COPD pharmacogenetics.

Moreover, in the asthma and COPD drug pathways multiple genes are involved, and it is unlikely that only one polymorphism in one gene causes an altered response to treatment. Multiple genes can be involved, and the eventual pharmacogenetic effect may be an addition of all these separate polymorphisms in different genes. Besides variation in genes in the anti-asthma pathway, polymorphisms in genes encoding drug metabolizing enzymes such as CYP enzymes may contribute to the differential response of patients to antiasthma drugs. CYP3A4 is involved in glucocorticoid, $\beta 2$-agonist, and leukotriene receptor antagonist metabolism [81–84]. Furthermore, CYP2C9 and CYP1A2 are suggested to be involved in asthma and COPD drug metabolism [85,86]. These multiple gene–drug interactions call for a different statistical approach; conventional methods are not sufficient to perform statistical analyses in these large genetic databases.

9.6 FUTURE DIRECTIONS

During the past few decades, the incidence of asthma and COPD has increased and this has led to an increase in medication use. Pharmacogenetics aims to maximise the benefit from drug therapy by prescribing only to patients in whom there is a high probability of efficacy without significant risk of adverse events. Many asthma and

COPD pharmacogenetic studies have been carried out. At present, however, the magnitude of effect of known polymorphisms in asthma and COPD treatment suggests that routine genotyping of all patients before treatment is unlikely to be clinically relevant and cost-effective. It is, however, possible when new data become available and novel therapies are developed, that knowledge of a patient's genotype will be necessary to optimize disease management. Some of the variation in treatment response can be explained by genetic factors, and with the decreasing cost of genotyping, in the future it may be cost-effective to screen individuals before starting therapy. Focus should be on children, in whom asthma is one of the most common chronic diseases [3], and antiasthmatic drugs are the most widely chronic used drugs in children [87]. Furthermore, in children the relation between genotype and phenotype (treatment response) is not biased to the same extent as in adults by environmental factors such as smoking or years of (possible) suboptimal drug use.

In conclusion, to reach the goal of individualized prescribing in asthma or COPD, more knowledge of genetic influences on drug response will be necessary. Expanding the research area using gene expression studies and genomewide association (GWA) scans promises to identify new loci that contribute to the variability in individual treatment response. Furthermore, not only focusing on genes but also expanding the research field to the molecular level will offer a better approach; differences in protein expression (proteomics) and transcription activity (transcriptomics) will add substantially to our knowledge. Furthermore, there is need for correct diagnosis (especially in children) and a good definition of response phenotypes (subtypes) and the development of new statistical methods for the integration and analysis of all these data (clinical diagnosis, genetic variation on DNA, RNA, and protein level). Together, this could lead to a more complete and realistic representation and could help us achieve the ultimate goal, that of individualised therapy.

REFERENCES

1. Masoli M, Fabian D, Holt S, Beasley R. The global burden of asthma: Executive summary of the GINA Dissemination Committee report. *Allergy* 2004; **59**(5):469–478.
2. Rabe KF, Hurd S, Anzueto A, Barnes PJ, Buist SA, Calverley P, et al. Global strategy for the diagnosis, management, and prevention of chronic obstructive pulmonary disease: GOLD executive summary. *Am. J. Respir. Crit. Care Med.* 2007; **176**(6):532–555.
3. Newacheck PW, Taylor WR. Childhood chronic illness: Prevalence, severity, and impact. *Am. J. Public Health* 1992; **82**(3):364–371.
4. Drazen JM, Silverman EK, Lee TH. Heterogeneity of therapeutic responses in asthma. *Br. Med. Bull.* 2000; **56**(4):1054–1070.
5. Duiverman EJ, Brackel HJ, Merkus PJ, Rottier BL, Brand PL. Guideline "treating asthma in children" for pediatric pulmonologists [2nd rev. ed.]. II. Medical treatment (in Dutch). *Ned. Tijdschr Geneeskd.* 2003; **147**(39):1909–1913.
6. Bindels PJE, van der Wouden JC, Ponsioen BP, Brand PL, Salome PL, van Hensbergen W, et al. NHG-Standaard Astma bij kinderen. *Huisarts Wetenschap* 2006; **49**(11):557–572.

7. Courtney AU, McCarter DF, Pollart SM. Childhood asthma: Treatment update. *Am. Fam. Physician* 2005; **71**(10):1959–1968.
8. Streetman DD, Bhatt-Mehta V, Johnson CE. Management of acute, severe asthma in children. *Ann. Pharmacother.* 2002; **36**(7–8):1249–1260.
9. Smeele IJM, van Weel C, van Schayck CP, van der Molen T, Thoonen BP, Schermer T, et al. NHG-Standaard COPD. *Huisarts Wetenschap* 2007; **50**(8):362–379.
10. Weiss ST, Litonjua AA, Lange C, Lazarus R, Liggett SB, Bleecker ER, et al. Overview of the pharmacogenetics of asthma treatment. *Pharmacogenomics J.* 2006; **6**(5):311–326.
11. Buist AS.Definitions. In Barnes PJ, Drazen J, Rennard S, Thomson NC, eds.: *Asthma and COPD*. London: Elsevier Science, 2002; pp. 3–6.
12. Mauad T, Dolhnikoff M. Pathologic similarities and differences between asthma and chronic obstructive pulmonary disease. *Curr. Opin. Pulm. Med.* 2008; **14**(1):31–38.
13. Falk JA, Minai OA, Mosenifar Z. Inhaled and systemic corticosteroids in chronic obstructive pulmonary disease. *Proc. Am. Thorac. Soc.* 2008; **5**(4):506–512.
14. Saha S, Siva R, Brightling CE, Pavord ID. COPD: An inhaled corticosteroid-resistant, oral corticosteroid-responsive condition. *Eur. Respir. J.* 2006; **27**(4):863–865.
15. Busse WW, Lemanske RF Jr. Asthma. *N. Engl. J. Med.* 2001; **344**(5):350–362.
16. Busse WW, Rosenwasser LJ. Mechanisms of asthma. *J. Allergy Clin. Immunol.* 2003; **111**(3 Suppl):S799–S804.
17. GINA report. Global strategy for asthma management and prevention (updated 2010). Available from `www.ginasthma.org`.
18. Barnes PJ. Chapter 254: Asthma. In: *Harrinson's Principles of Internal Medicine*, 18e. McGraw-Companies.
19. GOLD report. Global stratetegy for diagnosis, management and prevention of COPD (updated 2010). Available from `www.goldcopd.nl`.
20. Larj MJ, Bleecker ER. Therapeutic responses in asthma and COPD. *Corticosteroids. Chest* 2004; **126** (2 Suppl.): 138S–149S; discussion pp. 159S–161S.
21. Duiverman EJ, Jobsis Q, van Essen-Zandvliet EE, van Aalderen WM, de Jongste JC. Guideline "treating asthma in children" for pediatric pulmonologists (2nd rev. ed.). I. Diagnosis and prevention (in Dutch). *Ned. Tijdschr. Geneeskd.* 2003; **147**(39):1905–1908.
22. Sin DD, Man J, Sharpe H, Gan WQ, Man SF. Pharmacological management to reduce exacerbations in adults with asthma: A systematic review and meta-analysis. *JAMA* 2004; **292**(3):367–376.
23. Celli BR, Thomas NE, Anderson JA, Ferguson GT, Jenkins CR, Jones PW, et al. Effect of pharmacotherapy on rate of decline of lung function in chronic obstructive pulmonary disease: Results from the TORCH study. *Am. J. Respir. Crit. Care Med.* 2008; **178** (4):332–338.
24. Brodde OE, Leineweber K. Beta2-adrenoceptor gene polymorphisms. *Pharmacogenet. Genomics* 2005; **15**(5):267–275.
25. Bleecker ER, Postma DS, Lawrance RM, Meyers DA, Ambrose HJ, Goldman M. Effect of ADRB2 polymorphisms on response to longacting beta2-agonist therapy: A pharmacogenetic analysis of two randomised studies. *Lancet* 2007; **370**(9605):2118–2125.
26. Hall IP, Blakey JD, Al Balushi KA, Wheatley A, Sayers I, Pembrey ME, et al. Beta2-adrenoceptor polymorphisms and asthma from childhood to middle age in the British 1958 birth cohort: A genetic association study. *Lancet* 2006; **368**(9537):771–779.

27. Green SA, Turki J, Hall IP, Liggett SB. Implications of genetic variability of human beta 2-adrenergic receptor structure. *Pulm. Pharmacol.* 1995; **8**(1):1–10.

28. Migita O, Noguchi E, Jian Z, Shibasaki M, Migita T, Ichikawa K, et al. ADRB2 polymorphisms and asthma susceptibility: Transmission disequilibrium test and meta-analysis. *Int. Arch. Allergy Immunol.* 2004; **134**(2):150–157.

29. Liggett SB. Polymorphisms of adrenergic receptors: Variations on a theme. *Assay Drug Devel. Technol.* 2003; **1**(2):317–326.

30. Cho SH, Oh SY, Bahn JW, Choi JY, Chang YS, Kim YK, et al. Association between bronchodilating response to short-acting beta-agonist and non-synonymous single-nucleotide polymorphisms of beta-adrenoceptor gene. *Clin. Exp. Allergy* 2005; **35** (9):1162–1167.

31. Martinez FD, Graves PE, Baldini M, Solomon S, Erickson R. Association between genetic polymorphisms of the beta2-adrenoceptor and response to albuterol in children with and without a history of wheezing. *J. Clin. Invest.* 1997; **100**(12):3184–3188.

32. Wechsler ME, Lehman E, Lazarus SC, Lemanske RF Jr, Boushey HA, Deykin A, et al. Beta-adrenergic receptor polymorphisms and response to salmeterol. *Am. J. Respir. Crit. Care Med.* 2006; **173**(5):519–526.

33. Tan S, Hall IP, Dewar J, Dow E, Lipworth B. Association between beta 2-adrenoceptor polymorphism and susceptibility to bronchodilator desensitisation in moderately severe stable asthmatics. *Lancet* 1997; **350**(9083):995–999.

34. Israel E, Drazen JM, Liggett SB, Boushey HA, Cherniack RM, Chinchilli VM, et al. Effect of polymorphism of the beta(2)-adrenergic receptor on response to regular use of albuterol in asthma. *Int. Arch. Allergy Immunol.* 2001; **124**(1-3): 183–186.

35. Hawkins GA, Tantisira K, Meyers DA, Ampleford EJ, Moore WC, Klanderman B, et al. Sequence, haplotype, and association analysis of ADRbeta2 in a multiethnic asthma case-control study. *Am. J. Respir. Crit. Care Med.* 2006; **174**(10):1101–1109.

36. Drysdale CM, McGraw DW, Stack CB, Stephens JC, Judson RS, Nandabalan K, et al. Complex promoter and coding region beta 2-adrenergic receptor haplotypes alter receptor expression and predict in vivo responsiveness. *Proc. Natl. Acad. Sci. USA* 2000; **97**(19):10483–10488.

37. Israel E, Chinchilli VM, Ford JG, Boushey HA, Cherniack R, Craig TJ, et al. Use of regularly scheduled albuterol treatment in asthma: Genotype-stratified, randomised, placebo-controlled cross-over trial. *Lancet* 2004; **364**(9444):1505–1512.

38. Lee DK, Currie GP, Hall IP, Lima JJ, Lipworth BJ. The arginine-16 beta2-adrenoceptor polymorphism predisposes to bronchoprotective subsensitivity in patients treated with formoterol and salmeterol. *Br. J. Clin. Pharmacol.* 2004; **57**(1):68–75.

39. Bleecker ER, Yancey SW, Baitinger LA, Edwards LD, Klotsman M, Anderson WH, et al. Salmeterol response is not affected by beta2-adrenergic receptor genotype in subjects with persistent asthma. *J. Allergy Clin. Immunol.* 2006; **118**(4):809–816.

40. Kim WJ, Oh YM, Sung J, Kim TH, Huh JW, Jung H, et al. Lung function response to 12-week treatment with combined inhalation of long-acting beta(2) agonist and glucocorticoid according to ADRB2 polymorphism in patients with chronic obstructive pulmonary disease. *Lung* 2008; **186**(6):381–386.

41. Mokry M, Joppa P, Slaba E, Zidzik J, Habalova V, Kluchova Z, et al. Beta2-adrenergic receptor haplotype and bronchodilator response to salbutamol in patients with acute exacerbations of COPD. *Med. Sci. Monit.* 2008; **14**(8):CR392–CR398.

42. Hizawa N, Makita H, Nasuhara Y, Betsuyaku T, Itoh Y, Nagai K, et al. Beta2-adrenergic receptor genetic polymorphisms and short-term bronchodilator responses in patients with COPD. *Chest* 2007; **132**(5):1485–1492.

43. Scott MG, Swan C, Wheatley AP, Hall IP. Identification of novel polymorphisms within the promoter region of the human beta2 adrenergic receptor gene. *Br. J. Pharmacol.* 1999; **126**(4):841–844.

44. Benovic JL. Novel beta2-adrenergic receptor signaling pathways. *J. Allergy Clin. Immunol.* 2002; **110** (6 Suppl.):S229–S235.

45. Tantisira KG, Small KM, Litonjua AA, Weiss ST, Liggett SB. Molecular properties and pharmacogenetics of a polymorphism of adenylyl cyclase type 9 in asthma: Interaction between beta-agonist and corticosteroid pathways. *Hum. Mol. Genet.* 2005; **14** (12):1671–1677.

46. Ricciardolo FL, Sterk PJ, Gaston B, Folkerts G. Nitric oxide in health and disease of the respiratory system. *Physiol. Rev.* 2004; **84**(3):731–765.

47. Litonjua AA, Lasky-Su J, Schneiter K, Tantisira KG, Lazarus R, Klanderman B, et al. ARG1 is a novel bronchodilator response gene: Screening and replication in four asthma cohorts. *Am. J. Respir. Crit. Care Med.* 2008; **178**(7):688–694.

48. Barnes PJ. Corticosteroid effects on cell signalling. *Eur. Respir. J.* 2006; **27**(2):413–426.

49. Payne DN, Adcock IM. Molecular mechanisms of corticosteroid actions. *Paediatr. Respir. Rev.* 2001; **2**(2):145–150.

50. Pelaia G, Vatrella A, Cuda G, Maselli R, Marsico SA. Molecular mechanisms of corticosteroid actions in chronic inflammatory airway diseases. *Life Sci.* 2003; **72**(14):1549–1561.

51. Bray PJ, Cotton RG. Variations of the human glucocorticoid receptor gene (NR3C1): Pathological and in vitro mutations and polymorphisms. *Hum. Mutat.* 2003; **21** (6):557–568.

52. Ruiz M, Lind U, Gafvels M, Eggertsen G, Carlstedt-Duke J, Nilsson L, et al. Characterization of two novel mutations in the glucocorticoid receptor gene in patients with primary cortisol resistance. *Clin. Endocrinol. (Oxford)* 2001; **55**(3):363–371.

53. Koper JW, Stolk RP, de Lange P, Huizenga NA, Molijn GJ, Pols HA, et al. Lack of association between five polymorphisms in the human glucocorticoid receptor gene and glucocorticoid resistance. *Hum. Genet.* 1997; **99**(5):663–668.

54. Koyano S, Saito Y, Nagano M, Maekawa K, Kikuchi Y, Murayama N, et al. Functional analysis of three genetic polymorphisms in the glucocorticoid receptor gene. *J. Pharmacol. Exp. Ther.* 2003; **307**(1):110–116.

55. Stevens A, Ray DW, Zeggini E, John S, Richards HL, Griffiths CE, et al. Glucocorticoid sensitivity is determined by a specific glucocorticoid receptor haplotype. *J. Clin. Endocrinol. Metab.* 2004; **89**(2):892–897.

56. Malchoff DM, Brufsky A, Reardon G, McDermott P, Javier EC, Bergh CH, et al. A mutation of the glucocorticoid receptor in primary cortisol resistance. *J. Clin. Invest.* 1993; **91**(5):1918–1925.

57. Hurley DM, Accili D, Stratakis CA, Karl M, Vamvakopoulos N, Rorer E, et al. Point mutation causing a single amino acid substitution in the hormone binding domain of the glucocorticoid receptor in familial glucocorticoid resistance. *J. Clin. Invest.* 1991; **87**(2):680–686.

58. De Iudicibus S, Stocco G, Martelossi S, Drigo I, Norbedo S, Lionetti P, et al. Association of BclI polymorphism of the glucocorticoid receptor gene locus with response to glucocorticoids in inflammatory bowel disease. *Gut* 2007; **56**(9):1319–1320.

59. Tantisira KG, Lake S, Silverman ES, Palmer LJ, Lazarus R, Silverman EK, et al. Corticosteroid pharmacogenetics: Association of sequence variants in CRHR1 with improved lung function in asthmatics treated with inhaled corticosteroids. *Hum. Mol. Genet.* 2004; **13**(13):1353–1359.

60. Weiss ST, Lake SL, Silverman ES, Silverman EK, Richter B, Drazen JM, et al. Asthma steroid pharmacogenetics: A study strategy to identify replicated treatment responses. *Proc. Am. Thorac. Soc.* 2004; **1**(4):364–367.

61. Dijkstra A, Koppelman GH, Vonk JM, Bruinenberg M, Schouten JP, Postma DS. Pharmacogenomics and outcome of asthma: No clinical application for long-term steroid effects by CRHR1 polymorphisms. *J. Allergy Clin. Immunol.* 2008; **121**(6):1510–1513.

62. Tantisira KG, Hwang ES, Raby BA, Silverman ES, Lake SL, Richter BG, et al. TBX21: A functional variant predicts improvement in asthma with the use of inhaled corticosteroids. *Proc. Natl. Acad. Sci. USA* 2004; **101**(52):18099–18104.

63. Tantisira KG, Silverman ES, Mariani TJ, Xu J, Richter BG, Klanderman BJ, et al. FCER2: A pharmacogenetic basis for severe exacerbations in children with asthma. *J. Allergy Clin. Immunol.* 2007; Dec; **120**(6):1285–91.

64. Peters-Golden M, Henderson WR. Leukotrienes. New Engl. *J. Med.* 2007; **357**:1841–1854.

65. Wechsler ME, Israel E. Pharmacogenetics of treatment with leukotriene modifiers. *Curr. Opin. Allergy Clin. Immunol.* 2002; **2**(5):395–401.

66. Drazen JM, Yandava CN, Dube L, Szczerback N, Hippensteel R, Pillari A, et al. Pharmacogenetic association between ALOX5 promoter genotype and the response to anti-asthma treatment. *Nat. Genet.* 1999; **22**(2):168–170.

67. Telleria JJ, Blanco-Quiros A, Varillas D, Armentia A, Fernandez-Carvajal I, Jesus Alonso M, et al. ALOX5 promoter genotype and response to montelukast in moderate persistent asthma. *Respir. Med.* 2008; **102**:857–861.

68. Klotsman M, York TP, Pillai SG, Vargas-Irwin C, Sharma SS, van den Oord EJ, et al. Pharmacogenetics of the 5-lipoxygenase biosynthetic pathway and variable clinical response to montelukast. *Pharmacogenet. Genomics* 2007; **17**(3):189–196.

69. Silverman E, Yandava C, Drazen JM, et al. Pharmacogenetics of the 5-lipoxygenase pathway in asthma. *Clin. Exp. Allergy* 1998; **28**(Suppl 5):*164–170; discussion* pp. 171–173.

70. Lima JJ, Zhang S, Grant A, Shao L, Tantisira KG, Allayee H, et al. Influence of leukotriene pathway polymorphisms on response to montelukast in asthma. *Am. J. Respir. Crit. Care Med.* 2006; **173**(4):379–385.

71. Mastalerz E, Nizankowska E, Sanak M, Mejza F, Pierzchalska M, Bazan-Socha S, et al. Clinical and genetic features underlying the response of patients with bronchial asthma to treatment with a leukotriene recpetor antagonist. *Eur. J. Clin. Invest.* 2002; **32**(12):949–955.

72. Sampson AP, Siddiqui S, Buchanan D, Howarth PH, Holgate ST, Holloway JW, et al. Variant LTC(4) synthase allele modifies cysteinyl leukotriene synthesis in eosinophils and predicts clinical response to zafirlukast. *Thorax* 2000; **55**(Suppl 2):S28–S31.

73. Asano K, Shiomi T, Hasegawa N, Nakamura H, Kudo H, Matsuzaki T, et al. Leukotriene C4 synthase gene A(-444)C polymorphism and clinical response to a CYS-LT(1) antagonist, pranlukast, in Japanese patients with moderate asthma. *Pharmacogenetics* 2002; **12**(7):565–570.

74. Kang MJ, Lee SY, Kim HB, Yu J, Kim BJ, Choi WA, et al. Association of IL-13 polymorphisms with leukotriene receptor antagonist drug responsiveness in Korean children with exercise-induced bronchoconstriction. *Pharmacogenet. Genomics* 2008; **18**(7):551–558.

75. Kim JH, Lee SY, Kim HB, Jin HS, Yu JH, Kim BJ, et al. TBXA2R gene polymorphism and responsiveness to leukotriene receptor antagonist in children with asthma. *Clin. Exp. Allergy* 2008; **38**(1):51–59.

76. Barnes PJ. Muscarinic receptor subtypes in airways. *Life Sci.* 1993; **52**(5-6): 521–527.

77. Joos L, Sandford AJ. Genotype predictors of response to asthma medications. *Curr. Opin. Pulm. Med.* 2002; **8**(1):9–15.

78. Fenech A, Hall IP. Pharmacogenetics of asthma. *Br. J. Clin. Pharmacol.* 2002; **53**(1):3–15.

79. Fenech AG, Ebejer MJ, Felice AE, Ellul-Micallef R, Hall IP. Mutation screening of the muscarinic M(2) and M(3) receptor genes in normal and asthmatic subjects. *Br. J. Pharmacol.* 2001; **133**(1):43–48.

80. Fenech AG, Billington CK, Swan C, Richards S, Hunter T, Ebejer MJ, et al. Novel polymorphisms influencing transcription of the human CHRM2 gene in airway smooth muscle. *Am. J. Respir. Cell. Mol. Biol.* 2004; **30**(5):678–686.

81. Pearce RE, Leeder JS, Kearns GL. Biotransformation of fluticasone: In vitro characterization. *Drug Metab. Dispos.* 2006; **34**(6):1035–1040.

82. Kuperman AV, Kalgutkar AS, Marfat A, Chambers RJ, Liston TE. Pharmacokinetics and metabolism of a cysteinyl leukotriene-1 receptor antagonist from the heterocyclic chromanol series in rats: In vitro-in vivo correlation, gender-related differences, isoform identification, and comparison with metabolism in human hepatic tissue. *Drug Metab. Dispos.* 2001; **29**(11):1403–1409.

83. Manchee GR, Eddershaw PJ, Ranshaw LE, Herriott D, Park GR, Bayliss MK, et al. The aliphatic oxidation of salmeterol to alpha-hydroxysalmeterol in human liver microsomes is catalyzed by CYP3A. *Drug Metab. Dispos.* 1996; **24**(5):555–559.

84. Jonsson G, Astrom A, Andersson P. Budesonide is metabolized by cytochrome P450 3A (CYP3A) enzymes in human liver. *Drug Metab. Dispos.* 1995; **23**(1):137–142.

85. Dekhuijzen PN, Koopmans P.P. Pharmacokinetic profile of zafirlukast. *Clin. Pharmacokinet.* 2002; **41**(2):105–114.

86. Obase Y, Shimoda T, Kawano T, Saeki S, Tomari SY, Mitsuta-Izaki K, et al. Polymorphisms in the CYP1A2 gene and theophylline metabolism in patients with asthma. *Clin. Pharmacol. Ther.* 2003; **73**(5):468–474.

87. Schirm E, van den Berg P, Gebben H, Sauer P, De Jong-van den Berg L. Drug use of children in the community assessed through pharmacy dispensing data. *Br. J. Clin. Pharmacol.* 2000; **50**(5):473–478.

CHAPTER 10

Pharmacogenetics of Adverse Drug Reactions

ANN K. DALY
Newcastle University, Newcastle upon Tyne, UK

MARTIN ARMSTRONG
Shire AG, Geneva, Switzerland

MUNIR PIRMOHAMED
University of Liverpool, Liverpool, UK

10.1 INTRODUCTION

The development of many potentially valuable drugs has to be discontinued during the later stages of the development process if evidence of idiosyncratic adverse reactions or serious adverse events emerges. There are also a number of important examples of licensed drugs that were withdrawn from the market following the emergence of serious, sometimes fatal, adverse events. Idiosyncratic reactions, often classified as type B adverse drug reactions (ADRs), which are not directly predictable from drug concentration (see Table 10.1) [1], are difficult to study because of their rarity, but their potentially very serious consequences for the patient makes them an important current research area in pharmacogenetics. The immune system, especially the products of class I and class II HLA genes, often contributes to idiosyncratic reactions, but this is not the case for all reactions of this type [2]. ADRs linked to drug concentration (type A reactions) are more common than idiosyncratic reactions and are also important clinically. This type of reaction is not discussed further in this chapter, but some examples are mentioned briefly in Chapters 2 and 3.

More recent developments in pharmacogenetics suggest that genotyping tests may be developed to identify individuals for whom certain medicines will be unsuitable because of susceptibility to idiosyncratic reactions. It is also hoped that such

Pharmacogenetics and Individualized Therapy, First Edition.
Edited by Anke-Hilse Maitland-van der Zee and Ann K. Daly.

TABLE 10.1 Characteristics of Type A and Type B Adverse Drug Reactions (ADRs)

Characteristics	Type A	Type B
Frequency	Common	Rare
Dose dependence	Generally dose-dependent	No simple relationship
Severity	Usually mild	Variable but often severe
Predictable from drug pharmacology	Yes	Seldom
Host factors (including genetics)	Often important and some clear genetic associations now identified	Likely to be important but current knowledge especially on genetics more limited

developments can be applied to the drug development process, although associations reported up to the present are generally quite drug-specific, and devising general strategies that can be used during drug development to detect potential for idiosyncratic toxicity still represents a considerable challenge.

As summarized in Table 10.2, there are a number of different types of idiosyncratic ADR. Usually particular drugs are associated with one class of toxicity, although there are some examples where more than one type of toxicity can occur with the same drug. Examples of commonly prescribed drugs linked to the different toxicities are also provided.

10.2 DRUG-INDUCED LIVER INJURY

10.2.1 Background

Drug-induced liver injury (DILI) is a rare but clinically important problem. A US study suggested that DILI accounted for 20% of all hospital admissions due to severe liver injury and 50% of acute liver failure cases, 75% of whom required a liver transplant [3]. DILI is also the most common cause of termination of clinical trials of new therapeutic agents [4]. Many different drugs can cause DILI, with the precise

TABLE 10.2 Common Idiosyncratic (Type B) ADRs

Type	Drug Examples
Drug-induced liver injury	Coamoxiclav, flucloxacillin, isoniazid
Drug-induced QT prolongation	Thioridazine, clarithromycin, terfenadine
Drug-induced hypersensitivity	Abacavir
Drug-induced muscle toxicity	Statins, chloroquine, penicillamine
Drug-induced serious skin rash	Carbamazepine

pattern of injury varying between drugs. Typically, DILI reactions are classified as *hepatocellular* when the injury is focused on the hepatocyte and *cholestatic* when the damage occurs at the hepatocyte canalicular membrane or further downstream in the biliary tree. The underlying mechanism by which DILI develops is likely to be complex but may involve (1) direct toxic effects by the drug, for example, involving oxidative stress or cellular damage, and, (2) for some drugs, formation of reactive intermediates resulting ultimately in an inappropriate immune response.

Pharmacogenetic studies on DILI have proved difficult for a number of reasons, including the range of drugs associated with toxicity, the number of different disease phenotypes, and the relative rarity of severe toxicity, which makes assembling sufficient individuals to perform well-powered genetic studies difficult. As with other adverse drug reactions, a number of different genes and environmental factors are likely to contribute. The genes involved may encode proteins with diverse cellular roles, including drug metabolism and transport, apoptosis, the acquired and innate immune responses, and cellular repair and regeneration. Candidates from several of these pathways have now been identified, and although the majority of published studies involve small numbers of cases, a few genetic associations have now been independently replicated. A summary of the best established associations is provided in Table 10.3.

TABLE 10.3 Gene Associations in Drug-Induced Liver Injury

Gene	Allele	Drug	Effect	Reference
ABCB11	Exon 13	Various	Increased incidence of cholestatic injury	32
ABCC2	C-24T	Diclofenac	Increased DILI incidence	25
ABCC2	G-1549A/ C-24T	Various	Increased incidence of hepatocellular injury	34
CYP2E1	*5, *1B	Isoniazid	Increased DILI incidence	22,32
GSTM1	Null	Tacrine	Unclear	26,27
GSTM1	Null	Troglitazone	Increased DILI incidence	100
GSTT1	Null	Tacrine	Unclear	28
GSTT1	Null	Troglitazone	Increased DILI incidence	100
HLA-DRB1	*15	Coamoxiclav	Increased DILI incidence	5–7
	*07	Ximelagatran	Increased incidence of elevated ALT	12
HLA-B	*5701	Flucloxacillin	Increased incidence of cholestatic injury	10
HLA-A	*3303	Ticlopidine	Increased incidence of cholestatic injury	13
NAT2	Slow	Isoniazid	Increased DILI incidence	17–22
SOD2	C47T	Various	Increased incidence of hepatocellular injury	35
UGT1A	Various	Tolcapone	Increased DILI incidence	24
UGT2B7	*2	Diclofenac	Increased DILI incidence	25

10.2.2 HLA Associations in DILI

Although the extent of the immune component in DILI is still not completely clear, a number of associations with particular HLA genotypes have now been reported. HLA molecules play a central role in presentation of antigens (usually peptides from infectious agents) to T lymphocytes and are therefore biologically plausible candidates in determining genetic susceptibility to DILI. HLA class I molecules are expressed on many different cell types and are particularly important in CD8-positive cytotoxic T cell responses, whereas the expression of HLA class II molecules is mainly on antigen-presenting cells where they are important in CD4-positive T helper cell responses. HLA class I and II genes are subject to extensive polymorphism and are located in the MHC region on chromosome 6. This region is subject to strong linkage disequilibrium resulting in a series of common haplotypes including specific class I and II genes.

Initial reports of possible HLA associations with DILI appeared during the 1980s in relation to injury associated with nitrofurantoin, halothane, and clometacin but none were statistically significant, possibly due to small numbers of cases being studied. More recently, two separate studies considered the relationship between HLA class II genotype and susceptibility to co-amoxiclav-induced liver injury [5,6]. Both studies described an association with the HLA *DRB1**1501* allele. These findings were highly significant despite small numbers in both patient groups. A more recent study involving more cases has confirmed the *DRB1**1501* association [7]; a separate study of Spanish patients failed to find a significant increase in the *DRB1**1501* allele, but did report a significantly higher frequency of another class II allele, *DQB1**06* [8]. This may reflect the fact that *DRB1**1501* is less common in Spain than in northern Europe.

Flucloxacillin is used widely in Europe and Australia in the treatment of staphylococcal infections. Its use has been associated with characteristic cholestatic hepatitis, which appears to be more common in females, in the elderly, and after prolonged courses of treatment [9]. Until recently, no studies had been reported on genetic susceptibility to this form of DILI, but candidate gene and genomewide association studies (GWAS) have been performed on a UK cohort. Using both approaches (see GWAS profile in Fig. 10.1), a strong class I HLA association was detected with possession of the HLA-*B**5701* allele associated with an 80-fold increased risk of disease development [10]. This finding was replicated in a small additional cohort. The *B**5701* association has also been reported for another adverse drug reaction, abacavir-related hypersensitivity[11] (see Section 10.5.2), but has not been previously associated with DILI. The genomewide association study also suggested that a second non-HLA gene with a possible role in B cell immune responses also contributed to flucloxacillin toxicity but not as strongly as did *B**5701* [10].

Two other HLA associations with liver toxicity have also been described. One of these relates to the drug ximelagatran, which was found to be linked to liver toxicity in some patients during its development. From both GWAS and candidate gene studies with additional replication, liver toxicity with this drug appears to be

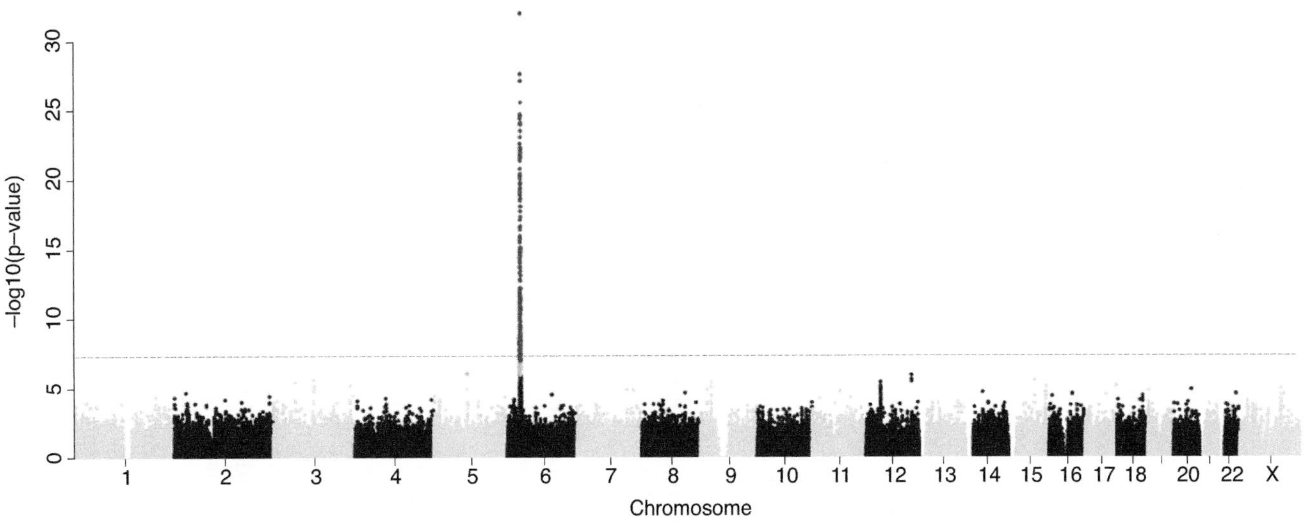

FIGURE 10.1 Genomewide association study on flucloxacillin-induced liver injury. This Manhattan plot of chromosomal location against −log p value indicates that a number of polymorphisms in the MHC region show genomewide significance. The polymorphism (rs2395029) showing the most significant difference in frequency between cases and controls is in complete linkage disequilibrium with the HLA class I *HLA-B*5701* allele. (Reproduced with permission from Daly et al. [10]). (See insert for color representation.)

associated with the class II HLA allele *DRB1*0701* [12]. This allele is more common among Europeans than in East Asians, and the liver toxicity was also more common in Europe than in Asia. On the other hand, hepatotoxicity with ticlopidine appears to be more common among Japanese patients than Europeans, and it has been shown that this is due in part to an association with *HLA-A*3303*, a class I HLA allele seen predominantly in East Asian populations [13].

These findings of HLA associations that seem to be drug-specific point to an important role for T cell responses, possibly to drug complexed with peptides, in the toxicity process. The fact that DILI typically develops several weeks after the start of drug treatment is consistent with this immune component, but it is likely that other factors also contribute and that not all DILI relates to HLA genotype.

10.2.3 Metabolic and Transporter Genes

The most widely investigated genes in relation to susceptibility to DILI are those encoding proteins that contribute to drug disposition, including cytochrome P450 genes, various genes affecting phase II metabolism such as UDP glucuronosyltransferases and drug transporters (for background on these genes, see Chapters 3–5).

The possible association that has been studied most widely relates to the antituberculosis drug isoniazid and the gene encoding *N*-acetyltransferase 2 (NAT2). The reasons why this has received the most attention include the facts that (1) isoniazid is an old drug compared with many of the other currently prescribed drugs known to be hepatotoxic, (2) metabolism by NAT2 is a major pathway of isoniazid metabolism, (3) isoniazid-induced injury is relatively common (possibly affecting up to 3% of patients [14]) compared with other drug toxicities, and (4) a functionally significant polymorphism in NAT2 that leads to absence of activity in approximately 50% of the population is well understood (see Chapter 4). Despite these observations, the relationship between NAT2 genotype and susceptibility to isoniazid-induced DILI remains rather unclear.

It has generally been proposed that the metabolite responsible for isoniazid-related DILI is acetylhydrazine, which can undergo further metabolism by cytochrome P450 to a toxic metabolite or by NAT2 to the less toxic diacetylhydrazine. It has been hypothesised that rapid acetylators (those with NAT2 activity in the normal range) will form diacetylhydrazine efficiently and therefore will have low levels of both acetylhydrazine and the toxic P450 metabolites [15]. It has also been suggested that slow acetylators (those with NAT2 deficiency) may form higher concentrations of hydrazine, another toxic compound, by cleavage of the amide bond on isoniazid to form isonicotinic acid [16]. There have been at least six published studies on isoniazid toxicity and *NAT2* genotype. Five of these studies showed an increased risk of DILI in slow acetylators, although this increase in risk was generally quite small and would explain only a small proportion of the total risk [17–21]. The sixth, a large study based in Europe, showed no effect [22].

Genes encoding cytochrome P450 enzymes have been relatively well studied as candidate genes for DILI because of the key role of these enzymes in oxidative metabolism of drugs and their ability to form reactive intermediates. However, overall, the effect of P450 on DILI susceptibility seems limited, with the main example relating to CYP2E1 and isoniazid hepatotoxicity. CYP2E1 is believed to activate acetylhydrazine, forming various hepatotoxins. Although genetic polymorphism in CYP2E1 is well studied and there is evidence that CYP2E1 levels show considerable interindividual variation, the precise effect of individual noncoding polymorphisms remains rather unclear and published studies on whether they are risk factors for DILI are contradictory [22,23].

Phase II metabolism by enzymes such as the UDP glucuronosyltransferases is generally considered to be detoxicating, although they also play roles in the formation of reactive intermediates such as acylglucuronides, which may be very relevant to DILI. In a study on tolcapone, a selective catechol-*O*-methyltransferase inhibitor, which was associated with DILI in some patients during the development process, it was found that polymorphisms in the main metabolizing enzyme UGT1A6 were significantly associated with elevated transaminase levels [24]. This finding suggested that toxicity might be linked to slow metabolism of the parent drug. In a study on the role of another UDP-glucuronosyltransferase gene UGT2B7 in susceptibility to diclofenac-induced DILI, possession of the variant *UGT2B7*2*, which is believed to be associated with higher glucuronidating activity, was associated with a significantly increased risk of toxicity [25]. This effect may be due to increased hepatic levels of the toxic diclofenac acylglucuronide, which may form covalent adducts with proteins.

The glutathione *S*-transferases (GSTs) are another family of phase II enzymes that conjugate a number of drugs implicated in hepatotoxicity. In addition, some GSTs have a role in the metabolism of toxic compounds generated when reactive-oxygen species are formed and could therefore have a more general role in protecting against DILI. The GSTM1 and GSTT1 genes are subject to common deletion polymorphisms that lead to complete absence of activity. Tacrine, a cholinesterase inhibitor, was one of the first drugs developed for Alzheimer's disease treatment, but its use was commonly associated with mild DILI. Two separate studies investigating whether GSTT1 or GSTM1-null patients were more susceptible to this problem have been performed, both on European populations. One of these found a significantly higher than expected frequency of patients null for both alleles [26], but the other failed to find any genetic association [27,28]. The reason for the discrepancy remains unclear, but a problem with the association is that there is no definitive evidence that tacrine or its metabolites are subject to conjugation by GST [29]. Troglitazone is a more recent example of a drug found to give rise to rare but serious DILI, which resulted in its withdrawal from the market. The genetic basis for this is still very unclear, but a study of 25 patients who had suffered liver toxicity with the drug reported a significantly increased frequency of the double null GSTM1-GSTT1 genotype. No associations were seen with 49 other candidate genes tested.

Drug transporter genes of the ABC transporter superfamily are biologically plausible candidates for a role in DILI susceptibility, especially because some ABC transporter family gene products transport bile acids in addition to drugs [30]. Also, some inherited forms of cholestasis have been demonstrated to result from specific mutations in the ABCB4 (MDR3) and ABCB11 (BSEP) genes [31]. In a study on patients who had suffered DILI related to a range of different drugs, an association between cholestatic injury and a polymorphism in exon 13 of ABCB11 that had previously been deemed associated with cholestasis of pregnancy was reported [32]. Overall, this polymorphism does not appear to be a major risk factor for cholestatic disease as it is quite common and the effect on disease risk is small, but the possibility of a larger association with individual causative drugs warrants further investigation.

The ABC transporters are also important in the biliary excretion of drugs generally and their metabolites. ABCC2 (MRP2) has a major role in the biliary excretion of a variety of glucuronide conjugates. In the study on diclofenac hepatotoxicity discussed above in the section on UDP glucuronosyltransferases, carriage of an upstream polymorphism in ABCC2 (C-24T) was more common among hepatotoxicity cases [25]. This finding is consistent with the association between higher UGT2B7 activity leading to increased levels of the reactive diclofenac acylglucuronide since there is evidence that C-24T results in lower expression of the MRP2 protein, which would favor cellular accumulation of the glucuronide [33,34]. In a Korean study on DILI caused by a range of drugs, a polymorphism at position −1549 of ABCC2 in linkage disequilibrium with C-24T was a significant risk factor for the development of hepatocellular toxicity [34]. These findings are in broad agreement with the data on diclofenac toxicity, although the lower level of statistical significance in the Korean study may reflect the fact that the DILI was due to a number of drugs, some of which may not be relevant to ABCC2.

10.2.4 Oxidative Stress Genes

Some individuals may have a poorer ability to deal with reactive-oxygen species generated from prescribed drugs, due to polymorphisms in genes encoding the relevant detoxicating enzymes. The resulting cellular damage could give rise to DILI. The relationship between genotype and susceptibility to DILI for enzymes that protect cells against reactive oxygen species has not been investigated in detail. However, in one 2007 study, a common polymorphism in the *SOD2* gene, which encodes the mitochondrial protein MnSOD, was found to be a predictor of hepatocellular damage, particularly that related to antituberculosis drugs, but also in relation to other drugs [35]. Unexpectedly, the association between DILI and *SOD2* genotype was with an allele predicted to be associated with higher MnSOD activity. The authors suggested that this finding might reflect the fact that the byproduct of MnSOD activity, hydrogen peroxide, is also toxic in addition to the superoxide substrate [35].

10.3 DRUG-INDUCED QT INTERVAL PROLONGATION

The cardiac depolarization–repolarization cycle, as measured on a surface electrocardiogram, is depicted in Figure 10.2a,b. Of particular relevance to the subject of drug-induced ADRs is the feature annotated as the "QT interval." Measured from the

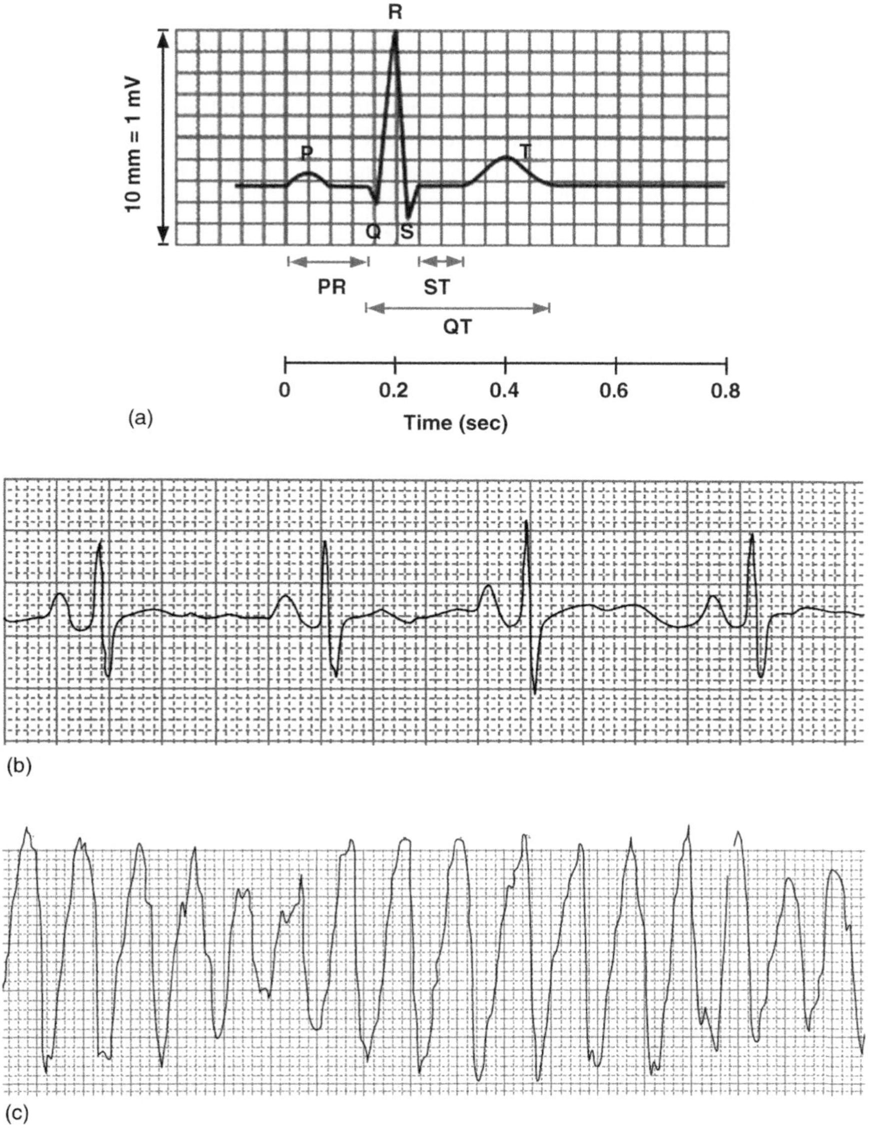

FIGURE 10.2 (a) Diagrammatic representation of normal sinus rhythm for a human heart as seen on an electrocardiogram (ECG), (b) ECG trace of a subject during normal sinus rhythm; (c) ECG trace of a subject during torsades de pointes episode.

beginning of the QRS complex to end of the T wave, the QT interval represents the time it takes for one complete cycle of ventricular depolarization and repolarization. While there is a normal distribution of QT intervals within a population, generally in the range of 200–480 ms, there are specific familial syndromes, termed *congenital long QT syndrome* (cLQTS) and clinical situations, termed *acquired long QT* (aLQT), in which the interval can become excessively prolonged (generally accepted as being >550 ms). In these circumstances ventricular myocytes continue progression through further phases of depolarization before repolarization is complete. This sets up the potential for the cardiac cycle to degenerate into ventricular tachycardia, of which *Torsade des pointes* (TdP) is that most classically associated with QT prolongation (Fig. 10.2c). While this ventricular arrhythmia can self-terminate, it also has the potential to degenerate into potentially fatal arrhythmias such as ventricular fibrillation.

Genetic analysis has shed light on some of the underlying mechanisms of QT prolongation, particularly in the rare monogenic arrhythmia syndromes characteristic of cLQT, where analyses of multiply affected family members have identified a number of associated genes (Table 10.4). Presently around 80% of affected families link to one of these genes, suggesting that other genes or/mechanisms remain to be determined [36].

Despite increasing regulatory requirements and more stringent preclinical and clinical cardiac toxicity screening strategies and monitoring, drug-induced arrhythmias related to excessive QT prolongation have been the single leading cause of drug withdrawal or restriction of use since the 1990s [37]. It is worth noting that QT prolongation itself is an imperfect surrogate biomarker for the arrhythmic potential of a drug, with many drugs prolonging the QT interval but not progressing to arrhythmia. Nevertheless, until better biomarkers are identified and validated, QT prolongation remains the accepted regulatory biomarker for arrhythmia.

Drugs from multiple classes are known to cause QT prolongation, and certain risk factors have been associated with the event (e.g., gender, preexisting heart disease, electrolyte disturbances) [38]. As with other idiosyncratic ADRs the reasons why only some individuals experience these events remains incompletely understood, although the supposition is that individual genetic variation and its interaction with the drug and the environment may play a role in determining individual susceptibility.

Because of the similarities in phenotype and the low penetrance of mutant alleles associated with cLQT, it was hypothesised that individuals presenting with aLQT may carry clinically in-apparent mutations within the cLQT genes [39]. Under normal circumstances these individuals are asymptomatic, presenting with no clinical features of QT prolongation and, potentially, QT intervals within the normal ranges. It is proposed that pharmacological challenge with trigger drugs may unmask reduced repolarization reserves, or that the variant ion channels themselves may be more sensitive to pharmacological blockade, rendering individuals more susceptible to QT prolongation and arrhythmia.

Individual case studies have appeared that support these hypothesis and have led to the study of cLQT genes in "larger" aLQT cohorts (see Table 10.5) [40,41]. Despite the limitations of these studies (related mostly to heterogeneous sample sets of cases triggered by multiple drugs, thereby assuming a common underlying mechanism across drug classes; small sample sizes; varying screening strategies and case ascertainment), these studies indicate that 5–12% of aLQT cases carry mutations in one of their cLQT genes [41].

TABLE 10.4 Genes Shown to be Associated with cLQT

Disease Subtype	Gene	Protein	Function	Ion Current Affected	Reference:
LQTS1	KCNQ1	KvLQT1	Principal subunit of the cardiac, voltage-activated potassium channel I_{Ks}	Potassium, I_{Ks}	100
LQTS2	KCNH2	HERG	Principal subunit of the cardiac voltage-activated K^+ channel I_{Kr}	Potassium, I_{Kr}	101
LQTS3	SCN5A	Nav1.5	Pore-forming subunit of the cardiac sodium channel, I_{Na}.	Sodium, I_{Na}	102
LQTS4	ANK2	Ankyrin B	Adapter protein, linking integral membrane proteins to spectrin-based cytoskeleton	Sodium, potassium and calcium	103
LQTS5	KCNE1	MinK, Isk	Auxillary subunit, co-assembles with KCNQ1 to form I_{Ks}	Potassium, IKs	104
LQTS6	KCNE2	MiRP1	Auxiliary subunit of Kv or eag channels; co-assembles with HERG to form I_{Kr}; other α partners are Kv4.2, HCN	Potassium, I_{Kr}	105
LQTS7	KCNJ2	Kir2.1, IRK1	Inward rectifier potassium (K^+) channel, I_{K1}/Kir2.1	Potassium, I_{K1}	106
LQTS8	CACNA1C	Cav1.2	Cardiac L-type calcium channel	Calcium, $I_{Ca\text{-}L\alpha}$	107
LQTS9	C_{AV3}	Calveolin 3	Muscle-specific protein and major component of calveolae	Sodium, I_{Na}	108
LQTS10	SCN4B	Nav β4	β_4 auxiliary subunit of the I_{Na} sodium channel	Sodium, I_{Na}	109
LQTS11	AKAP9	AKAP9/yotiao	The α-kinase anchoring protein	Potassium, I_{Ks}	110
LQTS12	SNTA1	α1-syntrophin	A dystrophin-associated cytoskeletal protein	Sodium, I_{Na}	111

TABLE 10.5 Number of aLQTS Patients in Whom a Disease Associated Mutation was Detected by Screening of cLQT Genes

Genes Screened	Abbott et al. [105]	Sesti et al. [112], Yang et al. [113]	Chevalier et al. [114]	Paulussen et al. [41]
ANKB (ankyrin B)	NS[a]	NS	NS	NS
KCNE1 (mink)	NS	0	0	2
KCNE2 (MiRP1)	1	4	0	1
KCNH2 (HERG)	NS	1	1	1
KCNQ1 (KvLQT1)	NS	1	0	0
SCN5A (SCN5A)	NS	3	NS	0
Number of aLQTS patients screened	20	92	16	32
Number of cases explained	1	9	1	4
Percentage of investigated aLQTS patient population	5	9	6	12

[a]Not studied.
Source: Adapted from Paulussen et al. [41].

These studies also indicate that there are factors beyond SNPs in the cLQT genes that are responsible for determining individual susceptibility to aLQT. While factors other than genetics will certainly be involved, these studies were limited in their selection of candidate genes by the level of information available at the time.

Whereas the original genetic studies focused on families presenting with rare monogenic arrhythmia syndromes, the emergence of whole-genome analysis technologies has allowed the exploration of the role of more common DNA variants in unrelated general populations showing variance in QT intervals. These studies have identified additional genes that are implicated in determining QT interval, and while the biological plausibility of some of these genes is apparent from their known ontology and biological function, the role of other genes in the cardiac cycle remains unclear [42,43]. Nevertheless, there is emerging evidence that this approach could have some utility since it has already been used to identify a variant in the *KCR1* gene as a potential modulator of risk of drug-induced TdP [44]. Future work on aLQT cases should include the expansion of gene lists to include these candidates.

For drugs with QT prolonging liabilities, their ability to elicit this response is increased at higher plasma concentrations. Therefore any factors impacting drug exposure could influence susceptibility to QT prolongation, including drug–drug interactions, inappropriate dosing, and genetic variability in drug metabolising enzymes. Thioridazine is an antipsychotic that has a QT liability and is metabolized by the polymorphic cytochrome P450 CYP2D6 [45]. With 5–10% of Caucasian populations genetically determined to be CYP2D6-poor metabolisers, the FDA has included labeling warnings for an increased risk of TdP in this subgroup (http://www.fda.gov/Drugs/ScienceResearch/ResearchAreas/Pharmacogenetics/ucm116034.htm). Thus genes influencing drug exposure should be assessed as additional risk factors.

Other approaches are also shedding light on the genetics of cLQT and could ultimately translate into an increased understanding of aLQT. Large deletions and duplications in the major cLQT genes, which would go undetected with the use of some screening technologies, were found to account for a further 10% of *genotype-negative* familial cases [46]. Their frequencies within a general population and any association with aLQT remains to be explored, but moving away from simple SNP analysis to copy number variation and epigenetics might provide further avenues of exploration.

The ultimate aim of understanding the mechanisms of ADRs is to mitigate against them. This could be achieved by either backtranslating the clinical findings into defining new or refining existing preclinical screens, or by exploiting personalized healthcare approaches.

Preclinical assessment of the QT liability of a drug is a regulatory requirement and is determined by measuring the potential of a drug to block the cardiac potassium channel hERG (*KCNH2*), heterologously expressed in an *in vitro* system (to date there are no known examples of drugs that cause QT prolongation and arrhythmia that do not block the hERG channel) [47]. Since the expressed channel invariably represents the population wild-type channel, more recent work has assessed whether increased risk in a genetically diverse population could be identified pre-clinically by screening against variant ion channels that have been associated with cases of aLQT/TdP [48]. Although the variant channels showed no differences in the *in vitro* test system used, the approach of backtranslating clinical findings is one that will be worthy of pursuit when the mechanisms of QT prolongation (and other ADRs) are better understood. Furthermore, there is also the likelihood that the *in vitro* results will not necessarily reflect the *in vivo* situation.

Personalized healthcare approaches based on genetics alone would not presently be feasible for aLQT, primarily because of the low predictive power of any genetic information to predict outcomes. Additionally, since most individuals present with novel or low frequency mutations not restricted to a single gene, there are technical challenges associated with developing comprehensive screening strategies amenable to personalized healthcare strategies.

As is likely to be the situation for most ADRs, the majority of cases are likely to result from a number of interacting factors, of which genetics will be just one component. The ability to integrate information from different sources and to build algorithms that can predict susceptibility is likely to provide the way forward. For aLQT, a limited example exists that highlights the utility of this approach.

A case study was presented of a single subject presenting with TdP, which was attributed to concomitant use of cisapride, an arrhythmogenic trigger drug, and the antibiotic clarithromycin. Since both cisapride and clarithromycin are CYP3A4 substrates, it was proposed that this drug–drug interaction raised the plasma levels of cisparide, triggering TdP [40]. Subsequent genetic analysis identified a SNP in the hERG gene that had previously been reported to be associated with aLQT [41]. It is now possible to piece together information relating to this individual ADR case, specifically, a potentially high circulating plasma level of cisapride, due to concomitant use of clarithromycin, acting on a pharmacologically sensitive hERG channel to elicit an arrhythmia.

Further work is still required to fully understand the causes of aLQT. This work needs to include an understanding of individual susceptibility and what causes some drugs to move from a QT prolongation to an arrhythmia. This is likely to be multifactorial with genetics contributing to risk, and the ultimate aim will be to translate this understanding into preclinical screens to identify and eliminate, or allow the management of, a drug's risk. In the interim the ability to develop more predictive biomarkers would represent a significant step forward. While there is still much work to be done in this area, initial work indicates that genetics plays a role in determining susceptibility and has the potential to help delineate mechanisms and contribute to biomarker identification and development. Ultimately this will be most easily achieved via an integrated holistic approach to the problem.

10.4 DRUG-INDUCED MUSCLE TOXICITY

A number of different drugs are known to be associated with myopathy, which usually involves subacute manifestation of myopathic symptoms such as muscle weakness, myalgia, creatine phosphokinase (CPK) elevation, or myoglobinuria. The precise disease phenotype is somewhat dependent on the individual drug ([49]). Most cases are not serious and are readily reversible by drug withdrawal, but a more severe form of disease resulting in rhabdomyolysis followed by death also occurs rarely.

Although statins are very effective drugs that are used widely worldwide (see Chapter 6), they can cause muscle toxicity. In most cases, this manifests as an asymptomatic rise in CPK but can be more serious (see Fig. 10.3). The mechanism by which statins give rise to toxicity is still not completely clear, but there is increasing evidence for induction of expression of the protein atrogin 1 in affected muscle tissue leading to muscular atrophy, possibly because of inhibition of geranylgeranyl isoprene unit transfer by statins [50]. The ability of different statins to cause myopathy varies, but an overall estimate of an incidence of 0.1% has been made on the basis of several different studies [51]. Cerivastatin was withdrawn in 2001

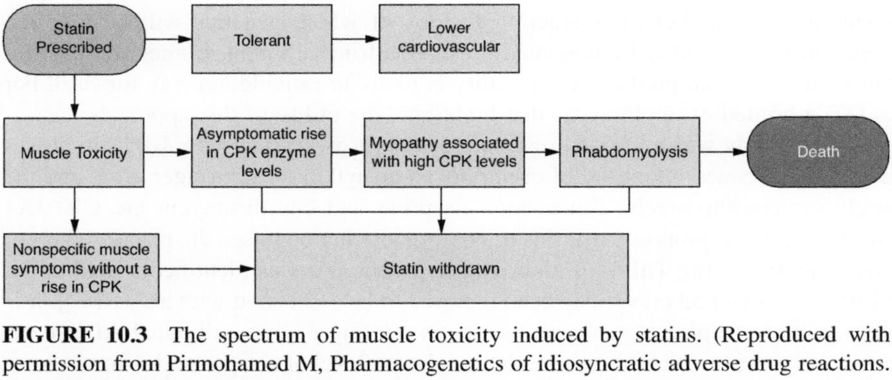

FIGURE 10.3 The spectrum of muscle toxicity induced by statins. (Reproduced with permission from Pirmohamed M, Pharmacogenetics of idiosyncratic adverse drug reactions. In Uetrecht J, ed.: *Handbook of Experimental Pharmacology, Adverse Drug Reactions*. Berlin: Springer-Verlag, 2010),

because of a relatively large number of deaths and serious injury [52]. Individual statins have been shown to vary in their liability to cause myopathy, with cerivastatin classed as the most toxic, followed by simvastatin, lovostatin, pravastatin, atorvastatin, and fluvastatin [53]. Drug interactions seem to be an important contributor to statin-induced myopathy, but there is also increasing evidence for a role for genetic polymorphisms relevant to their metabolism and transport in susceptibility to toxicity (see Table 10.6). There is also more limited evidence that genes encoding proteins relevant to muscular function may contribute [54,55]. Unlike the case in DILI, there is currently no evidence for a role of the immune system.

Statins are generally subject to metabolism by the cytochromes P450, especially CYP3A4/5, but also CYP2C8 and CYP2C9. There is some limited evidence that CYP2C8 genotype may affect susceptibility to cerivastatin myopathy [56], and carriage of the wild-type *CYP3A5*1* allele (which predicts expression of CYP3A5) was reported to increase susceptibility to atorvastatin myalgia [57]. A role for CYP2D6 in susceptibility to atorvastatin myalgia has also been suggested [58], but previous data suggest that any role for this enzyme in atorvastatin metabolism is quite limited [59,60], rendering the biological basis for a CYP2D6 association unclear.

Drug transporters from the OATP and ABC families are also good candidate genes for toxicity since roles for both in disposition of statins are well established. There is some limited evidence that genotype for ABCB1 is a risk factor for simvastatin myalgia, but evidence for a role for members of the OATP family is stronger. In particular, genetic polymorphisms affecting members of this family have been well characterized, and some have been clearly shown to be functionally significant. In the case of OATP1B1 (SLCO1B1), a major inward transporter of anionic drugs into hepatocytes, a coding region polymorphism is well established to affect activity toward a number of drugs, including some statins. It was originally suggested [61] that rare mutations in OATP1B1 were associated with susceptibility to myopathy induced by pravastatin and atorvastatin. More recently, a GWAS on a subgroup of patients suffering from elevated CPK in a large clinical trial involving use of simvastatin found a signal for a SNP in OATP1B1 in complete linkage disequilibrium with the well-studied rs4149056 (*SLCO1B1*15*; Val174Ala) SNP, which had been shown previously to affect transport activity with several statins [62]. A gene dose effect was seen with an odds ratio of 16.9 for disease development in homozygous mutants compared with homozygous wild-type subjects. This is an interesting

TABLE 10.6 Genes Relevant to Drug Metabolism and Transport that Are Risk Factors for Statin-Induced Myopathy

Drug	Gene variant	Reference
Cerivastatin	CYP2C8 (frameshift variant)	56
Pravastatin	SLCO1B1*15	61
Simvastatin	SLCO1B1*15, ABCB1 (wild type for 1236C > T, 2677G > A/T, and 3435C > T)	62,115
Atorvastatin	CYP3A5*1, CYP2D6*4	57,58,87

finding, but replication is needed with other statins and with simvastatin doses lower than those used in the patients studied by GWAS.

10.5 HYPERSENSITIVITY REACTIONS (INCLUDING SEVERE SKIN RASH)

10.5.1 Background

Hypersensitivity in the present context refers to an inappropriate immune reaction to an otherwise nontoxic agent. The manifestations of hypersensitivity reactions are broad; indeed, certain forms of DILI, covered in Section 10.2, can be regarded as hypersensitivity reactions, for example, coamoxiclav-induced hepatotoxicity. DILI will not be covered further in this section, but we focus on skin reactions where there may or may not be involvement of extracutaneous organs such as liver, lungs or kidneys.

There is a great deal of variability in the manifestations of hypersensitivity reactions. The mildest form consists of maculopapular exanthema (MPE), where the skin rash is not accompanied by any systemic symptoms, and withdrawal of the drug is all that is needed to alleviate the reaction. More severe than MPE is drug-induced hypersensitivity syndrome, which is also known as *DRESS* (drug rash with eoinophilia and systemic symptoms). In this condition, the skin rash is accompanied by eosinophilia, fever, and extracutaneous involvement such as hepatitis, pneumonitis, bone marrow involvement, myocarditis, and interstitial nephritis.

However, it is important to note that not every patient has significant extracutaneous involvement [63], and the reasons why some patients develop multiorgan manifestations, while others do not with the same drug, are unclear. Some patients develop blistering skin reactions, which are perhaps the most severe manifestation of drug hypersensitivity reactions affecting the skin, with involvement of $<10\%$, 10–30%, and $>30\%$ of the skin surface area, together with involvement of at least two mucous membranes, termed *Stevens–Johnson syndrome* (SJS), *overlap syndrome*, and *toxic epidermal necrolysis* (TEN), respectively [64].

The same drug can cause different forms of hypersensitivity reactions in different patients—the reasons for this are unclear. There are, however, some drugs that have been particularly implicated in the causation of TEN (Table 10.7), the form of hypersensitivity that is associated with the highest degree of morbidity and mortality.

TABLE 10.7 Drugs Most Frequently Implicated in Causing Stevens–Johnson Syndrome (SJS) and Toxic Epidermal Necrolysis (TEN)

Allopurinol
Anticonvulsants (carbamazepine, lamotrigine, phenytoin, phenobarbital)
β-Lactam antibiotics (penicillins, cephalosporins)
Cotrimoxazole
Nonnucleoside reverse transcriptase inhibitors (nevirapine, etravirine)
NSAIDs (particularly oxicam NSAIDs)

As with DILI, the most prominent genetic associations in this area have been identified in the MHC on the short arm of chromosome 6. To date, there have been no convincing associations in the genes determining drug disposition—although some have been reported [65], they have not been seen in other populations [66], and are certainly not of a magnitude that would be suitable for clinical implementation.

10.5.2 Abacavir Hypersensitivity

Abacavir, a potent HIV1 reverse transcriptase inhibitor, causes hypersensitivity in 5% of patients [67]. These reactions are characterized by skin rash, and gastrointestinal and respiratory manifestations, and can be fatal, particularly on rechallenge. An association between abacavir hypersensitivity and the haplotype comprising HLA-B*5701, HLA-DR7, and HLA-DQ3 was initially demonstrated by Mallal et al. [68]. It was replicated in two other cohorts by GlaxoSmithKline Pharmaceuticals, the manufacturer of the drug, and independently in a cohort of patients from the UK [69–71]. Subsequent studies have shown that this haplotype resides on the ancestral haplotype 57.1 [72], and immunological studies have implicated HLA-B*5701 as the causative allele [73]. The findings from the cohort and case–control studies have been confirmed in a large randomized controlled trial (PREDICT-1); in immunologically confirmed hypersensitivity reactions, no cases of hypersensitivity were seen in the prospective screening group but were seen in 2.7% of the comparator control group, providing a negative predictive value of 100% and a positive predictive value of 47.9% for HLA-B*5701 testing [11]. The association of HLA-B*5701 with immunologically confirmed abacavir hypersensitivity reactions has also been shown in black patients [74]. The frequency of abacavir hypersensitivity is lower in African patients than in Caucasians, and seems to reflect the population prevalence of HLA-B*5701. The result in black patients [74] is extremely important (unlike the scenario with other drugs; see discussion below) because it shows that HLA-B*5701 can be used predictively in all patient groups irrespective of ethnicity.

The prevention of abacavir hypersensitivity using HLA-B*5701 genetic testing represents the prime example of translational research. Not only has the association been convincingly demonstrated in several populations [69–71], and shown to be clinically valid in a randomized controlled trial [11]; its use in clinical settings decreases the frequency of hypersensitivity in Australia [75], the UK [76], and France [77], and it is a cost-effective approach [70,78]. In 2008, this evidence was evaluated by the regulators, and both the FDA and EMEA changed the drug label for abacavir.

10.5.3 Carbamazepine Hypersensitivity

Carbamazepine (CBZ), a widely used anticonvulsant, can cause rashes in up to 10% of patients, and in occasional cases, this may be the precursor to the development of a hypersensitivity syndrome [79,80]. Rarely, CBZ can induce blistering skin reactions such as Stevens–Johnson syndrome (SJS) and toxic epidermal necrolysis [81].

TABLE 10.8 Associations between Carbamazepine-Induced Stevens–Johnson Syndrome and Toxic Epidermal Necrolysis and HLA-B*1502 in Different Populations

Ethnic Population	Population Frequency of HLA-B*1502	Association with CBZ-Induced SJS/TEN	Reference
Han Chinese	0.07	Yes	82,116
Thai	0.08	Yes	83
Caucasians	0-0.001	No	84,85,95
Japanese	0.0001	No	86,117

A study in a Han Chinese patients from Taiwan has shown a strong association between HLAB*1502 and CBZ-induced SJS, with an odds ratio that was greater than 2504 [82]. The association seems to reflect the underlying frequency of the HLA-B*1502 allele (Table 10.8). Thus, in Thai patients, where the population frequency of the allele is similar to that seen in Han Chinese, an association between CBZ-induced SJS and HLA-B*1502 has also been demonstrated [odds ratio (OR) 25.5, 95% confidence interval(CI) 2.68–242.61] [83]. However, in Caucasians [84,85] and Japanese patients with CBZ-induced SJS [86], the allele frequency is lower, and no association has yet been shown with HLA-B*1502. Also, the association seems to be phenotype-specific in that it is observed with SJS, but not in patients with CBZ hypersensitivity syndrome, irrespective of whether they are Han Chinese [87] or Caucasian [84]. The predisposition to CBZ hypersensitivity syndrome also seems (at least partly) to lie within the MHC, with associations having been demonstrated with the haplotype TNF2-DR3-DQ2 [88], and with three SNPs in the class III region, in the HSP-70 locus, two in HSP70-1 and one in HSP-Hom [89]. It is important to note that this association was observed with the hypersensitivity syndrome, but not with the milder MPE.

Interestingly, despite extensive investigations, no association has been identified with respect to those genes involved in the metabolism of CBZ, including its activation to toxic metabolites and detoxication [80,90–93]. CBZ is extensively metabolized, and despite the involvement of several genes in its disposition that are polymorphically expressed, it is possible that even when the formation of the antigenic moiety is greatly reduced, the immune response, in those who are predisposed, is so sensitive that it can still identify the signal, leading to a full-blown immune response.

The findings with CBZ-induced SJS in Han Chinese patients and HLA-B*1502 prompted the FDA to change the drug label for CBZ stating that it should be tested in "most patients of Asian ancestry." The European label has different wording in stating that testing should be performed in patients of Han Chinese and Thai origin. Interestingly, in Thai patients, an association was also demonstrated between HLA-B*1502 and phenytoin-induced SJS (OR 18.5, 95% CI 1.82–188.40) [83]. Confusingly, however, some patients, who were HLA-B*1502 and suffered from CBZ-induced SJS, were tolerant to phenytoin and vice versa, suggesting either that HLA-B*1502 is not the causative allele or that other factors in addition to HLA-B*1502 are necessary to result in SJS.

Unlike abacavir hypersensitivity, because SJS is relatively rare, the positive predictive value of HLA-B*1502 testing, even in Han Chinese patients, is less than 10%, and no formal cost-effective analysis has been undertaken, Moreover, data on the uptake of testing are lacking.

In summary, the situation with CBZ hypersensitivity seems to be extraordinarily complex, with the associations demonstrated being not only ethnic-specific but also phenotype-specific. The underlying mechanistic reasons for these differences, particularly in phenotype specificity, remain to be elucidated.

10.5.4 Allopurinol Hypersensitivity

Allopurinol is an agent used for the treatment of gout. It is associated with hypersensitivity reactions, in the form of hypersensitivity syndrome and the blistering cutaneous reactions (SJS and TEN). In a study in Han Chinese patients, a strong association was demonstrated between allopurinol severe cutaneous adverse reactions (SCARs; which included hypersensitivity syndrome and SJS/TEN) and HLA-B*5801, the allele being found in all 51 patients with allopurinol-SCAR, but only in 20 (15%) of 135 tolerant patients (OR 580) [94]. Thus, unlike the association with CBZ, the association with allopurinol is not dependent on the phenotype of the severe cutaneous reaction, as it is seen in patients with both hypersensitivity syndrome and the blistering cutaneous reactions. A further distinction from CBZ is that the association with HLA-B*5801 and allopurinol-induced SCAR has been observed in several populations, including Caucasians [95], Japanese [86], and Thai [96].

Analysis of the results observed with CBZ and allopurinol highlight the complexity of the genetic associations observed to date with drug-induced hypersensitivity; for some drugs (e.g., allopurinol), the transition from the mild reactions (e.g., MPE) to the most severe reactions (e.g., TEN) seems to be part of the same disease spectrum dependent on the same genetic factor, while for other drugs (e.g., CBZ), the different phenotypic manifestations seem to represent different disease phenotypes. This makes it difficult to predict what spectrum new drugs found to cause hypersensitivity reactions will follow, and therefore emphasizes the need to (1) carefully phenotype patients who develop such reactions and (2) collect biological samples from all patients.

10.6 CONCLUDING REMARKS

Our understanding of genetic factors underlying serious adverse drug reactions has increased, due, at least in part, to our improved knowledge of the human genome and to the development of new approaches such as GWAS. This chapter has concentrated on the four best studied types of adverse reactions, although others exist including, for example, nephrotoxicity, a common cause of drug withdrawal in the United States between 1976 and 2005 [51], hematological toxicity (e.g., clozapine-induced agranulocytosis, which is a well-established clinical problem limiting the use of this antipsychotic drug [97]), and bisphosphonate-induced osteonecrosis of the jaw (BONJ) [98], a disabling condition seen in patients undergoing treatment with bisphosphonates. A GWAS on BONJ revealed an apparent association with a particular haplotype of CYP2C8 [99], although this finding needs replication in a larger cohort and further studies on the underlying mechanism.

REFERENCES

1. Rawlins MD, Thompson JW: Mechanisms of adverse drug reactions. In Davies DM, ed.: *Textbook of Adverse Drug Reactions*. Oxford UK: Oxford Univ. Press, 1991, pp. 18–45.
2. Pirmohamed M, Breckenridge AM, Kitteringham NR, Park BK. Adverse drug reactions. *Br Med.* 1998;**316**:1295–1298.
3. Lee WM. Medical progress: Drug-induced hepatotoxicity. *New Engl. J. Med.* 2003;**349**:474–485.
4. Spriet-Pourra C, Auriche M. Drug Withdrawal from Sales, 2nd ed. Richmond, VA: PJB Publications, 1994.
5. Hautekeete ML, Horsmans Y, van Waeyenberge C, Demanet C, Henrion J, Verbist L, et al. HLA association of amoxicillin-clavulanate-induced hepatitis. *Gastroenterology* 1999;**117**:1181–1186.
6. O'Donohue J, Oien KA, Donaldson P, Underhill J, Clare M, MacSween RM, et al. Co-amoxiclav jaundice: Clinical and histological features and HLA class II association. *Gut* 2000;**47**:717–720.
7. Donaldson PT, Bhatnagar P, Graham J, Henderson J, Leathart JB, Pirmohamed M, et al. Susceptibility to drug induced liver injury determined by hla class II genotype. *Proc. 59th Annual Meeting of the American Association for the Study of Liver Diseases*, Oct. 31–Nov. 04, 2008, p. 345.
8. Andrade RJ, Lucena MI, Alonso A, Garcia-Cortes M, Garcia-Ruiz E, Benitez R, et al. HLA class II genotype influences the type of liver injury in drug-induced idiosyncratic liver disease. *Hepatology* 2004;**39**:1603–1612.
9. Russmann S, Kaye JA, Jick SS, Jick H. Risk of cholestatic liver disease associated with flucloxacillin and flucloxacillin prescribing habits in the UK: Cohort study using data from the UK General Practice Research Database. *Br. J. Clin. Pharmacol.* 2005;**60**:76–82.
10. Daly AK, Donaldson PT, Bhatnagar P, Shen Y, Pe'er I, Floratos A, et al. HLA-B*5701 genotype is a major determinant of drug-induced liver injury due to flucloxacillin. *Nature Genet.* 2009;**41**:816–819.
11. Mallal S, Phillips E, Carosi G, Molina JM, Workman C, Tomazic J, et al. HLA-B*5701 screening for hypersensitivity to abacavir. *New Engl. J. Med.* 2008;**358**:568–579.
12. Kindmark A, Jawaid A, Harbron CG, Barratt BJ, Bengtsson OF, Andersson TB, et al. Genome-wide pharmacogenetic investigation of a hepatic adverse event without clinical signs of immunopathology suggests an underlying immune pathogenesis. *Pharmacogenomics J.* 2008;**8**:186–195.
13. Hirata K, Takagi H, Yamamoto M, Matsumoto T, Nishiya T, Mori K, et al. Ticlopidine-induced hepatotoxicity is associated with specific human leukocyte antigen genomic subtypes in Japanese patients: A preliminary case-control study. *Pharmacogenomics J.* 2008;**8**:29–33.

14. Yee D, Valiquette C, Pelletier M, Parisien I, Rocher I, Menzies D. Incidence of serious side effects from first-line antituberculosis drugs among patients treated for active tuberculosis. *Am. J. Respir. Crit. Care Med.* 2003;**167**:1472–1477.
15. Eichelbaum M, Musch E, Castroparra M, Vonsassen W. Isoniazid hepatotoxicity in relation to acetylator phenotype and isoniazid metabolism. *Br. J. Clin. Pharmacol.* 1982;**14**:P575–P576.
16. Sarich TC, Adams SP, Petricca G, Wright JM. Inhibition of isoniazid-induced hepatotoxicity in rabbits by pretreatment with an amidase inhibitor. *J. Pharmacol. Exp. Ther.* 1999;**289**:695–702.
17. Ohno M, Yamaguchi I, Yamamoto I, Fukuda T, Yokota S, Maekura R, et al. Slow N-acetyltransferase 2 genotype affects the incidence of isoniazid and rifampicin-induced hepatotoxicity. *Int. J. Tubercul Lung Dis.* 2000;**4**:256–261.
18. Huang YS, Chern HD, Su WJ, Wu JC, Lai SL, Yang SY, et al. Polymorphism of the N-acetyltransferase 2 gene as a susceptibility risk factor for antituberculosis drug-induced hepatitis. *Hepatology* 2002;**35**:883–889.
19. Cho HJ, Koh WJ, Ryu YJ, Ki CS, Nam MH, Kim JW, et al. Genetic polymorphisms of NAT2 and CYP2E1 associated with antituberculosis drug-induced hepatotoxicity in Korean patients with pulmonary tuberculosis. *Tuberculosis (Edinburgh)* 2007;**87**:551–556.
20. Possuelo LG, Castelan JA, de Brito TC, Ribeiro AW, Cafrune PI, Picon PD, et al. Association of slow N-acetyltransferase 2 profile and anti-TB drug-induced hepatotoxicity in patients from southern Brazil. *Eur. J. Clin. Pharmacol.* 2008;**64**:673–681.
21. Bozok Cetintas V, Erer OF, Kosova B, Ozdemir I, Topcuoglu N, Aktogu S, et al. Determining the relation between N-acetyltransferase-2 acetylator phenotype and antituberculosis drug induced hepatitis by molecular biologic tests. *Tuberk. Toraks.* 2008;**56**:81–86.
22. Vuilleumier N, Rossier MF, Chiappe A, Degoumois F, Dayer P, Mermillod B, et al. CYP2E1 genotype and isoniazid-induced hepatotoxicity in patients treated for latent tuberculosis. *Eur. J. Clin. Pharmacol.* 2006;**62**:423–429.
23. Huang YS, Chern HD, Su WJ, Wu JC, Chang SC, Chiang CH, et al. Cytochrome p450 2E1 genotype and the susceptibility to antituberculosis drug-induced hepatitis. *Hepatology* 2003;**37**:924–930.
24. Acuna G, Foernzler D, Leong D, Rabbia M, Smit R, Dorflinger E, et al. Pharmacogenetic analysis of adverse drug effect reveals genetic variant for susceptibility to liver toxicity. *Pharmacogenomics J.* 2002;**2**:327–334.
25. Daly AK, Aithal GP, Leathart JB, Swainsbury RA, Dang TS, Day CP. Genetic susceptibility to diclofenac-induced hepatotoxicity: contribution of UGT2B7, CYP2C8, and ABCC2 genotypes. *Gastroenterology* 2007;**132**:272–281.
26. Simon T, Becquemont L, Mary-Krause M, de Waziers I, Beaune P, Funck-Brentano C, et al. Combined glutathione-S-transferase M1 and T1 genetic polymorphism and tacrine hepatotoxicity. *Clini. Pharmacol. & Ther.* 2000;**67**:432–437.
27. Green VJ, Pirmohamed M, Kitteringham NR, Knapp MJ, Park BK. Glutathione S-transferase mu genotype (GSTM1*0) in Alzheimer's patients with tacrine transaminitis. *Br. J. Clin. Pharmacol.* 1995;**39**:411–415.

28. De Sousa M, Pirmohamed M, Kitteringham NR, Woolf T, Park BK. No association between tacrine transaminitis and the glutathione transferase theta genotype in patients with Alzheimer's disease. *Pharmacogenetics* 1998;**8**:353–355.

29. Madden S, Woolf TF, Pool WF, Park BK. An investigation into the formation of stable, protein-reactive and cytotoxic metabolites from tacrine in vitro. Studies with human and rat liver microsomes. *Biochem. Pharmacol.* 1993;**46**:13–20.

30. Geier A, Wagner M, Dietrich CG, Trauner M. Principles of hepatic organic anion transporter regulation during cholestasis, inflammation and liver regeneration. *Biochim. Biophys. Acta* 2007;**1773**:283–308.

31. Noe J, Kullak-Ublick GA, Jochum W, Stieger B, Kerb R, Haberl M, et al. Impaired expression and function of the bile salt export pump due to three novel ABCB11 mutations in intrahepatic cholestasis. *J. Hepatol.* 2005;**43**:536–543.

32. Lang C, Meier Y, Stieger B, Beuers U, Lang T, Kerb R, et al. Mutations and polymorphisms in the bile salt export pump and the multidrug resistance protein 3 associated with drug-induced liver injury. *Pharmacogenet. Genomics* 2007;**17**: 47–60.

33. Haenisch S, Zimmermann U, Dazert E, Wruck CJ, Dazert P, Siegmund W, et al. Influence of polymorphisms of ABCB1 and ABCC2 on mRNA and protein expression in normal and cancerous kidney cortex. *Pharmacogenomics J.* 2007;**7**:56–65.

34. Choi JH, Ahn BM, Yi J, Lee JH, Nam SW, Chon CY, et al. MRP2 haplotypes confer differential susceptibility to toxic liver injury. *Pharmacogenet. Genomics* 2007;**17**:403–415.

35. Huang YS, Su WJ, Huang YH, Chen CY, Chang FY, Lin HC, et al. Genetic polymorphisms of manganese superoxide dismutase, NAD(P)H:quinone oxidoreductase, glutathione S-transferase M1 and T1, and the susceptibility to drug-induced liver injury. *J. Hepatol.* 2007;**47**:128–134.

36. Tester D, Ackerman D. Novel gene and mutation discovery in congenital LQT: Let's keep looking where the street lamp standeth *Heart Rhythm* 2008;**5**:1282–1284.

37. Lasser KE, Allen PD, Woolhandler SJ, Himmelstein DU, Wolfe SM, Bor DH. Timing of new black box warnings and withdrawals for prescription medications. *JAMA* 2002;**287**:2215–2220.

38. Redfern WS, Carlsson L, Davis AS, Lynch WG, MacKenzie I, Palethorpe S, et al. Relationships between preclinical cardiac electrophysiology, clinical QT interval prolongation and torsade de pointes for a broad range of drugs: Evidence for a provisional safety margin in drug development. *Cardiovasc. Res.* 2003;**58**:32–45.

39. Priori SG, Napolitano C, Schwartz PJ. Low penetrance in the long-QT syndrome: Clinical impact. *Circulation* 1999;**99**:529–533.

40. Piquette RK. Torsade de pointes induced by cisapride/clarithromycin interaction. *Ann. Pharmacother.* 1999;**33**:22–26.

41. Paulussen AD, Gilissen RA, Armstrong M, Doevendans PA, Verhasselt P, Smeets HJ, et al. Genetic variations of KCNQ1, KCNH2, SCN5A, KCNE1, and KCNE2 in drug-induced long QT syndrome patients. *J. Mol. Med.* 2004;**82**:182–188.

42. Pfeufer A, Sanna S, Arking DE, Muller M, Gateva V, Fuchsberger C, et al. Common variants at ten loci modulate the QT interval duration in the QTSCD study. *Nat. Genet.* 2009;**41**:407–414.

43. Newton-Cheh C, Eijgelsheim M, Rice KM, de Bakker PI, Yin X, Estrada K, et al. Common variants at ten loci influence QT interval duration in the QTGEN study. *Nat. Genet.* 2009;**41**:399–406.

44. Petersen CI, McFarland TR, Stepanovic SZ, Yang P, Reiner DJ, Hayashi K, et al. In vivo identification of genes that modify ether-a-go-go-related gene activity in Caenorhabditis elegans may also affect human cardiac arrhythmia. *Proc. Natl. Acad. Sci. USA* 2004;**101**:11773–11778.

45. Llerena A, Berecz R, de la Rubia A, Dorado P. QTc interval lengthening is related to CYP2D6 hydroxylation capacity and plasma concentration of thioridazine in patients. *J. Psychopharmacol.* 2002;**16**:361–364.

46. Eddy CA, MacCormick JM, Chung SK, Crawford JR, Love DR, Rees MI, et al. Identification of large gene deletions and duplications in KCNQ1 and KCNH2 in patients with long QT syndrome. *Heart Rhythm* 2008;**5**:1275–1281.

47. Fenichel RR, Malik M, Antzelevitch C, Sanguinetti M, Roden DM, Priori SG, et al. Drug-induced torsades de pointes and implications for drug development. *J. Cardiovasc. Electrophysiol.* 2004;**15**:475–495.

48. Pollard CE, Mannikko R, Overend G, Perrey C, Gavaghan C, Valentin J-P, et al. Pharmacological and electrophysiological characterisation of nine, single nucleotide polymorphisms of the hERG-encoded potassium channel. *Br. J. Pharmacol.* 2009.

49. Dalakas MC. Toxic and drug-induced myopathies. *J. Neurol. Neurosurg. Psychiatry.* 2009;**80**:832–838.

50. Cao P, Hanai JI, Tanksale P, Imamura S, Sukhatme VP, Lecker SH. Statin-induced muscle damage and atrogin-1 induction is the result of a geranylgeranylation defect. *FASEB J.* 2009;**23**:2844–2854.

51. Wilke RA, Lin DW, Roden DM, Watkins PB, Flockhart D, Zineh I, et al. Identifying genetic risk factors for serious adverse drug reactions: Current progress and challenges. *Nat. Rev. Drug Discov.* 2007;**6**:904–916.

52. Marwick C. Bayer is forced to release documents over withdrawal of cerivastatin. *Br. Med. J.* 2003;**326**:518.

53. Thompson PD, Clarkson P, Karas RH. Statin-associated myopathy. *JAMA* 2003;**289**:1681–1690.

54. Vladutiu GD, Simmons Z, Isackson PJ, Tarnopolsky M, Peltier WL, Barboi AC, et al. Genetic risk factors associated with lipid-lowering drug-induced myopathies. *Muscle Nerve* 2006;**34**:153–162.

55. Oh J, Ban MR, Miskie BA, Pollex RL, Hegele RA. Genetic determinants of statin intolerance. *Lipids Health Dis.* 2007;**6**:7.

56. Ishikawa C, Ozaki H, Nakajima T, Ishii T, Kanai S, Anjo S, et al. A frameshift variant of CYP2C8 was identified in a patient who suffered from rhabdomyolysis after administration of cerivastatin. *J. Hum. Genet.* 2004;**49**:582–585.

57. Kivisto KT, Niemi M, Schaeffeler E, Pitkala K, Tilvis R, Fromm MF, et al. Lipid-lowering response to statins is affected by CYP3A5 polymorphism. *Pharmacogenetics* 2004;**14**:523–525.

58. Frudakis TN, Thomas MJ, Ginjupalli SN, Handelin B, Gabriel R, Gomez HJ. CYP2D6*4 polymorphism is associated with statin-induced muscle effects. *Pharmacogenet. Genomics* 2007;**17**:695–707.

59. Geisel J, Kivisto KT, Griese EU, Eichelbaum M. The efficacy of simvastatin is not influenced by CYP2D6 polymorphism. *Clin. Pharmacol. Ther.* 2002;**72**:595–596.
60. Prueksaritanont T, Ma B, Yu N. The human hepatic metabolism of simvastatin hydroxy acid is mediated primarily by CYP3A, and not CYP2D6. *Br. J. Clin. Pharmacol.* 2003;**56**:120–124.
61. Morimoto K, Oishi T, Ueda S, Ueda M, Hosokawa M, Chiba K. A novel variant allele of OATP-C (SLCO1B1) found in a Japanese patient with pravastatin-induced myopathy. *Drug Metab. Pharmacokinet.* 2004;**19**:453–455.
62. Link E, Parish S, Armitage J, Bowman L, Heath S, Matsuda F, et al. SLCO1B1 variants and statin-induced myopathy—a genomewide study. *New Engl. J. Med.* 2008;**359**:789–799.
63. Peyriere H, Dereure O, Breton H, Demoly P, Cociglio M, Blayac JP, et al. Variability in the clinical pattern of cutaneous side-effects of drugs with systemic symptoms: Does a DRESS syndrome really exist? *Br. J. Dermatol* 2006;**155**:422–428.
64. Bastuji-Garin S, Rzany B, Stern RS, Shear NH, Naldi L, Roujeau JC. Clinical classification of cases of toxic epidermal necrolysis, Stevens-Johnson syndrome, and erythema multiforme. *Arch. Dermatol.* 1993;**129**:92–96.
65. Wolkenstein P, Loriot MA, Flahault A, Cadilhac M, Caumes E, Eliaszewicz M, et al. Association analysis of drug metabolizing enzyme gene polymorphisms in AIDS patients with cutaneous reactions to sulfonamides. *J. Invest. Dermatol.* 2005;**125**:1080–1082.
66. Pirmohamed M, Alfirevic A, Vilar J, Stalford A, Wilkins EGL, Sim E, et al. Association analysis of drug metabolizing enzyme gene polymorphisms in HIV-positive patients with co-trimoxazole hypersensitivity. *Pharmacogenetics* 2000;**10**:705–713.
67. Hetherington S, McGuirk S, Powell G, Cutrell A, Naderer O, Spreen B, et al. Hypersensitivity reactions during therapy with the nucleoside reverse transcriptase inhibitor abacavir. *Clin. Ther.* 2001;**23**:1603–1614.
68. Mallal S, Nolan D, Witt C, Masel G, Martin AM, Moore C, et al. Association between presence of *HLA-B**5701*, *HLA-DR7*, and *HLA-DQ3* and hypersensitivity to HIV-1 reverse transcriptase inhibitor abacavir. *Lancet* 2002;**359**:727–732.
69. Hetherington S, Hughes AR, Mosteller M, Shortino D, Baker KL, Spreen W, et al. Genetic variations in HLA-B region and hypersensitivity reactions to abacavir. *Lancet* 2002;**359**:1121–1122.
70. Hughes DA, Vilar FJ, Ward CC, Alfirevic A, Park BK, Pirmohamed M. Cost-effectiveness analysis of HLA B*5701 genotyping in preventing abacavir hypersensitivity. *Pharmacogenetics* 2004;**14**:335–342.
71. Hughes AR, Mosteller M, Bansal AT, Davies K, Haneline SA, Lai EH, et al. Association of genetic variations in HLA-B region with hypersensitivity to abacavir in some, but not all, populations. *Pharmacogenomics* 2004;**5**:203–211.
72. Martin AM, Nolan D, Gaudieri S, Almeida CA, Nolan R, James I, et al. Predisposition to abacavir hypersensitivity conferred by HLA-B*5701 and a haplotypic Hsp70-Hom variant. *Proc. Natl. Acad. Sci. USA* 2004;**101**:4180–4185.
73. Chessman D, Kostenko L, Lethborg T, Purcell AW, Williamson NA, Chen Z, et al. Human leukocyte antigen class I-restricted activation of CD8 + T cells provides the immunogenetic basis of a systemic drug hypersensitivity. *Immunity* 2008;**28**:822–832.

74. Saag M, Balu R, Phillips E, Brachman P, Martorell C, Burman W, et al. High sensitivity of human leukocyte antigen-B*5701 as a marker for immunologically confirmed abacavir hypersensitivity in white and black patients. *Clin. Infect. Dis.* 2008;**46**:1111–1118.
75. Rauch A, Nolan D, Martin A, McKinnon E, Almeida C, Mallal S. Prospective genetic screening decreases the incidence of abacavir hypersensitivity reactions in the Western Australian HIV cohort study. *Clin. Infect. Dis.* 2006;**43**:99–102.
76. Waters LJ, Mandalia S, Gazzard B, Nelson M. Prospective HLA-B*5701 screening and abacavir hypersensitivity: A single centre experience. *AIDS* 2007;**21**:2533–2534.
77. Zucman D, Truchis P, Majerholc C, Stegman S, Caillat-Zucman S. Prospective screening for human leukocyte antigen-B*5701 avoids abacavir hypersensitivity reaction in the ethnically mixed French HIV population. *J. AIDS* 2007;**45**:1–3.
78. Schackman BR, Scott CA, Walensky RP, Losina E, Freedberg KA, Sax PE. The cost-effectiveness of HLA-B*5701 genetic screening to guide initial antiretroviral therapy for HIV. *AIDS* 2008;**22**:2025–2033.
79. Vittorio CC, Muglia JJ. Anticonvulsant hypersensitivity syndrome. *Arch. Intern. Med.* 1995;**155**:2285–2290.
80. Leeder JS. Mechanisms of idiosyncratic hypersensitivity reactions to antiepileptic drugs. *Epilepsia* 1998; **39** (Suppl. 7): S8–S16.
81. Rzany B, Correia O, Kelly JP, Naldi L, Auquier A, Stern R. Risk of Stevens-Johnson syndrome and toxic epidermal necrolysis during first weeks of antiepileptic therapy: A case-control study. Study group of the international case control study on severe cutaneous adverse reactions. *Lancet* 1999;**353**:2190–2194.
82. Chung WH, Hung SI, Hong HS, Hsih MS, Yang LC, Ho HC, et al. Medical genetics: A marker for Stevens-Johnson syndrome. *Nature* 2004;**428**:486.
83. Locharernkul C, Loplumlert J, Limotai C, Korkij W, Desudchit T, Tongkobpetch S, et al. Carbamazepine and phenytoin induced Stevens-Johnson syndrome is associated with HLA-B*1502 allele in Thai population. *Epilepsia* 2008;**49**:2087–2091.
84. Alfirevic A, Jorgensen AL, Williamson PR, Chadwick DW, Park BK, Pirmohamed M. HLA-B locus in Caucasian patients with carbamazepine hypersensitivity. *Pharmacogenomics* 2006;**7**:813–818.
85. Lonjou C, Thomas L, Borot N, Ledger N, de Toma C, LeLouet H, et al. A marker for Stevens-Johnson syndrome ... Ethnicity matters. *Pharmacogenomics J.* 2006; **6**:265–268.
86. Kaniwa N, Saito Y, Aihara M, Matsunaga K, Tohkin M, Kurose K, et al. HLA-B locus in Japanese patients with anti-epileptics and allopurinol-related Stevens-Johnson syndrome and toxic epidermal necrolysis. *Pharmacogenomics* 2008;**9**:1617–1622.
87. Hung SI, Chung WH, Jee SH, Chen WC, Chang YT, Lee WR, et al. Genetic susceptibility to carbamazepine-induced cutaneous adverse drug reactions. *Pharmacogenet. Genomics* 2006;**16**:297–306.
88. Pirmohamed M, Lin K, Chadwick D, Park BK. TNFalpha promoter region gene polymorphisms in carbamazepine- hypersensitive patients. *Neurology* 2001;**56**:890–896.
89. Alfirevic A, Mills T, Harrington P, Pinel T, Sherwood J, Jawaid A, et al. Association between serious carbamazepine hypersensitivity reactions and the HSP70 gene cluster. *Toxicology* 2005;**213**:264–265.
90. Shear NH, Spielberg SP, Cannon M, Miller M. Anticonvulsant hypersensitivity syndrome: In vitro risk assessment. *J. Clin. Invest.* 1988;**82**:1826–1832.

91. Pirmohamed M, Graham A, Roberts P, Smith D, Chadwick D, Breckenridge AM, et al. Carbamazepine hypersensitivity: Assessment of clinical and in vitro chemical cross-reactivity with phenytoin and oxcarbazepine. *Br. J. Clin. Pharmacol.* 1991;**32**:741–749.
92. Gaedigk A, Spielberg SP, Grant DM. Characterization of the microsomal epoxide hydrolase gene in patients with anticonvulsant adverse drug reactions. *Pharmacogenetics* 1994;**4**:142–153.
93. Green VJ, Pirmohamed M, Kitteringham NR, Gaedigk A, Grant DM, Boxer M, et al. Genetic analysis of microsomal epoxide hydrolase in patients with carbamazepine hypersensitivity. *Biochem. Pharmacol.* 1995;**50**:1353–1359.
94. Hung SI, Chung WH, Liou LB, Chu CC, Lin M, Huang HP, et al. HLA-B*5801 allele as a genetic marker for severe cutaneous adverse reactions caused by allopurinol. *Proc. Natl. Acad. Sci. USA* 2005;**102**:4134–4139.
95. Lonjou C, Borot N, Sekula P, Ledger N, Thomas L, Halevy S, et al. A European study of HLA-B in Stevens-Johnson syndrome and toxic epidermal necrolysis related to five high-risk drugs. *Pharmacogenet. Genomics* 2008;**18**:99–107.
96. Tassaneeyakul W, Jantararoungtong T, Chen P, Lin PY, Tiamkao S, Khunarkornsiri U, et al. Strong association between HLA-B*5801 and allopurinol-induced Stevens-Johnson syndrome and toxic epidermal necrolysis in a Thai population. *Pharmacogenet. Genomics* 2009;**19**:704–709.
97. Opgen-Rhein C, Dettling M. Clozapine-induced agranulocytosis and its genetic determinants. *Pharmacogenomics* 2008;**9**:1101–1111.
98. Allen MR, Burr DB. The pathogenesis of bisphosphonate-related osteonecrosis of the jaw: so many hypotheses, so few data. *J. Oral. Maxillofac. Surg.* 2009;**67**:61–70.
99. Sarasquete ME, Garcia-Sanz R, Marin L, Alcoceba M, Chillon MC, Balanzategui A, et al. Bisphosphonate-related osteonecrosis of the jaw is associated with polymorphisms of the cytochrome P450 CYP2C8 in multiple myeloma: A genome-wide single nucleotide polymorphism analysis. *Blood* 2008;**112**:2709–2712.
100. Watanabe I, Tomita A, Shimizu M, Sugawara M, Yasumo H, Koishi R, et al. A study to survey susceptible genetic factors responsible for troglitazone-associated hepatotoxicity in Japanese patients with type 2 diabetes mellitus. *Clin. Pharmacol. & Ther.* 2003;**73**:435–455.
101. Curran ME, Splawski I, Timothy KW, Vincent GM, Green ED, Keating MT. A molecular basis for cardiac arrhythmia: HERG mutations cause long QT syndrome. *Cell* 1995;**80**:795–803.
102. Wang Q, Shen J, Splawski I, Atkinson D, Li Z, Robinson JL, et al. SCN5A mutations associated with an inherited cardiac arrhythmia, long QT syndrome. *Cell* 1995;**80**:805–811.
103. Mohler PJ, Schott JJ, Gramolini AO, Dilly KW, Guatimosim S, duBell WH, et al. Ankyrin-B mutation causes type 4 long-QT cardiac arrhythmia and sudden cardiac death. *Nature* 2003;**421**:634–639.
104. Splawski I, Tristani-Firouzi M, Lehmann MH, Sanguinetti MC, Keating MT. Mutations in the hminK gene cause long QT syndrome and suppress IKs function. *Nat. Genet.* 1997;**17**:338–340.
105. Abbott GW, Sesti F, Splawski I, Buck ME, Lehmann MH, Timothy KW, et al. MiRP1 forms IKr potassium channels with HERG and is associated with cardiac arrhythmia. *Cell* 1999;**97**:175–187.

106. Plaster NM, Tawil R, Tristani-Firouzi M, Canun S, Bendahhou S, Tsunoda A, et al. Mutations in Kir2.1 cause the developmental and episodic electrical phenotypes of Andersen's syndrome. *Cell* 2001;**105**:511–519.

107. Splawski I, Timothy KW, Sharpe LM, Decher N, Kumar P, Bloise R, et al. Ca(V)1.2 calcium channel dysfunction causes a multisystem disorder including arrhythmia and autism. *Cell* 2004;**119**:19–31.

108. Vatta M, Ackerman MJ, Ye B, Makielski JC, Ughanze EE, Taylor EW, et al. Mutant caveolin-3 induces persistent late sodium current and is associated with long-QT syndrome. *Circulation* 2006;**114**:2104–2112.

109. Medeiros-Domingo A, Kaku T, Tester DJ, Iturralde-Torres P, Itty A, Ye B, et al. SCN4B-encoded sodium channel beta4 subunit in congenital long-QT syndrome. *Circulation* 2007;**116**:134–142.

110. Chen L, Marquardt ML, Tester DJ, Sampson KJ, Ackerman MJ, Kass RS. Mutation of an A-kinase-anchoring protein causes long-QT syndrome. *Proc. Natl. Acad. Sci. USA* 2007;**104**:20990–20995.

111. Ueda K, Valdivia C, Medeiros-Domingo A, Tester DJ, Vatta M, Farrugia G, et al. Syntrophin mutation associated with long QT syndrome through activation of the nNOS-SCN5A macromolecular complex. *Proc. Natl. Acad. Sci. USA* 2008;**105**:9355–9360.

112. Sesti F, Abbott GW, Wei J, Murray KT, Saksena S, Schwartz PJ, et al. A common polymorphism associated with antibiotic-induced cardiac arrhythmia. *Proc. Natl. Acad. Sci. USA* 2000;**97**:10613–10618.

113. Yang P, Kanki H, Drolet B, Yang T, Wei J, Viswanathan PC, et al. Allelic variants in long-QT disease genes in patients with drug-associated torsades de pointes. *Circulation* 2002;**105**:1943–1948.

114. Chevalier P, Rodriguez C, Bontemps L, Miquel M, Kirkorian G, Rousson R, et al. Non-invasive testing of acquired long QT syndrome: Evidence for multiple arrhythmogenic substrates. *Cardiovasc. Res.* 2001;**50**:386–398.

115. Fiegenbaum M, da Silveira FR, Van der Sand CR, Van der Sand LC, Ferreira ME, Pires RC, et al. The role of common variants of ABCB1, CYP3A4, and CYP3A5 genes in lipid-lowering efficacy and safety of simvastatin treatment. *Clin. Pharmacol. Ther.* 2005;**78**:551–558.

116. Man CB, Kwan P, Baum L, Yu E, Lau KM, Cheng AS, et al. Association between HLA-B*1502 allele and antiepileptic drug-induced cutaneous reactions in Han Chinese. *Epilepsia* 2007;**48**:1015–1018.

117. Ikeda H, Takahashi Y, Yamazaki E, Fujiwara T, Kaniwa N, Saito Y, et al. HLA Class I markers in Japanese patients with carbamazepine-induced cutaneous adverse reactions. *Epilepsia* 2009.

CHAPTER 11

Pharmacogenomics of Inflammatory Bowel Diseases

ALEXANDER TEML, SUSANNE KARNER, and ELKE SCHAEFFELER
Dr. Margarete Fischer-Bosch Institute of Clinical Pharmacology, Stuttgart, Germany

MATTHIAS SCHWAB
Dr. Margarete Fischer-Bosch Institute of Clinical Pharmacology, Stuttgart, Germany and Department of Clinical Pharmacology, Institute of Experimental and Clinical Pharmacology, University Hospital, Tuebingen, Germany

11.1 INTRODUCTION

Crohn's disease (CD) and ulcerative colitis (UC) represent the two main forms of inflammatory bowel diseases (IBD) [1]. CD is a relapsing, transmural inflammatory disease of the gastrointestinal mucosa. Typical presentations include the patchy and discontinuous involvement of potentially any portion of the gastrointestinal tract (Figs 11.1a) with subsequent development of complications such as stenoses or fistulas. The clinical presentation is dependent on disease location and behavior and includes diarrhea, abdominal pain, obstructive symptoms, malnutrition, fever, and perianal disease [2]. UC is a relapsing inflammatory disease of the rectal and colonic mucosa and superficial submucosa (Fig. 11.1b), extending typically in a continuous manner proximally from the rectum [1]. The typical symptoms are diarrhea, urgent bowel movements, abdominal cramps, rectal bleeding, and passage of pus and mucus [3]. IBD incidence and prevalence vary substantially depending on geographic location and racial or ethnic background. In Europe and North America, prevalence ranges from 8 to 214 cases per 100,000 persons for CD and from 21 to 246 cases per 100,000 persons for UC [4].

Disease pathogenesis is multifactorial, including genetic, environmental, and social factors. The relevance of genetic factors was indicated by the observation that

Pharmacogenetics and Individualized Therapy, First Edition.
Edited by Anke-Hilse Maitland-van der Zee and Ann K. Daly.

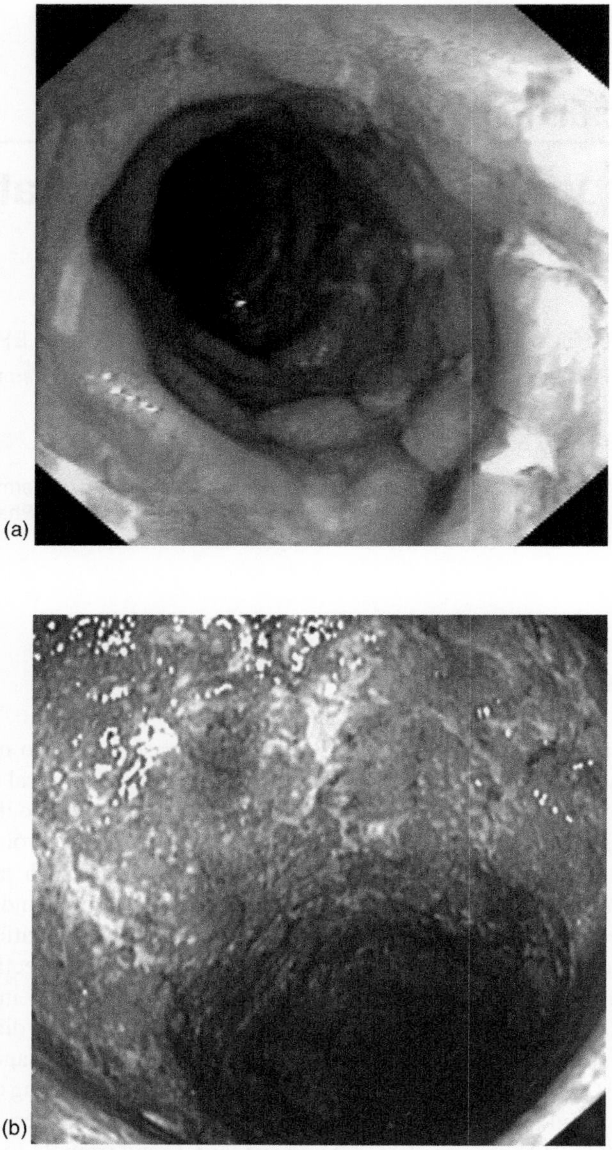

FIGURE 11.1 (a) Typical endoscopic image in Crohn's disease, showing discontinuous involvement, with linear and serpinguous ulcerations resulting in cobblestone pattern; (b) typical endoscopic view in ulcerative colitis, exhibiting continuous involvement, absent vascular pattern, greatly increased vulnerability of the mucosa with spontaneous bleeding, and pronounced mucosal damage with fibrin and ulcerations. (Endoscopic images provided by W. Reinisch, Medical University of Vienna, Austria.)

cases of IBD tend to cluster within families and by twin concordance studies. The concordance rate for CD in monozygotic twins is higher (20–50%) than for UC (14–19%), implying a weaker heritable component and a relatively greater role of nongenetic factors in UC pathogenesis than in CD [5]. These complex genetic disorders do not follow a simple Mendelian trait but instead exhibit a complex mode of inheritance.

For treatment, highly efficacious medical therapies have been approved for both CD and UC, including corticosteroids (e.g., prednisolone, budesonide), thiopurines (azathioprine, 6-mercaptopurine), other immunosuppressants (e.g., methotrexate, cyclosporine), and antitumor necrosis factor alpha (TNFα) antibodies (e.g., infliximab, adalimumab, certolizumab) [6]. However, these medications may potentially lead to serious adverse drug reactions (ADR) and even mortality [7,8]. Furthermore, drug failure by onset of or during maintenance therapy is an important clinical issue in a substantial proportion of patients [9]. Thus, as a consequence of drug failure, up to 57% of patients with CD require one or more gastrointestinal resections [10], and 30% of patients with UC eventually require colectomy [11], both potentially causing morbidity, a decrease in health-related quality of life [12,13], and high socioeconomic expenditures [14].

In the first part of this chapter (Section 11.2), we present current knowledge on IBD genetics and pathogenesis from genetic linkage studies, candidate gene association studies, and, most recently, from genomewide association studies, and subsequent basic research. It is common sense that better understanding of disease pathophysiology might be helpful for future drug development processes to establish a more tailored drug therapy for IBD based on specific molecular drug targets. In Section 11.3, we focus on currently available medical therapeutics in IBD. We summarize knowledge on the genetic basis of drug response and toxicity. There is a significant need to individualize the currently available therapeutics to minimize treatment failure and ADR. In both sections we discuss the goals of pharmacogenomics, which aims to concentrate on new insights to discover new therapeutic targets and interventions and to elucidate the constellation of genes that determine the efficacy and toxicity of specific medications.

11.2 SUSCEPTIBILITY GENES IN IBD

11.2.1 Nucleotide Oligomerization Domain 2

In 2001, three working groups identified single-nucleotide polymorphisms (SNPs, R702W and G908R) and a frameshift mutation (L1007fsinsC) in the nulceotide oligomerization domain (NOD)2 [location 16q21; also known as *caspase activating recruitment domain* (CARD15)] within the IBD1 susceptibility locus [15], which confer susceptibility to CD but not to UC [16–18]. NOD2 is involved in the innate immunity as an intracellular sensor of muramyldipeptide, a component of bacterial cell wall peptidoglycan of both Gram-positive and Gram-negative bacteria [19,20]. The NOD2 protein is composed of a central nucleotide oligomerization domain, two

CARD domains, and a leucine-rich repeat (LRR) domain [21]. The LRR domain is particularly significant in that it mediates host response to microbial stimulation and all three CD-associated variants are located in or near the LRR. NOD2 is expressed in intestinal epithelial cells [22,23], particularly in Paneth cells [24], monocyte-derived cells [25] including macrophages, intestinal myofibroblasts [26], and endothelial cells [27]. Activation of NOD2 with muramyldipeptide results in activation of multiple signaling pathways, including the nuclear factor (NF)κB and mitogen-activated protein kinases pathways, and ultimately leads to a variety of immune responses [28–31]. Nevertheless, the exact mechanism of NOD2 polymorphisms to CD pathogenesis has not been unraveled so far. Nod2 knockout mice did not develop spontaneous colitis [32], but showed a decrease in α-defensin (cryptidin) mRNA expression in intestinal Paneth cells and were unable to detect muramyldipeptide. Most interestingly, these mice were more susceptible to oral, but not systemic, infection with *Listeria monocytogenes*, supporting the fact that NOD2 is important in epithelial antimicrobial function. In patients with CD, a decrease in the mRNA and protein levels of the α-defensins, human defensin (HD)5 and HD6, was observed [30,33]. Decreased expression was more pronounced in patients with the frameshift NOD2 mutation L1007fsinsC resulting in a diminished bactericidal activity [30,34]. Thus, a compromise in innate immunity of the ileal mucosa may initiate and perpetuate an inflammatory response to intestinal microbes, thus leading to CD (loss-of-function model). Maeda et al., in contrast, demonstrated that Nod2 mutant mice exhibited an elevated NFκB activation in response to muramyl-dipeptide and more efficient processing and secretion of IL1β [29]. These effects favoring a gain-of-function model of NOD2 were linked to an increased susceptibility to bacterial induced intestinal inflammation.

In populations of European ancestry, around 35–45% of CD patients [35] and 5% of healthy individuals [36] carry at least one NOD2 variant. In African-American patients NOD2 variants are rare [37] and in different Asian populations they are completely absent [38,39]. A meta-analysis of 42 studies revealed that NOD2 heterozygosity had an odds ratio for CD of 2.39 (95% CI 2.00–2.86) and homozygosity or compound heterozygosity of 17.1 (95% CI 10.7–27.2) [40]. In phenotype–genotype association studies NOD2 carriage was associated with ileal location [40,41], stricturing behavior [40,42], and an aggressive course of disease [43]. In a pharmacogenetic approach, patients with perianal fistulas who had a wild-type NOD2 genotype responded better to antibiotic treatment than did patients with NOD2 variants [44]. This finding needs further confirmation in larger CD cohorts.

11.2.2 Autophagy Pathway

Hampe et al. [45] performed the first genomewide association study in IBD and identified a coding SNP (T300A) in the autophagy-related 16-like 1 (ATG16L1, location 2q37.1) gene as a susceptibility factor for CD but not for UC. Subsequent studies confirmed these findings [46–49]. Moreover, in further genomewide approaches, the immunity related guanosine triphosphatase M (IRGM) gene (location 5q33.1), encoding a GTP binding protein that induces autophagy and is involved in elimination of intracellular bacteria, was found to be a risk factor for CD, implicating the autophagy pathway as being significant in CD pathogenesis [47,50,51]. The hallmark of autophagy is the formation of double-membrane vesicles that sequester cytoplasmic contents and deliver them to the lysosome for subsequent degradation [52]. Autophagy has an important role in cell and tissue homeostasis, including elimination of microbial pathogens from host cells [53].

Cadwell et al. [54,55] and Saitoh et al. [56] revealed how ATG16L1 and autophagy may contribute to the development of CD. In mouse models Paneth cells deficient for the autophagy complex proteins Atg16l1 and Atg5 showed notable abnormalities in the granule exocytosis pathway. CD patients homozygous for the disease-associated variant (T300A) displayed morphologic Paneth cell abnormalites similar to those in the mouse models. Moreover, Saitoh et al. [56] demonstrated that Atg16l1 deficiency resulted in impairment of authophagosome formation and degradation of longlived proteins. Stimulation of Atg16l1-deficient macrophages with lipopolysaccharide induced high amounts of the cytokines IL1β and IL18. Chimeric mice lacking Atg16l1 in hematopoetic cells were highly susceptible to dextran sodium sulfate (DSS)-induced colitis, which could be ameliorated by anti-IL1β and anti-IL18 antibodies, indicating the importance of the inappropriate secretion of these cytokines by dysfunctional hematopoetic cells.

In European populations the allele frequency of the risk-conferring G allele was 57–64% in CD patients versus 50–57% in healthy controls [48,57,58]. Homozygous carriers of the GG allele (300AA) had an increased risk for CD (OR 1.65, 95% CI 1.32–2.07). Interestingly, no association between the ATG16L1 variant and CD in Asians was observed [59]. Phenotype–genotype analyses demonstrated an association of the ATG16L1 risk allele with ileal disease [48,60], which is in line with experimental findings of alterations in Paneth cells. However, this association is not described unequivocally [57,61].

11.2.3 Interleukin 23 Pathway

Duerr et al. [62] identified a highly significant association between ileal CD as well as UC and a nonsynonymous SNP (Arg381Gly) as well as nine other markers in the interleukin 23 receptor (IL23R, location 1p31.3) and in the intergenic region between IL23R and IL12 receptor β2 gene (IL12RB2). Subsequent studies confirmed these findings [47,63–65,129]. In a more recent meta-analysis and replication study four genes (IL23R, IL12B, STAT3, and JAK2) playing a role in IL23 signaling were identified or replicated to be in association with CD.

Most IL23 is secreted by activated dendritic cells, monocytes, and macrophages in response to microbial ligands that bind to toll-like receptors [66]. Studies in animal models of IBD have showed that IL23 plays a key role in chronic intestinal inflammation. Thus, the findings from genomewide association studies as well as those from animal models [67,68] support the relevance of IL23 in IBD. The role of IL23 as drug target in IBD was already evaluated in two studies. Mannon et al. investigated the efficacy of a human anti-p40 antibody directed against the subunit of IL12 and IL23 in active CD in a randomized, placebo-controlled, double-blind phase

II study [69]. The antibody ABT-874/J695 may induce response and remission, but the differences to placebo were largely statistically insignificant. In a randomized, placebo-controlled, double-blind cross over phase II trial ($n = 104$) as well as in an open-label trial including nonresponders to infliximab ($n = 27$), another human anti-p40 antibody (ustekinumab) was investigated in patients with moderate to severe CD [70]. Although the results failed to definitely show that induction therapy with ustekinumab was superior to placebo, the data demonstrated beneficial treatment effects, especially in infliximab nonresponders. Further controlled, sufficiently powered trials for efficacy analysis in CD as well as in UC patients are needed to better understand the relevance of antagonizing IL23 in IBD treatment.

The nonsynomymous SNP Arg381Gln showing the strongest association with IBD has an allele frequency of 0.8–4.0% in patients with CD, 1.9–4.6% in patients with UC, and 5.9–7.0 in healthy controls [57,58,62,64], thus conferring protection against the development of CD (OR 0.38, 95% CI 0.29–0.50) and UC (OR 0.73, 95% CI 0.55–0.96) [64]. In the listed studies no associations of IL23R variants with a certain disease phenotype were observed, suggesting that IL23R variants rather exert a generalized effect on chronic intestinal inflammation than on development of a specific phenotype.

11.2.4 Defensins

As indicated above, in CD, and also in UC, intestinal microbes are assumed to trigger intestinal inflammation in genetically susceptible individuals. Therefore, the possible role of diminished antimicrobial peptides, in particular the human α- and β-defensins in the pathogenesis of IBD, has been the focus of more recent research. Wehkamp et al. demonstrated that patients with ileal CD had dimished HD5 as well as HD6 mRNA as well as protein level [30,33] and that patients with the NOD2 frameshift mutation L1007fsinsC even had a pronounced decrease in HD5 and HD6 [30]. In a 2007 study, a high correlation between mRNA levels of the Wnt signaling pathway transcription factor (TCF)4 (location 10q25.3), a regulator of Paneth cell differentiation and expression of HD5 ($r_s = 0.68, p < 0.0001$) and HD6 ($r_s = 0.68, p < 0.0001$) was reported [71]. Since TCF4 binds to and directly regulates the promoter regions of HD5 and HD6, it was speculated that genetic variants of TCF4 resulting in reduced expression could account for a decrease of both defensins. Subsequently, the authors found that a TCF4 promoter variant was associated with ileal CD (OR 1.23, 95% CI 1.07–1.41) but not with colonic CD or UC [72]. The observed link between TCF4 and ileal CD suggests that impaired differentiation in Paneth cells might predispose to this phenotype. The same working group disclosed an attenuation of the human β-defensin (HBD) 2 induction in patients with colonic CD [73,74], which was related to a lower HBD2 gene (location 8p23.1) copy number compared to controls [75]. Individuals with ≤ 3 copies were shown to have a significantly higher risk for developing colonic CD than were individuals with ≥ 4 copies (OR 3.06, 95% CI 1.46–6.45). Thus, defective β-defensin induction seems to predispose to colonic CD.

11.2.5 Toll-Like Receptor 4

In a candidate gene approach, several working groups investigated a potential association of variants in the toll-like receptor (TLR)4 gene (location 9q32-33) and IBD. The TLR4 is a transmembrane protein with the extracellular domain consisting of a LRR [76,77]. It recognizes conserved pathogenic motifs of Gram-negative bacteria, mainly lipopolysaccharide (LPS), and results in the activation of NFκB and subsequent induction of an inflammatory response [78,79]. Data from animal models suggest a role of TLR4 in IBD pathogenesis [80,81] since mouse strains defective for LPS signaling due to loss of function mutation in the TLR4 gene are highly susceptible to DSS-induced or spontaneous colitis. One polymorphism, Asp299Gly, is functionally relevant as it is responsible for airway hypo-responsiveness to LPS [82], leading to an increased risk of Gram-negative infections [83]. Franchimont et al. [84] demonstrated for the first time that the allele frequency of the Asp299Gly variant was significantly higher in two independent CD populations (10.9% and 11.5%) and a UC population (9.8%) compared to a control population (5.0%). However, subsequent association studies yielded inconsistent results. A meta-analysis eventually revealed an increased risk of the Asp299Gly polymorphism for CD (OR 1.45, 95% CI 1.11–1.90) and IBD in general (OR 1.36, 95% CI 1.01–1.84) but not for UC (OR 1.14, 95% CI 0.79–1.63) [85]. Most recently, Ungaro et al. examined the effect of an antibody against the TLR4/MD2 complex in two murine models of IBD. This study suggests that the anti-TLR4 antibody may decrease inflammation in IBD but results in defective mucosal healing [86], challenging the role of TLR4 as drug target in IBD.

11.2.6 Disks Large Homolog 5 (*Drosophila*)

Stoll et al. initially described an association between IBD and variants in the Drosophila disks large homolog 5 (DLG5) gene on chromosome 10q23 [87]. In particular, R30Q was found to be associated with IBD. DLG5 belongs to the membrane associated guanylate kinase (MAGUK) family and is ubiquitously expressed in human tissue, including large and small intestines [87]. The protein is involved in the formation of cell junctions, maintenance of cell shape, and clustering of channel proteins at the cell surface [88]. The variants were hypothesized to interfere with the epithelial barrier function thus predisposing to IBD.

Daly et al. confirmed the association of variant R30Q and CD in one of two case–control cohorts and in a family cohort [89]. However, subsequent studies and a meta-analysis [90] failed to replicate the association between R30Q and IBD. On observing male–female allele frequency differences [91], Browning et al. performed a gender-stratified analysis of the DLG5 R30Q variant in 4707 patients with CD and 4973 controls [92]. In that large cohort, no male–female allele frequency differences in the control population were observed. The R30Q variant was associated with a decreased risk for CD in women (OR 0.86, 95% CI 0.76–0.97) but not in men.

11.2.7 Solute Carrier Family 22, Member (SLC22A) 4 Gene

Rioux et al. described another CD susceptibility locus on chromosome 5 in a genomewide linkage study, denoted as IBD5 locus [93]. Fine mapping of this area has identified a single, highly conserved 250-kb risk haplotype of 11 SNPs spanning a cytokine gene cluster in association with CD. In 2004, Peltekova et al. [94] postulated that functional polymorphisms, L503F in the solute carrier family 22, member (SLC22A)4 gene (location 5q31.1, coding for the novel organic cation transporter OCTN1) and G-207C in the SLC22A5 gene (coding for OCTN2), comprised a two-locus risk haplotype that accounted for the association findings at IBD5. OCTN1 is strongly expressed in kidney, trachea, bone marrow, and small bowel and has been characterized as a carnitine transporter [95]. OCTN2 is about 75% homologous to OCTN1, and is a high-affinity sodium carnitine transporter that is expressed in kidney, smooth muscle, and heart tissue [95]. The variants might reduce carnitine transport leading to an impairment of fatty acid β-oxidation, which causes colitis in animal models [96]. Several subsequent studies confirmed the association between the two-locus risk haplotype and CD [97,98]. However, when an additional number of surrounding SNPs comprising the IBD5 haplotype were examined, no independent association between OCTN variants and CD were found [99–101]. Taubert et al. demonstrated that the polymorphism L503F resulted in a 50% higher intrinsic transport efficiency of the food ingredient ergothioneine [102]. Accordingly, ergothineine levels were significantly higher in 503F than in 503L carriers without differences between patients and controls [103]. The authors hypothesized that an increased tissue accumulation of ergothioneine, which is suggested to inhibit apoptosis, might contribute to a defective innate immunity by prolonging immune cell survival or by impairing removal of intracellular bacteria.

11.2.8 ATP Binding Cassette, Subfamily B, Member 1

Satsangi et al. found evidence for linkage to markers on chromosome 7q in siblings with UC [104]. At this region (7q21.1) interestingly the ATP-binding cassette B1 gene (ABCB1; formerly multidrug resistance gene 1, MDR1) encoding P-glycoprotein 170 (P-gp) is located. P-gp is a transmembrane protein, expressed in several human tissues, including the apical surfaces of epithelial colonic and ileal cells and lymphocytes. P-gp functions as trans-membrane efflux pump for a chemically diverse array of xenobiotics [105]. Development of spontaneous colitis resembling UC in mdr1a knockout mice has been shown, which can be prevented or is reversible by administration of antibiotics [106,107]. In a candidate gene approach, Schwab et al. demonstrated for the first time an association of the C3435T variant and UC in a German population [105]. C3435T is a silent polymorphism, and it is hypothesized that the presence of a rare codon affects the timing of cotransitional folding and insertion of P-gp into the membrane, thereby altering the structure of substrate and inhibitor interaction sites [108]. Hoffmeyer et al. observed a significant correlation of the C3435T polymorphism with decreased intestinal expression levels and function of P-gp [109]. The lower P-gp expression and function might impair the defense against intestinal bacteria and so represent a risk factor for development of IBD. C3435T is more prevalent in patients with UC (42.9–58.2%) compared to controls (35.7–56.1%). Two meta-analyses, including studies showing conflicting results [110–114], confirmed the association between the C3435T polymorphism and UC (3435T allele, OR 1.12, $p = 0.013$ [115]; 3435T allele, OR = 1.17, $p = 0.003$ and 3435TT genotype, OR = 1.36, $p = 0.017$ [116]). Another polymorphism, G2677T/A, which has also been shown to affect expression and activity of P-gp [117] and is in part in linkage with C3435T, was reported to be associated also with IBD [118], UC [115] but was also refractory CD [113]. However, association studies again showed contradictory results, and a meta-analysis could not confirm such an association [116].

Interindividual variability in ABCB1 expression and/or ABCB1 geno/haplotypes alter pharmacokinetics of drugs that are substrates of P-gp (e.g., steroids [119,120], immunosuppressants [121,122]). Therefore, ABCB1 genetics may explain differences in treatment response. Whereas several retrospective studies did not show a relationship between ABCB1 genetics and steroid resistance [123–125], an association between ABCB1 variants and refractory disease [113] as well as an increased expression of P-gp in lymphocytes of IBD patients failing medical treatment [120] were reported. For a definite conclusion on the impact of ABCB1 genetics, well-designed, prospective studies are required. For thiopurine therapy in CD patients, homozygous carriers for the 2677T allele as well as the 3435T allele showed a lower frequency of drug response [126]. In addition, the 2677TT, but not the 3435TT genotype, was significantly associated with an increased risk for cyclosporine failure in patients with steroid resistant UC [127]. A plausible explanation therefore is still lacking.

11.2.9 Genomewide Association Studies

Because the effect of single variants is so small, the major determinant in the identification of novel genetic risk factors by genomewide association studies (GWASs) generally depends on the sample size of index patients and controls [128]. For instance, the first genomewide association studies identified eight thus far unknown genetic risk loci for CD. In a large meta-analysis including three studies on Crohn's disease (3230 cases and 4829 controls) and additional replication in 3664 independent cases, the results strongly confirm 11 previously reported loci and provide evidence for 21 additional loci, including the regions containing STAT3, JAK2, ICOSLG, CDKAL1, and ITLN1 [129]. An updated summary of GWAS in IBD (CD and UC) is available at `http://www.genome.gov/26525384`. Of note, the functional relevance of most of these genetic variants as well as underlying mechanisms related to the pathophysiology of IBD is currently unknown.

11.3 PHARMACOGENETICS IN IBD

A broad variety of individual factors may influence pharmacokinetics, commonly referred to by the acronym *ADME* (drug absorption, distribution, metabolism, and elimination) of a drug and must, therefore, be taken into account when determining dosage for a given patient. Drug concentration at its target will, in many cases, represent a mere fraction of the systemic concentration. Active transport processes, however, may influence local target concentrations. It has become increasingly clear that hereditary variances in drug metabolizing enzymes and drug transporters can exert considerable influence on drug concentrations. However, in addition to inherited variants, it should be mentioned that many other factors (e.g., age, sex, weight, body fat, alcohol consumption, concomitant drugs, nutritional status, liver and renal function, cardiovascular function, environmental pollutants) are important so-called non-genetic factors possibly influencing ADME processes of drugs [130].

11.3.1 Azathioprine/6-Mercaptopurine

The thiopurines azathioprine and 6-mercaptopurine are indicated for the maintenance of remission in IBD and corticosteroid-sparing in chronic active disease [6,131–133]. Several anabolic and catabolic pathways are involved in the metabolism of thiopurines (Fig. 11.2), resulting in the formation of most important metabolites, the 6-thioguanine nucleotides (6-TGN) and 6-methylmercaptopurine

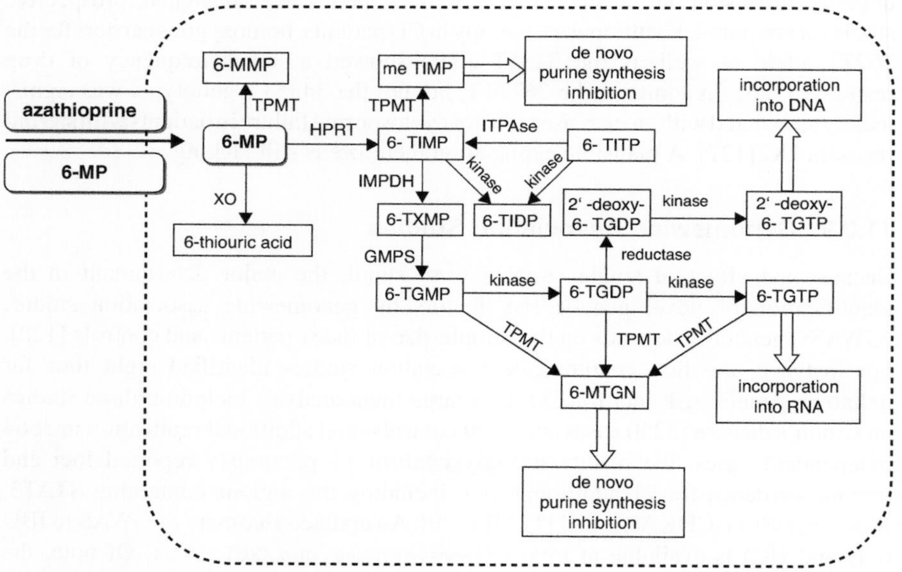

FIGURE 11.2 Metabolic scheme of thiopurine metabolism (6-MP — mercaptopurine; 6-MMP — 6-methylmercaptopurine; 6-MMPR — 6-methylmercaptopurine ribonucleotides; 6-MTGN — 6-methyl-thioguanine nucleotides; 6-TG — 6-thioguanine; 6-TGDP — 6-thioguanosine 5-diphosphate; 6-TGMP — 6-thioguanosine 5-monophosphate; 6-TGTP — 6-thioguanosine 5′-triphosphate; 6-TIMP — 6-thioinosine 5′-monophosphate; 6-TX — 6-thioxanthine; 6-TXMP — 6-thioxanthine monophosphate; GMPS — guanosine monophosphate synthetase; HPRT — hypoxanthine guanine phosphoribosyltransferase; IMPDH — inosine monophosphate dehydrogenase; TPMT — thiopurine S-methyltransferase; XO — xandine oxidase).

ribonucleotides (6MMPR). 6TGN are incorporated into DNA and RNA, thereby inhibiting replication, DNA repair mechanisms, and protein synthesis [134,135]. The 6-thio-GTP leads to apoptosis of activated T cells and to a suppression of T-cell-dependent pathogenic immune responses [136–138]. The meTIMP inhibits the purine *de novo* synthesis, thus interfering with replication [139]. Moreover, thiopurines have been shown to arrest the proliferation of stimulated T cells, but despite proliferation arrest, T cells were able to differentiate into effector cells [140]. Thiopurines do not enhance apoptosis of T cells until day 5 postexposition, and thus prolonged treatment may result in depletion of antigen-specific memory T cells depending on repeated encounters with the antigen over a prolonged timecourse.

The enzyme thiopurine *S*-methyltransferase (TPMT) catalyzes the *S*-adenosyl-L-methionine dependent *S*-methylation of mercaptopurine and its metabolites (Fig. 11.2). Weinshilboum et al. [141] for the first time described large inherited variations in TMPT activity with a trimodal frequency distribution (very low, intermediate, and normal/high activity). In a large population of more than 1200 Caucasians, very low TPMT activity was determined in 0.6%, and about 10% and 90% were found to be intermediate and normal/high methylators, respectively [142]. Family studies considered the inheritance of TPMT activity, and after characterization of the human TPMT gene located on chromosome 6p22.3, the phenotypic variation of TPMT activity could be explained by genetic variants. To date (2011), at least 25 allelic variants (TPMT*2–*25) with pronounced effects on expression/function associated with altered enzyme activity have been identified [142–145]. There are substantial interethnic differences in the occurrence and frequency of allelic variants. In Caucasians, the most common variant alleles showing decreased activity are TPMT*3A (4.5%) and TPMT*3C (0.4%); all other mutations are rare (TPMT*2 0.17%) or have been described only in single cases [142,146,147]. In subjects with African or Asian ancestry, TPMT*3C is the predominant allele [146]. On the basis of several comprehensive phenotype–genotype correlation studies [142,148], TPMT genotyping can be recommended to replace measurement of TPMT activity in red blood cells [149].

In general, TPMT serves as a model for pharmacogenetic research because patients with TPMT deficiency treated with standard doses of azathioprine/6-mercaptopurine are at approximately 100% risk of developing severe myelosuppression within a few weeks after commencing drug therapy independently of the underlying disease [150–152]. This can be explained by an 8–15-fold increase of 6TGN levels in RBCs compared with wild-type patients, subsequently leading to an exaggerated cytotoxic effect [153]. TPMT deficiency is not a contraindication of thiopurine therapy. An initial dose reduction to 10–15% of the standard dose of azathioprine is a reliable approach for treatment of TPMT-deficient IBD patients [154]. Although data from prospective trials in IBD are still lacking, dose reduction to approximately 50% of standard dosage in TMPT heterozygous IBD patients is recommended [155]. To avoid hematotoxicity in TPMT-deficient patients treated with thiopurines, pretreatment TPMT testing is reasonable as a routine clinical measure with subsequent pharmacogenetically guided dosing [156]. However, since nongenetic factors may predispose patients to ADR independent of

TPMT (e.g., viral infection, comedication), repeated laboratory controls are required during thiopurine therapy.

The inosine triphosphate pyrophosphohydrolase (ITPAse), a cytosolic enzyme, catalyzes the pyrophosphohydrolysis of ITP/deoxy-ITP and xanthosine triphosphate, thereby preventing accumulation of nucleotides and incorporation into RNA and DNA. Polymorphisms in the ITPA gene correlate excellently with decreased ITPase activity in RBCs [157,158]. More recently, a relationship between the C94A polymorphism in the ITPA gene and an increased risk for ADR under thiopurine therapy was reported [159,160]. However, these findings are currently controversially discussed [161–163]. Stocco et al. [164] investigated the effects of the ITPA variant C94A on the 6-mercaptopurine metabolism and toxicity in children with ALL. Children with the variant C94A had significantly higher concentrations of 6MMPR.

Among patients whose 6MP dose had been adjusted for TPMT genotype, those with the variant allele had a significantly higher probability of severe febrile neutropenia. The authors tentatively attributed the inconsistentcy of results in earlier studies to the fact that the thiopurine doses were systematically adjusted on the basis of the TPMT genotype in only a few of these studies. In another study, Stocco et al. [165] demonstrated an association between wild-type glutathion *S*-tranferase M1 and an increased probability of adverse events and increased incidence of lymphopenia during azathioprine treatment in IBD patients. Hawwa et al. [166] correlated XO polymorphisms with metabolite concentrations (6TU, 6MP, and 6-TGN) and myelotoxicity in a small population of patients with IBD and childhood ALL resulting in statistically in significant effects. Since these study populations were small, larger studies are needed to elucidate the impact of ITPA genetics.

11.3.2 Methotrexate

The immunosuppressant methotrexate (MTX) is indicated for induction and maintenance of remission in CD [204], preferentially in patients intolerant of or resistant to thiopurines [131]. The metabolism of MTX is complex (Fig. 11.3), and, for instance, inhibition of thymidylate synthase by MTX polyglutamates interferes with DNA synthesis in actively dividing cells. Furthermore, MTX polyglutamates have an indirect inhibitory influence on several enzymes within the adenosine pathway leading to the release of adenosine, a potent antiinflammatory mediator. The metabolism of MTX involves several polymorphically expressed enzymes representing promising candidates for a pharmacogenetic/genomic approach. In one retrospective pilot study, 102 patients receiving MTX for steroid-dependent or unresponsive IBD were studied. Patients homozygous for the methylene tetrahydrofolate reductase (MTHFR) 1298C variant have had a higher risk for developing overall toxicity, particularly nausea and vomiting, compared to controls [167]. None of the other candidate genes (reduced folate carrier 1, γ-glutamylhydrolase) were associated with MTX toxicity or response to treatment. Most reports investigating MTX pharmacogenetics included cancer or rheumatic patient cohorts, and their somewhat contradicatory results have been extensively summarized elsewhere [168,169].

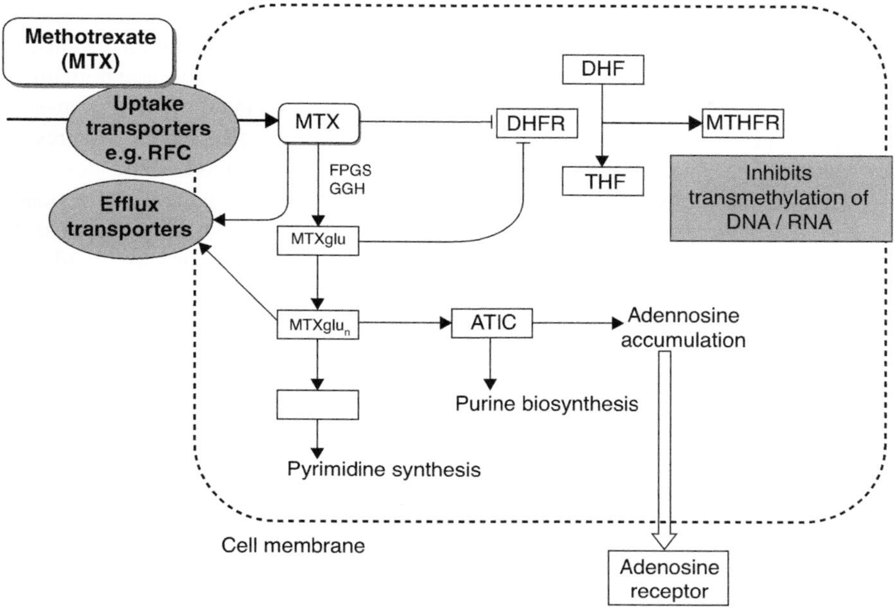

FIGURE 11.3 Simplified scheme of methotrexate metabolism (RFC1 — reduced folate carrier 1; MTX-PGs — polyglutamated MTX; FPGS — folylpolyglutamate synthase; GGH — γ-glutamylhydrolase; DHF, dihydrofolate; THF — tetrahydrofolate; TS — thymidylate synthase; DHFR — dihydrofolate reductase; MTHFR — methylenetetrahydrofolate reductase; ATIC — 5-aminoimidazole-4-carboxamide ribonucleotide transformylase).

11.3.3 Infliximab

Infliximab is indicated for induction and maintenance of remission in patients with moderate to severe IBD, with draining perianal, abdominal, or rectovaginal fistulas, steroid sparing, as well as extraintestinal manifestations of IBD [170]. Infliximab is a high-molecular-weight chimeric monoclonal IgG1 antibody against soluble and membrane-bound human TNFα. Once TNFα has been blocked by infliximab, clinical benefit in responding patients with IBD is achieved by downregulation of local and systemic proinflammatory cytokines, reduction of lymphocyte and leukocyte migration to sites of inflammation, induction of apoptosis of TNF-producing cells (e.g., activated monocytes and T lymphocytes), increase in NKκB inhibitor levels, and reduction of endothelial adhesion molecules and acute-phase proteins [171,172]. Specific biomarkers for better prediction of clinical efficacy and/or for avoidance of ADR are currently missing [173]. As the induction of apoptosis is an important action mechanism of infliximab, Hlavaty et al. investigated the association between infliximab response and polymorphisms in genes of the extrinsic and intrinsic apoptotic pathways [174]. The authors identified three polymorphisms in apoptosis genes (Fas ligand C-843T, Fas G-670A, and Caspase9 C93T) potentially influencing the response to infliximab. On the basis of these data, the authors proposed an apoptotic pharmacogenetic index for prediction of low, medium, and high response to infliximab [175]. Moreover, a haplotype for the ADAM metallopeptidase domain 17 gene, which cleaves membrane-bound TNFα, was associated with response to infliximab [176] as well as a variant in the IgG1 Fcγ receptor IIIa, which is expressed on macrophages and natural killer cells and is involved in antibody-dependent cell-mediated cytotoxicity [177]. Urcelay et al. [178] reported an increased frequency of the IBD5 homozygous mutant genotype in CD patients lacking response to infliximab. Finally, the distribution of variants in the TNF receptor superfamily 1A and 1B showed significant differences in Japanese responders versus nonresponders [179] but not in Caucasians [180,181]. Several other pharmacogenetic studies failed to identify an association between additional candidate genes such as NOD2, lymphotoxin α, C-reactive protein, and clinical outcome of infliximab use in IBD [176,180,182–186].

11.3.4 Corticosteroids

Corticosteroids such as prednisone or budesonide are indicated for moderate to severe IBD [6,131,187]. Corticosteroids exert their effect on immune cells by activating the intracytoplasmic corticosteroid receptor (CR) to regulate the expression of certain target genes important in the inflammatory process [188] such as proinflammatory cytokines, adhesion molecules, chemokines, and inflammatory enzymes. About 32–49% of IBD patients treated with corticosteroids are steroid responders, whereas 22–36% and 16–20% are steroid-dependent or steroid-resistant, respectively [189,190]. Predictive genetic markers for steroid dependence or steroid resistance are lacking. As mentioned above, a relationship between genetic variants of the efflux transporter protein P-gp (ABCB1) and reduced steroid responsiveness is controversially discussed [113,123–125]. De et al. [191] investigated the impact of variants in the CR gene on treatment response to glucocorticoids in 119 patients with IBD since it was previously reported that sensitivity to glucocorticoids may be explained by CR polymorphisms [192–194]. Patients homozygous for the intronic BclI variant responded better to steroid treatment compared to wild-type or heterozygous patients. Cucchiara et al. [124] reported that CD patients carrying the TNFα –308A allele showed more frequent resistance to steroids compared to noncarriers (OR = 0.29; $p = 0.032$). A promoter polymorphism in the CD14 gene (T/C at position –159) of UC patients, playing a role in recognition of lipopolysaccharide, was associated with cumulative steroid doses reflecting steroid unresponsiveness [195]. Furthermore, in patients with CD, a variation (G/C at position –173) in the macrophage migration inhibitory factor gene, which is involved in the regulation of the innate immune system, was associated with cumulative steroid doses [196]. In a study investigating the relevance of DLG5 in IBD, Lakatos et al. [197] found an association between the DLG5 allele 113A and steroid resistance in patients with CD. Altogether, these results are based on small study populations and therefore replication in larger prospective studies is warranted.

11.3.5 Cyclosporine

Cyclosporine (CsA) is recommended in patients with severe steroid-refractory UC to avoid colectomy [6,131]. CsA isolated from the fungus *Tolypocladium inflatum* is a calcineurin inhibitor. Normally, presentation of antigen to T cells leads to an increase of intracellular calcium, and subsequently the calcium–calmodulin-dependent serine/threonine phosphatase calcineurin is activated. Calcineurin dephosphorylates the cytosolic nuclear factor of activated T cells, which is subsequently able to translocate into the nucleus and stimulate production of cytokines [198,199]. CsA binds to the cyclophilins and exerts an immunosuppressive effect by inhibiting the dephosphorylation of nuclear factor of activated T cells by binding to calcineurin. Conseqeuntly, expression of cytokines such as IL2, IL3, IL4, TNFα, and interferon γ from T lymphocytes is inhibited. CsA is a substrate of P-gp and also of cytochrome P450 (CYP) isoenzymes, which are the major cyclosporine-metabolizing enzymes in humans (e.g., CYP3A4, CYP3A5) [200]. In IBD studies investigating the impact of genetic polymorphisms on CsA response including ADR are limited. Palmieri et al. investigated the association between ABCB1 variants and IBD drug response [123]. Since only 11 IBD patients on CsA had been included, no definite conclusion can be drawn. A French study group investigated the frequency distribution of ABCB1 variants in 154 patients who had received CsA for steroid-resistant UC [127]. A significant association between the G2677T variant and CsA treatment failure has been reported, which remained significant after multivariate analysis (2677TT, OR 6.75, 95% CI 1.53–29.71). Of note, most CsA pharmacogenetic studies, including ABCB1, CYP3A4, and CYP3A5 genetic variants, are performed in transplantation medicine since here CsA is the drug of choice [201,202]. On the basis of these data, only a minor impact of ABCB1 and CYP3A genotypes on CsA response in IBD patients is expected, although substantial data for IBD patients are still missing.

11.4 CONCLUSION

In parallel with the ongoing elucidation of the genetic basis of IBD, there is an increasing awareness that genetic information may be helpful in improving drug therapy and identifying patients at risk for ADR by selecting individual groups according to their specific genetic make-up. In spite of several promising examples, the use of pharmacogenetic information for individualized prescription of drugs in treatment of IBD is still in its infancy. TPMT is the best recognized example of genetic variants that can provide an explanation of the severe hematotoxicity in patients treated with azathioprine/6-mercaptopurine under standard dosage. Thus this polymorphism serves as a model for pharmacogenetic research. TPMT has accessed clinical practice, and the FDA recommends that individuals be tested for TPMT (genotyping or phenotyping) before initiation of thiopurine therapy. In contrast, pharmacogenetic findings are less convincing for other drugs used in treatment of IBD. New strategies are therefore needed to identify, for a given drug, the relevant genes that are involved in pharmacokinetic and pharmacodynamic processes. Various strategies are now being used, including genomewide association studies, gene expression analyses, proteomics, metabolomics, and epigenomics [129,130,203,204]. Completion of the HapMap project, together with the development of new genotyping technologies, provides powerful tools for a comprehensive search for relevant genetic variants. Several novel disease susceptibility genes have been reported, but their functional relevance for pathogenesis of IBD is still poorly understood. The most promising candidates seem to be NOD2, ATG16L1, and IL23R. Alltogether, pharmacogenomics in IBD will hopefully help in the future to improve drug therapy in clinical practice by providing novel drug targets and/or relevant biomarkers for better prediction of drug response, including ADR.

ACKNOWLEDGMENTS

This work has been funded by the Robert Bosch Foundation, Stuttgart, Germany. The work by MS is supported in part by the Deutsche Forschungsgemeinschaft Grant A9 SFB685-2009 and the BMBF grant 03IS2061C.

REFERENCES

1. Podolsky DK. Inflammatory bowel disease. *New Engl. J. Med.* 2002;**347**:417–429.
2. Nikolaus S, Schreiber S. Diagnostics of inflammatory bowel disease. *Gastroenterology* 2007;**133**:1670–1689.
3. Waljee AK, Joyce JC, Wren PA, Khan TM, Higgins PD. Patient reported symptoms during an ulcerative colitis flare: A qualitative focus group study. *Eur. J. Gastroenterol. Hepatol.* 2009;**21**:558–564.
4. Loftus EV Jr. Clinical epidemiology of inflammatory bowel disease: Incidence, prevalence, and environmental influences. *Gastroenterology* 2004;**126**:1504–1517.
5. Halfvarson J, Bodin L, Tysk C, Lindberg E, Järnerot G. Inflammatory bowel disease in a Swedish twin cohort: A long-term follow-up of concordance and clinical characteristics. *Gastroenterology* 2003;**124**:1767–1773.
6. Lichtenstein GR, Abreu MT, Cohen R, Tremaine W. American Gastroenterological Association Institute medical position statement on corticosteroids, immunomodulators, and infliximab in inflammatory bowel disease. *Gastroenterology* 2006;**130**:935–939.
7. Lichtenstein GR, Feagan BG, Cohen RD, Salzberg BA, Diamond RH, Chen DM, et al. Serious infections and mortality in association with therapies for Crohn's disease: TREAT registry. *Clin. Gastroenterol. Hepatol.* 2006;**4**:621–630.
8. Moore TJ, Cohen MR, Furberg CD. Serious adverse drug events reported to the Food and Drug Administration, 1998–2005. *Arch. Intern. Med.* 2007;**167**:1752–1759.
9. Peyrin-Biroulet L, Deltenre P, de SN, Branche J, Sandborn WJ, Colombel JF. Efficacy and safety of tumor necrosis factor antagonists in Crohn's disease: Meta-analysis of placebo-controlled trials. *Clin. Gastroenterol. Hepatol.* 2008;**6**:644–653.
10. Silverstein MD, Loftus EV, Sandborn WJ, Tremaine WJ, Feagan BG, Nietert PJ, et al. Clinical course and costs of care for Crohn's disease: Markov model analysis of a population-based cohort. *Gastroenterology* 1999;**117**:49–57.

11. Caprilli R, Viscido A, Latella G. Current management of severe ulcerative colitis. *Nat. Clin. Pract. Gastroenterol. Hepatol.* 2007;**4**:92–101.

12. Waljee A, Waljee J, Morris AM, Higgins PD. Threefold increased risk of infertility: A meta-analysis of infertility after ileal pouch anal anastomosis in ulcerative colitis. *Gut* 2006;**55**:1575–1580.

13. Ananthakrishnan AN, Weber LR, Knox JF, Skaros S, Emmons J, Lundeen S, et al. Permanent work disability in Crohn's disease. *Am. J. Gastroenterol.* 2008;**103**:154–161.

14. Odes S. How expensive is inflammatory bowel disease? A critical analysis. *World J. Gastroenterol.* 2008;**14**:6641–6647.

15. Hugot JP, Laurent-Puig P, Gower-Rousseau C, Olson JM, Lee JC, Beaugerie L, et al. Mapping of a susceptibility locus for Crohn's disease on chromosome 16. *Nature* 1996;**379**:821–823.

16. Hugot JP, Chamaillard M, Zouali H, Lesage S, Cezard JP, Belaiche J, et al. Association of NOD2 leucine-rich repeat variants with susceptibility to Crohn's disease. *Nature* 2001;**411**:599–603.

17. Ogura Y, Bonen DK, Inohara N, Nicolae DL, Chen FF, Ramos R, et al. A frameshift mutation in NOD2 associated with susceptibility to Crohn's disease. *Nature* 2001;**411**:603–606.

18. Hampe J, Cuthbert A, Croucher PJ, Mirza MM, Mascheretti S, Fisher S, et al. Association between insertion mutation in NOD2 gene and Crohn's disease in German and British populations. *Lancet* 2001;**357**:1925–1928.

19. Inohara N, Ogura Y, Fontalba A, Gutierrez O, Pons F, Crespo J, et al. Host recognition of bacterial muramyl dipeptide mediated through NOD2. Implications for Crohn's disease. *J. Biol. Chem.* 2003;**278**:5509–5512.

20. Girardin SE, Boneca IG, Viala J, Chamaillard M, Labigne A, Thomas G, et al. Nod2 is a general sensor of peptidoglycan through muramyl dipeptide (MDP) detection. *J. Biol. Chem.* 2003;**278**:8869–8872.

21. Inohara N, Nunez G. NODs: Intracellular proteins involved in inflammation and apoptosis. *Nat. Rev. Immunol.* 2003;**3**:371–382.

22. Berrebi D, Maudinas R, Hugot JP, Chamaillard M, Chareyre F, De Lagausie P, et al. Card15 gene overexpression in mononuclear and epithelial cells of the inflamed Crohn's disease colon. *Gut* 2003;**52**:840–846.

23. Rosenstiel P, Fantini M, Brautigam K, Kuhbacher T, Waetzig GH, Seegert D, et al. TNF-alpha and IFN-gamma regulate the expression of the NOD2 (CARD15) gene in human intestinal epithelial cells. *Gastroenterology* 2003;**124**:1001–1009.

24. Lala S, Ogura Y, Osborne C, Hor SY, Bromfield A, Davies S, et al. Crohn's disease and the NOD2 gene: A role for paneth cells. *Gastroenterology* 2003;**125**:47–57.

25. Ogura Y, Inohara N, Benito A, Chen FF, Yamaoka S, Nunez G: Nod2, a Nod1/Apaf-1 family member that is restricted to monocytes and activates NF-kappaB. _*J. Biol. Chem.* 2001;**276**:4812–4818.

26. Otte JM, Rosenberg IM, Podolsky DK. Intestinal myofibroblasts in innate immune responses of the intestine. *Gastroenterology* 2003;**124**:1866–1878.

27. Davey MP, Martin TM, Planck SR, Lee J, Zamora D, Rosenbaum JT. Human endothelial cells express NOD2/CARD15 and increase IL-6 secretion in response to muramyl dipeptide. *Microvasc. Res.* 2006;**71**:103–107.

28. Fritz JH, Girardin SE, Fitting C, Werts C, Mengin-Lecreulx D, Caroff M, et al. Synergistic stimulation of human monocytes and dendritic cells by Toll-like receptor 4 and. *Eur. J. Immunol.* 2005;**35**:2459–2470.
29. Maeda S, Hsu LC, Liu H, Bankston LA, Iimura M, Kagnoff MF, et al. Nod2 mutation in Crohn's disease potentiates NF-kappaB activity and IL-1beta processing. *Science* 2005;**307**:734–738.
30. Wehkamp J, Salzman NH, Porter E, Nuding S, Weichenthal M, Petras RE, et al. Reduced Paneth cell alpha-defensins in ileal Crohn's disease. *Proc. Natl. Acad. Sci. USA* 2005;**102**:18129–18134.
31. Fishbein T, Novitskiy G, Mishra L, Matsumoto C, Kaufman S, Goyal S, et al. NOD2-expressing bone marrow-derived cells appear to regulate epithelial innate immunity of the transplanted human small intestine. *Gut* 2008;**57**:323–330.
32. Kobayashi KS, Chamaillard M, Ogura Y, Henegariu O, Inohara N, Nunez G, et al. Nod2-dependent regulation of innate and adaptive immunity in the intestinal tract. *Science* 2005;**307**:731–734.
33. Wehkamp J, Harder J, Weichenthal M, Schwab M, Schaffeler E, Schlee M, et al. NOD2 (CARD15) mutations in Crohn's disease are associated with diminished mucosal alpha-defensin expression. *Gut* 2004;**53**:1658–1664.
34. Nuding S, Fellermann K, Wehkamp J, Stange EF. Reduced mucosal antimicrobial activity in Crohn's disease of the colon. *Gut* 2007;**56**:1240–1247.
35. Vermeire S. NOD2/CARD15: Relevance in clinical practice. *Best Pract. Res. Clin. Gastroenterol.* 2004;**18**:569–575.
36. Hugot JP, Zaccaria I, Cavanaugh J, Yang H, Vermeire S, Lappalainen M, et al. Prevalence of CARD15/NOD2 mutations in Caucasian healthy people. *Am. J. Gastroenterol.* 2007;**102**:1259–1267.
37. Kugathasan S, Loizides A, Babusukumar U, McGuire E, Wang T, Hooper P, et al. Comparative phenotypic and CARD15 mutational analysis among African American, Hispanic, and White children with Crohn's disease. *Inflamm. Bowel Dis.* 2005;**11**:631–638.
38. Inoue N, Tamura K, Kinouchi Y, Fukuda Y, Takahashi S, Ogura Y, et al. Lack of common NOD2 variants in Japanese patients with Crohn's disease. *Gastroenterology* 2002;**123**:86–91.
39. Leong RW, Armuzzi A, Ahmad T, Wong ML, Tse P, Jewell DP, et al. NOD2/CARD15 gene polymorphisms and Crohn's disease in the Chinese population. *Aliment. Pharmacol. Ther.* 2003;**17**:1465–1470.
40. Economou M, Trikalinos TA, Loizou KT, Tsianos EV, Ioannidis JP. Differential effects of NOD2 variants on Crohn's disease risk and phenotype in diverse populations: A metaanalysis. *Am. J. Gastroenterol.* 2004;**99**:2393–2404.
41. Ahmad T, Armuzzi A, Bunce M, Mulcahy-Hawes K, Marshall SE, Orchard TR, et al. The molecular classification of the clinical manifestations of Crohn's disease. *Gastroenterology* 2002;**122**:854–866.
42. Lesage S, Zouali H, Cezard JP, Colombel JF, Belaiche J, Almer S, et al. CARD15/NOD2 mutational analysis and genotype-phenotype correlation in 612 patients with inflammatory bowel disease. *Am. J. Hum. Genet.* 2002;**70**:845–857.
43. Helio T, Halme L, Lappalainen M, Fodstad H, Paavola-Sakki P, Turunen U, et al. CARD15/NOD2 gene variants are associated with familially occurring and complicated forms of Crohn's disease. *Gut* 2003;**52**:558–562.

44. Angelberger S, Reinisch W, Dejaco C, Miehsler W, Waldhoer T, Wehkamp J, et al. NOD2/CARD15 gene variants are linked to failure of antibiotic treatment in perianal fistulating Crohn's disease. *Am. J. Gastroenterol.* 2008;**103**:1197–1202.
45. Hampe J, Franke A, Rosenstiel P, Till A, Teuber M, Huse K, et al. A genome-wide association scan of nonsynonymous SNPs identifies a susceptibility variant for Crohn disease in ATG16L1. *Nat. Genet.* 2007;**39**:207–211.
46. Rioux JD, Xavier RJ, Taylor KD, Silverberg MS, Goyette P, Huett A, et al. Genome-wide association study identifies new susceptibility loci for Crohn disease and implicates autophagy in disease pathogenesis. *Nat. Genet.* 2007;**39**:596–604.
47. Wellcome Trust Case Control, Consortium. Genome-wide association study of 14,000 cases of seven common diseases and 3,000 shared controls. *Nature* 2007;**447**:661–678.
48. Prescott NJ, Fisher SA, Franke A, Hampe J, Onnie CM, Soars D, et al. A nonsynonymous SNP in ATG16L1 predisposes to ileal Crohn's disease and is independent of CARD15 and IBD5. *Gastroenterology* 2007;**132**:1665–1671.
49. Baldassano RN, Bradfield JP, Monos DS, Kim CE, Glessner JT, Casalunovo T, et al. Association of the T300A non-synonymous variant of the ATG16L1 gene with susceptibility to paediatric Crohn's disease. *Gut* 2007;**56**:1171–1173.
50. Parkes M, Barrett JC, Prescott NJ, Tremelling M, Anderson CA, Fisher SA, et al. Sequence variants in the autophagy gene IRGM and multiple other replicating loci contribute to Crohn's disease susceptibility. *Nat. Genet.* 2007;**39**:830–832.
51. McCarroll SA, Huett A, Kuballa P, Chilewski SD, Landry A, Goyette P, et al. Deletion polymorphism upstream of IRGM associated with altered IRGM expression and Crohn's disease. *Nat. Genet.* 2008;**40**:1107–1112.
52. Levine B, Kroemer G. Autophagy in the pathogenesis of disease. *Cell* 2008;**132**:27–42.
53. Klionsky DJ. Crohn's disease, autophagy, and the Paneth cell. *New Engl. J. Med.* 2009;**360**:1785–1786.
54. Cadwell K, Patel KK, Komatsu M, Virgin HW, Stappenbeck TS. A common role for Atg16L1, Atg5 and Atg7 in small intestinal Paneth cells and Crohn disease. *Autophagy* 2009;**5**:250–252.
55. Cadwell K, Liu JY, Brown SL, Miyoshi H, Loh J, Lennerz JK, et al. A key role for autophagy and the autophagy gene Atg16l1 in mouse and human intestinal Paneth cells. *Nature* 2008;**456**:259–263.
56. Saitoh T, Fujita N, Jang MH, Uematsu S, Yang BG, Satoh T, et al. Loss of the autophagy protein Atg16L1 enhances endotoxin-induced IL-1beta production. *Nature* 2008;**456**:264–268.
57. Latiano A, Palmieri O, Valvano MR, D'Inca R, Cucchiara S, Riegler G, et al. Replication of interleukin 23 receptor and autophagy-related 16-like 1 association in adult- and pediatric-onset inflammatory bowel disease in Italy. *World J. Gastroenterol.* 2008;**14**:4643–4651.
58. Weersma RK, Zhernakova A, Nolte IM, Lefebvre C, Rioux JD, Mulder F, et al. ATG16L1 and IL23R are associated with inflammatory bowel diseases but not with celiac disease in the Netherlands. *Am. J. Gastroenterol.* 2008;**103**:621–627.
59. Yamazaki K, Onouchi Y, Takazoe M, Kubo M, Nakamura Y, Hata A. Association analysis of genetic variants in IL23R,ATG16L1 and 5p13.1 loci with Crohn's disease in Japanese patients. *J. Hum. Genet.* 2007;**52**:575–583.

60. Van LJ, Russell RK, Nimmo ER, Drummond HE, Smith L, Anderson NH, et al. Autophagy gene ATG16L1 influences susceptibility and disease location but not childhood-onset in Crohn's disease in Northern Europe. *Inflamm. Bowel Dis.* 2008;**14**:338–346.

61. Glas J, Konrad A, Schmechel S, Dambacher J, Seiderer J, Schroff F, et al. The ATG16L1 gene variants rs2241879 and rs2241880 (T300A) are strongly associated with susceptibility to Crohn's disease in the German population. *Am. J. Gastroenterol.* 2008;**103**:682–691.

62. Duerr RH, Taylor KD, Brant SR, Rioux JD, Silverberg MS, Daly MJ, et al. A genome-wide association study identifies IL23R as an inflammatory bowel disease gene. *Science* 2006;**314**:1461–1463.

63. Raelson JV, Little RD, Ruether A, Fournier H, Paquin B, Van EP, et al. Genome-wide association study for Crohn's disease in the Quebec Founder population identifies multiple validated disease loci. *Proc. Natl. Acad. Sci. USA* 2007;**104**:14747–14752.

64. Tremelling M, Cummings F, Fisher SA, Mansfield J, Gwilliam R, Keniry A, et al. IL23R variation determines susceptibility but not disease phenotype in inflammatory bowel disease. *Gastroenterology* 2007;**132**:1657–1664.

65. Cummings JR, Ahmad T, Geremia A, Beckly J, Cooney R, Hancock L, et al. Contribution of the novel inflammatory bowel disease gene IL23R to disease susceptibility and phenotype. *Inflamm. Bowel Dis.* 2007;**13**:1063–1068.

66. McKenzie BS, Kastelein RA, Cua DJ. Understanding the IL-23-IL-17 immune pathway. *Trends Immunol.* 2006;**27**:17–23.

67. Hue S, Ahern P, Buonocore S, Kullberg MC, Cua DJ, McKenzie BS, et al. Interleukin-23 drives innate and T cell-mediated intestinal inflammation. *J. Exp. Med.* 2006;**203**:2473–2483.

68. Kullberg MC, Jankovic D, Feng CG, Hue S, Gorelick PL, McKenzie BS, et al. IL-23 plays a key role in Helicobacter hepaticus-induced T cell-dependent colitis. *J. Exp. Med.* 2006;**203**:2485–2494.

69. Mannon PJ, Fuss IJ, Mayer L, Elson CO, Sandborn WJ, Present D, et al. Anti-interleukin-12 antibody for active Crohn's disease. *New Engl. J. Med.* 2004;**351**:2069–2079.

70. Sandborn WJ, Feagan BG, Fedorak RN, Scherl E, Fleisher MR, Katz S, et al. A randomized trial of Ustekinumab, a human interleukin-12/23 monoclonal antibody, in patients with moderate-to-severe Crohn's disease. *Gastroenterology* 2008;**135**:1130–1141.

71. Wehkamp J, Wang G, Kubler I, Nuding S, Gregorieff A, Schnabel A, et al. The Paneth cell alpha-defensin deficiency of ileal Crohn's disease is linked to Wnt/Tcf-4. *J. Immunol.* 2007;**179**:3109–3118.

72. Koslowski MJ, Kubler I, Chamaillard M, Schaeffeler E, Reinisch W, Wang G, et al. Genetic variants of Wnt transcription factor TCF-4 (TCF7L2) putative promoter region are associated with small intestinal Crohn's disease. *PLoS ONE* 2009;**4**:e4496.

73. Wehkamp J, Fellermann K, Herrlinger KR, Baxmann S, Schmidt K, Schwind B, et al. Human beta-defensin 2 but not beta-defensin 1 is expressed preferentially in colonic mucosa of inflammatory bowel disease. *Eur. J. Gastroenterol. Hepatol.* 2002;**14**:745–752.

74. Wehkamp J, Harder J, Weichenthal M, Mueller O, Herrlinger KR, Fellermann K, et al. Inducible and constitutive beta-defensins are differentially expressed in Crohn's disease and ulcerative colitis. *Inflamm. Bowel Dis.* 2003;**9**:215–223.

75. Fellermann K, Stange DE, Schaeffeler E, Schmalzl H, Wehkamp J, Bevins CL, et al. A chromosome 8 gene-cluster polymorphism with low human beta-defensin 2 gene copy number predisposes to Crohn disease of the colon. *Am. J. Hum. Genet.* 2006;**79**:439–448.

76. Medzhitov R. Toll-like receptors and innate immunity. *Nat. Rev. Immunol.* 2001;**1**:135–145.

77. Medzhitov R, Janeway CA Jr., Innate immunity: Impact on the adaptive immune response. *Curr. Opin. Immunol.* 1997;**9**:4–9.

78. Barton GM, Medzhitov R. Toll-like receptor signaling pathways. *Science* 2003;**300**:1524–1525.

79. Palsson-McDermott EM, O'Neill LA. Signal transduction by the lipopolysaccharide receptor, toll-like receptor-4. *Immunology* 2004;**113**:153–162.

80. Mahler M, Bristol IJ, Leiter EH, Workman AE, Birkenmeier EH, Elson CO, et al. Differential susceptibility of inbred mouse strains to dextran sulfate sodium-induced colitis. *Am. J. Physiol.* 1998;**274**:G544–G551.

81. Sundberg JP, Elson CO, Bedigian H, Birkenmeier EH. Spontaneous, heritable colitis in a new substrain of C3H/HeJ mice. *Gastroenterology* 1994;**107**:1726–1735.

82. Arbour NC, Lorenz E, Schutte BC, Zabner J, Kline JN, Jones M, et al. TLR4 mutations are associated with endotoxin hyporesponsiveness in humans. *Nat. Genet.* 2000;**25**:187–191.

83. Agnese DM, Calvano JE, Hahm SJ, Coyle SM, Corbett SA, Calvano SE, et al. Human toll-like receptor 4 mutations but not CD14 polymorphisms are associated with an increased risk of gram-negative infections. *J. Infect. Dis.* 2002;**186**:1522–1525.

84. Franchimont D, Vermeire S, El HH, Pierik M, Van SK, Gustot T, et al. Deficient host-bacteria interactions in inflammatory bowel disease? The toll-like receptor (TLR)-4 Asp299gly polymorphism is associated with Crohn's disease and ulcerative colitis. *Gut* 2004;**53**:987–992.

85. Browning BL, Huebner C, Petermann I, Gearry RB, Barclay ML, Shelling AN, Ferguson LR. Has toll-like receptor 4 been prematurely dismissed as an inflammatory bowel disease gene? Association study combined with meta-analysis shows strong evidence for association. *Am. J. Gastroenterol.* 2007;**102**:2504–2512.

86. Ungaro R, Fukata M, Hsu D, Hernandez Y, Breglio K, Chen A, et al. A novel toll-like receptor 4 antagonist antibody ameliorates inflammation but impairs mucosal healing in murine colitis. *Am. J. Physiol. Gastrointest. Liver Physiol.* 2009;**296**:G1167–G1179.

87. Stoll M, Corneliussen B, Costello CM, Waetzig GH, Mellgard B, Koch WA, et al. Genetic variation in DLG5 is associated with inflammatory bowel disease. *Nat. Genet.* 2004;**36**:476–480.

88. Shah G, Brugada R, Gonzalez O, Czernuszewicz G, Gibbs RA, Bachinski L, et al. The cloning, genomic organization and tissue expression profile of the human DLG5 gene. *BMC Genomics* 2002;**3**:6.

89. Daly MJ, Pearce AV, Farwell L, Fisher SA, Latiano A, Prescott NJ, Forbes A, Mansfield J, Sanderson J, Langelier D, Cohen A, Bitton A, Wild G, Lewis CM, Annese V, Mathew CG, Rioux JD. Association of DLG5 R30Q variant with inflammatory bowel disease. *Eur. J. Hum. Genet.* 2005;**13**:835–839.

90. Browning BL, Huebner C, Petermann I, Demmers P, McCulloch A, Gearry RB, et al. Association of DLG5 variants with inflammatory bowel disease in the New Zealand

Caucasian population and meta-analysis of the DLG5 R30Q variant. *Inflamm. Bowel Dis.* 2007;**13**:1069–1076.

91. Friedrichs F, Brescianini S, Annese V, Latiano A, Berger K, Kugathasan S, et al. Evidence of transmission ratio distortion of DLG5 R30Q variant in general and implication of an association with Crohn disease in men. *Hum. Genet.* 2006;**119**:305–311.
92. Browning BL, Annese V, Barclay ML, Bingham SA, Brand S, Buning C, et al. Gender-stratified analysis of DLG5 R30Q in 4707 patients with Crohn disease and 4973 controls from 12 Caucasian cohorts. *J. Med. Genet.* 2008;**45**:36–42.
93. Rioux JD, Silverberg MS, Daly MJ, Steinhart AH, McLeod RS, Griffiths AM, et al. Genomewide search in Canadian families with inflammatory bowel disease reveals two novel susceptibility loci. *Am. J. Hum. Genet.* 2000;**66**:1863–1870.
94. Peltekova VD, Wintle RF, Rubin LA, Amos CI, Huang Q, Gu X, et al. Functional variants of OCTN cation transporter genes are associated with Crohn disease. *Nat. Genet.* 2004;**36**:471–475.
95. Tamai I, Yabuuchi H, Nezu J, Sai Y, Oku A, Shimane M, et al. Cloning and characterization of a novel human pH-dependent organic cation transporter, OCTN1. *FEBS Lett.* 1997;**419**:107–111.
96. Roediger WE, Nance S. Metabolic induction of experimental ulcerative colitis by inhibition of fatty acid oxidation. *Br. J. Exp. Pathol.* 1986;**67**:773–782.
97. Torok HP, Glas J, Tonenchi L, Lohse P, Muller-Myhsok B, Limbersky O, et al. Polymorphisms in the DLG5 and OCTN cation transporter genes in Crohn's disease. *Gut* 2005;**54**:1421–1427.
98. Newman B, Gu X, Wintle R, Cescon D, Yazdanpanah M, Liu X, et al. A risk haplotype in the solute carrier family 22A4/22A5 gene cluster influences phenotypic expression of Crohn's disease. *Gastroenterology* 2005;**128**:260–269.
99. Noble CL, Nimmo ER, Drummond H, Ho GT, Tenesa A, Smith L, et al. The contribution of OCTN1/2 variants within the IBD5 locus to disease susceptibility and severity in Crohn's disease. *Gastroenterology* 2005;**129**:1854–1864.
100. Babusukumar U, Wang T, McGuire E, Broeckel U, Kugathasan S. Contribution of OCTN variants within the IBD5 locus to pediatric onset Crohn's disease. *Am. J. Gastroenterol.* 2006;**101**:1354–1361.
101. Silverberg MS, Duerr RH, Brant SR, Bromfield G, Datta LW, Jani N, et al. Refined genomic localization and ethnic differences observed for the IBD5 association with Crohn's disease. *Eur. J. Hum. Genet.* 2007;**15**:328–335.
102. Taubert D, Grimberg G, Jung N, Rubbert A, Schomig E. Functional role of the 503F variant of the organic cation transporter OCTN1 in Crohn's disease. *Gut* 2005;**54**:1505–1506.
103. Taubert D, Jung N, Goeser T, Schomig E. Increased ergothioneine tissue concentrations in carriers of the Crohn's disease risk-associated 503F variant of the organic cation transporter OCTN1. *Gut* 2009;**58**:312–314.
104. Satsangi J, Parkes M, Louis E, Hashimoto L, Kato N, Welsh K, et al. Two stage genome-wide search in inflammatory bowel disease provides evidence for susceptibility loci on chromosomes 3, 7 and 12. *Nat. Genet.* 1996;**14**:199–202.
105. Schwab M, Schaeffeler E, Marx C, Fromm MF, Kaskas B, Metzler J, et al. Association between the C3435T MDR1 gene polymorphism and susceptibility for ulcerative colitis. *Gastroenterology* 2003;**124**:26–33.

106. Panwala CM, Jones JC, Viney JL. A novel model of inflammatory bowel disease: Mice deficient for the multiple drug resistance gene, mdr1a, spontaneously develop colitis. *J. Immunol.* 1998;**161**:5733–5744.

107. Wilk JN, Bilsborough J, Viney JL. The mdr1a-/- mouse model of spontaneous colitis: A relevant and appropriate animal model to study inflammatory bowel disease. *Immunol. Res.* 2005;**31**:151–159.

108. Kimchi-Sarfaty C, Oh JM, Kim IW, Sauna ZE, Calcagno AM, Ambudkar SV, et al. A "silent" polymorphism in the MDR1 gene changes substrate specificity. *Science* 2007;**315**:525–528.

109. Hoffmeyer S, Burk O, von RO, Arnold HP, Brockmoller J, Johne A, et al. Functional polymorphisms of the human multidrug-resistance gene: Multiple sequence variations and correlation of one allele with P-glycoprotein expression and activity in vivo. *Proc. Natl. Acad. Sci. USA* 2000;**97**:3473–3478.

110. Glas J, Torok HP, Schiemann U, Folwaczny C. MDR1 gene polymorphism in ulcerative colitis. *Gastroenterology* 2004;**126**:367.

111. Ho GT, Nimmo ER, Tenesa A, Fennell J, Drummond H, Mowat C, et al. Allelic variations of the multidrug resistance gene determine susceptibility and disease behavior in ulcerative colitis. *Gastroenterology* 2005;**128**:288–296.

112. Croucher PJ, Mascheretti S, Foelsch UR, Hampe J, Schreiber S. Lack of association between the C3435T MDR1 gene polymorphism and inflammatory bowel disease in two independent Northern European populations. *Gastroenterology* 2003;**125**:1919–1920.

113. Potocnik U, Ferkolj I, Glavac D, Dean M. Polymorphisms in multidrug resistance 1 (MDR1) gene are associated with refractory Crohn disease and ulcerative colitis. *Genes Immun.* 2004;**5**:530–539.

114. Ardizzone S, Maconi G, Bianchi V, Russo A, Colombo E, Cassinotti A, Penati C, Tenchini ML, Bianchi Porro G. Multidrug resistance 1 gene polymorphism and susceptibility to inflammatory bowel disease. *Inflamm. Bowel Dis.* 2007;**13**:516–523.

115. Onnie CM, Fisher SA, Pattni R, Sanderson J, Forbes A, Lewis CM, et al. Associations of allelic variants of the multidrug resistance gene (ABCB1 or MDR1) and inflammatory bowel disease and their effects on disease behavior: A case-control and meta-analysis study. *Inflamm. Bowel Dis.* 2006;**12**:263–271.

116. Annese V, Valvano MR, Palmieri O, Latiano A, Bossa F, Andriulli A. Multidrug resistance 1 gene in inflammatory bowel disease: A meta-analysis. *World J. Gastroenterol.* 2006;**12**:3636–3644.

117. Kim RB, Leake BF, Choo EF, Dresser GK, Kubba SV, Schwarz UI, et al. Identification of functionally variant MDR1 alleles among European Americans and African Americans. *Clin. Pharmacol. Ther.* 2001;**70**:189–199.

118. Brant SR, Panhuysen CI, Nicolae D, Reddy DM, Bonen DK, Karaliukas R, et al. MDR1 Ala893 polymorphism is associated with inflammatory bowel disease. *Am. J. Hum. Genet.* 2003;**73**:1282–1292.

119. Dilger K, Schwab M, Fromm MF. Identification of budesonide and prednisone as substrates of the intestinal drug efflux pump P-glycoprotein. *Inflamm. Bowel Dis.* 2004;**10**:578–583.

120. Farrell RJ, Murphy A, Long A, Donnelly S, Cherikuri A, O'Toole D, et al. High multidrug resistance (P-glycoprotein 170) expression in inflammatory bowel disease patients who fail medical therapy. *Gastroenterology* 2000;**118**:279–288.

121. Lown KS, Mayo RR, Leichtman AB, Hsiao HL, Turgeon DK, Schmiedlin-Ren P, et al. Role of intestinal P-glycoprotein (mdr1) in interpatient variation in the oral bioavailability of cyclosporine. *Clin. Pharmacol. Ther.* 1997;**62**:248–260.

122. Buchman AL, Paine MF, Wallin A, Ludington SS. A higher dose requirement of tacrolimus in active Crohn's disease may be related to a high intestinal P-glycoprotein content. *Digest. Dis. Sci.* 2005;**50**:2312–2315.

123. Palmieri O, Latiano A, Valvano R, D'Inca R, Vecchi M, Sturniolo GC, et al. Multidrug resistance 1 gene polymorphisms are not associated with inflammatory bowel disease and response to therapy in Italian patients. *Aliment. Pharmacol. Ther.* 2005;**22**:1129–1138.

124. Cucchiara S, Latiano A, Palmieri O, Canani RB, D'Inca R, Guariso G, et al. Polymorphisms of tumor necrosis factor-alpha but not MDR1 influence response to medical therapy in pediatric-onset inflammatory bowel disease. *J. Pediatr. Gastroenterol. Nutr.* 2007;**44**:171–179.

125. Fischer S, Lakatos PL, Lakatos L, Kovacs A, Molnar T, Altorjay I, et al. ATP-binding cassette transporter ABCG2 (BCRP) and ABCB1 (MDR1) variants are not associated with disease susceptibility, disease phenotype response to medical therapy or need for surgeryin Hungarian patients with inflammatory bowel diseases. *Scand. J. Gastroenterol.* 2007;**42**:726–733.

126. Mendoza JL, Urcelay E, Lana R, Martin MC, Lopez N, Guijarro LG, et al. MDR1 polymorphisms and response to azathioprine therapy in patients with Crohn's disease. *Inflamm. Bowel Dis.* 2007;**13**:585–590.

127. Daniel F, Loriot MA, Seksik P, Cosnes J, Gornet JM, Lemann M, et al. Multidrug resistance gene-1 polymorphisms and resistance to cyclosporine A in patients with steroid resistant ulcerative colitis. *Inflamm. Bowel Dis.* 2007;**13**:19–23.

128. Lettre G, Rioux JD. Autoimmune diseases: Insights from genome-wide association studies. *Hum. Mol. Genet.* 2008;**17**:R116–R121.

129. Barrett JC, Hansoul S, Nicolae DL, Cho JH, Duerr RH, Rioux JD, et al. Genome-wide association defines more than 30 distinct susceptibility loci for Crohn's disease. *Nat. Genet.* 2008;**40**:955–962.

130. Kirchheiner J, Schwab M. Heterogeneity of drug responses and individualization of therapy. In Waldman SA, Terzic A, eds.: *Pharmacology and Therapeutics. Principles to Practice.* Philadelphia: Elsevier; 2008; pp. 225–238.

131. Travis SP, Stange EF, Lemann M, Oresland T, Chowers Y, Forbes A, et al. European evidence based consensus on the diagnosis and management of Crohn's disease: Current management. *Gut* 2006;**55** (Suppl. 1): i16–i35.

132. Brain O, Travis SP. Therapy of ulcerative colitis: state of the art. *Curr. Opin. Gastroenterol.* 2008;**24**:469–474.

133. Lichtenstein GR, Hanauer SB, Sandborn WJ. Management of Crohn's disease in adults. *Am. J. Gastroenterol.* 2009;**104**:465–483.

134. Swann PF, Waters TR, Moulton DC, Xu YZ, Zheng Q, Edwards M, et al. Role of postreplicative DNA mismatch repair in the cytotoxic action of thioguanine. *Science* 1996;**273**:1109–1111.

135. Somerville L, Krynetski EY, Krynetskaia NF, Beger RD, Zhang W, Marhefka CA, et al. Structure and dynamics of thioguanine-modified duplex DNA._*J. Biol. Chem.* 2003;**278**:1005–1011.

136. Tiede I, Fritz G, Strand S, Poppe D, Dvorsky R, Strand D, et al. CD28-dependent Rac1 activation is the molecular target of azathioprine in primary human CD4+ T lymphocytes. *J. Clin. Invest.* 2003;**111**:1133–1145.

137. Neurath MF, Kiesslich R, Teichgraber U, Fischer C, Hofmann U, Eichelbaum M, et al. 6-Thioguanosine diphosphate and triphosphate levels in red blood cells and response to azathioprine therapy in Crohn's disease. *Clin. Gastroenterol. Hepatol.* 2005;**3**:1007–1014.

138. Poppe D, Tiede I, Fritz G, Becker C, Bartsch B, Wirtz S, et al. Azathioprine suppresses ezrin-radixin-moesin-dependent T cell-APC conjugation through inhibition of Vav guanosine exchange activity on Rac proteins. *J. Immunol.* 2006;**176**:640–651.

139. Tidd DM, Kim SC, Horakova K, Moriwaki A, Paterson AR. A delayed cytotoxic reaction for 6-mercaptopurine. *Cancer Res.* 1972;**32**:317–322.

140. Ben-Horin S, Goldstein I, Fudim E, Picard O, Yerushalmi Z, Barshack I, et al. Early preservation of effector functions followed by eventual T cell memory depletion: A model for the delayed onset of the effect of thiopurines. *Gut* 2009;**58**:396–403.

141. Weinshilboum RM, Sladek SL. Mercaptopurine pharmacogenetics: Monogenic inheritance of erythrocyte thiopurine methyltransferase activity. *Am. J. Hum. Genet.* 1980;**32**:651–662.

142. Schaeffeler E, Fischer C, Brockmeier D, Wernet D, Moerike K, Eichelbaum M, et al. Comprehensive analysis of thiopurine S-methyltransferase phenotype-genotype correlation in a large population of German-Caucasians and identification of novel TPMT variants. *Pharmacogenetics* 2004;**14**:407–417.

143. Salavaggione OE, Wang L, Wiepert M, Yee VC, Weinshilboum RM. Thiopurine S-methyltransferase pharmacogenetics: Variant allele functional and comparative genomics. *Pharmacogenet. Genomics* 2005;**15**:801–815.

144. Ujiie S, Sasaki T, Mizugaki M, Ishikawa M, Hiratsuka M. Functional characterization of 23 allelic variants of thiopurine S-methyltransferase gene (TPMT*2 - *24). *Pharmacogenet. Genomics* 2008;**18**:887–893.

145. Garat A, Cauffiez C, Renault N, Lo-Guidice JM, Allorge D, Chevalier D, et al. Characterisation of novel defective thiopurine S-methyltransferase allelic variants. *Biochem. Pharmacol.* 2008;**76**:404–415.

146. Schaeffeler E, Zanger UM, Eichelbaum M, Sante-Poku S, Shin JG, Schwab M. Highly multiplexed genotyping of thiopurine s-methyltransferase variants using MALD-TOF mass spectrometry: Reliable genotyping in different ethnic groups. *Clin. Chem.* 2008;**54**:1637–1647.

147. Samochatova EV, Chupova NV, Rudneva A, Makarova O, Nasedkina TV, Fedorova OE, et al. TPMT genetic variations in populations of the Russian Federation. *Pediatr. Blood Cancer* 2009;**52**:203–208.

148. Yates CR, Krynetski EY, Loennechen T, Fessing MY, Tai HL, Pui CH, et al. Molecular diagnosis of thiopurine S-methyltransferase deficiency: Genetic basis for azathioprine and mercaptopurine intolerance. *Ann. Intern. Med.* 1997;**126**:608–614.

149. Teml A, Schaeffeler E, Herrlinger KR, Klotz U, Schwab M. Thiopurine treatment in inflammatory bowel disease: Clinical pharmacology and implication of pharmacogenetically guided dosing. *Clin. Pharmacokinet.* 2007;**46**:187–208.

150. Schwab M, Schaeffeler E, Marx C, Zanger U, Aulitzky W, Eichelbaum M. Shortcoming in the diagnosis of TPMT deficiency in a patient with Crohn's disease using phenotyping only. *Gastroenterology* 2001;**121**:498–499.

151. Schwab M, Schaffeler E, Marx C, Fischer C, Lang T, Behrens C, et al. Azathioprine therapy and adverse drug reactions in patients with inflammatory bowel disease: Impact of thiopurine S-methyltransferase polymorphism. *Pharmacogenetics* 2002;**12**:429–436.
152. Evans WE, Hon YY, Bomgaars L, Coutre S, Holdsworth M, Janco R, et al. Preponderance of thiopurine S-methyltransferase deficiency and heterozygosity among patients intolerant to mercaptopurine or azathioprine. *J. Clin. Oncol.* 2001;**19**:2293–2301.
153. Lennard L, Van Loon JA, Weinshilboum RM. Pharmacogenetics of acute azathioprine toxicity: Relationship to thiopurine methyltransferase genetic polymorphism. *Clin. Pharmacol. Ther.* 1989;**46**:149–154.
154. Kaskas BA, Louis E, Hindorf U, Schaeffeler E, Deflandre J, Graepler F, et al. Safe treatment of thiopurine S-methyltransferase deficient Crohn's disease patients with azathioprine. *Gut* 2003;**52**:140–142.
155. Sandborn WJ; Rational dosing of azathioprine and 6-mercaptopurine. *Gut* 2001;**48**:591–592.
156. Teml A, Schaeffeler E, Schwab M. Pretreatment determination of TPMT - state of the art in clinical practice. *Eur. J. Clin. Pharmacol.* 2009;**65**:219–221.
157. Shipkova M, Lorenz K, Oellerich M, Wieland E, von AN. Measurement of erythrocyte inosine triphosphate pyrophosphohydrolase (ITPA) activity by HPLC and correlation of ITPA genotype-phenotype in a Caucasian population. *Clin. Chem.* 2006;**52**:240–247.
158. Sumi S, Marinaki AM, Arenas M, Fairbanks L, Shobowale-Bakre M, Rees DC, et al. Genetic basis of inosine triphosphate pyrophosphohydrolase deficiency. *Hum. Genet.* 2002;**111**:360–367.
159. Marinaki AM, Ansari A, Duley JA, Arenas M, Sumi S, Lewis CM, et al. Adverse drug reactions to azathioprine therapy are associated with polymorphism in the gene encoding inosine triphosphate pyrophosphatase (ITPase). *Pharmacogenetics* 2004;**14**:181–187.
160. Zelinkova Z, Derijks LJ, Stokkers PC, Vogels EW, van Kampen AH, Curvers WL, et al. Inosine triphosphate pyrophosphatase and thiopurine s-methyltransferase genotypes relationship to azathioprine-induced myelosuppression. *Clin. Gastroenterol. Hepatol.* 2006;**4**:44–49.
161. Allorge D, Hamdan R, Broly F, Libersa C, Colombel JF. ITPA genotyping test does not improve detection of Crohn's disease patients at risk of azathioprine/6-mercaptopurine induced myelosuppression. *Gut* 2005;**54**:565.
162. Gearry RB, Roberts RL, Barclay ML, Kennedy MA. Lack of association between the ITPA 94C > A polymorphism and adverse effects from azathioprine. *Pharmacogenetics* 2004;**14**:779–781.
163. Van Dieren JM, Hansen BE, Kuipers EJ, Nieuwenhuis EE, Van der Woude CJ. Meta-analysis: Inosine triphosphate pyrophosphatase polymorphisms and thiopurine toxicity in the treatment of inflammatory bowel disease. *Aliment. Pharmacol. Ther.* 2007;**26**:643–652.
164. Stocco G, Cheok MH, Crews KR, Dervieux T, French D, Pei D, et al. Genetic polymorphism of inosine triphosphate pyrophosphatase is a determinant of mercaptopurine metabolism and toxicity during treatment for acute lymphoblastic leukemia. *Clin. Pharmacol. Ther.* 2009;**85**:164–172.
165. Stocco G, Martelossi S, Barabino A, Decorti G, Bartoli F, Montico M, et al. Glutathione-S-transferase genotypes and the adverse effects of azathioprine in young patients with inflammatory bowel disease. *Inflamm. Bowel Dis.* 2007;**13**:57–64.

166. Hawwa AF, Millership JS, Collier PS, Vandenbroeck K, McCarthy A, Dempsey S, et al. Pharmacogenomic studies of the anticancer and immunosuppressive thiopurines mercaptopurine and azathioprine. *Br. J. Clin. Pharmacol.* 2008;**66**:517–528.

167. Herrlinger KR, Cummings JR, Barnardo MC, Schwab M, Ahmad T, Jewell DP. The pharmacogenetics of methotrexate in inflammatory bowel disease. *Pharmacogenet. Genomics* 2005;**15**:705–711.

168. Hider SL, Bruce IN, Thomson W. The pharmacogenetics of methotrexate. *Rheumatology* (Oxford, UK) 2007;**46**:1520–1524.

169. Davidsen ML, Dalhoff K, Schmiegelow K. Pharmacogenetics influence treatment efficacy in childhood acute lymphoblastic leukemia. *J. Pediatr. Hematol. Oncol.* 2008;**30**:831–849.

170. Clark M, Colombel JF, Feagan BC, Fedorak RN, Hanauer SB, Kamm MA, et al. American gastroenterological association consensus development conference on the use of biologics in the treatment of inflammatory bowel disease, June 21–23, 2006. *Gastroenterology* 2007;**133**:312–339.

171. Nahar IK, Shojania K, Marra CA, Alamgir AH, Anis AH. Infliximab treatment of rheumatoid arthritis and Crohn's disease. *Ann. Pharmacother.* 2003;**37**:1256–1265.

172. Klotz U, Teml A, Schwab M. Clinical pharmacokinetics and use of infliximab. *Clin Pharmacokinet.* 2007;**46**:645–660.

173. Hyrich KL, Watson KD, Silman AJ, Symmons DP. Predictors of response to anti-TNF-alpha therapy among patients with rheumatoid arthritis: Results from the British Society for Rheumatology Biologics Register. *Rheumatology* (Oxford UK) 2006;**45**:1558–1565.

174. Hlavaty T, Pierik M, Henckaerts L, Ferrante M, Joossens S, van SN, et al. Polymorphisms in apoptosis genes predict response to infliximab therapy in luminal and fistulizing Crohn's disease. *Aliment. Pharmacol. Ther.* 2005;**22**:613–626.

175. Hlavaty T, Ferrante M, Henckaerts L, Pierik M, Rutgeerts P, Vermeire S. Predictive model for the outcome of infliximab therapy in Crohn's disease based on apoptotic pharmacogenetic index and clinical predictors. *Inflamm. Bowel Dis.* 2007;**13**:372–379.

176. Dideberg V, Theatre E, Farnir F, Vermeire S, Rutgeerts P, Vos MD, et al. The TNF/ADAM 17 system: Implication of an ADAM 17 haplotype in the clinical response to infliximab in Crohn's disease. *Pharmacogenet. Genomics* 2006;**16**:727–734.

177. Louis E, El GZ, Vermeire S, Dall'Ozzo S, Rutgeerts P, Paintaud G, et al. Association between polymorphism in IgG Fc receptor IIIa coding gene and biological response to infliximab in Crohn's disease. *Aliment. Pharmacol. Ther.* 2004;**19**:511–519.

178. Urcelay E, Mendoza JL, Martinez A, Fernandez L, Taxonera C, az-Rubio M, et al. IBD5 polymorphisms in inflammatory bowel disease: Association with response to infliximab. *World J. Gastroenterol.* 2005;**11**:1187–1192.

179. Matsukura H, Ikeda S, Yoshimura N, Takazoe M, Muramatsu M. Genetic polymorphisms of tumour necrosis factor receptor superfamily 1A and 1B affect responses to infliximab in Japanese patients with Crohn's disease. *Aliment. Pharmacol. Ther.* 2008;**27**:765–770.

180. Mascheretti S, Hampe J, Croucher PJ, Nikolaus S, Andus T, Schubert S, et al. Response to infliximab treatment in Crohn's disease is not associated with mutations in the CARD15 (NOD2) gene: An analysis in 534 patients from two multicenter, prospective GCP-level trials. *Pharmacogenetics* 2002;**12**:509–515.

181. Pierik M, Vermeire S, Steen KV, Joossens S, Claessens G, Vlietinck R, et al. Tumour necrosis factor-alpha receptor 1 and 2 polymorphisms in inflammatory bowel disease and

their association with response to infliximab. *Aliment. Pharmacol. Ther.* 2004;**20**:303–310.

182. Vermeire S, Louis E, Rutgeerts P, De VM, Van GA, Belaiche J, et al. NOD2/CARD15 does not influence response to infliximab in Crohn's disease. *Gastroenterology* 2002;**123**:106–111.

183. Louis E, Vermeire S, Rutgeerts P, De VM, Van GA, Pescatore P, et al. A positive response to infliximab in Crohn disease: Association with a higher systemic inflammation before treatment but not with −308 TNF gene polymorphism. *Scand. J. Gastroenterol.* 2002;**37**:818–824.

184. Mascheretti S, Hampe J, Kuhbacher T, Herfarth H, Krawczak M, Folsch UR, et al. Pharmacogenetic investigation of the TNF/TNF-receptor system in patients with chronic active Crohn's disease treated with infliximab. *Pharmacogenomics J.* 2002;**2**:127–136.

185. Taylor KD, Plevy SE, Yang H, Landers CJ, Barry MJ, Rotter JI, et al. ANCA pattern and LTA haplotype relationship to clinical responses to anti-TNF antibody treatment in Crohn's disease. *Gastroenterology* 2001;**120**:1347–1355.

186. Willot S, Vermeire S, Ohresser M, Rutgeerts P, Paintaud G, Belaiche J, et al. No association between C-reactive protein gene polymorphisms and decrease of C-reactive protein serum concentration after infliximab treatment in Crohn's disease. *Pharmacogenet. Genomics* 2006;**16**:37–42.

187. Brain O, Travis SP. Therapy of ulcerative colitis: State of the art. *Curr. Opin. Gastroenterol.* 2008;**24**:469–474.

188. Yang YX, Lichtenstein GR. Corticosteroids in Crohn's disease. *Am. J. Gastroenterol.* 2002;**97**:803–823.

189. Munkholm P, Langholz E, Davidsen M, Binder V. Frequency of glucocorticoid resistance and dependency in Crohn's disease. *Gut* 1994;**35**:360–362.

190. Faubion WA Jr, Loftus EV Jr, Harmsen WS, Zinsmeister AR, Sandborn WJ. The natural history of corticosteroid therapy for inflammatory bowel disease: A population-based study. *Gastroenterology* 2001;**121**:255–260.

191. De IS, Stocco G, Martelossi S, Drigo I, Norbedo S, Lionetti P, et al. Association of BclI polymorphism of the glucocorticoid receptor gene locus with response to glucocorticoids in inflammatory bowel disease. *Gut* 2007;**56**:1319–1320.

192. Buemann B, Vohl MC, Chagnon M, Chagnon YC, Gagnon J, Perusse L, et al. Abdominal visceral fat is associated with a BclI restriction fragment length polymorphism at the glucocorticoid receptor gene locus. *Obes. Res.* 1997;**5**:186–192.

193. Lin RC, Wang WY, Morris BJ. High penetrance, overweight, and glucocorticoid receptor variant: Case-control study. *Br. Med. J.* 1999;**319**:1337–1338.

194. van Rossum EF, Koper JW, Huizenga NA, Uitterlinden AG, Janssen JA, Brinkmann AO, et al. A polymorphism in the glucocorticoid receptor gene, which decreases sensitivity to glucocorticoids in vivo, is associated with low insulin and cholesterol levels. *Diabetes* 2002;**51**:3128–3134.

195. Griga T, Wilkens C, Schmiegel W, Folwaczny C, Hagedorn M, Duerig N, et al. Association between the promoter polymorphism T/C at position -159 of the CD14 gene and anti-inflammatory therapy in patients with inflammatory bowel disease. *Eur. J. Med. Res.* 2005;**10**:183–186.

196. Griga T, Wilkens C, Wirkus N, Epplen J, Schmiegel W, Klein W. A polymorphism in the macrophage migration inhibitory factor gene is involved in the genetic predisposition of

Crohn's disease and associated with cumulative steroid doses. *Hepatogastroenterology* 2007;**54**:784–786.

197. Lakatos PL, Fischer S, Claes K, Kovacs A, Molnar T, Altorjay I, et al. DLG5 R30Q is not associated with IBD in Hungarian IBD patients but predicts clinical response to steroids in Crohn's disease. *Inflamm. Bowel Dis.* 2006;**12**:362–368.
198. Ruhlmann A, Nordheim A. Effects of the immunosuppressive drugs CsA and FK506 on intracellular signalling and gene regulation. *Immunobiology* 1997;**198**:192–206.
199. Wiederrecht G, Lam E, Hung S, Martin M, Sigal N. The mechanism of action of FK-506 and cyclosporin A. *Ann NY Acad. Sci.* 1993;**696**:9–19.
200. Kronbach T, Fischer V, Meyer UA. Cyclosporine metabolism in human liver: Identification of a cytochrome P-450III gene family as the major cyclosporine-metabolizing enzyme explains interactions of cyclosporine with other drugs. *Clin. Pharmacol. Ther.* 1988;**43**:630–635.
201. Thervet E, Anglicheau D, Legendre C, Beaune P. Role of pharmacogenetics of immunosuppressive drugs in organ transplantation. *Ther. Drug Monit.* 2008;**30**:143–150.
202. Mourad M, Wallemacq P, De MM, Malaise J, De PL, Eddour DC, et al. Biotransformation enzymes and drug transporters pharmacogenetics in relation to immunosuppressive drugs: Impact on pharmacokinetics and clinical outcome. *Transplantation* 2008;**85**: S19–S24.
203. Clayton TA, Lindon JC, Cloarec O, Antti H, Charuel C, Hanton G, et al. Pharmacometabonomic phenotyping and personalized drug treatment. *Nature* 2006;**440**:1073–1077.
204. Gomez A, Ingelman-Sundberg M. Pharmacoepigenetics: Its role in interindividual differences in drug response. *Clin. Pharmacol. Ther.* 2009;**85**:426–430.

CHAPTER 12

Pharmacogenetics of Pain Medication

JÖRN LÖTSCH

Johann Wolfgang Goethe-University Hospital, Frankfurt, Germany

12.1 INTRODUCTION

A fifth of adults in Europe have moderate or severe chronic pain [1], and successful analgesia is still one of the main healthcare issues. The identification of functional genetic polymorphisms modulating the individual response to nociceptive input or to analgesic therapy has fueled expectations that genotyping of patients recalcitrant to treatment may provide (1) explanations for the poor responses and (2) guidelines for personalized therapy to obtain the intended responses.

In complex settings such as pain management, several genetic factors [2–4] (Fig. 12.1) contribute to the patient's phenotype by controlling (1) the local availability of analgesic molecules at the action site, (2) their interaction with target structures, (3) the clinical picture of pain, (4) factors modulating the risk for development of a pain-producing disease or its clinical course and severity, or (5) factors modulating the opioid dosage requirements by conferring a risk for drug addiction. The local availability of active molecules at the site of their pharmacodynamic action may be influenced by genetic polymorphisms of drug metabolizing enzymes causing changes in either inactivation or activation of the administered drugs [5,6], or by polymorphisms of transmembrane transporters causing changes in the absorption of orally administered analgesics or accumulation of active molecules in the brain [7]. The interaction between analgesic molecules and their target structures may be influenced by genetic polymorphisms of opioid receptors causing altered agonist affinity of receptor signaling [8,9]. Nociception may be altered by changes in transmitter production [10,11] or transmission of nociceptive input [12]. From increased methadone requirements for substitution therapy in carriers of dopamine D_2 receptor variants [13], a role of genetics for high opioid doses in the context of pain therapy appears to be conceivable.

Pharmacogenetics and Individualized Therapy, First Edition.
Edited by Anke-Hilse Maitland-van der Zee and Ann K. Daly.

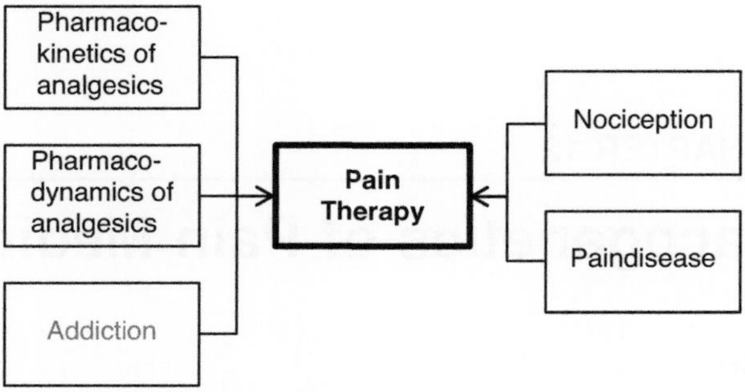

FIGURE 12.1 Influences with genetic contribution on the individual phenotype met during pain therapy.

In this chapter, the limited number of human genetic variants that have so far been identified to modulate the pharmacotherapy of pain are summarized (see Table 12.1). However, the focus will be on evidence for a modulation of pain pharmacotherapy rather than the underlying disease, with a specific focus on the clinical effects of analgesics. Most of the candidate polymorphisms that could theoretically modulate pain because of biologically plausible associations due to their functional consequences in other contexts, but that lack actual clinical evidence of pain control, will not be discussed here.

12.2 GENETIC MODULATION OF THE EFFECTS OF CLASSICAL ANALGESICS

The main classical groups of analgesics are (1) opioids; (2) antipyretic non-opioid analgesics, which include classical nonselective cyclooxygenase (COX) inhibitors (e.g., ibuprofen, diclofenac, non-low-dose acetylsalicylic acid), selective COX2 inhibitors (e.g., celecoxib, parecoxib, etoricoxib) and also metamizol (dipyrone) and acetaminophen acting via involvement of COX inhibition [14,15]; and (3) triptans. Their effects are based on their local availability at the target site. When the drug molecules have reached their action, sites, of their effects may be modulated by altered interaction with their targets or by altered consequences of this interaction.

12.2.1 Pharmacokinetics

By altering the local availability of analgesic molecules at the action site, pharmacokinetics plays a role in pain therapy. Drug metabolism or drug transport mainly governs the timecourse of the analgesic' s concentration at the action site (i.e., the site at which the drug's effect is produced). Clinically this is most often detectable in plasma and modified drug metabolism or transport and leads to changes in drug clearance or distribution. However, due to the therapeutic range of analgesics, not all measurable genetically caused changes in the drug's plasma concentrations impact the drug's effect. Therefore, the focus here will be on those genetic polymorphisms that, by altering the analgesic's pharmacokinetics, have been shown to alter its clinical effects.

12.2.1.1 Drug Metabolizing Enzymes

Analgesics are subject to metabolic clearance by several enzymes. When the administered compound is the main active agent (also known as the *active principle*), decreased metabolism may lead to increased effects due to slower systemic elimination. In contrast, when a prodrug is administered, decreased effects due to reduced production of the active metabolite are the consequence.

12.2.1.2 Prodrug Activation

Prodrugs are substances that are administered in a generally inactive form and need to be activated in order to produce a clinical effect. Typical prodrugs among analgesics are codeine, tilidine, and parecoxib. Less typical is tramadol, which is metabolically activated but exerts its own clinical pharmacodynamic activity [16]. In contrast, the existence of an active metabolite such as morphine-6-glucuronide does not necessarily render the parent a prodrug such as morphine, which exerts the main clinical effects itself unless the metabolite accumulates in special populations [17].

Codeine and tramadol are activated via cytochrome P450 (CYP)2D6. However, codeine is extensively metabolized (Fig. 12.2), and in one study, after a single oral dose of 30 mg, 81% of the codeine was transformed to codeine-6-glucuronide, 2.2% to norcodeine, 0.6% to free morphine, 2.1% to morphine-3-glucuronide, 0.8% to morphine-6-glucuronide, and 2.4% to normorphine [19]. Adding the morphine metabolites to morphine, this amounts to approximately 6% of codeine metabolized into morphine. The clinical effects of codeine are attributed mainly to its transformation to morphine, which has 200 times higher affinity and 50 times higher intrinsic activity at μ-opioid receptors than does codeine itself [20,21]. Morphine is therefore considered the active principle of codeine despite some evidence that codeine or codeine-6-glucuronide contribute to the pharmacodynamic effects [18,22–25]. Since CYP2D6 [26] is known to be genetically highly polymorphic [27], the effects of codeine are under pharmacogenetic control [28]. Genetically altered codeine effects may occur in subjects with either decreased to absent or highly increased CYP2D6 activity as compared to the population average. Decreased codeine effects may occur in approximately 7–11% of the Caucasian population in whom CYP2D6 is inactive for genetic reasons [29–31] [CYP2D6 poor metabolizer phenotype (PM)], with interethnic differences [27], leading to very low or absent morphine formation from codeine.

Relevant known *CYP2D6* polymorphisms in Caucasians include the nonfunctional alleles **3, *4, *5, *6, *7, *8* [6] and the reduced-function **41* allele [32]. On the other hand, increased codeine effects may involve $\leq$7% of the Caucasian population in whom CYP2D6 is extremely active [33] [CYP2D6 ultrafast metabolizer phenotype (UM)] leading to very high morphine formation from codeine. For example, life-threatening opioid intoxication developed in a 62-year-old man after he was given 25 mg oral codeine 3 times a day for 4 days. Then, 12 h after the last dose had been administered, the patient's level of consciousness deteriorated and he

TABLE 12.1 Evidence for Pharmacogenetic Modulation of Pharmacodynamic Effects of Analgesic Drugs in Humans

Gene	Variant	Minor Allele Frequency	Affected Analgesic	Clinical Effect	Study Population	Gene	Reference
OPRM1 (μ-opioid receptor)	118A>G (rs1799971)	13.5 % for minor allele	Morphine-6-glucuronide	Decreased miotic effects	Healthy volunteers	12	84
				Decreased miotic effects	Healthy volunteers	12	76
				Decreased side effects	Single case	1	128
				Decreased analgesia	Healthy volunteers	20	77
				Decreased analgesia	Healthy volunteers	16	78
			Morphine	Decreased miotic effects	Healthy volunteers	12	76
				Increased opioid requirements	Single case	1	89
				Increased opioid requirements	Cancer pain patients	207	80, 90
				Increased opioid requirements	Postoperative patients	80	81
				Increased opioid requirements	Postoperative patients	147	88
				Increased opioid requirements	Postoperative patients	588	82
				Increased opioid requirements	Chronic pain patients	352	91

			Alfentanil	Decreased analgesia and respiratory depression	Healthy volunteers	20	79
				Decreased analgesia	Healthy volunteers	25	86
			Fentanyl	Decreased opioid requirements	Women in labor	223	83
			Levomethadone	Decreased miotic effects	Healthy volunteers	51	85
				Increased opioid requirements	Postoperative patients	138	129
KCNJ6 (potassium inwardly-rectifying channel, subfamily J, member 6)	rs2070995G > A	21–46%	Fentanyl or morphine	Increased opioid requirements	Postoperative patients	129	94
COMT (cathecol-*O*-methyl transferase)	472 G > A (rs4680)	48.1% for minor allele	Morphine	Decreased morphine requirements	Cancer pain patients	207	98
MC1R (melanocortin 1 receptor)	29insA, 451C >T (rs1805007), 478C > T (rs1805008), 880G > C (rs1805009), other	0–8.5 %; 2.2% with two variant alleles	M6G	Increased analgesia	Healthy volunteers	47	102
			Pentazocine	Increased analgesia in women	Healthy volunteers	42	100
ABCB1 (P-glycoprotein)	3435 C > T (rs1045642)	50.4% for minor[a] allele	Several	Decreased opioid doses	Chronic pain patients	352	91
			Fentanyl	Respiratory depression	Postoperative patients	126	7
	1236TT/2677TT/3435TT	35.7% for minor[a] allele					

(*continued*)

TABLE 12.1 (*Continued*)

Gene	Variant	Minor Allele Frequency	Affected Analgesic	Clinical Effect	Study Population	Gene	Reference
CYP2D6 (cytochrome P450 2D6)	Only non-functional alleles	5.3% of patients	Codeine	Decreased analgesia	Healthy volunteers	24	130
				Decreased analgesia	Healthy volunteers	18	22
				Decreased respiratory, psychomotor and miotic effects	Healthy volunteers	16	131
			Oxycodone	Insufficient or inadequate clinical responses	Pain patients	Each 1	63, 64
			Tramadol	Decreased analgesia	Healthy volunteers	27	52
				Decreased analgesia	Postoperative patients	300	54
	>2 copies of functional alleles	1.7% of patients	Codeine	Increased effects up to toxicity	Single cases	Each 1	34–38
			Tramadol	Increased effects up to toxicity	Single case	1	132
UGT2B7 (UDP glucuronosyl transferase 2B7)	*2 allele[b]	—	Codeine	Increased effects up to toxicity	Single cases	2	47
PTGS2 (cyclooxygenase 2)	−765C>G (rs20417)	17	Rofecoxib	Increased analgesia	Postmolar surgery pain	72	107
Combinations of genes							

OPRM1 and COMT	Group 1: OPRM1 118AA and COMT 472AA Group 2: OPRM1 118 AA and COMT 472G Group 3: OPRM1 118G and COMT 472 AA Group 4: OPRM1 118G and COMT 472G	15.9% of patients 57.1% of patients 7.1% of patients 18.2% of patients		Morphine	Morphine requirements increasing from group 1 to group 4	Cancer pain patients 207	90
OPRM1 and ABCB1	Group 1: OPRM1 118AA and ABCB1 3435TT Group 2: OPRM1 118AA and ABCB1 3435C or OPRM1 118G and ABCB1 3435TT Group 3: OPRM1 118G and ABCB1 3435C	19.9% of patients 59.6% of patients 20.5% of patients	Morphine	Opioid analgesia decreasing from group 1 to group 3	Cancer pain patients	145	[42]

[a]Allele frequency reported as *minor* refers to an allele reported to be minor in gene databases. When its reported allelic frequency is close to 50%, the so-called minor allele may have a frequency of >50% in the actual cohort. We nevertheless preserved the denomination *minor* for consistency with the literature.
[b]The distribution of homozygous, heterozygous, and noncarriers of the minor alleles of the selected variants agreed with χ^2 the expectations from the Hardy–Weinberg law (χ^2 goodness-of-fit tests: $p \geq 0.17$).

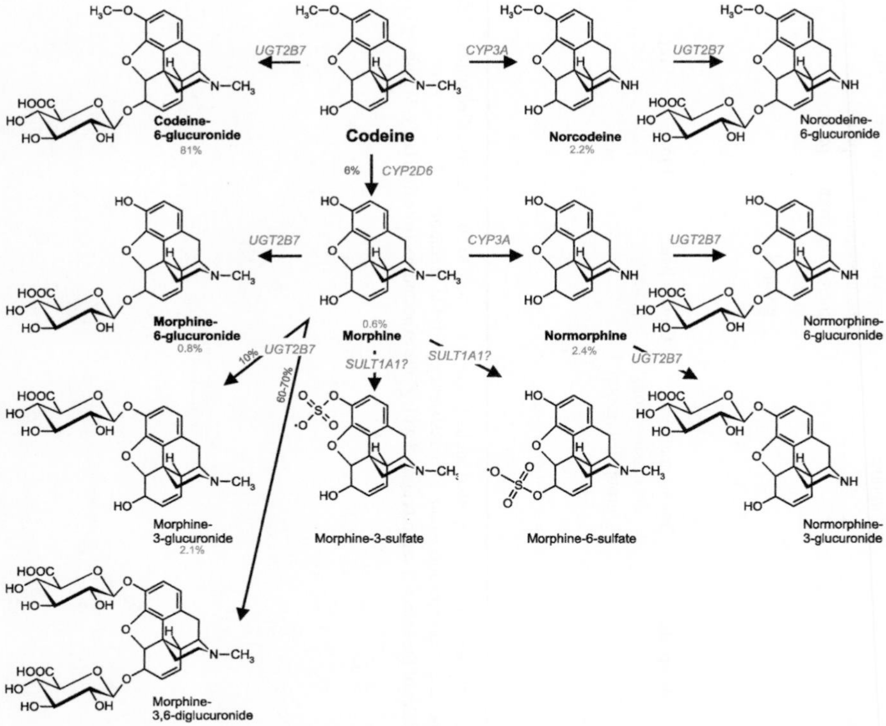

FIGURE 12.2 The metabolism of codeine including that of morphine [18]. Key enzymes are indicated. The respective fractions of a 30 mg codeine dose found in the form of the major metabolites [19] are indicated below the respective metabolites.

became unresponsive [34]. A 33-year-old woman took 60 mg codeine prophylactically to avoid pain in connection with tooth extraction. Within 30 min she experienced euphoria, dizziness, and severe epigastric pain [35]. A 29-month-old child experienced apnea resulting in brain injury following codeine administration for pain relief after tonsillectomy [36]. A newborn died from morphine poisoning when his mother used codeine while breastfeeding [37]. Another newborn also died on day 13 after his mother had been prescribed codeine for postepisiotomy pain. The mother was diagnosed as an ultrarapid metabolizer [38]. Relevant known *CYP2D6* polymorphisms in Caucasians include gene amplification [39], which, however, is present only in the 1–3% who are phenotypic ultrafast metabolizers.

Thus, roughly one in seven of Caucasians [40] is at risk for either failure or toxicity of codeine therapy due to CYP2D6-dependent extremely low or high morphine formation, respectively. Nevertheless, the fraction of 7–11% CYP2D6 PMs among Caucasians [29–31] is too low to explain the high numbers needed to treat (50) to achieve at least 50% relief of dental or postsurgical pain, respectively, by administration of 60 mg codeine [41]. Nongenetic factors such as pain characteristics or simply the low morphine dose resulting from codeine probably play a role. In addition, codeine analgesia is probably modulated by additional genetic factors affecting the effects of morphine such as variants altering drug transport [42], opioid receptor expression [43] or signaling [44], nociception or pain [2,45], and genetic variants in other enzymes such as CYP3A [46] or UGT2B7 [47], accounting for approximately 70–80% of the metabolism of codeine [19,48]. Similarly, high morphine formation is probably a prerequisite but not a sufficient single cause of severe codeine side effects. Codeine toxicity is documented in only a few case reports [34–38,47] and therefore rarer than expected from the $\leq$7% Caucasian phenotypic UMs and also rarer than in 1–3% carriers of *CYP2D6* amplification. The clinical diagnosis of altered codeine effects is still not satisfactorily possible. While low morphine formation can be predicted by genotyping in some ethnic groups such as Caucasians at a reasonable hit rate, extremely high morphine formation cannot, and requires additional phenotyping [49].

Tramadol has a lower affinity at μ-opioid receptors than its metabolite *O*-desmethyltramadol (M1). Specifically, the K_i values for the racemic mixture of tramadol, its (+) and (−) enantiomers, the racemic mixture of M1, and its (+) and (−) enantiomers at μ-opioid receptors expressed in transfected HN9.10 neuroblastoma cells, were 17,000, 15,700, 28,800, 3190, 153, and 9680 nM, respectively, compared to 7.1 nM for morphine [50]. Therefore, CYP2D6 activity is a major determinant of the antinociception elicited after (+)-tramadol administration [51]. Indeed, due to the lack of formation of the active metabolite *O*-desmethyltramadol in CYP2D6 PMs, the analgesic effects of tramadol on experimental pain were decreased [52]. Moreover, the pupillary response to systemic tramadol administration differed between extensive CYP2D6 metabolizers (EMs; i.e., subjects with "normal" CYP2D6 function) and PMs [53]. In the patients, observed, the percentage of nonresponders to postoperative tramadol administration was higher in poor metabolizers than in patients with functional CYP2D6 [54], which agreed with the formation of *O*-desmethyltramadol stratified according to the CYP2D6 genotype and phenotype [55]. However, tramadol was not completely devoid of analgesic effects in persons without functional CYP2D6 [56] because it possesses opioid activity and acts also through non-opioid-dependent mechanisms [57]. For example, concomitant administration of the serotonin $5HT_3$ receptor antagonist ondansetron diminished the analgesic effects of tramadol [58].

For other CYP2D6 substrates with active metabolites, evidence for altered analgesic effects with altered CYP2D6 function is either negative, such as for dihydrocodeine [21,59,60] or, at least at a nongenetic level, for oxycodone [61]; or evidence may be available only from animal research such as for hydrocodone [62], or restricted to single case reports communicating a reasonable mechanism-based interpretation of ineffectiveness [63] or inadequate responses to oxycodone administration [64] rather than systematic evidence.

Tilidine is activated (transformed) to nortilidine and parecoxib is activated to valdecoxib via CYP3A. CYP3A is phenotypically highly variable, but only a minor part of this variability can be attributed to genetics. Individuals with at least one *CYP3A5*1* allele copy (adenine in position 6986) produce high levels of full-length *CYP3A5* mRNA and express active CYP3A5 [5]. However, the majority (95%) of

Caucasians have no active CYP3A5, due to a premature stop codon [65]. Positive associations in the context of analgesics, prodrug activation in and analgesic actions have not been reported so far.

12.2.1.3 Transmembrane Transporters

P-glycoprotein coded by the *ABCB1* gene is located mainly in organs with excretory functions such as liver, kidney, and gastrointestinal tract [66] and has also been found at the blood–brain barrier, where it forms an outward transporter [67]. Therefore, functional impairment of P-glycoprotein transport may be expected to result in increased bioavailability of orally administered drug or in increased brain concentrations of its substrates. Both mechanisms give rise to the expectation of decreased dose requirements or increased clinical effects of analgesics that are substrates of P-glycoprotein. Fentanyl is a substrate of P-glycoprotein [68,69]. A diplotype consisting of three single-nucleotide polymorphic positions in the *ABCB1* gene (1236TT, 2677TT, and 3435TT) was associated with increased susceptibility to clinical fentanyl effects [7]. Moreover, the opioid loperamide, clinically prescribed as antidiarrheic because it does not produce effective CNS concentrations because of its rapid excretion from the CNS by P-gp [68], produced CNS opioid effects associated with an *ABCB1* 3435TT genotype [70]. Together with the *OPRM1* 118A > G variant, the *ABCB1* 3435C > T predicted the response to morphine in cancer patients with sensitivity close to 100% and specificity of >70% [42].

12.2.2 Pharmacodynamics

Decreased effects of analgesics may result from pharmacodynamic irregularities such as insufficient receptor binding, activation or signaling, or decreased expression of the drug's target such as opioid receptors or cyclooxygenases. Genetic factors have been found to act via any of these mechanisms.

12.2.2.1 Opioid Receptors

The μ-opioid receptor is the clinically most relevant target of opioid analgesics. The *OPRM1* gene is highly polymorphic [71,72], with 1799 human single-nucleotide polymorphisms (SNPs) currently listed in the NCBI SNP database (`www.ncbi.nlm.nih.gov/SNP/`; accessed 1/18/09). Coding mutations affecting the third intracellular loop of the μ-opioid receptor (e.g., 779G > A, 794G > A, 802T > C) have been shown to result in reduced G-protein coupling, receptor signaling, and receptor desensitization [9,73,74], leading to the expectation that opioids are almost ineffective in patients carrying those polymorphisms, which, however, has not been shown and, due to their extremely low allele frequency ($<<1\%$), is restricted to rare single cases. Of the few more frequently found ($>5\%$) SNPs (e.g., -172G > T, 17C > T, 118A > G, IVS2-31G > A, IVS2-691G > A), substantial evidence for a functional consequence for the effects of endogenous or exogenous opioids is available for the 118A > G SNP [75]. This causes an amino acid exchange of the aspartate into an asparagine at position 40 of the receptor protein deleting a putative extracellular glycosylation site.

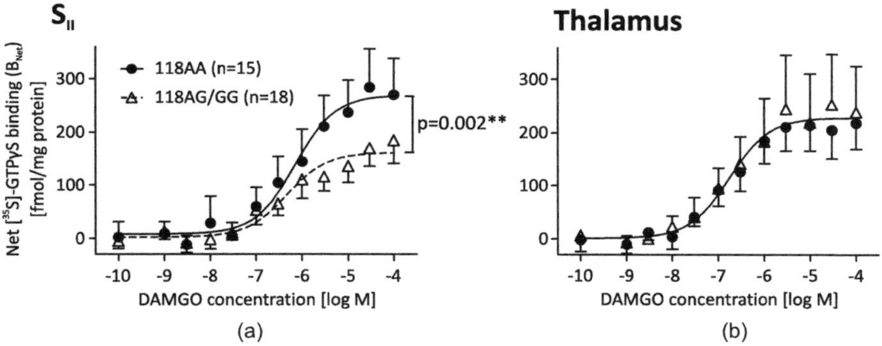

FIGURE 12.3 Decreased μ-opioid receptor agonist D-Ala^2,N-MePhe^4,Gly-ol^5-enkephalin (DAMGO) induced signaling in the presence of the *OPRM1* 118G allele in human brain tissue is seen in the secondary somatosensory area S_{II} but not in the thalamus. (Reproduced from Oertel et al. [44].)

This may cause decreased μ-opioid receptor expression [43] or signaling [44] (Fig. 12.3).

The molecular effects translate into decreased clinical effects of various opioids in experimental [76–79] and clinical [42,80–82] settings, except for a single opposite report [83]. The consequence of the 118A > G SNP have consistently been observed to be a decrease in opioid potency for pupil constriction, which resulted in a rightshift of pupil size versus opioid concentration. Evidence for this is available for various opioids such as morphine [76], M6G [76,84], or methadone [85]. For analgesia, the SNP decreased the concentration effects of alfentanil on experimental pain [79]. Specifically, the variant decreases the effects of opioids on pain-related activation mainly in those regions of the brain that are processing the sensory dimension of pain [86]. In the clinical setting, greater postoperative requirements of alfentanil [87] and morphine [80,81,88] have been reported for carriers of the variant, and higher concentrations of alfentanil [79] or M6G [77,78] were needed to produce analgesia in experimental pain models. In addition, a single case of a patient heterozygously carrying the variant 118G allele was reported in whom a daily oral dose of 2 g morphine was necessary for satisfactory pain relief [89].

The *OPRM1* 118A > G SNP resulted in a broadened therapeutic range of alfentanil in healthy homozygous carriers because it decreased opioid induced respiratory depression more than opioid induced analgesia [79] (Fig. 12.4), whereas such an effect was not present in heterozygous carriers [78,79]. Finally, the variant is involved in joint genetic consequences for opioid effects together with *COMT* [90] or *ABCB1* [42] variants, with clinical consequences according to the expectations from the single SNPs (see discussion below). However, lower opioid requirements are also possible [83,91], and with all the functional evidence and the molecular support, the clinical consequences of this SNP seem modest, as it failed a meta-analysis of its opioid effect modulation in clinical settings [92].

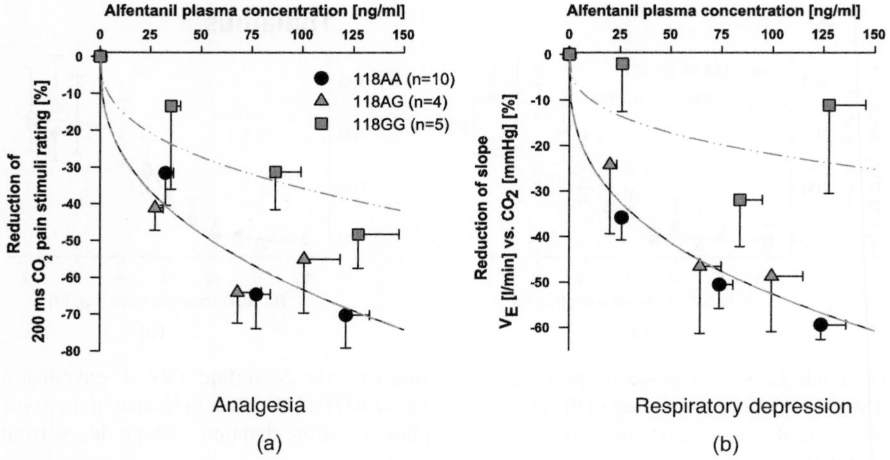

FIGURE 12.4 Consequences of the OPRM1 118A>G single-nucleotide polymorphism (dbSNP accession number: rs1799971, see `http://www.ncbi.nlm.nih.gov/SNP/`) for analgesia (a) and respiratory depression (b) after intravenous infusion of alfentanil establishing different plasma (and brain) concentration levels in healthy young volunteers [79]. The effects of alfentanil on pain and further on respiratory depression are significantly reduced in homozygous carriers of the variant G allele.

12.2.2.2 GIRK2

Opioid receptors along with α-adrenergic, muscarinic cholinergic, γ-aminobutyric acid B, and cannabinoid receptors, are coupled with postsynaptic GIRK2 channels (Kir3.2). This pathway accounts for essentially all of the antinociceptive effects in males, although females appear to recruit additional signal transduction mechanisms for some analgesic drugs [93]. Genetic variants in *KCNJ6* have been shown to increase opioid requirements in Japanese patients after abdominal surgery [94].

12.2.2.3 Catechol-O-Methyl Transferase

Catechol-*O*-methyl transferase (COMT) degrades catecholamine neurotransmitters such as norepinephrine and dopamine. Increased dopamine concentrations have been shown to suppress the production of endogenous opioid peptides [95]. Opioid receptor expression is compensatorily upregulated. For the V158M variant of COMT coded by the 472G>A SNP of the *COMT* gene, this has been shown both in human postmortem brain tissue [96] and *in vivo* by assessing the binding of the μ-opioid receptor selectively radiolabeled ^{11}C-carfentanil using positron emission tomography (PET) [97]. The variant leads to a low-function COMT enzyme that fails to degrade dopamine, which may cause a depletion of encephalin. Cancer pain patients carrying the V158M variant needed less morphine than did patients not carrying this variant [98]. Finally, the variant interacts with the OPRM1 118A>G variant [90].

12.2.2.4 Melanocortin 1 Receptors

The major melanocortin 1 receptor gene (*MC1R*) variants that have been associated with altered opioid analgesia are 451C>T coding for R151C MC1 receptors, 479G>A coding for R160W MC1 receptors, and 880G>C coding for D294H MC1 receptors. They result in functionally impaired melanocortin 1 receptors and a red hair color and fair skin [99]. Women with two nonfunction variant alleles (n=5) of the melanocortin 1 receptor gene (*MC1R*) displayed significantly greater analgesia by the κ-opioid agonist pentazocine than did women carrying only one or no *MC1R* variant (n=13) or than men (n=24) [100]. The consequence of *MC1R* variants for analgesia was related to the binding of endogenous κ-opioid receptor ligand, dynorphin, which binds at nonmutated MC1 receptors [101]. When hypothesizing that MC1R activation by endogenous neuromodulators exerts antiopioid actions [100], the greater effect of pentazocine in carriers of those mutations may be explained by an omission of this antiopioid effect. The observation of greater analgesic effects of κ-opioids in female carriers of *MC1R* nonfunctional variants suggests that this neurochemical pain modulation has a sex-specific regulation when the κ-opioid system is involved [100]. However, the consequences of inactive MC1 receptors appear to be non-sex-specific for μ-opioid-related enhanced analgesic effects of morphine-6-glucuronide [102].

12.2.2.5 Cyclooxygenases

Polymorphisms in the *PTGS2* gene coding for cyclooxygenase 2 may modulate the development of inflammation as well as the response to treatment with inhibitors of cyclooxygenases, especially of those with a COX2 preference [103]. This has been proposed for the *PTGS2* -765G>C SNP, which was reported to be associated with a >2-fold decrease in COX2 expression [104]. By altering a putative Sp1 binding site [105], this *PTGS2* gene variant was found to decrease the promoter activity by 30% [106]. This was associated with a net decrease in COX2 function, quantified by prostaglandin E2 production from peripheral blood monocytes after stimulation with bacterial LPS [104]. This condition was reported to cause absence of rofecoxib analgesia in carriers of the –765C variant allele [107]. However, neither the –765G>C-associated lower COX2 expression nor reduced effects of COX2 inhibitors were reproduced in a subsequent study in healthy volunteers having received celecoxib [108].

12.3 GENETICS OF DRUG ADDICTION

Substance abuse and addiction include complex genetic causes. It is conceivable to hypothesize that high opioid doses may include an addiction component in some pain patients. Some of genetic variants have implications for both pain therapy and addiction, such as an association between the OPRM1 118A>G SNP and opiate addiction [109–111]. However, other genetic polymorphisms add to the pain-related variants such as an association of the minor T allele of the ankyrin repeat and kinase domain containing one gene [112] (*ANKK1*) variant (rs1800497C>T) with poor treatment outcomes of methadone substitution [113], a higher nonresponse rate to methadone substitution therapy in carriers of the wild-type C allele *DRD2* rs6277 C > T SNP [114], or increased methadone dosage requirements in carriers of the *DRD2* rs6275C > T SNP [13]. These and other addiction-related genetic variants may add to the genetic reasons for high opioid dosage requirements in some pain patients. However, evidence supporting this hypothesis is thus far not available.

12.4 PHARMACOGENETICS OF DRUG INTERACTIONS

Pharmacogenetic variants might be compensated unless a second factor additionally challenges the affected system. By inhibiting CYP2D6, paroxetine was found to increase the steady-state plasma concentrations of (*R*)-methadone in extensive but not in poor metabolizers of debrisoquine/sparteine [115]. Inhibition of CYP2D6 by methadone might also contribute to exaggerated response or unexpected toxicity from drugs that are substrates of this enzyme [116]. CYP2C9 nonfunctional variants might increase the plasma concentrations of COX inhibitors [117–119], but because of the broad therapeutic range, this might not translate into altered clinically effects unless warfarin, also a CYP2C9 substrate, is coadministered, which then may result in an increased bleeding risk [120,121]. Life-threatening intoxication to dextromethorphan was seen in a 60-year-old man who had developed postsurgical neuropathic cervical pain, which was treated by hydromorphone, gabapentin, clonazepam, and amitriptyline [122]. Two days after he received a dextromethorphan preparation for a catarrhal syndrome, he was admitted into an emergency department in a profound coma. He had a CYP2D6*4 variant leading to a PM phenotype, potentially aggravated by intake of the CYP2D6 inhibitor amitriptyline.

12.5 CONCLUSIONS AND FUTURE PERSPECTIVES

Genetic differences undoubtedly account for a part of the variability of pain [123] and the response to analgesic treatment [2–4,45]. Genetic research in pain and its therapy has identified several relevant polymorphisms. In some cases such as codeine administration [124] or postoperative morphine treatment [42], genetics has been shown to predict the individual responses, albeit only retrospectively by statistical association. Genetic variants may help explain uncommonly high opioid dosage requirements in some patients such as daily morphine doses of > 2 g [89] or severe side effects following codeine administration [38]. However, this is still limited to specific analgesic drugs or clinical settings, and pain therapy treatment cannot yet be satisfactorily personalized on the patient's genotype. In addition, the clinical consequences are still known from only a few clinical studies, and the only meta-analysis showed that one of the promising SNPs, *OPRM1* 118A > G, has a modest to absent effect in clinical practice [92]. Moreover, most of the functional genetic variants have a frequency of 10–50% and are therefore rarely present alone in an individual. In contrast, they interact with each other in the same subject with partly counterbalancing, effects [125]. For this reason, and given the complex nature of pain involving various mechanisms of nociception [126], a multigenic approach is required. Whether this will improve the thus far modest contribution of genetics to pain therapy [127] remains to be seen.

REFERENCES

1. Breivik H, Collett B, Ventafridda V, Cohen R, Gallacher D. Survey of chronic pain in Europe: Prevalence, impact on daily life, and treatment. *Eur. J. Pain* 2006;**10**:287–333.
2. Lötsch J, Geisslinger G. Current evidence for a modulation of nociception by human genetic polymorphisms. *Pain* 2007;**132**:18–22.
3. Lötsch J, Geisslinger G. Current evidence for a genetic modulation of the response to analgesics. *Pain* 2006;**121**:1–5.
4. Somogyi AA, Barratt DT, Coller JK. Pharmacogenetics of opioids. *Clin. Pharmacol. Ther.* 2007;**81**:429–444.
5. Kuehl P, Zhang J, Lin Y, et al. Sequence diversity in CYP3A promoters and characterization of the genetic basis of polymorphic CYP3A5 expression. *Nat. Genet.* 2001;**27**:383–391.
6. Ingelman-Sundberg M. Genetic polymorphisms of cytochrome P450 2D6 (CYP2D6): Clinical consequences, evolutionary aspects and functional diversity. *Pharmacogenomics J.* 2005;**5**:6–13.
7. Park HJ, Shinn HK, Ryu SH, Lee HS, Park CS, Kang JH. Genetic polymorphisms in the ABCB1 gene and the effects of fentanyl in Koreans. *Clin. Pharmacol. Ther.* 2007;**81**:539–546.
8. Bond C, LaForge KS, Tian M, et al. Single-nucleotide polymorphism in the human mu opioid receptor gene alters beta-endorphin binding and activity: Possible implications for opiate addiction. *Proc. Natl. Acad. Sci. USA* 1998;**95**:9608–9613.
9. Befort K, Filliol D, Decaillot FM, Gaveriaux-Ruff C, Hoehe MR, Kieffer BL. A single-nucleotide polymorphic mutation in the human mu-opioid receptor severely impairs receptor signaling. *J. Biol. Chem.* 2001;**276**:3130–3137.
10. Tegeder I, Costigan M, Griffin RS, et al. GTP cyclohydrolase and tetrahydrobiopterin regulate pain sensitivity and persistence. *Nat. Med.* 2006;**12**:1269–1277.
11. Solovieva S, Leino-Arjas P, Saarela J, Luoma K, Raininko R, Riihimaki H. Possible association of interleukin 1 gene locus polymorphisms with low back pain. *Pain* 2004;**109**:8–19.
12. Cox JJ, Reimann F, Nicholas AK, et al. An SCN9A channelopathy causes congenital inability to experience pain. *Nature* 2006;**444**:894–898.
13. Doehring A, Hentig N, Graff J, et al. Genetic variants altering dopamine D2 receptor expression or function modulate the risk of opiate addiction and the dosage requirements of methadone substitution. *Pharmacogenet. Genomics* 2009;**19**:407–414.
14. Hinz B, Cheremina O, Brune K. Acetaminophen (paracetamol) is a selective cyclooxygenase-2 inhibitor in man. *FASEB J.* 2008;**22**:383–390.
15. Pierre SC, Schmidt R, Brenneis C, Michaelis M, Geisslinger G, Scholich K. Inhibition of cyclooxygenases by dipyrone. *Br. J. Pharmacol.* 2007;**151**:494–503.

16. Gillen C, Haurand M, Kobelt DJ, Wnendt S. Affinity, potency and efficacy of tramadol and its metabolites at the cloned human mu-opioid receptor. *Naunyn. Schmiedebergs Arch. Pharmacol.* 2000;**362**:116–121.

17. Lötsch J, Geisslinger G. Morphine-6-glucuronide: An analgesic of the future? *Clin. Pharmacokinet.* 2001;**40**:485–499.

18. Lötsch J, Skarke C, Schmidt H, et al. Evidence for morphine-independent central nervous opioid effects after administration of codeine: Contribution of other codeine metabolites. *Clin. Pharmacol. Ther.* 2006;**79**:35–48.

19. Vree TB, Verwey-van Wissen CP. Pharmacokinetics and metabolism of codeine in humans. *Biopharm. Drug Dispos.* 1992;**13**:445–460.

20. Mignat C, Wille U, Ziegler A. Affinity profiles of morphine, codeine, dihydrocodeine and their glucuronides at opioid receptor subtypes. *Life Sci.* 1995;**56**:793–799.

21. Schmidt H, Vormfelde SV, Walchner-Bonjean M, et al. The role of active metabolites in dihydrocodeine effects. *Int. J. Clin. Pharmacol. Ther.* 2003;**41**:95–106.

22. Eckhardt K, Li S, Ammon S, Schanzle G, Mikus G, Eichelbaum M. Same incidence of adverse drug events after codeine administration irrespective of the genetically determined differences in morphine formation. *Pain* 1998;**76**:27–33.

23. Vree TB, van Dongen RT, Koopman-Kimenai PM. Codeine analgesia is due to codeine-6-glucuronide, not morphine. *Int. J. Clin. Pract.* 2000;**54**:395–398.

24. Srinivasan V, Wielbo D, Simpkins J, Karlix J, Sloan K, Tebbett I. Analgesic and immunomodulatory effects of codeine and codeine 6- glucuronide. *Pharm. Res.* 1996;**13**:296–300.

25. Srinivasan V, Wielbo D, Tebbett IR. Analgesic effects of codeine-6-glucuronide after intravenous administration. *Eur. J. Pain* 1997;**1**:185–190.

26. Dayer P, Desmeules J, Leemann T, Striberni R. Bioactivation of the narcotic drug codeine in human liver is mediated by the polymorphic monooxygenase catalyzing debrisoquine 4-hydroxylation (cytochrome P-450 dbl/bufI). *Biochem. Biophys. Res. Commun.* 1988;**152**:411–416.

27. Cascorbi I. Pharmacogenetics of cytochrome p4502D6: Genetic background and clinical implication. *Eur. J. Clin. Invest.* 2003;**33** (Suppl. 2):17–22.

28. Fagerlund TH, Braaten O. No pain relief from codeine...? An introduction to pharmacogenomics. *Acta Anaesthesiol. Scand.* 2001;**45**:140–149.

29. Lovlie R, Daly AK, Molven A, Idle JR, Steen VM. Ultrarapid metabolizers of debrisoquine: Characterization and PCR-based detection of alleles with duplication of the CYP2D6 gene. *FEBS Lett.* 1996;**392**:30–34.

30. Bertilsson L, Dahl ML, Dalen P, Al-Shurbaji A. Molecular genetics of CYP2D6: Clinical relevance with focus on psychotropic drugs. *Br. J. Clin. Pharmacol.* 2002;**53**:111–122.

31. Tamminga WJ, Wemer J, Oosterhuis B, et al. Polymorphic drug metabolism (CYP2D6) and utilisation of psychotropic drugs in hospitalised psychiatric patients: A retrospective study. *Eur. J. Clin. Pharmacol.* 2003;**59**:57–64.

32. Raimundo S, Toscano C, Klein K, et al. A novel intronic mutation, 2988G> A, with high predictivity for impaired function of cytochrome P450 2D6 in white subjects. *Clin. Pharmacol. Ther.* 2004;**76**:128–138.

33. Steijns LS, Van Der Weide J. Ultrarapid drug metabolism: PCR-based detection of CYP2D6 gene duplication. *Clin. Chem.* 1998;**44**:914–917.

34. Gasche Y, Daali Y, Fathi M, et al. Codeine intoxication associated with ultrarapid CYP2D6 metabolism. *New. Engl. J. Med.* 2004;**351**:2827–2831.
35. Dalen P, Frengell C, Dahl ML, Sjoqvist F. Quick onset of severe abdominal pain after codeine in an ultrarapid metabolizer of debrisoquine. *Ther. Drug Monit.* 1997;**19**:543–544.
36. Voronov P, Przybylo HJ, Jagannathan N. Apnea in a child after oral codeine: A genetic variant—an ultra-rapid metabolizer. *Paediatr. Anaesth.* 2007;**17**:684–687.
37. Madadi P, Koren G, Cairns J, et al. Safety of codeine during breastfeeding: Fatal morphine poisoning in the breastfed neonate of a mother prescribed codeine. *Can. Fam. Physician.* 2007;**53**:33–35.
38. Koren G, Cairns J, Chitayat D, Gaedigk A, Leeder SJ. Pharmacogenetics of morphine poisoning in a breastfed neonate of a codeine-prescribed mother. *Lancet* 2006;**368**:704.
39. Johansson I, Lundqvist E, Bertilsson L, Dahl ML, Sjoqvist F, Ingelman-Sundberg M. Inherited amplification of an active gene in the cytochrome P450 CYP2D locus as a cause of ultrarapid metabolism of debrisoquine. *Proc. Natl. Acad. Sci. USA* 1993;**90**:11825–11829.
40. Zanger UM, Raimundo S, Eichelbaum M. Cytochrome P450 2D6: Overview and update on pharmacology, genetics, biochemistry. *Naunyn. Schmiedebergs Arch. Pharmacol.* 2004;**369**:23–37.
41. Moore RA, McQuay HJ. Single-patient data meta-analysis of 3453 postoperative patients: Oral tramadol versus placebo, codeine and combination analgesics. *Pain* 1997;**69**:287–294.
42. Campa D, Gioia A, Tomei A, Poli P, Barale R. Association of ABCB1/MDR1 and OPRM1 gene polymorphisms with morphine pain relief. *Clin. Pharmacol. Ther.* 2008;**83**:559–566.
43. Zhang Y, Wang D, Johnson AD, Papp AC, Sadee W. Allelic expression imbalance of human mu opioid receptor (OPRM1) caused by variant A118G. *J. Biol. Chem.* 2005;**280**:32618–32624.
44. Oertel BG, Kettner M, Scholich K, et al. A common human mu-opioid receptor genetic variant diminishes the receptor signaling efficacy in brain regions processing the sensory information of pain. *J. Biol. Chem.* 2009;**284**:6530–6535.
45. Kim H, Dionne RA. *Genetics, Pain, and Analgesia*, Pain: Clinical Updates (series), International Association for the Study of Pain 2005; Vol. 8
46. Lalovic B, Phillips B, Risler LL, Howald W, Shen DD. Quantitative contribution of CYP2D6 and CYP3A to oxycodone metabolism in human liver and intestinal microsomes. *Drug Metab. Dispos.* 2004;**32**:447–454.
47. Madadi P, Ross CJ, Hayden MR, et al. Pharmacogenetics of neonatal opioid toxicity following maternal use of codeine during breastfeeding: A case-control study. *Clin. Pharmacol. Ther.* 2009;**85**:31–35.
48. Chen ZR, Somogyi AA, Reynolds G, Bochner F. Disposition and metabolism of codeine after single and chronic doses in one poor and seven extensive metabolisers. *Br. J. Clin. Pharmacol.* 1991;**31**:381–390.
49. Lötsch J, Rohrbacher M, Schmidt H, Doehring A, Brockmöller J, Geisslinger G. Can extremely low or high morphine formation from codeine be predicted prior to therapy initiation? *Pain* 2009;**144**:119–124.

50. Lai J, Ma SW, Porreca F, Raffa RB. Tramadol, M1 metabolite and enantiomer affinities for cloned human opioid receptors expressed in transfected HN9. 10 neuroblastoma cells. *Eur. J. Pharmacol.* 1996;**316**:369–372.

51. Garrido MJ, Sayar O, Segura C, et al. Pharmacokinetic/pharmacodynamic modeling of the antinociceptive effects of (+)-tramadol in the rat: role of cytochrome P450 2D activity. *J. Pharmacol. Exp. Ther.* 2003;**305**:710–718.

52. Poulsen L, Arendt-Nielsen L, Brosen K, Sindrup SH. The hypoalgesic effect of tramadol in relation to CYP2D6. *Clin. Pharmacol. Ther.* 1996;**60**:636–644.

53. Fliegert F, Kurth B, Gohler K. The effects of tramadol on static and dynamic pupillometry in healthy subjects—the relationship between pharmacodynamics, pharmacokinetics and CYP2D6 metaboliser status. *Eur. J. Clin. Pharmacol.* 2005;**61**:257–266.

54. Stamer UM, Lehnen K, Hothker F, et al. Impact of CYP2D6 genotype on postoperative tramadol analgesia. *Pain* 2003;**105**:231–238.

55. Stamer UM, Musshoff F, Kobilay M, Madea B, Hoeft A, Stuber F. Concentrations of tramadol and O-desmethyltramadol enantiomers in different CYP2D6 genotypes. *Clin. Pharmacol. Ther.* 2007;**82**:41–47.

56. Collart L, Luthy C, Favario-Constantin C, Dayer P. Duality of the analgesic effect of tramadol in humans. *Schweiz. Med. Wochenschr.* 1993;**123**:2241–2243.

57. Enggaard TP, Poulsen L, Arendt-Nielsen L, Brosen K, Ossig J, Sindrup SH. The analgesic effect of tramadol after intravenous injection in healthy volunteers in relation to CYP2D6. *Anesth. Analg.* 2006;**102**:146–150.

58. De Witte JL, Schoenmaekers B, Sessler DI, Deloof T. The analgesic efficacy of tramadol is impaired by concurrent administration of ondansetron. *Anesth. Analg.* 2001;**92**:1319–1321.

59. Platten HP, Schweizer E, Dilger K, Mikus G, Klotz U. Pharmacokinetics and the pharmacodynamic action of midazolam in young and elderly patients undergoing tooth extraction. *Clin. Pharmacol. Ther.* 1998;**63**:552–560.

60. Webb JA, Rostami-Hodjegan A, Abdul-Manap R, Hofmann U, Mikus G, Kamali F. Contribution of dihydrocodeine and dihydromorphine to analgesia following dihydrocodeine administration in man: A PK-PD modelling analysis. *Br. J. Clin. Pharmacol.* 2001;**52**:35–43.

61. Heiskanen T, Olkkola KT, Kalso E. Effects of blocking CYP2D6 on the pharmacokinetics and pharmacodynamics of oxycodone. *Clin. Pharmacol. Ther.* 1998;**64**:603–611.

62. Lelas S, Wegert S, Otton SV, Sellers EM, France CP. Inhibitors of cytochrome P450 differentially modify discriminative-stimulus and antinociceptive effects of hydrocodone and hydromorphone in rhesus monkeys. *Drug Alcohol Depend.* 1999;**54**:239–249.

63. Susce MT, Murray-Carmichael E, de Leon J. Response to hydrocodone, codeine and oxycodone in a CYP2D6 poor metabolizer. *Prog. Neuropsychopharmacol. Biol. Psychiatry* 2006;**30**:1356–1358.

64. Foster A, Mobley E, Wang Z. Complicated pain management in a CYP450 2D6 poor metabolizer. *Pain Pract.* 2007;**7**:352–356.

65. Hustert E, Haberl M, Burk O, et al. The genetic determinants of the CYP3A5 polymorphism. *Pharmacogenetics* 2001;**11**:773–779.

66. Fromm MF, Kim RB, Stein CM, Wilkinson GR, Roden DM. Inhibition of P-glycoprotein-mediated drug transport: A unifying mechanism to explain the interaction between digoxin and quinidine. *Circulation* 1999;**99**:552–557.

67. Cordon-Cardo C, O'Brien JP, Casals D, et al. Multidrug-resistance gene (P-glycoprotein) is expressed by endothelial cells at blood-brain barrier sites. *Proc. Natl. Acad. Sci. USA* 1989;**86**:695–698.

68. Wandel C, Kim R, Wood M, Wood A. Interaction of morphine, fentanyl, sufentanil, alfentanil, and loperamide with the efflux drug transporter P-glycoprotein. *Anesthesiology* 2002;**96**:913–920.

69. Kharasch ED, Hoffer C, Altuntas TG, Whittington D. Quinidine as a probe for the role of p-glycoprotein in the intestinal absorption and clinical effects of fentanyl. *J. Clin. Pharmacol.* 2004;**44**:224–233.

70. Skarke C, Jarrar M, Schmidt H, et al. Effects of ABCB1 (multidrug resistance transporter) gene mutations on disposition and central nervous effects of loperamide in healthy volunteers. *Pharmacogenetics* 2003;**13**:651–660.

71. Thony B, Blau N. Mutations in the BH4-metabolizing genes GTP cyclohydrolase I, 6-pyruvoyl-tetrahydropterin synthase, sepiapterin reductase, carbinolamine-4a-dehydratase, and dihydropteridine reductase. *Hum. Mutat.* 2006;**27**:870–878.

72. Shabalina SA, Zaykin DV, Gris P, et al. Expansion of the human mu-opioid receptor gene architecture: Novel functional variants. *Hum. Mol. Genet.* 2009;**18**(6):1037–1051.

73. Wang D, Quillan JM, Winans K, Lucas JL, Sadee W. Single nucleotide polymorphisms in the human mu opioid receptor gene alter basal G protein coupling and calmodulin binding. *J. Biol. Chem.* 2001;**276**:34624–34630.

74. Koch T, Kroslak T, Averbeck M, et al. Allelic variation S268P of the human mu-opioid receptor affects both desensitization and G protein coupling. *Mol. Pharmacol.* 2000;**58**:328–334.

75. Lötsch J, Geisslinger G. Relevance of frequent mu-opioid receptor polymorphisms for opioid activity in healthy volunteers. *Pharmacogenomics J.* 2006;**6**:200–210.

76. Skarke C, Darimont J, Schmidt H, Geisslinger G, Lötsch J. Analgesic effects of morphine and morphine-6-glucuronide in a transcutaneous electrical pain model in healthy volunteers. *Clin. Pharmacol. Ther.* 2003;**73**:107–121.

77. Romberg R, Olofsen E, Sarton E, den Hartigh J, Taschner PE, Dahan A. Pharmacokinetic-pharmacodynamic modeling of morphine-6-glucuronide-induced analgesia in healthy volunteers: Absence of sex differences. *Anesthesiology* 2004;**100**:120–133.

78. Romberg RR, Olofsen E, Bijl H, et al. Polymorphism of mu-opioid receptor gene (OPRM1: c.118A>G) does not protect against opioid-induced respiratory depression despite reduced analgesic response. *Anesthesiology* 2005;**102**:522–530.

79. Oertel BG, Schmidt R, Schneider A, Geisslinger G, Lötsch J. The mu-opioid receptor gene polymorphism 118A>G depletes alfentanil-induced analgesia and protects against respiratory depression in homozygous carriers. *Pharmacogenet. Genomics* 2006;**16**:625–636.

80. Klepstad P, Rakvag TT, Kaasa S, et al. The 118 A > G polymorphism in the human mu-opioid receptor gene may increase morphine requirements in patients with pain caused by malignant disease. *Acta Anaesthesiol. Scand.* 2004;**48**:1232–1239.

81. Chou WY, Wang CH, Liu PH, Liu CC, Tseng CC, Jawan B. Human opioid receptor A118G polymorphism affects intravenous patient-controlled analgesia morphine consumption after total abdominal hysterectomy. *Anesthesiology* 2006;**105**:334–337.

82. Sia AT, Lim Y, Lim EC, et al. A118G single nucleotide polymorphism of human mu-opioid receptor gene influences pain perception and patient-controlled intravenous

morphine consumption after intrathecal morphine for postcesarean analgesia. *Anesthesiology* 2008;**109**:520–526.

83. Landau R, Kern C, Columb MO, Smiley RM, Blouin JL. Genetic variability of the mu-opioid receptor influences intrathecal fentanyl analgesia requirements in laboring women. *Pain* 2008;**139**:5–14.
84. Lötsch J, Skarke C, Grösch S, Darimont J, Schmidt H, Geisslinger G. The polymorphism A118G of the human mu-opioid receptor gene decreases the clinical activity of morphine-6-glucuronide but not that of morphine. *Pharmacogenetics* 2002;**12**:3–9.
85. Lötsch J, Skarke C, Wieting J, et al. Modulation of the central nervous effects of levomethadone by genetic polymorphisms potentially affecting its metabolism, distribution, and drug action. *Clin. Pharmacol. Ther.* 2006;**79**:72–89.
86. Oertel BG, Preibisch C, Wallenhorst T, et al. Differential opioid action on sensory and affective cerebral pain processing. *Clin. Pharmacol. Ther.* 2008;**83**:577–588.
87. Caraco Y, Maroz Y, Davidson E. Variability in alfentanil analgesia maybe attributed to polymorphism in the mu-opiod receptor gene. *Clin. Pharmacol. Ther.* 2001;**69**:63.
88. Chou WY, Yang LC, Lu HF, et al. Association of mu-opioid receptor gene polymorphism (A118G) with variations in morphine consumption for analgesia after total knee arthroplasty. *Acta Anaesthesiol. Scand.* 2006;**50**:787–792.
89. Hirota T, Ieiri I, Takane H, et al. Sequence variability and candidate gene analysis in two cancer patients with complex clinical outcomes during morphine therapy. *Drug Metab. Dispos.* 2003;**31**:677–680.
90. Reyes-Gibby CC, Shete S, Rakvag T, et al. Exploring joint effects of genes and the clinical efficacy of morphine for cancer pain: OPRM1 and COMT gene. *Pain* 2007;**130**:25–30.
91. Lötsch J, von Hentig N, Freynhagen R, et al. Cross-sectional analysis of the influence of currently known pharmacogenetic modulators on opioid therapy in outpatient pain centers. *Pharmacogenet. Genomics* 2009;**19**:429–436.
92. Walter C, Lötsch J. Meta-analysis of the relevance of the OPRM1 118A>G genetic variant for pain treatment. *Pain* 2009.
93. Blednov YA, Stoffel M, Alva H, Harris RA. A pervasive mechanism for analgesia: Activation of GIRK2 channels. *Proc. Natl. Acad. Sci. USA* 2003;**100**:277–282.
94. Nishizawa D, Nagashima M, Katoh R, et al. Association between KCNJ6 (GIRK2) gene polymorphisms and postoperative analgesic requirements after major abdominal surgery. *PLoS ONE* 2009;**4**:e7060.
95. George SR, Kertesz M. Met-enkephalin concentrations in striatum respond reciprocally to alterations in dopamine neurotransmission. *Peptides* 1987;**8**:487–492.
96. Berthele A, Platzer S, Jochim B, et al. COMT Val108/158Met genotype affects the mu-opioid receptor system in the human brain: Evidence from ligand-binding, G-protein activation and preproenkephalin mRNA expression. *Neuroimage* 2005;**28**:185–193.
97. Zubieta JK, Heitzeg MM, Smith YR, et al. COMT val158met genotype affects mu-opioid neurotransmitter responses to a pain stressor. *Science* 2003;**299**:1240–1243.
98. Rakvag TT, Klepstad P, Baar C, et al. The Val158Met polymorphism of the human catechol-O-methyltransferase (COMT) gene may influence morphine requirements in cancer pain patients. *Pain* 2005;**116**:73–78.

99. Beaumont KA, Newton RA, Smit DJ, Leonard JH, Stow JL, Sturm RA. Altered cell surface expression of human MC1R variant receptor alleles associated with red hair and skin cancer risk. *Hum. Mol. Genet.* 2005;**14**:2145–2154.
100. Mogil JS, Wilson SG, Chesler EJ, et al. The melanocortin-1 receptor gene mediates female-specific mechanisms of analgesia in mice and humans. *Proc. Natl. Acad. Sci. USA* 2003;**100**:4867–4872.
101. Quillan JM, Sadee W. Dynorphin peptides: Antagonists of melanocortin receptors. *Pharm. Res.* 1997;**14**:713–719.
102. Mogil JS, Ritchie J, Smith SB, et al. Melanocortin-1 receptor gene variants affect pain and mu-opioid analgesia in mice and humans. *J. Med. Genet.* 2005;**42**:583–587.
103. Esser R, Berry C, Du Z, et al. Preclinical pharmacology of lumiracoxib: A novel selective inhibitor of cyclooxygenase-2. *Br. J. Pharmacol.* 2005;**144**:538–550.
104. Cipollone F, Patrono C. Cyclooxygenase-2 polymorphism: Putting a brake on the inflammatory response to vascular injury? *Arterioscler. Thromb. Vasc. Biol.* 2002;**22**:1516–1518.
105. Hernandez-Avila CA, Covault J, Gelernter J, Kranzler HR. Association study of personality factors and the Asn40Asp polymorphism at the mu-opioid receptor gene (OPRM1). *Psychiatr. Genet.* 2004;**14**:89–92.
106. Papafili A, Hill MR, Brull DJ, et al. Common promoter variant in cyclooxygenase-2 represses gene expression: Evidence of role in acute-phase inflammatory response. *Arterioscler. Thromb. Vasc. Biol.* 2002;**22**:1631–1636.
107. Lee YS, Kim H, Wu TX, Wang XM, Dionne RA. Genetically mediated interindividual variation in analgesic responses to cyclooxygenase inhibitory drugs. *Clin. Pharmacol. Ther.* 2006;**79**:407–418.
108. Skarke C, Reus M, Schmidt R, et al. The cyclooxygenase 2 genetic variant -765G>C does not modulate the effects of celecoxib on prostaglandin E2 production. *Clin. Pharmacol. Ther.* 2006;**80**:621–632.
109. Szeto CY, Tang NL, Lee DT, Stadlin A. Association between mu opioid receptor gene polymorphisms and Chinese heroin addicts. *Neuroreport* 2001;**12**:1103–1106.
110. Tan EC, Tan CH, Karupathivan U, Yap EP. Mu opioid receptor gene polymorphisms and heroin dependence in Asian populations. *Neuroreport* 2003;**14**:569–572.
111. Shi J, Hui L, Xu Y, Wang F, Huang W, Hu G. Sequence variations in the mu-opioid receptor gene (OPRM1) associated with human addiction to heroin. *Hum. Mutat.* 2002;**19**:459–460.
112. Neville MJ, Johnstone EC, Walton RT. Identification and characterization of ANKK1: A novel kinase gene closely linked to DRD2 on chromosome band 11q23.1. *Hum. Mutat.* 2004;**23**:540–545.
113. Lawford BR, Young RM, Noble EP, et al. The D(2) dopamine receptor A(1) allele and opioid dependence: Association with heroin use and response to methadone treatment. *Am. J. Med. Genet.* 2000;**96**:592–598.
114. Crettol S, Besson J, Croquette-Krokar M, et al. Association of dopamine and opioid receptor genetic polymorphisms with response to methadone maintenance treatment. *Prog. Neuropsychopharmacol. Biol. Psychiatry* 2008;**32**(7):1722–1727.
115. Begre S, von Bardeleben U, Ladewig D, et al. Paroxetine increases steady-state concentrations of (R)-methadone in CYP2D6 extensive but not poor metabolizers. *J. Clin. Psychopharmacol.* 2002;**22**:211–215.

116. Wu D, Otton SV, Sproule BA, et al. Inhibition of human cytochrome P450 2D6 (CYP2D6) by methadone. *Br. J. Clin. Pharmacol.* 1993;**35**:30–34.
117. Kirchheiner J, Stormer E, Meisel C, Steinbach N, Roots I, Brockmöller J. Influence of CYP2C9 genetic polymorphisms on pharmacokinetics of celecoxib and its metabolites. *Pharmacogenetics* 2003;**13**:473–480.
118. Kirchheiner J, Meineke I, Steinbach N, Meisel C, Roots I, Brockmöller J. Pharmacokinetics of diclofenac and inhibition of cyclooxygenases 1 and 2: No relationship to the CYP2C9 genetic polymorphism in humans. *Br. J. Clin. Pharmacol.* 2003;**55**:51–61.
119. Kirchheiner J, Meineke I, Freytag G, Meisel C, Roots I, Brockmöller J. Enantiospecific effects of cytochrome P450 2C9 amino acid variants on ibuprofen pharmacokinetics and on the inhibition of cyclooxygenases 1 and 2. *Clin. Pharmacol. Ther.* 2002;**72**:62–75.
120. Rordorf CM, Choi L, Marshall P, Mangold JB. Clinical pharmacology of lumiracoxib: A selective cyclo-oxygenase-2 inhibitor. *Clin. Pharmacokinet.* 2005;**44**:1247–1266.
121. Malhi H, Atac B, Daly AK, Gupta S. Warfarin and celecoxib interaction in the setting of cytochrome P450 (CYP2C9) polymorphism with bleeding complication. *Postgrad. Med. J.* 2004;**80**:107–109.
122. Forget P, le Polain de Waroux B, Wallemacq P, Gala JL. Life-threatening dextromethorphan intoxication associated with interaction with amitriptyline in a poor CYP2D6 metabolizer: A single case re-exposure study. *J. Pain. Symptom Manage.* 2008;**36**:92–96.
123. Mogil JS. The genetic mediation of individual differences in sensitivity to pain and its inhibition. *Proc. Natl. Acad. Sci. USA* 1999;**96**:7744–7751.
124. Sindrup SH, Brosen K. The pharmacogenetics of codeine hypoalgesia. *Pharmacogenetics* 1995;**5**:335–346.
125. Lötsch J, Flühr K, Neddermayer T, Doehring A, Geisslinger G. The consequence of concomitantly present functional genetic variants for the identification of functional genotype-phenotype associations in pain. *Clin. Pharmacol. Ther.* 2009;**85**:25–30.
126. Julius D, Basbaum AI. Molecular mechanisms of nociception. *Nature* 2001;**413**:203–10.
127. Mogil JS. Are we getting anywhere in human pain genetics? *Pain* 2009.
128. Lötsch J, Zimmermann M, Darimont J, et al. Does the A118G polymorphism at the mu-opioid receptor gene protect against morphine-6-glucuronide toxicity? *Anesthesiology* 2002;**97**:814–819.
129. Hayashida M, Nagashima M, Satoh Y, et al. Analgesic requirements after major abdominal surgery are associated with OPRM1 gene polymorphism genotype and haplotype. *Pharmacogenomics* 2008;**9**:1605–1616.
130. Sindrup SH, Brosen K, Bjerring P, et al. Codeine increases pain thresholds to copper vapor laser stimuli in extensive but not poor metabolizers of sparteine. *Clin. Pharmacol. Ther.* 1990;**48**:686–693.
131. Caraco Y, Sheller J, Wood AJ. Pharmacogenetic determination of the effects of codeine and prediction of drug interactions. *J. Pharmacol. Exp. Ther.* 1996;**278**:1165–1174.
132. Stamer UM, Stuber F, Muders T, Musshoff F. Respiratory depression with tramadol in a patient with renal impairment and CYP2D6 gene duplication. *Anesth. Analg.* 2008;**107**:926–929.

PART III

PHARMACOGENETICS: IMPLEMENTATION IN CLINICAL PRACTICE

CHAPTER 13

Ethical and Social Issues in Pharmacogenomics Testing

SUSANNE VIJVERBERG
Utrecht University, Utrecht, The Netherlands

TOINE PIETERS
Utrecht University, Utrecht, The Netherlands and VU University Medical Center, Amsterdam, The Netherlands

MARTINA CORNEL
VU University Medical Center, Amsterdam, The Netherlands and Center for Society and Genomics, Radboud University, Nijmegen, The Netherlands

13.1 INTRODUCTION

From the 1950s onward human disease has increasingly been treated on a one-size-fits-all blockbuster basis; patients suffering from hypertension receive prescriptions for antihypertensive drugs, diabetic patients take oral medication or insulin injections on a daily basis, and standard care for patients enduring psychotic disorders includes antipsychotic drug treatment. The choice of a specific drug is guided, among other things, by evidence-based information, professional guidelines, and a trial-and-error approach in the consulting room. A physician might adjust the dose or change to another drug when a patient shows substantial adverse drug reactions (ADRs) or does not seem to respond adequately to the prescribed drug therapy. However, through unraveling molecular pathways of disease processes, genomics research is producing new insights that will open doors to more tailored forms of drug treatment based on individual-specific factors underlying disease and drug response. It has become clear that for most common complex disorders, many genes and many environmental factors play an etiological role. As part of this new genetic horizon of personalized

Pharmacogenetics and Individualized Therapy, First Edition.
Edited by Anke-Hilse Maitland-van der Zee and Ann K. Daly.

medicine, interest in pharmacogenetics and more recently pharmacogenomics has grown exponentially in the first decade of the 21st century [1].

Pharmacogenomics investigates the relationship between one's drug response and one's genetic constitution and promises to improve the safety and efficacy of drug treatment and putting an end to the trial-and-error era in drug medication. To meet these high expectations, much more translational research is needed and, most importantly, ethical and social questions should be addressed. To what extent are we able to safeguard a healthy balance between individual and collective interests, rights, and duties? Tensions between the interests and rights of researchers and human subjects have already been identified with regard to the issue of informed consent and the research practice of data sharing. In this chapter we will address and discuss in a systematic way the social and ethical issues that emerge in the area of pharmacogenomics. First, we will focus on pharmacogenomics in a research context, and then we will take a closer look at the use and translation of pharmacogenomics knowledge in a treatment context. In addition, recent experiences with direct-to-consumer (DTC) testing are assessed. Finally, we will focus on health equity and the use of pharmacogenomics in low-resource settings.

13.2 THE RISE OF GENOMICS RESEARCH

The release of the "complete" human genome sequence occurred in April 2003 to coincide with the 50th anniversary of the Watson–Crick publication on the double–helix structure in 1953. In the intervening years, biomedical research production has accelerated by orders of magnitude brought about by associated advances in laboratory technology, computing, and bioinformatics. From 2003 onward, data production in the field of genomics has continued to grow exponentially, and instead of focusing on the human genome as an end in itself, genomic researchers turned their attention toward the role of DNA, RNA, proteins, and metabolites in disease etiology. As part of this trend toward more complexity, interest shifted from the relatively rare monogenic diseases to the more common complex diseases, including cardiovascular disorders, diabetes, cancer, depression, and Alzheimer's disease. When studying a monogenic disorder, the researcher may perform linkage studies in families with few affected relatives, and a study including less than 100 individuals is usual. However, genomics demands large numbers of cases to identify small effects of common gene variants. The results of genomewide association studies (GWASs) have become available where both large numbers of participants and large numbers of single-nucleotide polymorphisms (SNPs) were studied. An example is the Wellcome Trust Case Control Consortium study on seven common diseases (bipolar disorder, coronary artery disease, Crohn's disease, hypertension, rheumatoid arthritis, type 1 and type 2 diabetes) using 14,000 cases and 3000 shared controls [2]. While this was a study performed in one country–(the UK), the large number of cases and the need for replication implies a need for pooling of data from several countries and several studies. The global scale of genomic research challenges conventional biomedical ethical principles.

13.3 ETHICAL PRINCIPLES IN THE ERA OF GENOMICS

Biomedical ethics is a specialized field of ethics, which focuses on a wide array of emerging ethical issues raised by medicine and biomedical research: from debates over the boundaries of life to the allocation of scarce healthcare resources, to human subject research in medicine, and the limits of consent. As such, it provides an international platform for critical reflection on moral obligations of biomedical researchers, health professionals, and society in preventing disease and injury and meeting the needs of the sick and injured. This includes reflection on the changing relationships between the professional and the patient in modern medicine and on problems of truthfulness, privacy, justice, and communal responsibility [3].

The classical principles of biomedical ethics are built on four clusters of norms originally presented by Beauchamp and Childress [3]:

- *Respect for autonomy*—the decisionmaking capacities of autonomous persons should be respected.
- *Nonmaleficence*—do not harm.
- *Beneficence*—do good.
- *Justice*—people should be treated equally and fairly, and it should be ensured that they are accorded their full rights.

These classical principles were conceived to deal with the relationship between the individual patient and the physician in clinical practice, as well as the relationships in clinical research. However, debate has emerged concerning whether these principles are still appropriate for dealing with questions that arise in the rather dynamic genomic era. Early in the Human Genome Project (HGP) era, Knoppers and Chadwick identified five basic principles underlying the international consensus on the need for harmonization of national regulation on topics related to human genome research [4]:

- *Autonomy*—participating in genetic testing should be an autonomous choice of an informed participant.
- *Privacy*—the privacy of the individual and the confidentiality of genetic information should be respected.
- *Justice*—people should be treated equally and fairly, and it should be ensured that they are accorded their full rights.
- *Equity*—equity of access to genetic research, testing, and information; equal costs; equal resources; and equal sharing of information should be ensured.
- *Quality out of respect for human dignity*—accredited and licensed laboratories and personnel, professional oversight and monitoring and ethical review are required.

During the completion of the HGP, the focus of genomics research shifted from a clinical genetics perspective toward a more population-orientated viewpoint [5]. This has tipped the balance scale from the individual perspective to the collective perspective in genomics and more recently also in research ethics. Chadwick and Knoppers have proposed a novel set of ethical principles to address research in human genetics and genomics [5,6]:

- *Reciprocity*—the contribution of the research participant should be recognized. Communication and transparency between researchers and participants are required, also concerning possible commercialization.
- *Mutuality*—genetic information and DNA are regarded as family property. An ethical duty to warn at-risk family members exists.
- *Solidarity*—there should be a willingness to share information for the benefit of others.
- *Citizenry*—the public should be kept informed of science (policy); this principle also involves the concept of a collective identity.
- *Universality*—the human genome is shared by all (common heritage of humanity); therefore, we have obligations towards future generations, and benefits should be shared.

Knoppers and Chadwick do not intend to give up old values, but state that "ethical thinking will inevitably evolve as science does." Following the release of the sequence of the human genome, the era of genomics raised previously unknown questions related to the scale and pace of research. The dynamic nature of genomics research challenges ethical thinking. We will discuss here some changing aspects of genomics research and consider the possible ethical and social implications that these may have at both the individual and communal levels.

13.4 "INFORMED" CONSENT?

The concept of informed consent is a cornerstone in modern medical research ethics and part of most national legislation concerning medical research. This is not without good reason. History shows us (Nazi war crimes and also, e.g., the Tuskegee syphilis study (1932–1972)) not only the necessity for consent but that the adoption of consent practices in biomedical research was a hard-fought battle. The basic idea of informed consent is that a researcher is (ethically and/or legally) justified in using a research subject in a project only if the research subject has consented to being so used [7].

For a consent to be a valid informed consent, four elements must be present [7];

1. The relevant information has been given.
2. The relevant information has been understood.
3. The person is capable of consenting.
4. The person is uncoerced.

In order to be considered sufficient, information disclosed to subjects must generally include in a comprehensible way the research procedure, its purpose, anticipated benefits and harms, alternative treatments (if available), an invitation to ask any questions, and a statement that the subject may withdraw from the study at any time. The two last elements make an often tacit assumption explicit by pointing out that a valid consent has to be voluntary, and it has to be given by somebody who is psychologically capable of consenting. The text in the consent form usually also includes possible implications for the research participant concerning issues such as privacy, confidentiality, and re-contacting.

In the pregenomics area, the researcher involved would be a single person or a member of a small group. The research question was often a clear hypothesis. A typical question on an informed-consent form would mention by which researcher (s) and in what department the potential role of a specific gene in the metabolism of a specific drug would be investigated. Today, consent may cover a wide range of issues, and many participants may be involved in setting up the framework for consent [7]. Current research often has a global character and can be performed only if large numbers of participants consent to the use of their biological material for a hypothesis-free study by a large number of researchers. Large databases and biobanks have emerged to store biological specimens and genetic information. Furthermore, data sharing is considered to be an essential part of the current genomic research process. Many people are prepared to voluntarily share their health data as long as they do not experience any negative effects from participating in the study. This can be regarded as a form of health information altruism [8]. However, in the current genomic era, participants may be unaware of the true extent of the researcher's promise of privacy, confidentiality, and anonymity when giving their consent. As a result of extensive data sharing, the emergence of large-scale research platforms, and the unique fingerprint nature of DNA, the significance of those promises should be reconsidered. Within this research context the role of consent will become additionally burdened and those involved will experience growing demands with regard to the decisionmaking process. Can ethically and legally justified consent still be obtained in practice? When the genome of Dr. James Watson (discoverer of the double helix) was sequenced, he agreed to release it to public databases, except for the information on apolipoprotein E (ApoE) because of its association with late-onset Alzheimer's disease. Even James Watson had not foreseen that his genotype could be imputed with more than 99% certainty, due to the linkage disequilibrium that exists between polymorphisms flanking *APOE* [9]. Hiding genetic information is far from simple or straightforward.

In medical research, a key-coded or reversibly anonymized approach is commonly used to store data. A sample is coded and stored separately from the identifying information. However, it remains possible to link the sample with the identifying information through a code. Keeping genetic information in complete anonymity is not technically feasible, nor desirable, should the participant wish to withdraw from the study [10]. Several biobanks currently use a broad, general consent. For example, participants to the UK Biobank. consent to "participate in the UK Biobank." In cases where ethically and scientifically approved purposes do not fall within the scope of the original consent, a participant would be recontacted and requested to give consent again [11]. The question emerges concerning whether participants realize what they are authorizing and whether this approach to consent does justice to the principle of reciprocity. Is it possible to inform the participants in a truthful and comprehensive way?

Lunshof and colleagues have proposed an open-consent model in which veracity (telling the truth and bringing information in a comprehensive and objective way) is the leading moral principle, and in which confidentiality, privacy, and anonymity are not warranted [12]. This approach to consent has been devised for the *Personal Genome Project* (PGP)[1], a study initiated by professor George M. Church (Harvard Medical School/MIT) that aims to publish the genomes and medical records of several volunteers. Participants consent to unconstrained redisclosure of their medical health details, and to the unrestricted publication of information that emerges from any future research on their genotype–phenotype dataset. Although the open consent model might be considered a very genuine approach, it is likely that broad implementation of the open-consent model might scare off a large group of potential research volunteers. Furthermore, this form of individualistic consent also has implications for the family or community members of research participants when genomic data are published in publicly accessible databases. Genomic data obtained from a research participant may also hold information about family members who did not consent [13]—which also brings us to the issue of feedback. Should participants receive feedback on their individual research results? It has been argued that validated, verified, and clinically useful research data should be returned to the participant (if requested by the participant), based on the classical biomedical ethical principles of respect for the person, beneficence, and justice [10]. In addition to the costs that this individual feedback might incur, the question arises as to how to include informed decisionmaking for recontacting in the consent. How does one know in advance what information a participant would want to be provided with and what not? Especially concerning clinically relevant data that may emerge during the study but that do not address the main research question (secondary information), this is a complex matter. For example, it has been shown that some genetic variants associated with drug response can also be associated with disease predispositions. How, then, should the researcher handle the feedback of this kind of unforeseen information? Or how to handle information that might not directly affect the risk profile of the participant, but might affect the risk profile of the offspring of the participant?

Undervaluation of consent in the governance of research undermines the integrity of consent as much as does overvaluation. The idea that a researcher can and should provide full and complete information on which a potential research participant will rationally decide whether to participate, is overly idealized. Participants may attach more value to general beliefs and assumptions (i.e., concerning the benefits of medical research) than to the process of informing and being informed during recruitment procedures. In addition, a rather strong culture of consent may create a

[1] Website of the Personal Genome Project: `http://www.personalgenomes.org/`.

climate of excessive caution that indirectly harms patients by hindering and even preventing promising research. Furthermore, overenthusiastic attempts to gain consent can disturb and alienate already stressed individuals for whom the act of discriminating between consent to treatment and research is rather challenging [13]. Liddell and Richards propose to improve consent practices by changing slightly the nature and process of consent [13].

The first thing one could do is to set apart consent forms, so that separate forms deal with consent to treatment, consent to research, and consent to storage of data and tissue for future research. A second step may be to recognize variability in consent practices and that the requirements for "valid" or "good enough" consent can vary according to the circumstances, without undermining the principles underlying the integrity of consent. At least legally valid consent must be sufficiently but not perfectly informed and voluntary. This provides room for maneuvering and designing qualitatively different consent procedures for particular categories of research and treatment. This may imply the development of procedures for family or community consent. The challenge will be to keep attuned to the tensions between the interests of the individuals and the community as well as between the researcher/healthcare professional and the patient, in particular, in genetic and tissue research when data sharing is involved [13].

13.5 INDIVIDUAL AND COLLECTIVE IMPLICATIONS

The emerging social and ethical issues raised by pharmacogenomics research can have an individual dimension (i.e., "Do I consent to participate in a clinical pharmacogenomics trial?") and a community dimension (i.e., the need for privacy protection in order to prevent the access to genetic information by insurers and employers). Friction may arise between the implications of "do good and do not harm" at both individual level and collective levels of a nation or community. For example; the use of an open-consent model in the context of research participation might benefit the individual, but it might not benefit the community. It is likely that with the introduction of the open consent model, fewer volunteers will participate in pharmacogenomics research, which will make it more difficult to generate and validate data.

Another implication on a collective level is the fear among some scholars that new groups of "orphan patients" will be created: groups of patients for whom no treatment is available [14]. The concern is that classifying patients according to their phenotypic and genotypic information may lead to new small subgroups of disease populations, some with rare genotypes. Pharmaceutical companies might find it unattractive to invest in drug development for these small subgroups. These groups will then be "orphaned" by the economic laws of the international therapeutic drug market.

In The Netherlands, the Dutch Steering Committee for Orphan Drugs launched an initiative in January 2009 in order to encourage translation in the field of rare diseases by supporting companies to submit an *orphan designation dossier* (ODD) to the

European Medicines Agency (EMA) [15]. Similar public–private partnerships are needed to stimulate research on rare genotypes. Especially in the field of rare diseases, both research and treatment will often take place in one setting, which implies that the boundaries between research ethics and clinical ethics will necessarily blur. This might raise specific problems concerning the interests of the researcher/healthcare professional and the patient, and as a consequence for informed consent. In addition, all those involved have to make decisions in the context of larger uncertainty than in the "normal" therapeutic context. A possible solution to these problems is to follow a similar in-process feedback-learning trajectory as is practiced in pediatric oncology.

Furthermore, developments in pharmacogenomics have lead to a renewed discussion on the geneticalization of race or ethnicity [14]. In 2005 the FDA approved BiDil® a drug for the treatment of heart failure in self-identified black patients. Early clinical studies of BiDil, showed no compelling efficacy in the general public, however, *post hoc* analysis showed that a small subsample of African Americans did seem to benefit from the drug [16]. In 2001, the FDA therefore approved a full-scale clinical trial with 1050 African American men and women with severe heart failure, which showed that BiDil was significantly more effective than a placebo concerning hospitalization rates and heart failure-related symptoms [17]. Nevertheless, a clinical study designed to investigate the efficacy of BiDil in people of different races never took place. The mechanisms underlying the different drug response were never identified. There has been much concern as to whether the approval of ethnic drugs, such as BiDil, would promote the re-biologization of race within medical research and practice, which could potentially lead to stigmatization and discrimination.

Participation by disease communities and ethnic minorities in research, policymaking, and the development of services might be a safeguard against misfits between bench and bedside. For instance, race and ethnicity are not the key to unlocking the secrets of the causes of disease, but constantly evolving conceptual tools for assessing needs and inequality and guiding health policy and practical action. As such, racial and ethnic differences and similarities in the susceptibility of specific diseases might even provide the basis for reinventing community-based public health.

Having said this, we should take seriously weigh and address public fears concerning the misuse of genetic information by third parties. Access to genetic information by employers and insurers might lead to discrimination or stigmatization of individuals with an "unfavorable" genetic constitution. For example, individuals with a genetic predisposition for a certain condition, or who would tolerate only expensive drugs, might be charged higher insurance premiums. This fear might discourage people from participating in pharmacogenomics research [18]. In order to prevent misuse of genetic information, most European countries have adopted genetic antidiscrimination legislation. Belgium was the first European country to introduce genetic nondiscrimination legislation in 1990, and many countries followed. In addition, in 2008, after several years of pending in Congress, the United States adopted the Genetic Information Nondiscrimination Act (GINA), which promised to provide extensive protection against the misuse of genetic information by employers and insurers, and was intended to encourage US citizens to participate in clinical research and genetic testing. However, there is an ongoing debate on how well these antidiscrimination laws actually protect the privacy and confidentiality of individuals. Belgian insurance companies may still use genetic test results or genetic information derived from physician records or insurance questionnaires [19]. This practice is caused mainly by ignorance, confusion, and misunderstanding, but is also the result of a lack of clear legal definitions of genetic data and genetic tests. The definitions of *genetic testing* used by a wide range of organisations and entities (e.g., professional genetics organizations, insurance companies, pharmaceutical companies, and law firms) are extremely varied and—especially in the legislation area—often very inconsistent [20].

Furthermore, employers in the United States are still permitted to require potential employees to undergo a medical examination and are allowed access to the health records of these candidates [20]. These health records may still include genetic information. In addition, GINA only protects asymptomatic individuals from genetic discrimination by health insurers. In most US states, an insurer can still decide not to renew the policy, or to increase the premiums when a predisposed individual becomes affected [21].

Rapid advances in technology and the scale on which current research is being performed threaten protection of the privacy of research volunteers. With the development of new approaches to consent and proper data protection, this does not need to be problematic. However, effective antidiscrimination legislation that protects not only genetic information but all predictive health-related information is essential to protect research participants.

Yet another concern is a general reserve of pharmaceutical companies to invest in and use pharmacogenetic technology and information. This raises some uncomfortable issues for the industry as a whole, and those responsible for regulating its practices. How might companies be stimulated to perform pharmacogenetic studies that may lead to important, but commercially damaging, health findings? For example, if a company were to discover that one of its products was unsafe or ineffective in specific genotype groups, how might governments be able to safeguard that such information would be shared with regulators and the public? Also, what might be a company's legal responsibilities with respect to pharmacogenetic studies? Worryingly, such potential problems may mean that companies are simply disinclined to undertake such studies in the first place, because the results may turn out to be detrimental to their commercial interests. Aligning commercial interests with the potential public health benefits of pharmacogenetics thus presents a real challenge for policymakers and regulators. Stimulating public–private partnerships may be a way to prevent the industry from opting out due to sound fears for liability risks [22].

13.6 PHARMACOGENOMICS APPLICATIONS IN HEALTHCARE

Powerful analytical and computing technologies are producing information on genetic variation and related health problems at an extremely rapid pace. Both useful and less useful applications are becoming available, either in theory or in practice. The need for translational research is now more pressing than ever. Before a certain drug is prescribed, one might imagine that all patients would be tested to assess whether they metabolize the drug quickly or slowly, so that the dosage can be determined or information on the risk of side effects can be established. In order to decide what could be offered to the general population or to specific disease communities or groups of individual patients, there is a need for a framework for an integral assessment of large-scale genetic testing possibilities.

In a 2008 report of the Health Council of The Netherlands [23], a distinction was proposed for screening tests that might also be useful for pharmacogenomic tests: high-quality responsible screening leading to health gains, screening that does not convincingly lead to health gains and is not harmful, and risky or unsound screening. In this report *genetic screening* was defined as the testing of the DNA, RNA, proteins, or metabolites of healthy individuals in order to detect a hereditary disease at an early stage, or to detect the predisposition for a hereditary disease. Regardless of the definition of genetic screening, governments and health institutions have often built on the screening principles of Wilson and Jungner as guiding principles (Table 13.1).

The central idea was that potential benefits of screening should outweigh the harm that is also always inflicted by a screening program, and the model mentions several aspects to be evaluated in order to assess pros and cons [24]. In more recent decades, several sets of criteria have been derived from this original set. The report of the Health Council of The Netherlands [23] recommended that high-quality, responsible forms of screening ought to be available and (financially) accessible. Governments can comply with their duty to care by ensuring that these facilities are made available and accessible by incorporating them in the basic healthcare package. An important condition for collective funding is that health gain results from the service provision. At the other end of the spectrum, the government has a duty to protect against health damage that might result from risky or unsound screening. Information provided on test possibilities should be true, clear, and comprehensible. Independent scientific evidence should be available to show the effectiveness of the test. The right to privacy

TABLE 13.1 Wilson and Jungner Criteria

1. The condition sought should be an important public health problem
2. There should be an effective treatment for patients with recognized disease
3. Facilities for diagnosis and treatment should be available
4. There should be a recognizable latent or early symptomatic stage
5. There should be a suitable test or examination
6. The test should be acceptable to the population
7. The natural history of the condition, including development from latent to declared disease, should be adequately understood
8. There should be an unanitnously agreed-to policy on whom to treat as patients
9. The cost of case finding (including diagnosis and treatment of patients diagnosed) should be economically balanced in relation to possible expenditure on medical care as a whole
10. Case finding should be a continuous process and not a once-and-for-all project

should be guaranteed. Testing offers not complying with these requirements should not be allowed onto the market. Between these two ends of the spectrum, one could imagine that some testing possibilities neither have clinical utility nor are unsound. Tests could be available for recreational purposes, to obtain information on ancestry or nonmedical characteristics such as the risk of baldness (alopecia). With the decreasing price of genomic information [25], the need to evaluate what could be useful and what is probably of less use is rather urgent. This demands that a strategy for translational research be developed in which the evidence is built to allow incorporation of some tests in healthcare practice within several years, while for other tests it will become clear that they lack either clinical utility or cost-effectiveness. Building evidence will take place in several phases, similar to phases of pharmacological research. A framework for translational research was proposed by Khoury and colleagues [26]. The "continuum of translational research" that they propose includes four phases, starting from phase I translation research, which seeks to move a basic genome-based discovery into a health application. An example could be the construction of a genomic profile that predicts individual reactions to drugs. Phase II translation research leads to the development of evidence-based guidelines. A study showing that the genomic profile in a large group of people of, say, $N=1000$–3000 is effective in avoiding side effects would fit in this phase. Phase III attempts to move evidence-based guidelines into health practice. An implementation project designed to ensure that all people to whom a certain drug is being prescribed in an entire country are first tested using the genomic profile to determine their risk of side effects would fit in phase III. Phase IV seeks to evaluate the real-world health outcomes of a genomic application in practice. Evaluation of the occurrence of the side effect to show that fewer people are affected after implementation of the genomic profile would be the phase IV study of our example. The authors estimate that no more than 3% of published genomics research focuses on Phase II and beyond, implying that evidence-based guidelines are rare in the field of genomics. They also argue that adequate support for the continuum of translational research is needed to realize the promise of genomics for human health. We filled out the model for HER2/neu testing and trastuzumab treatment as an example where translation has progressed to the highest phases of translation (Table 13.2). What is sometimes considered as *translation* or *valorization* in genomics, is gene patenting, starting spinoff companies, and other new economic activities [27]. For genomics to reach the bedside, these economic activities are not sufficient but will need to be accompanied by clinical trials, the development of clinical guidelines, dissemination, and implementation research, as well as outcomes research.

13.7 LOST IN TRANSLATION

Although there are some potentially useful pharmacogenomics tests utilized in clinical healthcare, few are currently used in routine practice (Table 13.3). Many applications need further phase II research to develop evidence-based guidelines. Other applications (such as *HLA-B*5701, HLA-B*1502,* and *HER2/neu* testing)

TABLE 13.2 Example Application of Phases of Translation Research to Trastuzumab Treatment after *HER2/neu* Testing

Description of Phase	Research Question or Activity	Recommendation
Phase I	Discovery of health application	Determine how cancer cells with HER2/neu overexpression respond to trastuzumab therapy
Phase II	Development of evidence-based guideline	Develop guideline specifying to whom to offer HER2/neu testing and to whom to prescribe trastuzumab in cancer clinic in research setting
Phase III	Move guideline into health practice	Instruct oncologists nationwide to use guideline
Phase IV	Evaluate health outcome	Study survival of breast cancer patients after stratified application of trastuzumab according to HER2/neu status

require phase III and IV research to evaluate whether the implementation of guidelines has been successful and leads to reduction of morbidity and mortality. Furthermore, pharmacogenomics remains limited to a few clinical fields, such as oncology and psychiatry [28]. In 2008 Scheuner et al. performed a systematic review to synthesize current information on genetic health services for common adult-onset conditions [29]. Their systematic review started with more than 10,000 papers on genetics/genomics and some potentially relevant health issues, only 16 of which were related to an outcome of genomic medicine. Only one of the papers was a randomized controlled trial of a genetic testing intervention for a common condition that measured clinical outcomes: a pharmacogenomic study on warfarin dose and *CYP2CP* and *VKORC1* genotypes [30]. The authors concluded that many gaps in knowledge about organization, clinician, and patient needs must be filled to translate basic and clinical science advances in genomics of common chronic diseases into practice. Although more RCTs have been performed (see Table 13.3), there is also a need for cost-effectiveness analyses in which, besides the impact on healthcare costs, the impact on patients is included [31]. It is only with this information that policy-makers will be able to decide whether the introduction of a specific pharmacogenomics test in clinical practice will have an added value in comparison to current practice.

The lack of translation was already apparent before the age of genomics (see Table 13.4 for examples). Some knowledge based on classical genetics could have been applied for decades, but still has not utilized to its full clinical potential. Approximately 10% of the world population suffers from glucose-6-phosphate dehydrogenase (G6PD) deficiency, and is at risk of acute hemolysis when exposed to an oxidative drug (such as the antimalaria agent primaquine). Regions where G6PD deficiency is more prevalent include Africa and Asia, which are also malaria-endemic areas. Knowledge of *G6PD* status might lead to fewer side effects. Although screening of G6PD deficiency does occur on a case-by-case basis in countries where

TABLE 13.3 Various Pharmacogenomics Applications and Their Implementation Status

Drug Name	Drug Type	Marker	Goal	Implementation
Trastuzumab	Chemotherapy agent directed against HER2/neu	HER2/neu overexpression in tumor tissue	Predict drug response	Evidence-based guidelines for clinical practice exist; testing is required according to drug label
Cetuximab	Chemotherapy agent directed against EGFR	EGFR expression in tumor tissue	Predict drug response	Testing is required for colorectal carcinoma patients participating in clinical studies according to drug label; colorectal clinical studies have shown no correlation between amount of EGFR expression and response rate
		KRAS mutation in tumor tissue	Predict drug response	Retrospective studies have shown a correlation between presence of *KRAS* mutation status in tumor tissue and poorer outcome of cetuximab therapy; lack of prospective validation
Gefinitib	Chemotherapy agent directed against EGFR	EGFR overexpression in tumor	Predict drug response	Drug label includes information on testing (no recommendation); some retrospective studies have shown a correlation between EGFR expression and gefinitib response, others have not (prospective data are lacking)
Irinotecan	Chemotherapy agent	*UGT1A1*28*	Guide drug dose and reduce incidence of ADRs (severe neutropenia)	In 2005 FDA approved a diagnostic test for UGT1A1 testing and recommended testing in drug label, based on a prospective study; cost-effectiveness study has been performed; data from RCTs are lacking

(Continued)

TABLE 13.3 ***(Continued)***

Drug Name	Drug Type	Marker	Goal	Implementation
Azathioprine and 6-mercaptopurine	Immunosuppressive agents	*TMPT* variants	Reduce incidence of ADRs (severe hematological toxicity)	In 2004 FDA approved a diagnostic phenotypic *TMPT* test; FDA recommends genetic testing in drug label; a RCT has been finished recently (TARGET study); routine use in some clinical settings (Spain, UK); economic evaluations have been performed, although all were based on retrospective studies; added clinical value is under debate
Warfarin	Anticoagulant	*CYP2C9* and *VKORC1* variants	Guide drug dose and avoid ADRs (major bleeding)	FDA recommends testing in drug label; meta-analysis and RCT have been performed; a prospective observational study to assess clinical and economical impact of pharmacogenomic testing for warfarin is ongoing
Imatinib mesylate	Chemotherapy agent	*C-KIT* mutation in tumor tissue	Predict drug response	Retrospective studies have shown a correlation between *C-KIT* mutation status in tumor tissue and drug response Drug label includes information on testing (no recommen-dation); lack of prospective validation

Tamoxifen	Chemotherapy agent	*CYP2D6* variants	Predict drug response	Some retrospective studies have shown a correlation between presence of a *CYP2D6* gene variant and poorer tamoxifen outcome; others have not (prospective studies are ongoing); in 2006 the Subcommittee for Clinical Pharmacology of the Advisory Committee for Pharmaceutical Science (FDA) recommended drug relabeling
Clopidogrel	Anti-platelet agent	*CYP2C19* variants	Predict drug response	Some observational studies have suggested a correlation between presence of a *CYP2C19* gene variant and clopidogrel responsiveness; others have not; no prospective clinical study results available yet
Abacavir	Nucleoside analog reverse transcriptase inhibitor	*HLA-B**5701*	Reduce the incidence of ADRs (abacavir hypersensitivity reactions)	In 2008 the results of a RCT were published; FDA recommends testing in drug label; there are no FDA-cleared tests for *HLA-B**5701*; rapid uptake of testing in some clinical settings (i.e., UK); cost-effectiveness analysis has been performed using a simulation model

(*Continued*)

TABLE 13.3 (*Continued*)

Drug Name	Drug Type	Marker	Goal	Implementation
Fluoxetine and other selective serotonin reuptake inhibitors (SSRIs)	Antidepressants	*CYP2D6*, *CYP2D19* and others	Predict response and guide drug dose	In 2004 FDA approved the Roche AmpliChip CYP450 microarray for identifying *CYP2D6* and *CYP2D19* genotype, based on test accuracy; drug label includes information on testing (not recommended); in 2007, EGAPP Working Group concluded that there were insufficient data to recommend testing for SSRIs; there is a lack of translation research in phases III and IV
Carbamazepine	Anticonvulsant	*HLA-B*1502*	Reduce incidence of ADRs (possibly fatal skin reactions; Stevens–Johnson syndrome and toxic epidermal necrolysis)	FDA recommends testing for individuals of Han Chinese, Hong Kong Chinese, or Thai origin in drug label; retrospective studies have shown a strong association between the presence of *HLA-B*1502* and the occurrence of ADRs

Sources: The information presented in this table has been adapted from: (1) an article by A. Pollack, Patient's DNA may be signal to tailor medication, *The New York Times*, Dec. 2008; (2) US FDA, *Genomics at FDA* (2008) (available at `http://www.fda.gov/cder/genomics/`); (3) National Guideline Clearinghouse™ (`www.guideline.gov`); and (4) US National Institutes of Health, Bethesda, MD (`www.ClinicalTrials.gov/`).

TABLE 13.4 Some Pregenomic Examples of Genetics-Based Pharmacotherapy

Gene or Disorder	Pharmacotherapeutic Choice	Potential Adverse Side Effect
G6PD deficiency	Avoid primaquine, sulfonamides, acetanilide (and certain food products such as fava beans)	Hemolytic anaemia
NAT2	Avoid isoniazid, hydralazine, procainamide, sulfonamides	Neuropathy, lupus erythematosus
Thalassemia	Take into account the possibility of non-iron–deficient anemia	Secondary hemochromatosis

antimalarial drugs are frequently prescribed [32], individuals worldwide who have ancestors from G6PD deficient regions could benefit from a systematic screening of *G6PD* variants, for instance, before a first prescription of oxidative drugs. For such a screening to be effective, the information would have to be stored in an electronic patient record, such as at the pharmacy. Similar considerations apply to an *N*-acetyltransferase (*NAT2*) polymorphism that is associated with side effects of isoniazid [33].

An even older example is thalassemia. Not only patients but also carriers experience anemias that may be mistaken for iron deficiency anemia. A screening—information storage system might help to avoid secondary hemochromatosis [34]. In all three of these examples, knowledge has been available for many years, but optimal translation into current pharmaceutical practice has not yet been achieved. Even without expensive DNA tests, it might be possible to use genomics knowledge simply by recognizing the pattern of side effects of, for instance, G6PD deficiency.

The core ethical principles of medicine—to do good (beneficence), or at least to do no harm (nonmaleficence)—requires that knowledge be used to improve health and to avoid adverse effects. Although genomics knowledge may perhaps have satisfied the curiosity of many researchers, it has hardly contributed to "do good" and "do no harm."

13.8 INTEGRATION INTO THE CLINIC AND PHARMACY

In order to successfully bring pharmacogenomics to the clinic and pharmacy counter, several challenges need to be faced [35–37]. In 2008, the US Secretary's Advisory Committee on Genetics, Health and Society (SACGHS) published an extensive report on the challenges and potentials of pharmacogenomics [38]. They listed a number of issues to be addressed in order to use pharmacogenomics in clinical practice to its full potential, including

- Assessment of the analytical validity, clinical validity, and clinical utility of pharmacogenomics diagnostics and therapies
- Regulation of pharmacogenomics products

- Coverage and reimbursement of pharmacogenetics technologies
- Necessity of a well-organised health information technology structure
- Need for education and training of health professionals

Concerning the latter, it is essential to train and educate healthcare providers, including physicians, pharmacists, dieticians, and nurses, to enable them to use pharmacogenomics and interpret test results correctly. Education should not only be part of the basic training, but also be included in postgraduate courses. Several initiatives are emerging. In 2007, the American Medical Association (AMA) and the Food and Drug Administration (FDA) developed an introductory online educational tool (pharmacogenomics and personalized medicine) to improve the basic knowledge of physicians on pharmacogenomics.[2] The American College of Clinical Pharmacy provides courses on the application of pharmacogenomics to patient healthcare for pharmacists. The Royal Dutch Association for the Advancement of Pharmacy (KNMP) has set up a similar initiative in The Netherlands. Although pharmacogenetics-literacy is a basic requirement for using pharmacogenomics in clinical practice, it is a rather naive idea that to get professionals to engage with this new technology, we just have to educate them about it. Professional acceptance, if it is to be stimulated, can be dealt with only by actually engaging with those ethical and social issues about which professionals are concerned. This engagement includes taking into account the local procedural and cultural norms in which tests are used, the economical drivers on the departmental or individual level (whether it saves the clinician/on department money), and more general aspects of clinical decisionmaking (e.g., whether clinical judgment takes precedence over decisions based on external, scientific information) [39].

Implementation of pharmacogenomics in clinical practice also requires that healthcare providers are prepared for the sometimes new, and often complex legal issues that the introduction of a new technology brings with it, for example, concerning liability [37]. A pharmacist has a professional duty to assess whether a certain drug type and dose is suitable for a patient. When an adverse drug reaction occurs in a patient, one that could have been avoided by the use of a pharmacogenomics test, the pharmacist could be held liable—in other words, legally responsible. Consider, for example, coumarin anticoagulants. A major side effect of coumarin anticoagulants is severe bleeding, with reported incidences of 1.5–5.0 per 100 patients a year [40]. It has been shown that especially individuals who have variant alleles of the *VKORC1* and *CYP2C9* genotypes are at increased risk of drug-induced bleeding. Therefore, if pharmacogenetic testing for *VKORC1* and *CYP2C9* were to be made standard care, and a pharmacist were to dispense warfarin in the absence of testing, the pharmacist could be held liable if drug-induced bleeding occurred. However, the extent of liability depends on accepted standards of care, as formulated in guidelines. According to the *Webster New World Medical Dictionary*, *standard care* is defined as "a diagnostic and treatment process that a clinician should

[2] Accessible via `http://ama.learn.com`.

follow for a certain type of patient, illness, or clinical circumstance." However, it is unclear whether any pharmacogenomics application is currently considered to be standard care [38]. Although there are some pharmacogenomics tests used in clinical care, clinical practice guidelines are rare, and labeling content is limited.

Health information technology guides the exchange of medical information between healthcare consumers and providers. A well-structured health information technology infrastructure needs to be developed to enable standardized data collection, and to link pharmacogenomics data to clinical information systems in order to facilitate surveillance and guide treatment decisions [38]. In The Netherlands, the Pharmacogenetics Working Party of the Royal Dutch Society for the Advancement of Pharmacy is currently working to implement pharmacogenomics in their automated medication control database in order to link pharmacogenomics test results to therapeutic recommendations. These databases are used by the majority of general practitioners and community and hospital pharmacists in The Netherlands [28]. However, a major limitation is the lack of genotyping data. There is limited evidence to justify prospective pharmacogenomic testing. Furthermore, the infrastructure for genotyping is available only in a subset of centers [28]. In order to bring pharmacogenomics successfully to the clinic and pharmacy counter, it is necessary to develop guidelines, register unfavorable gene variants, and implement signaling systems that trigger an alarm when drugs are dispensed for which pharmacogenomics tests are available.

13.9 DIRECT-TO-CONSUMER (DTC) PHARMACOGENETIC TESTING

Although the implementation of pharmacogenomics testing in clinical healthcare seems to be progressing at a very slow pace, the implementation of pharmacogenomics in the commercial health sector is progressing rather quickly. An increasing number of companies are starting to offer health-related genetic testing services directly to the public, particularly in the United States [41]. The tests offered may predict response to medication, such as *HER2/neu* testing prior to prescribing trastuzumab and *CYP450* gene testing related to liver metabolism of many commonly prescribed drugs. Critics have raised concerns regarding the limited access to genetic counselling, uncertain laboratory quality of the tests, the accuracy and adequacy of the information provided by companies, the protection of privacy, and the risk that consumers may be misled by false or misleading claims, resulting in these consumers making decisions that will cause harm on the basis of test results [38,41,42]. According to a commercial company, testing for trombophylia (factor V Leiden) might, for instance, be considered by everyone, before starting oral contraceptives or hormone replacement therapy (see `www.dnadirect.com`). However, the test is trivial in terms of disease prognosis, because the test is hardly better than flipping a coin (the area under the curve is 0.61, compared to 0.50 for flipping a coin) [43]. Although the company may be right to state that the risk of thrombosis is many times higher than the population risk for carriers of one or two factor V Leiden mutations, they do not mention the fact that the population risk is very low. While the information provided is not incorrect, one might argue that not all information that is needed for an informed decision is provided. The clinical utility of the test is probably close to zero. If a decision not to take birth control pills were based on such a test result, and unwanted pregnancy were to occur, the harm is probably greater than the good.

Regulation of DTC testing is under debate. Proponents of DTC argue that it empowers consumers to make independent medical decisions, and that it would be paternalistic to prevent individuals from accessing information about their genomes [41]. For genetic testing in a clinical setting, however, many quality criteria apply to guarantee that patient or consumer benefits outweigh drawbacks or risks. These include requirements for personnel training, analytical validity, recording of data, advertisement, and consumer information [41]. Quality criteria for DTC testing are needed, either by self-regulation or by governmental regulation [38,42,44].

13.10 THE NEED FOR PARTNERSHIPS TO BUILD THE NECESSARY EVIDENCE

Although applications of pharmacogenomics might be progressing rather quickly into the commercial sector, implementation of pharmacogenomics applications in the healthcare sector requires a joint standardized approach. Establishing evidence of the analytical and clinical validity, clinical utility, the cost-effectiveness of pharmacogenomics applications and the subsequent development of evidence-based guidelines, requires the standardized participation of large groups of patients. The use of a pharmacogenomics application in a single hospital or by a DTC company will not give rise to the necessary evidence-based rationale, nor will it do justice to the principle of equity, the equal access to genetic technology and information. Collaborations between public bodies and private companies (public–private partnerships) may facilitate the development and validation of pharmacogenomics applications [38].

Moreover, the implementation of pharmacogenomics in clinical healthcare requires an in-process feedback–learning trajectory in which new knowledge from the laboratory is used to assess, monitor, and fine-tune current clinical applications. The field of pharmacogenomics is rather dynamic. What might be the "best" pharmacogenomics test for a certain condition today, might not be so within 6 months. Therefore, it is important that validation and adaptation go hand in hand, for example, through a periodical revision of the test approval. Currently, pharmacogenetics tests can be divided into two groups; those provided through clinical laboratories (e.g., TMPT test) and those for which a product license has been granted in a way similar to new medicines (e.g., Third Wave Technologies' Invader® *UGT1A1* molecular assay) [45]. Laboratory-developed tests do need to meet external quality assessments standards, but do not need to undergo the licensing process in which the quality, safety, and efficacy of the test is evaluated by a regulatory body. A uniform regulatory system is needed to evaluate and assess the value of a new pharmacogenomics test.

The current regulatory drug approval process is under debate. There are concerns that the current system is inadequate, that it is highly focused on the rapid approval of new drugs, but does not include systematic provisions to obtain important data needed to guide clinical practice [46]. The ultimate benefit of a drug is often incompletely understood at the time of introduction. Several scholars have proposed an alternative regulatory approach, in which drugs are conditionally approved initially. During this period marketing is restricted until larger postmarketing studies have shown convincing evidence of health benefits. Pharmacogenomics technology might be very helpful in opening up new avenues for this conditional approval trajectory. However, it is important not to get carried away with the promise of a new regulatory tool without careful assessments of the consequences for drug governance within the wider context of (inter)national drug markets [46,47].

13.11 PHARMACOGENOMICS IN LOW-RESOURCE SETTINGS

Although some genomics initiatives have begun to emerge in developing countries such as Mexico and Gambia, for the majority of countries in the developing world (pharmaco)genomics seems to be far out of reach [48]. They lack the resources and infrastructure and cannot bear the costs. However, especially for developing countries, pharmacogenomics may hold promise in addressing their limited health resources as efficiently as possible [48]. Although the translation of pharmacogenomics might be more challenging in low-resource settings than in high-technology settings, they may still hold potential. In a report on personalized medicines from 2005, the Royal Society advocates the development and use of simple phenotypic tests in order to screen common genetic defects, so that the medical needs of countries with limited resources can be addressed [49]. For G6PD deficiency, there are simple enzyme-based tests available, but they are not widely applied in practice. Even more simple, rapid stick tests are currently under development. The use of genetic testing might not be cost-effective in developing countries where basic healthcare is limited and appropriate drugs are not always available. Further research is needed to address this matter [50].

13.12 CONCLUSIONS

Pharmacogenomics will lead to improved health and reduced side effects only if translation from bench to bedside is taken seriously. Data production is impressive, but the clinical evidence is often unclear and policymakers may find themselves under pressure to make decisions before they feel that the evidence is compelling. Promise and hope will materialize only if clinical evidence is built, translated into guidelines, incorporated into education, implemented in pharmacy databases, and evaluated. Public–private partnerships are needed to facilitate this process and to safeguard a healthy balance between individual and collective interests, rights, and duties. In addition, positive health effects will depend on a more specific focus on the special medical needs of both disease communities and individual patients. It is important to realize that for any pharmacogenetic test to be introduced, the clinical culture, and thus the ethical and social issues it raises, is quite different. As such, appreciating the ethical problems with developing pharmacogenetic products and the storage of genetic material is only a first step in creating a healthy and productive user environment for pharmacogenetic testing. Community engagement will at least help to incorporate the procedural and cultural norms in the user's environment and hence build public confidence and trust in the public regulation of pharmacogenetics research and development. More recent work in biomedical ethics has begun to consider this issue more seriously by proposing more sophisticated shared and unbundled models of consent that fit into the uncertainty picture of processing and sharing genetic information worldwide on, both (inter)national and community levels. The concept of "good enough" consent is a most valuable product of this approach and requires further elaboration. What is needed is not more forms and an emphasis on better information, but more personalized support for doctors and patients alike in the process of decisionmaking. Consent as a one-off permission holy grail should grow into a more sophisticated safeguard of patient and community interests that is part of an in-process feedback-learning trajectory between bench and bedside.

REFERENCES

1. van der Greef J, Hankemeier T, McBurney RN. Metabolomics-based systems biology and personalized medicine: moving towards n = 1 clinical trials? *Pharmacogenomics* 2006;**7**:1087–1094.
2. Consortium WTCC. Genome-wide association study of 14,000 cases of seven common diseases and 3,000 shared controls. *Nature* 2007;**447**:661–678.
3. Beauchamp TL, Childress JF. *Principles of Biomedical Ethics*, 6th ed. Oxford, UK: Oxford Univ. Press, 2008 (original edition published in 1979).
4. Knoppers BM, Chadwick R. The Human Genome Project: Under an international ethical microscope. *Science* 1994;**265**:2035–2036.
5. Lunshof JE. Personalized medicine: new perspectives—new ethics? *Personal. Med.* 2006;**3**:187–194.
6. Knoppers BM, Chadwick R. Human genetic research: Emerging trends in ethics. *Nat. Rev. Genet.* 2005;**6**:75–79.
7. Holm S, Madsen S. Informed consent in medical research–a procedure stretched beyond breaking point? In Corrigan O, Liddell K, McMillan J, Richards M, Weijer C, eds: *The Limits of Consent: A Socio-ethical Approach to Human Subject Research in Medicine*. Oxford, UK: Oxford Univ. Press, 2009, pp. 11–24.
8. Kohane IS, Altman RB. Health-information altruists—a potentially critical resource. *New Engl. J. Med.* 2005;**353**:2074–2077.
9. Nyholt DR, Yu C-E, Visscher PM. On Jim Watson's APOE status: Genetic information is hard to hide. *Eur. J. Hum. Genet.* 2008;**17**:147–149.
10. Joly Y, Knoppers BM. Pharmacogenomic data sample collection and storage: Ethical issues and policy approaches. *Pharmacogenomics* 2006;**7**:219–226.
11. Sampogna C. *Creation and Governance of Human Genetic Research Databases*. Paris: Organisation for Economic Co-operation and Development, 2006 (e-book available at `http://new.sourceoecd.org/`; accessed 2/09).

12. Lunshof JE, Chadwick R, Vorhaus DB, Church GM. From genetic privacy to open consent. *Nat. Rev. Genet.* 2008;**9**:406–411.
13. Liddell K, Richards M. Consent and beyond: some conclusions. In Corrigan O, Liddell K, McMillan J, Richards M, Weijer C, eds: *The Limits of Consent: A Socio-ethical Approach to Human Subject Research in Medicine*. Oxford, UK: Oxford Univ. Press, 2009, pp. 213–226.
14. Lee SS. Pharmacogenomics and the challenge of health disparities. *Public Health Genomics* 2009;**12**:170–179.
15. `http://www.weesgeneesmiddelen.nl/?id=558` (accessed 3/09).
16. Taylor AL, Cohn JN, Worcel M, Franciosa JA. The African-American heart failure trial: Background, rationale and significance. *J. Natl. Med. Assoc.* 2002;**94**:762–769.
17. Taylor AL. The African American heart failure trial: A clinical trial update. *Am. J. Cardiol.* 2005;**96**:44–48.
18. Wertz DC. Ethical, social and legal issues in pharmacogenomics. *Pharmacogenomics J.* 2003;**3**:194–196.
19. Van Hoyweghen I, Horstman K. European practices of genetic information and insurance: Lessons for the Genetic Information nondiscrimination Act. *JAMA* 2008;**300**:326–327.
20. Sequeiros J, and Guimarães B. Definitions of Genetic Testing, 3rd draft. EuroGentest, 2005 (available at `http://www.eurogentest.org/web/info/public/unit3/DefinitionsGeneticTesting-3rdDraf18Jan07.xhtml`; accessed 2/09).
21. Rothstein MA. Is GINA worth the wait? *J. Law Med. Ethics* 2008;**36**:174–178.
22. Smart A, Martin P. The promise of pharmacogenetics: Assessing the prospects for disease and patient stratification. *Studies in History and Philosophy of Science Part C: Studies in History and Philosophy of Biological and Biomedical Sciences*, 2006;**37**:583–601.
23. Health Council of The Netherlands. Screening: Between Hope and Hype. The Hague: Health Council of The Netherlands, 2008, publication. 2008/05E.
24. van El C, Pieters T, Cornel MC. The changing focus of screening criteria in the age of genomics: A brief history from the Netherlands. In Wieser B, Berger W., eds.: *Assessing Life: On the Organisation of Genetic Testing,* Science and Technology Studies Series Vol. 59, Munich/Vienna: Profil, 2009.
25. Service RF. Gene sequencing. The race for the $1000 genome. *Science* 2006;**311**:1544–1546.
26. Khoury MJ, Gwinn M, Yoon PW, Dowling N, Moore CA, Bradley L. The continuum of translation research in genomic medicine: how can we accelerate the appropriate integration of human genome discoveries into health care and disease prevention? *Genet. Med.* 2007;**9**:665–674.
27. `http://www.genomics.nl/Valorisation.aspx`; (accessed 3/09).
28. Swen JJ, Wilting I, Goede ALD, et al. Pharmacogenetics: From bench to byte. *Clin. Pharmacol. Ther.* 2008;**83**:781–787.
29. Scheuner MT, Sieverding P, Shekelle PG. Delivery of genomic medicine for common chronic adult diseases: A systematic review. *JAMA* 2008;**299**:1320–1334.
30. Anderson JL, Horne BD, Stevens SM, et al. Randomized trial of genotype-guided versus standard warfarin dosing in patients initiating oral anticoagulation. *Circulation* 2007;**116**:2563–2570.

31. Gurwitz D, Rodriguez-Antona C, Payne K, et al. Improving pharmacovigilance in Europe: TPMT genotyping and phenotyping in the UK and Spain. *Eur. J. Hum. Genet.* 2009;**17**:991–998.
32. The Advisory Committee on Health Research. *Genomics and World Health*. Geneva: World Health Organization, 2002.
33. Pompeo F, Brooke E, Kawamura A, Mushtaq A, Sim E. The pharmacogenetics of NAT: Structural aspects. *Pharmacogenomics* 2002;**3**:19–30.
34. Irwin JJ, Kirchner JT. Anemia in children. *Am. Fam. Physician* 2001;**64**:1379–1386.
35. Swen JJ, Huizinga TW, Gelderblom H, et al. Translating pharmacogenomics: Challenges on the road to the clinic. *PLoS Med.* 2007;**4**:e209.
36. Lunshof JE, Pirmohamed M, Gurwitz D. Personalized medicine: Decades away? *Pharmacogenomics* 2006;**7**:237–241.
37. Newman W, Payne K. Removing barriers to a clinical pharmacogenetics service. *Personal. Med.* 2008;**5**:471–480.
38. Secretary's Advisory Committee on Genetics, Health, and Society (SACGH). *Realizing the Potential of Pharmacogenomics: Opportunities and Challenges*. Bethesa, MD: US Department of Health and Human Services, 2008 (available at `http://oba.od.nih.gov/oba/SACGHS/reports/SACGHS_PGx_report.pdf`; accessed 2/09).
39. Hedgecoe A. From resistance to usefulness: Sociology and the clinical use of genetic tests. *BioSocieties* 2008;**3**:183–194.
40. Beinema M, Brouwers JR, Schalekamp T, Wilffert B. Pharmacogenetic differences between warfarin, acenocoumarol and phenprocoumon. *Thromb. Haemost.* 2008;**100**:1052–1057.
41. Hogarth S, Javitt G, Melzer D. The current landscape for direct-to-consumer genetic testing: Legal, ethical, and policy issues. *Annu. Rev. Genomics Human. Genet.* 2008;**9**:161–182.
42. Patch C, Sequeiros J, Cornel MC. Genetic horoscopes: Is it all in the genes? Points for regulatory control of direct-to-consumer genetic testing. *Eur. J. Hum. Genet.* 2009;**17**:857–859.
43. Reitsma P. No praise for folly: Genomics will never be useful in arterial thrombosis. *J. Thromb. Haemost.* 2007;**5**:454–457.
44. Gurwitz D, Bregman-Eschet Y. Personal genomics services: Whose genomes? *Eur. J. Hum. Genet.* 2009;**17**:883–889.
45. Payne K. Towards an economic evidence base for pharmacogenetics: Consideration of outcomes is key. *Pharmacogenomics* 2008;**9**:1–4.
46. Ray WA, Stein CM. Reform of drug regulation—beyond an independent drug-safety board. *New Engl. J. Med.* 2006;**354**:194–201.
47. Strom BL. How the US drug safety system should be changed. *JAMA* 2006;**295**:2072–2075.
48. Hardy B-J, Seguin B, Goodsaid F, Jimenez-Sanchez G, Singer PA, Daar AS. The next steps for genomic medicine: Challenges and opportunities for the developing world. *Nat. Rev. Genet.* 2008;**9**:S23–S27.
49. The Royal Society. Personalised medicines: Hopes and Realities. London: The Royal Society, 2005 (available at `http://royalsociety.org/displaypagedoc.asp?id=15874`; accessed 3/09).
50. Meyer UA. Pharmacogenetics—five decades of therapeutic lessons from genetic diversity. *Nat. Rev. Genet.* 2004;**5**:669–676.

PART IV

DEVELOPMENTS IN PHARMACOGENETIC RESEARCH

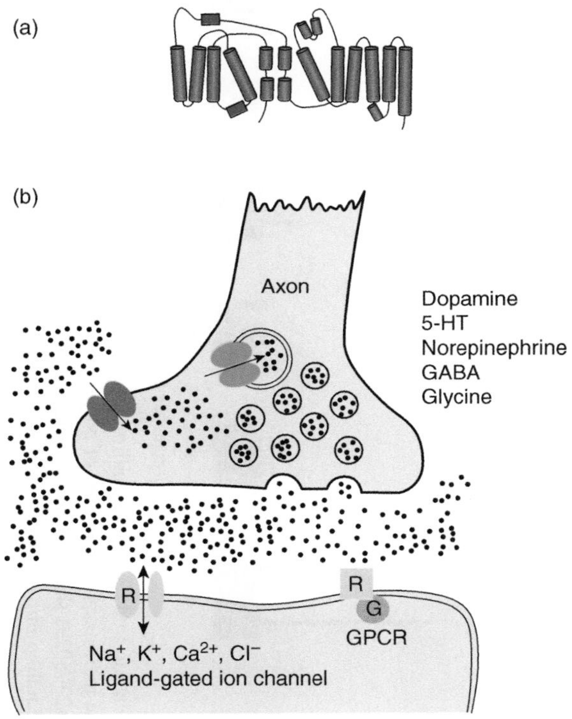

FIGURE 5.5 SLC6 gene family transporter structure: (a) the structure with transmembrane domains shown in red; (b) in the presynaptic nerve terminals of dopamine-, 5HT-, norepinephrine-, glycine-, and GABA-containing synapses, the vesicular transporters [shown in green (e.g., VMAT1 and VMAT2)] sequester neurotransmitters into synaptic vesicles. Released neurotransmitter exerts its effects via receptors such as dopamine receptors, adrenoceptors, and 5HT receptors (light blue, with associated G protein in gray). The plasma membrane transporters encoded by the SLC6 gene family (red) are located in the membrane of the presynaptic neuron (DAT, SERT, NET, GlyT2, GAT1, and GAT2). (Adapted from Gether et al. [177] and reproduced with permission.)

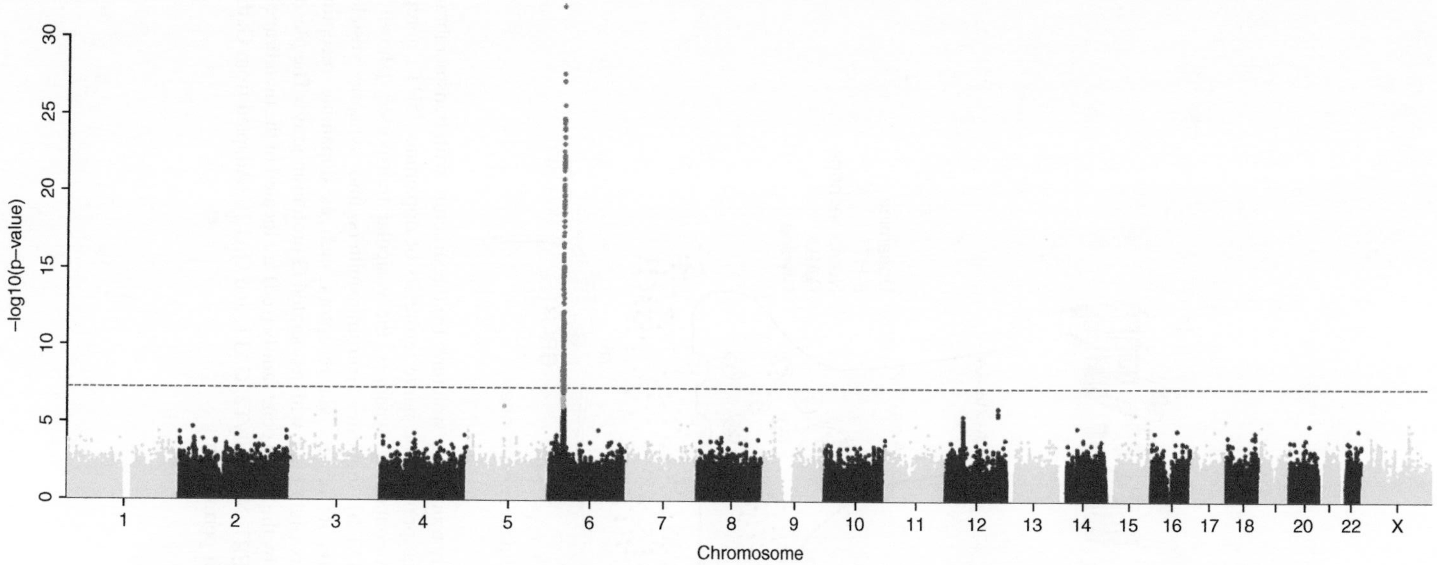

FIGURE 10.1 Genomewide association study on flucloxacillin-induced liver injury. This Manhattan plot of chromosomal location against −log *p* value indicates that a number of polymorphisms in the MHC region show genomewide significance. The polymorphism (rs2395029) showing the most significant difference in frequency between cases and controls is in complete linkage disequilibrium with the HLA class I *HLA-B*5701* allele. (Reproduced with permission from Daly et al. [10]).

CHAPTER 14

High-Throughput Genotyping Technologies for Pharmacogenetics

BEATRIZ SOBRINO and ANGEL CARRACEDO

University of Santiago de Compostela, Spain

14.1 INTRODUCTION

Various genetic tools are used to analyze the genetic component of a trait, each one with its domain of applicability. Thus, classical linkage analysis of families, although powerful for detecting loci involved in single gene disorders, is less effective for complex traits where association studies have demonstrated more power to detect genes with small effects. From the genetic perspective, the individual variation in the response to drugs is a complex trait.

Association studies were until recently hampered by the low density of classical short tandem repeat (STR) markers. The great jump in the field was the discovery of millions of SNP markers in the human genome when DNA from multiple donors was sequenced and compared for the genome sequencing projects. At the moment there are more than 11 million SNPs in the NCBI dbSNP database (http://www.ncbi.nlm.nih.gov/SNP/).

Genotyping technologies have also experienced a rapid evolution, and numerous throughput SNP typing approaches are now available, with various platforms and chemistries allowing researchers to use the most appropriate one for each specific purpose. In some countries national genotyping facilities have been set up. This is the case of Spain where the Spanish National Genotyping Center (GeGen: www.cegen.org) offers Spanish researchers a complete range of technologies for genotyping plus pre-genotyping (SNP selection) and postgenotyping (association study analysis) services. This provides a straightforward and very inexpensive facility for researchers to perform association studies of any size. In addition, experts can help with SNP assay designs and selection of the platform best suited for the characteristics of each project.

Pharmacogenetics and Individualized Therapy, First Edition.
Edited by Anke-Hilse Maitland-van der Zee and Ann K. Daly.

However, progress in technology would not be sufficient without a parallel advance in the HapMap project.

The question is that if we had to perform a whole-genome scan with 10 million SNPs in 1000 samples, a medium size for an association study, this would represent 10 billion genotypes, a difficult task in terms of workload and cost. The discovery [1] that clustering is observed in all the autosomes and that the human genome contains haplotype blocks—that is to say, regions with little evidence of recombination, separated by recombination hot spots—gave another perspective to association studies. The ability to identify the blocks and the tagSNPs defining all variations in the block would reduce the number of SNPs required to examine the entire genome for association with a phenotype from 10 million to 1 million tagSNPs improving the efficiency and thoroughness of genome scan approaches.

For this reason the HapMap project (`www.hapmap.org`) was launched and the third phase recently finished in 2010. Using HapMap software facilities such as Haploview, researchers can use HapMap information to design association studies.

From the pharmacogenetics perspective, copy number variation (CNV) is also of central interest since differences in response can be due to differences in the number of copies, and a continuous progress in the knowledge and analysis of these regions is being made [2].

Designing an association study is not easy, and for traits such as pharmacogenetic studies, there are requirements for a high number of samples (so the establishment of networks is usually a prerequisite), definition of the phenotype, definition of study populations, and decisions on whether to carry out a candidate gene approach or whole-genome scans (WGSs). WGSs have the advantage of being free of bias and they have demonstrated their ability with success in identifying many genes involved in complex diseases [3]. Both the approaches, the genomewide association study (GWAS) and candidate genes, are complementary, as are the technologies, since confirmation of GWAS results require replication in subsets of samples, with an increasing number of samples and with a progressively decreasing SNP set, so high-throughput technologies need to be complemented by technologies appropriate for a reduced SNP number.

The development of new genotyping technologies has improved throughput, performance, and costs over the last few yars. As a consequence of these advances, increasing amounts of information on genomic variability of the human genome have been generated. In this chapter we provide an overview of the most common technologies used for medium- and high-throughput genotyping.

14.2 TaqMan OpenArray GENOTYPING SYSTEM

A new system that enables researchers to perform high-throughput genotyping studies with TaqMan genotyping assays has been commercialized by Applied Biosystems from 2008, expanding the potential uses of TaqMan technology.

The TaqMan assay is based in the 5′-nuclease activity of Taq polymerase that displaces and cleaves the oligonucleotide probes hybridized to the target DNA, generating a fluorescent signal [4,5]. The assay includes two locus-specific PCR primers that flank the SNP of interest, and two allele-specific oligonucleotide TaqMan probes. These probes have a fluorescent reporter dye at the 5′ end, and a nonfluorescent quencher (NFQ) with a minor groove binder (MGB) at the 3′ end [6,7]. When the probes are intact, the quencher interacts with the fluorophore by FRET, quenching their fluorescence. During the PCR annealing step, the TaqMan probes hybridize to the target DNA. In the extension step, the 5′-fluorescent dye is cleaved by the 5′-nuclease activity of the Taq polymerase, leading to an increase in fluorescence of the reporter dye. Mismatch probes are displaced without fragmentation. The genotype of a sample is determined by measuring the signal intensity of the two different dyes.

An important number of SNPs of pharmaceutical and clinical value are known to be triallelic. For this situation, two paired conventional TaqMan SNP assays are used to detect all three alleles of a triallelic SNP [8].

There is a library of human and mouse assays that includes over 4.5 million predesigned SNP assays and over 2600 drug metabolism assays to genotype polymorphisms located in regulatory elements and coding regions for 220 drug metabolism and transporter genes. Additionally, it is also possible to design one's own custom SNP genotyping assays.

A new platform, the TaqMan OpenArray™ genotyping system, combines TaqMan genotyping assays and OpenArray technology, which uses nanoliter fluidics for massively parallel and low-volume solution-phase reaction analyses for higher sample throughput and lower cost per data point. The main components of the TaqMan OpenArray genotyping system are the TaqMan OpenArray genotyping plates (preloaded with predesigned or custom TaqMan SNP genotyping or drug metabolism assays) and the TaqMan OpenArray genotyping instrument platform [9]. Each TaqMan OpenArray genotyping plate contains 3072 through-holes arranged in 48 subarrays of 64 through-holes each. The OpenArray autoloader can precisely load one, two, or three samples onto each subarray. This result in a choice of six plate format options: from 16 assays in 192 samples per plate for up to 256 assays in 12 samples.

14.3 SEQUENOM

MassArray (Sequenom) technology is based on the detection of the products of an allelic discrimination reaction using matrix-assisted laser desorption-ionization/time-of-flight mass spectrometry (MALDI/TOF-MS). There are two genotyping strategies: hME and iPLEX Gold [10–12]. In both cases, the genotyping process involves two reactions. In the first reaction, which is carried out in the same way for both strategies, the fragments of DNA that contain the SNPs of interest are amplified by multiplex PCR. The second reaction, which is carried out differently for both strategies, is an allelic discrimination reaction.

With the ***hME*** strategy, the allelic discrimination is performed by a minisequencing reaction that generates allele-specific products generally around 1–4 bases longer than the original primer. The largest number of SNPs genotyped per assay using this strategy is 15, although the average number is around 8, as it greatly depends on the number of candidate SNPs available for the design of the project, and on the presence of sequence motifs, oligonucleotide interactions, and so on.

In the iPLEX Gold strategy, all the reactions finish after a single-base extension (SBE). In order to resolve the problem of the small mass difference between the SBE products, iPLEX Gold incorporates terminators of modified mass. The efficiency of the plex designs is increased with the use of a unique termination mixture. This modification enables the genotyping of up to 36 SNPs per assay, with an average genotyping of 24 SNPs.

The use of minisequencing probes of different lengths enables identification of the product peaks for each SNP. The reactions are carried out on 384-well plates, and the products are transferred in an automated fashion by a robot to the surface of the chip, to be read by the spectrophotometer. Up to 10 chips can be processed by the spectrometer at the same time.

14.4 COMMERCIAL HIGH-DENSITY ARRAYS

There are two main companies offering high-throughput genomewide genotyping technologies: Affymetrix and Illumina. Independently of the technology used for each company, an important point to consider is the marker selection strategy. Illumina SNP chips include tag SNPs derived from over 2 million common SNPs (Minimum Allele Frequency, MAF... ≥ 0.05) in the HapMap data. The Affymetrix SNP array 10, 100, 500K (500,000), and 5.0 include SNPs selected on the basis of sequence constraints when choosing the probes and this represents a set of quasirandom SNPs that ignores LD patterns. The additional SNPs in the SNP array 6.0 are mostly tag SNPs [13].

Both technologies offer prefixed design arrays but also custom arrays, where researchers can design the content of the array for specific applications. (Table 14.1)

14.4.1 Affymetrix Technology

Affymetrix GeneChip arrays are synthesized *in situ* by photolithography, allowing the location of millions of probes on a typical 1.28-cm^2 array. The highest-density array has 6.5 million probe locations spaced 5 μm apart [14–16]. Affymetrix has two classes of arrays for genotyping applications with different array design and allelic discrimination reactions: mapping arrays for whole-genome analysis and targeted genotyping arrays for specific application and custom arrays.

Affymetrix mapping arrays do not require site-specific primers, are highly scalable, and enable the creation of hybridization target starting with as little as 250 ng of gDNA. The assay involves five primary steps, starting with restriction digestion, ligation of adapter, amplification, fragmentation, and labeling, prior to hybridization to the oligonucleotide array. The complexity reduction occurs at the polymerase chain reaction (PCR) step, which preferentially amplifies restriction fragments that are between 250 and 1000 bp. The PCR is performed using a generic primer that recognizes the adapter and amplifies adapter-ligated DNA fragments. The

TABLE 14.1 Commercial Human Arrays Available from Affymetrix and Illumina

Array Name	Description	Technology
Affymetrix		
Genome-Wide Human SNP array 6.0	GWAS/CNV ~ 1M SNPs and ~ 1M nonpolymorphic probes	Mapping arrays
Genome-Wide Human SNP array 5.0.	GWAS/CNV 500K SNPs and ~ 420,000 non-polymorphic probes	Mapping arrays
GeneChip Human Mapping 500K array set	GWAS/CNV500K SNPs	Mapping arrays
Genechip Human Mapping 250K array.	GWAS/CNV 250K SNPs	Mapping arrays
GeneChip Human Mapping 100K array set	GWAS/CNV100K SNPs	Mapping arrays
Genechip Human Mapping 50K array	GWAS/CNV 50K SNPs	Mapping arrays
GeneChip Human Mapping 10K 2.0 array	GWAS/CNV 10K SNPs	Mapping arrays
GeneChip Human MALD 3K SNP kit	3000 MALD SNPs	Targeted genotyping
GeneChip Human Immune and Inflammation 9K SNP kit	9000 SNPs in 1000 genes implicated in immune and inflammatory process	Targeted genotyping
GeneChip Human 20K cSNP kit	20.000 cSNPs in > 10,000 genes	Targeted genotyping
Affymetrix custom oligos Custom Panel 3–20K SNPs	Custom panels 3–20K	Targeted genotyping
DMET Plus kit	1936 markers in 225 genes	Targeted genotyping
Illumina		
Human1M-Duo	GWAS/CNV analysis, > 1.1 m markers	Infinium
Human660W-Quad	GWAS/CNV analysis, >658,000	Infinium
HumanCytoSNP-12	GWAS/CNV analysis, ~300,000	Infinium
Human510S-Duo	GWAS/CNV analysis, > 510,000	Infinium
Semi-Custom Human1M-Duo +, and HumanHap550-Quad +	GWAS/CNV analysis, standard content and ≤60,800 customized SNPs per sample	Infinium
HumanLinkage-12	Linkage analysis, 6090 SNPs	Infinium
HumanCVD	Focused analysis, 49,000 SNPs in candidate genes for cardiovascular disease	Infinium
Infinium iSelect genotyping panels	Custom panels 6–60 K SNPs	Infinium
Golden Gate genotyping panels	Custom panels, 96–1536 SNPs	Golden Gate
HumanLinkage V	Linkage analysis 6056 SNPs	Golden Gate
African-American Admixture	1509 SNPs for admixture studies	Golden Gate
Cancer SNP	1421 SNPs in candidate genes in cancer	Golden Gate
MHC	SNPs for MHC mapping	Golden Gate
DNA test	360 validated SNPs	Golden Gate
VeraCode custom panel	Custom panels, 96–384 SNPs	VeraCode Golden Gate

choice of restriction enzyme determines the sequence content of the reduced fraction of the genome [17–19].

Earlier genotyping arrays (Affymetrix 10K, 100K, 500K) interrogated each SNP with 24–40 different 25-mer probes, designed to query both strands at multiple offsets with respect to each SNP. Affymetrix SNP 5.0 and 6.0 were designed using the best A/B probe pair, each in four copies. The reduction in the number of probes per SNP allows the researcher increase to the number of SNPs analyzed in one array. Affymetrix 6.0 arrays include almost 1 million SNPs and 940,000 copy number probes to directly interrogated copy number variation, unrestricted by the locations and sequence properties of SNPs [20].

Affymetrix targeted genotyping arrays are based on molecular inversion probe technology [21]. Molecular-inversion probe (MIP) genotyping uses circularizable probes with 5′ and 3′ ends that anneal upstream and downstream of the SNP site, leaving a 1 bp gap. Polymerase extension with dNTPs and a non-strand-displacing polymerase is used to fill in the gap. Ligation seals the nick, and exonuclease I (which has 3′ exonuclease activity) is used to remove excess unannealed and unligated circular probes. Finally, the circularized probe is released through restriction digestion at a consensus sequence, and the resultant product is PCR-amplified using common primers to built-in sites on the circular probe. The orientation of the primers ensures that only circularized probes will be amplified. Each amplified probe contains a unique tag sequence that is complementary to a sequence on the universal tag array. Amplicons are fluorescently labeled and the tag sequences are released from the genome homology regions using a restriction endonuclease treatment. The tags are then detected using a complementary tag array. A four-color scanner is used for detecting tag arrays. Targeted genotyping arrays are available for specific applications or for custom design (Table 14.1).

At the end of 2008, Affymetrix launched a new array for genotyping drug-metabolizing enzymes and transporters (DMET) markers: the ***DMET Plus array***. This chip provides coverage of 1936 drug metabolism markers in 225 genes, including common and rare SNPs, short insertion or deletion alleles, triallelic SNPs, and copy number variations (Table 14.2). In addition to known biomarkers such as common variants in CYP2D6, CYP2C19, and other cytochrome P450 genes, DMET Plus contains over 1000 variants in drug transporters and also performs quantitative assessment of genes with whole-gene deletions (including GSTT1, GSTM1, CYP2D6, CYP2A6, and UGT2B17) and reports allele names in both genotyping reports and translation reports. Markers on the DMET Plus chip are interrogated using MIP technology [22–26].

The design of the DMET Plus array differs somewhat from the designs of other targeted genotyping arrays because the DMET Plus array requires genotyping of triallelic as well as biallelic SNPs, insertions/deletions (indels), and copy number variation of some regions. In addition, some markers are first preamplified using multiplex PCR prior to joining the other markers in the DMET Plus assay flow, due to the presence of pseudogenes or other closely related genomic sequences. A previous version of this array known as *targeted human DMET 1.0 assay*, based on the same MIP technology, but with 1228 markers in 170 DMETs [27,28].

TABLE 14.2 Genes and Marker Types Included in DMET Plus Array (Affymetrix)

Gene Symbol	SNPs	in-del	CNV	Gene Symbol	SNPs	in-del	CNV	Gene Symbol	SNPs	in-del	CNV
ABCB1	40	—	—	CYP2C9	16	2	—	RXRA	4	—	—
ABCB11	31	2	—	CYP2D6	19	11	1	SEC15L1	1	—	—
ABCB4	25	—	—	CYP2E1	10	—	—	SERPINA7	7	—	—
ABCB7	6	—	—	CYP2F1	3	—	—	SETD4	2	—	—
ABCC1	17	1	—	CYP2J2	9	—	—	SLC10A1	7	—	—
ABCC2	44	1	—	CYP2S1	4	—	—	SLC10A2	8	—	—
ABCC3	6	—	—	CYP39A1	7	—	—	SLC13A1	7	—	—
ABCC4	15	1	—	CYP3A4	22	3	—	SLC15A1	18	1	—
ABCC5	8	1	—	CYP3A43	7	—	—	SLC15A2	10	—	—
ABCC6	7	—	—	CYP3A5	13	1	—	SLC16A1	7	—	—
ABCC8	5	2	—	CYP3A7	7	—	—	SLC19A1	5	—	—
ABCC9	6	—	—	CYP46A1	1	—	—	SLC22A1	24	1	—
ABCG1	7	—	—	CYP4A11	4	—	—	SLC22A11	6	—	—
ABCG2	8	—	—	CYP4B1	6	1	—	SLC22A12	2	—	—
ABP1	7	—	—	CYP4F11	4	—	—	SLC22A13	7	—	—
ADH1A	7	—	—	CYP4F12	6	—	—	SLC22A14	6	—	—
ADH1B	5	1	—	CYP4F2	11	—	—	SLC22A2	15	1	—
ADH1C	5	—	—	CYP4F3	7	—	—	SLC22A3	5	—	—
ADH4	6	—	—	CYP4F8	7	—	—	SLC22A4	6	1	—
ADH5	5	—	—	CYP4Z1	4	—	—	SLC22A5	8	—	—
ADH6	6	—	—	CYP51A1	6	—	—	SLC22A6	6	1	—
ADH7	5	—	—	CYP7A1	7	—	—	SLC22A7	7	—	—
AHR	6	—	—	CYP7B1	4	—	—	SLC22A8	11	—	—
AKAP9	4	—	—	CYP8B1	7	—	—	SLC28A1	27	—	—
ALB	7	—	—	DCK	4	—	—	SLC28A2	7	—	—
ALDH1A1	4	3	—	DPYD	16	2	—	SLC28A3	7	—	—
ALDH2	6	—	—	EPHX1	12	—	—	SLC29A1	9	—	—
ALDH3A1	4	1	—	EPHX2	4	1	—	SLC29A2	5	1	—
ALDH3A2	7	—	—	FAAH	2	—	—	SLC5A6	7	—	—
AOX1	7	—	—	FMO1	7	—	—	SLC6A6	7	—	—
ARNT	7	—	—	FMO2	17	4	—	SLC7A5	3	—	—
ARSA	5	—	—	FMO3	26	1	—	SLC7A7	7	—	—
ATP7A	7	—	—	FMO4	6	—	—	SLC7A8	7	—	—
ATP7B	10	—	—	FMO5	5	2	—	SLCO1A2	15	1	—
CBR1	4	—	—	FMO6	4	—	—	SLCO1B1	18	—	—
CBR3	6	—	—	G6PD	6	—	—	SLCO1B3	5	2	—
CDA	6	—	—	GSTA1	12	—	—	SLCO2B1	5	—	—
CES2	7	—	—	GSTA2	7	—	—	SLCO3A1	6	—	—
CGT_HUMAN// UGT8	1	—	—	GSTA3	6	1	—	SLCO4A1	5	—	—
CHST1	6	—	—	GSTA4	7	—	—	SLCO5A1	5	—	—
CHST10	14	—	—	GSTA5	7	—	—	SPG7	6	—	—
CHST11	7	—	—	GSTM1	3	—	1	SULT1A1	3	—	—
CHST13	6	—	—	GSTM2	5	—	—	SULT1A2	4	—	—

(Continued)

TABLE 14.2 ***(Continued)***

Gene Symbol	SNPs	in-del	CNV	Gene Symbol	SNPs	in-del	CNV	Gene Symbol	SNPs	in-del	CNV
CHST2	5	—	—	GSTM3	6	1	—	SULT1A2_A3	7	—	—
CHST3	13	1	—	GSTM4	4	—	—	SULT1A3	6	—	—
CHST4	3	—	—	GSTM5	5	—	—	SULT1B1	6	—	—
CHST5	7	—	—	GSTO1	5	—	—	SULT1C1	9	—	—
CHST6	3	—	—	GSTP1	5	—	—	SULT1C2	7	—	—
CHST7	7	—	—	GSTT1	6	—	1	SULT1E1	5	—	—
CHST8	3	—	—	GSTT2	4	—	—	SULT2A1	6	—	—
CHST9	5	—	—	GSTZ1	4	—	—	SULT2B1	7	—	—
COMT	5	—	—	HMGCR	6	—	—	SULT4A1	5	—	—
CROT	6	—	—	HNMT	5	1	—	TBXAS1	25	—	—
CYP11A1	7	—	—	MAOA	7	—	—	TPMT	8	—	—
CYP11B1	19	—	—	MAOB	6	—	—	TPSG1	1	1	—
CYP11B2	5	—	—	MAT1A	7	—	—	TYMS	5	—	—
CYP17A1	6	—	—	METTL1	4	—	—	UGT1A1	31	—	—
CYP19A1	11	—	—	NAT1	20	1	—	UGT1A10	3	—	—
CYP1A1	12	1	—	NAT2	16	—	—	UGT1A3	4	—	—
CYP1A2	16	1	—	NNMT	6	1	—	UGT1A4	2	2	—
CYP1B1	15	5	—	NQO1	7	—	—	UGT1A5	3	—	—
CYP20A1	5	—	—	NR1I2	15	—	—	UGT1A6	4	—	—
CYP21A2	3	—	—	NR1I3	7	—	—	UGT1A7	2	—	—
CYP24A1	7	1	—	NR3C1	12	—	—	UGT1A8	8	—	—
CYP26A1	5	—	—	ORM1	4	—	—	UGT1A9	11	1	—
CYP27A1	5	1	—	ORM2	2	—	—	UGT2A1	7	—	—
CYP27B1	7	—	—	PNMT	4	—	—	UGT2B11	5	—	—
CYP2A13	4	—	—	PON1	4	1	—	UGT2B15	7	—	—
CYP2A6	17	2	1	PON2	4	—	—	UGT2B17	4	—	1
CYP2A7	11	—	—	PON3	7	—	—	UGT2B28	3	—	—
CYP2B6	23	—	—	POR	3	—	—	UGT2B4	7	—	—
CYP2B7	2	—	—	PPARD	47	—	—	UGT2B7	7	—	—
CYP2B7P1	1	—	—	PPARG	6	—	—	UGT8	4	—	—
CYP2C18	5	1	—	PTGIS	12	—	—	VKORC1	23	—	—
CYP2C19	16	2	—	RALBP1	6	—	—	XDH	8	—	—
CYP2C8	9	2	—	RPL13	4	—	—	—	—	—	—

The first microarray-based pharmacogenomic test cleared by the FDA for clinical use was the ***AmpliChip CYP450 array*** (Roche). It includes gene variations for the CYP2D6 and CYP2C19 genes, which play a major role in the metabolism of an estimated 25% of all prescription drugs. The AmpliChip CYP450 array uses Affymetrix technology for the detection of the genotypes. The protocol include five major steps: PCR amplification of purified DNA, fragmentation and labelling of the amplified products, hybridization of the amplified products to the microarray and staining of the bound products, scanning of the microarray, and determination of the CYP450 genotype and predicted phenotype [29].

14.4.2 Illumina

Illumina's *BeadArray* technology is based on 3-μm silica beads that self-assemble in microwells on either of two substrates: fiberoptic bundles or planar silica slides. When randomly assembled on one of these two substrates, the beads have a uniform spacing of ~5.7 μm. Each bead is covered with hundreds of thousands of copies of a specific oligonucleotide that act as the capture sequences in one of Illumina's assays [30].

The ***Illumina Golden Gate genotyping assay*** uses a discriminatory DNA polymerase and ligase to interrogate 96, or from 384 to 1536, SNP loci simultaneously [31]. In this approach, during the liquid phase, allele-specific oligonucleotides (ASO) are hybridized to genomic DNA, extended, and ligated to a locus-specific oligonucleotide (LSO). All three oligonucleotide sequences contain regions of genomic complementarity and universal PCR primer sites, and the LSO also contains a unique address sequence complementary to a particular bead-type. The address sequence hybridizes to the universal bead-type probes in the last hybridization step. PCR is performed using universal primers. The multiplexed products ($\leq$ 1536) are hybridized to a universal Sentrix array for detection and analysis. Golden Gate products include predesigned panels for specific application as well as custom genotyping panels (Table 14.1).

The ***Illumina Infinium assay*** is based on direct hybridization of whole-genome-amplified (WGA) genomic DNA to a bead array of 50-mer locus-specific primers [32–37]. After locus-specific hybridization capture of each individual target to their bead, each SNP locus is "scored" by an enzyme-based extension assay using labeled nucleotides. After extension, these labels are visualized by staining with an immunohistochemistry assay that increases the overall sensitivity of the assay.

We employ two different primer extension assays: allele-specific primer extension (ASPE) for Infinium I assay and single-base extension (SBE) for Infinium II assay. The ASPE assay, a one-color format, is specifically designed to allow the detection of all SNP classes by employing two identical probes per SNP differing only at their 3′ base. One probe is the perfect match hybrid for allele A, and the other is the perfect match hybrid for allele B, creating allelic discrimination in the polymerase extension step. Probe sequences on a particular bead type will be extended and labeled only when hybridized to a perfectly matched allelic target. The genotype state of a given SNP locus (AA, AB, or BB) is determined by the intensity ratio between the two corresponding bead types.

The SBE assay format uses a single probe per SNP with two-color readout. This characteristic reduces the required number of oligonucleotides by half as compared to the ASPE assay, allowing WGG probe sets to be made more economically. The limitation of the two-color SBE assay design is that only 83% of common biallelic SNPs can be scored on a single slide. The A and T nucleotides are stained in one color and C and G in another, therefore, AT and GC polymorphisms cannot be detected. However, the remaining 17% of SNPs can be simultaneously genotyped on the same slide using a two-probe ASPE design with SBE biochemical scoring [38].

One of the most important advantages of this approach is the ability for virtually unlimited scalability, dependent only on the physical constraint of the number of array elements, but not by loci multiplexing constraints. Infinium products include whole-genome solutions (from 240K to 1M SNPs) and custom genotyping panels (from 6K to 60K SNPs) (Table 14.1). Illumina also has a platform for low–mid-throughput assays based on ***Veracode technology***, which, combined with Golden Gate genotyping assay, achieve the simultaneous genotyping of 96–384 SNPs in a standard 96-well plate [39].

14.5 CONCLUSION

The prospects for success have improved markedly with the development of an array of genomic and proteomics technologies and resources. Genetic association studies have proved to be an excellent tool for assessing the correlation between genetic variants and differences in traits on a population scale, and especially for pharmacogenetics. Genotyping technologies have also experienced an enormous evolution, and various high-throughput SNP typing technologies are available, with different platforms and chemistries, allowing the researchers to use the most appropriate one for each specific purpose.

REFERENCES

1. Gabriel SB, Schaffner SF, Nguyen H, Moore JM, Roy J, Blumenstiel B, Higgins J, DeFelice M, Lochner A, Faggart M, Liu-Cordero SN, Rotimi C, Adeyemo A, Cooper R, Ward R, et al. The structure of haplotype blocks in the human genome. *Science* 2002;**296**:2225–2259.
2. Kidd JM, Cooper GM, Donahue WF, Hayden HS, Sampas N, Graves T, Hansen N, Teague B, Alkan C, Antonacci F, Haugen E, Zerr T, Yamada NA, Tsang P, et al. Mapping and sequencing of structural variation from eight human genomes. *Nature* 2008;**453**:56–64.
3. Manolio TA, Brooks LD, Collins FS. A HapMap harvest of insights into the genetics of common disease. *J. Clin. Invest.* 2008;**118**:1590–1605.
4. Holland PM, Abramson RD, Watson R, Gelfand DH. Detection of specific polymerase chain reaction product by utilizing the 5′-3′ exonuclease activity of Thermus aquaticus DNA polymerase. *Proc. Natl. Acad. Sci. USA* 1991;**88**:7276–7280.
5. Livak KJ, Flood SJ, Marmaro J, Giusti W, Deetz K. Oligonucleotides with fluorescent dyes at opposite ends provide a quenched probe system useful for detecting PCR product and nucleic acid hybridization. *PCR Methods Appl.* 1995;**4**:357–362.
6. Livak KJ. Allelic discrimination using fluorogenic probes and the 5′ nuclease assay. *Genet. Analy. Biomol. Eng.* 1999;**14**:143–149.
7. Afonina M, Zivarts I, Kutyavin E, Lukhtanov H, Gamper Meyer RB. Efficient priming of PCR with short oligonucleotides conjugated to a minor groove binder. *Nucleic Acids Res.* 1997;**25**:2657–2660.
8. Aplication Note: TaqMan Drug Metabolism Assays for triallelic SNPs (`https://www.appliedbiosystems.com`).

9. https://info.appliedbiosystems.com/taqmanopenarray.
10. van den Boom D, Beaulieu M, Oeth P, Roth R, Honisch C, Nelson MR, Jurinke C, Cantor C. MALDI-TOF MS: A platform technology for genetic discovery. *Int. J. Mass Spectrom.* 2004;**238**(2):173–188.
11. Sequenom Brochure. MassARRAY iPLEX Gold–SNP genotyping (http://www.sequenom.com).
12. Gabriel S, Ziaugra L, Tabbaa D. SNP genotyping using the Sequenom MassARRAY iPLEX platform. *Curr. Protoc. Hum. Genet.* 2009;**2**:Unit 2. 12.
13. Barrett JC, Cardon LR. Evaluating coverage of genome-wide association studies. *Nat. Genet.* 2006;**38**(6):659–662.
14. Fodor SP, Read JL, Pirrung MC, Stryer L, Lu AT, Solas D. Light-directed, spatially addressable parallel chemical synthesis. *Science.* 1991;**251**:767–773.
15. Pease AC, Solas D, Sullivan EJ, Cronin MT, Holmes CP, Fodor SP. Light-generated oligonucleotide arrays for rapid DNA sequence analysis. *Proc. Natl. Acad. Sci. USA* 1994;**91**(11):5022–5026.
16. Barone AD, Beecher JE, Bury PA, Chen C, Doede T, Fidanza JA, McGall GH. Photolithographic synthesis of high-density oligonucleotide probe arrays. *Nucleos. Nucleot. Nucleic Acids* 2001;**20**(4–7):525–531.
17. Kennedy GC, Matsuzaki H, Dong S, Liu WM, Huang J, Liu G, Su X, Cao M, Chen W, Zhang J, Liu W, Yang G, Di X, Ryder T, He Z, Surti U, Phillips M S, Boyce-Jacino MT, Fodor SP, Jones KW. Large-scale genotyping of complex DNA. *Nat. Biotechnol.* 2003;**21**:1233–1237.
18. Matsuzaki H, Loi H, Dong S, Tsai YY, Fang J, Law J, Di X, Liu WM, Yang G, Liu G, Huang J, Kennedy GC, Ryder TB, Marcus GA, Walsh PS, Shriver MD, Puck JM, Jones KW, Mei R. Parallel genotyping of over 10,000 SNPs using a one-primer assay on a high-density oligonucleotide array. *Genome Res.* 2004;**14**:414–425.
19. Matsuzaki H, Dong S, Loi H, Di X, Liu G, Hubbell E, Law J, Berntsen T, Chadha M, Hui H, Yang G, Kennedy GC, Webster TA, Cawley S, Walsh PS, Jones KW, Fodor SP, Mei R. Genotyping over 100,000 SNPs on a pair of oligonucleotide arrays. *Nat. Methods* 2004;**1**(2):109–111.
20. McCarroll SA, Kuruvilla FG, Korn JM, Cawley S, Nemesh J, Wysoker A, Shapero MH, de Bakker PI, Maller JB, Kirby A, et al. Integrated detection and population-genetic analysis of SNPs and copy number variation. *Nat. Genet.* 2008;**40**(10):1166–1174.
21. Hardenbol P, Baner J, Jain M, Nilsson M, Namsaraev EA, Karlin-Neumann GA, Fakhrai-Rad H, Ronaghi M, Willis TD, Landegren U, et al. Multiplexed genotyping with sequence-tagged molecular inversion probes. *Nat. Biotechnol.* 2003;**21**:673–678.
22. Karlin-Neumann G, et al. Molecular inversion probes and universal tag arrays: Application to highplex targeted SNP genotyping. In Weiner MP, Gabriel SB, Stephens JC, eds.: *Genetic Variation: A Laboratory Manual.* Cold Spring Harbor Laboratory Press, 2007.
23. Wang Y, Moorhead M, Karlin-Neumann G, Wang NJ, Ireland J, Lin S, Chen C, Heiser LM, Chin K, Esserman L, Gray JW, Spellman PT, Faham M. Analysis of molecular inversion probe performance for allele copy number determination. *Genome Biol.* 2007;**8**:R246.
24. Wang Y, Moorhead M, Karlin-Neumann G, Falkowski M, Chen C, Siddiqui F, Davis RW, Willis TD, Faham M. Allele quantification using molecular inversion probes (MIP). *Nucleic Acids Res.* 2005;**33**:e183.

25. Moorhead M, Hardenbol P, Siddiqui F, Falkowski M, Bruckner C, Ireland J, Jones HB, Jain M, Willis TD, Faham M. Optimal genotype determination in highly multiplexed SNP data. *Eur. J. Hum. Genet.* 2006;**14**:207–215.
26. Affymetrix Inc. White Paper: Single-sample analysis methodology for the DMET™ Plus Product (`http://www.affymetrix.com/support/technical/whitepapers/dmet_plus_algorithm_whitepaperv1.pdf`).
27. Dumaual C, Miao X, Daly TM, Bruckner C, Njau R, Fu DJ, Close-Kirkwood S, Bauer N, Watanabe N, Hardenbol P, Hockett RD. Comprehensive assessment of metabolic enzyme and transporter genes using the affymetrix targeted genotyping system. *Pharmacogenomics* 2007;**8**(3):293–305.
28. Caldwell MD, Awad T, Johnson JA, Gage BF, Falkowski M, Gardina P, Hubbard J, Turpaz Y, Langaee TY, Eby C, et al. *CYP4F2* genetic variant alters required warfarin dose. *Blood* 2008;**111**:4106–4112.
29. AmpliChip CYP450 test. (`http://www.roche.com`).
30. Oliphant A, Barker DL, Stuelpnagel JR, Chee MS. BeadArray technology: Enabling an accurate, cost-effective approach to high-throughput genotyping. *Biotechniques* 2002;**56**(8):60–61.
31. Fan JB, Oliphant A, Shen R, Kermani BG, Garcia F, Gunderson KL, Hansen M, Steemers F, Butler SL, Deloukas P, et al. Highly parallel SNP genotyping. *Cold Spring Harb. Symp. Quant. Biol.* 2003;**68**:69–78.
32. Gunderson KL, Steemers FJ, Lee G, Mendoza LG, Chee MS. A genome-wide scalable SNP genotyping assay using microarray technology. *Nat. Genet.* 2005;**37**:549–554.
33. Steemers FJ, Chang W, Lee G, Barker DL, Shen R, Gunderson KL. Whole-genome genotyping with the single-base extension assay. *Nat. Methods* 2006;**3**:31–33.
34. Steemers FJ, Gunderson KL. Illumina, Inc. *Pharmacogenomics* 2005;**6**:777–782.
35. Gunderson KL, Kuhn KM, Steemers FJ, Ng P, Murray SS, Shen R. Whole-genome genotyping of haplotype tag single nucleotide polymorphisms. *Pharmacogenomics* 2006;**7**:641–648.
36. Gunderson KL, Steemers FJ, Ren H, Ng P, Zhou L, Tsan C, Chang W, Bullis D, Musmacker J, King C, Lebruska LL, Barker D, Oliphant A, Kuhn KM, Shen R. Whole-genome genotyping. *Methods Enzymol.* 2006;**410**:359–376.
37. Steemers FJ and Gunderson KL. Whole genome genotyping technologies on the BeadArray™ platform. *Biotechnol. J.* 2007;**2**:41–49.
38. Steemers FJ, Chang W, Lee G, Barker DL, Shen R, Gunderson KL. Whole-genome genotyping with the single-base extension assay. *Nat. Methods* 2006;**3**:31–33.
39. Lin CH, Yeakley JM, McDaniel TK, Shen R. Medium- to high-throughput SNP genotyping using VeraCode microbeads. *Methods Mol. Biol.* 2009;**496**:129–142.

CHAPTER 15

Developments in Analyses in Pharmacogenetic Datasets

ALISON A. MOTSINGER-REIF

North Carolina State University, Raleigh, North Carolina, USA

15.1 INTRODUCTION

As a crucial first step in pharmacogenetics and genomics, the identification and characterization of genetic variants that predict drug response phenotypes is an important challenge [1–3]. Such discoveries will allow the development of rational means to optimize drug therapy, with respect to the patient's genotype, to ensure maximum efficacy with minimal adverse effects [1]. The terms *pharmacogenetics* and *pharmacogenomics* are often used interchangeably, and clear distinctions are rarely possible, but these terms actually imply different scopes of genetic mapping, and in return require different statistical and computational analysis plans. *Pharmacogenetics* is generally regarded as the study or clinical testing of genetic variation that gives rise to differing response to drugs, while *pharmacogenomics* generally refers to the broader application of genomic technologies. Pharmacogenetics considers one or at most a few genes of interest, while pharmacogenomics generally considers the entire genome or its products (including proteomic and metabolomic data). In the case of pharmacogenetics, analysis is typically performed within a hypothesis testing framework, utilizing traditional statistical methodology to directly test for correlations between specific variants and drug response. In the case of pharmacogenomics, analysis often proceeds in a hypothesis generation framework, where high-throughput data are used to explore the whole genome for new regions of interest to pursue in future studies. In the current chapter, we will use the acronym PGX interchangeably to represent either term.

Statistical genetic risk mapping methods all rest on one biological phenomenon, recombination (crossover), which is exploited for the purposes of determining the

Pharmacogenetics and Individualized Therapy, First Edition.
Edited by Anke-Hilse Maitland-van der Zee and Ann K. Daly.

genetic distance—or at least the closeness—between two loci [4]. Crossovers between homologous chromosome strands occur semirandomly. Loci in close proximity to each other will rarely be separated by a recombination, whereas, for distant loci, recombinations occur as often as not. This phenomenon is used to derive a statistical measure of genetic distance. In family pedigrees, recombination may be seen more or less directly; on the other hand, the consequences of recombinations in previous generations can be observed in the form of linkage disequilibrium—that is, the preferential occurrence, in one gamete, of specific alleles at different loci [4].

The identification of such variants that predict complex phenotypes such as drug response is a major challenge, and has been generally less successful than for simple Mendelian disorders [5]. It is likely that this is due to many complicating factors such as an increased number of contributing loci and susceptibility alleles, incomplete penetrance, and contributing environmental and clinical effects [5–10]. Additionally, interactions are inherent components of pharmacogenomic outcomes [2]. Inherently, pharmacogenomic phenotypes represent gene–environment interactions, as the variation in phenotype can be viewed as the "plastic reaction" norm to the environmental exposure to the drug [2]. Additionally, underlying even these gene–environment interactions, gene–gene interaction, or epistasis, is hypothesized to play an important role in the underlying etiology of such complex phenotypes [8,11–13].

In this chapter, we discuss the tools available to pharmacogeneticists to detect predictors of drug response. First, we discuss the challenges and advances in quantifying drug response, in a range of study designs. Next, we discuss the traditional statistical tools available in genetic epidemiology for detecting interactions and how they can be applied to drug response outcomes. We then discuss novel computational approaches that have been developed for genetic mapping in complex phenotypes.

15.2 DEFINING DRUG RESPONSE PHENOTYPE

Whether pursuing a pharmacogenetics or pharmacogenomics approach, the process of *gene mapping*, through linkage or association analysis, is really *phenotype mapping* [14]. Regardless of the study design and analytical approach used, the importance of careful phenotype definition and delineation cannot be overemphasized [14]. While this is an important step in any gene mapping, there are particular challenges in defining a biologically relevant/meaningful phenotype in PGX.

Above, we defined PGX as an approach to detect genetic/genomic predictors for an individual's response to a drug. There are many aspects of response that may be outcomes of interest in phenotype mapping. Typically, PGX studies focus on aspects of efficacy or toxicity of a drug [15,16], but with the great diversity of experimental studies available to assess these aspects, narrowing down phenotype definitions is not straightforward. A variety of drug outcomes could be considered a success, including resolution of a medical condition of minimal adverse effects. The difficulty is determining what defines a successful drug response outcome (e.g. required dose, length of time that a patient is disease-free). A comprehensive approach to drug response phenomics [17] likely will entail the collection of data at the molecular, cellular, tissue, and whole-organism levels. There have been efforts standardize the representation of classes of phenotypes, organized in the pharmacogenomics-knowledge base (PharmGKB) [18]. With a great diversity of experimental study designs to approach PGX outcomes, initial categories of pharmacogenomics information include the following categories: studies focused on genotype (GN), molecular and cellular functional assays (FA), pharmacokinetics (PK), pharmacodynamics and drug response (PD), and clinical outcome (CO) [18]. While these categories will provide an important ontology for PGX data, there are various of summary measures within these categories that could be considered as the outcome variable for genetic mapping analysis.

An additional challenge that is common in PGX is that often phenotype definition not only concerns clinical considerations and selection of study participants but also requires statistical and mathematical modeling to summarize drug response prior to any genetic mapping. For example, under the broad category of pharmacokinetics (PK) outcomes, traditional PK modeling tools may need to be employed to summarize population data to calculate values including, but not exclusively, the following summary measures: loading dose, maintenance dose, volume of distribution, half-life, binding rates, phase 1 or 2 reaction, and therapeutic index [19,20]. While discussion of the modeling for each of these values is beyond the scope of this chapter, an excellent introduction and discussion of pharmacokinetic modeling can be found in the text by Reddy [20]. Similarly, in pharmacodynamics and drug response (PD) and clinical outcomes (CO) studies, summary measures of toxicity grades and rate, agonism and antagonism, adverse events, and relative measures of efficacy may need to be derived as outcomes for genetic mapping [21,22].

While this complex phenotype data can be challenging in narrowing down particular phenotypes for mapping, it offers a distinct advantage in dissecting the complex pathways that control drug response. Measuring *intermediate phenotypes* or *endophenotypes* assumed to be functionally related or potentially underlying the broader phenotype of drug response offers a great advantage in dissecting the genetic etiology of response as a whole, since these multiple phenotypes may have stronger genetic determinants than the more remote phenotype to which they relate [9,14].

It also should be noted that in many cases in PGX, the definition of a phenotype *dichotomizes* what is actually a *quantitative* or *continuous* physiological measurement [14]. For example, toxicity outcomes are often summarized in a yes/no-type measure, based on thresholds of toxicity grade levels [16]. While for clinical purposes this may be useful, in genetic studies it may reduce important variation and hence reduce the underlying genetic "signals" [23]. As a gene might affect not only one phenotype but rather an entire network of correlated biological systems, the joint analysis of multiple phenotypes can also increase the ability to detect genes [24].

Clear and clinically appropriate definitions of phenotype are a crucial component of any genetic study [14].

15.3 ESTABLISHING THE HERITABILITY OF DRUG RESPONSE PHENOTYPES

Evidence has shown that genetics contributes to almost every disease [25,26], so it is reasonable to assume that the same it true for variability to response pharmaceuticals. In fact, the inherent nature of chemical and metabolic responses was one of the first phenotypes demonstrated to be heritability in humans [27].

Generally, the first step of any disease mapping study is to establish the heritability of a given phenotype or disease, where heritability is the proportion of phenotypic variation in a population that is attributable to the genetic variation among individuals [28]. Variation among individuals may be due to genetic and/or environmental factors, and heritability analyses estimate the relative contributions of differences in genetic and nongenetic or environmental factors to the total phenotypic variance in a population. Again, because controlled experiments are not always possible for all phenotypes in human studies, heritability studies often rely on observational twin studies [29]. By contrasting identical twins that have been separated early in life and raised in different environments, the researcher can identify the effects of genotype and environment. If twin studies are not possible, data from closely related individuals—such as brothers, sisters, parents, and offspring—are used. Familial clustering of a phenotype, or the resemblance of relatives of any degree (siblings, cousins, etc.) with regard to a phenotype can provide further evidence that genetic factors contribute to a phenotype [30]. One has to keep in mind that, depending on the phenotype in question, this type of analysis has to be interpreted cautiously as familial resemblance can be caused by shared familial environmental factors, rather than overt, inherited genetic factors [31]. Details of traditional heritability studies and statistical methods to determine heritability can be found in Jorde et al. [30].

Often in pharmacogenomics, traditional familial genetic methods are not possible because of the rarity of simultaneous occurrence of a specific clinical events among family members and the inability to administer pharmaceutical agents to healthy, normal volunteer subjects. In order to overcome these limitations, novel utilization of *in vitro* cell-based assays have emerged as an important resource in assessing the heritability of dose response traits [32,33]. The Centre d'Etude du Polymorphisme Humain (CEPH) pedigree cell lines have been used to assess drug response phenotypes for a broad range of drugs. The CEPH cell lines are Epstein–Barr virus–transformed lymphoblastoid cell lines that include cell lines derived from individuals in a number of multigenerational families that are readily accessible and have genomewide microsatellite and polymorphisms markers freely available [34,35]. The use of these assays provides for the rigorous testing of samples while minimizing the influence of environmental conditions, and utilizes pedigree information to assess heritability of drug response phenotypes. A discussion of the utilization of these cell based assays for heritability assessment can be found in Walgren et al. [36].

15.4 APPROPRIATE STUDY DESIGNS FOR PHARMACOGENOMICS STUDIES

After a trait or disease has been established as heritable, genomic mapping is undertaken to begin to narrow in on the genetic regions or variants that cause the trait. Typically, observational studies are used to statistically relate genetics to the phenotype under study [37]. In addition to the cell-based assays mentioned above, there are several study designs appropriate for pharmacogenomic applications: (1) pharmacokinetics and pharmacodynamic outcomes can be evaluated in healthy volunteers, and PK–PD differences compared with proportions of genotyped variants; (2) genetic mapping can be performed in cohort design randomized clinical trials, where differences in clinical outcomes can be compared between/among genotype groups; (3) analysis of adverse events can be evaluated in nested case–control designs in clinical trials; and (4) prospective designs comparing genotype-adjusted to conventionally treated patients can also be used. While observational and clinical trials are not exclusively the only designs that can be used, they do represent the most popular designs used. A more complete discussion of the advantages and disadvantages within available study designs for pharmacogenomics can be found in Guessous et al. [37].

Within these study designs there are two broad types of genetic approached designs that may be used in genetic mapping in any of the study designs mentioned above: linkage analysis and association analysis [38]. *Linkage analysis* determines whether a chromosomal region is preferentially inherited by offspring with the trait of interest by using genotype and phenotype data from multiple biologically related family members. Linkage analysis capitalizes on the fact that, as a causative gene(s) segregates through a family kindred, other markers nearby on the same chromosome tend to segregate together (are in linkage) with the causative gene due to the lack of recombination in that region. *Association analysis*, on the other hand, describes the use of case–control, cohort, or even family data to statistically relate genetic variations to a specific disease or phenotype. Because association analysis directly examines the effect of a candidate locus, rather than an effect that is diffused across large regions of chromosomes, its greatest applicability is in fine localization and identification of causative loci [39].

Both linkage and association studies are used in genetic mapping in pharmacogenomics, and the choice of the analytical method used is dependent on the study design choice. Because of the practical limitations on collecting familial data for drug response outcomes, association studies represent the most commonly used mapping approach, and analytical methods for association analysis will be the focus of this chapter.

15.5 TRADITIONAL METHODS FOR GENETIC MAPPING

Traditional statistical approaches to detect genetic associations have been successful in identifying single-locus associations and in detecting interactions when properly applied. In any genetic analysis plan, particularly in pharmacogenomics studies, both single-locus and epistatic models should be considered. Below, we briefly outline the traditional methods most commonly used in genetic epidemiology and their application in the search for epistatic interactions. Then, we discuss some general concerns and limitations of these methods for detecting interaction effects such as drug response outcomes. A more detailed discussion of these methods and their application to finding epistasis can be found in the literature [40,41]. Table 15.1 lists many of the most commonly used traditional methods in genetic association analysis to detect gene–gene and gene–environment interactions. This list is certainly not exhaustive, but does list many of the most commonly used methods in three main categories: contingency table analysis, generalized linear models, and analysis of variance. This table is provided as a starting point in designing a genetic mapping data analysis plan.

Contingency tables provide a simple yet effective method for determining interactions. These methods compare the observed data to what would be expected under various genetic models. For case–control studies, Pearson's χ^2 and Fisher's exact test can be used. For family-based data, the transmission disequilibrium test (TDT) is commonly used to compare observed to expected transmitted alleles [42,43].

Generalized linear models, an extension of ordinary least-squares regression, encompasses a flexible class of regression methods that describe the relationship between response (dependent) and predictor (independent) variables. Multiple regression seeks to quantify the relationship between several independent variables (multiple genotypes) and a single dependent variable (phenotype), whereas multivariate regression extends to multiple dependent variables (multiple phenotypes). For continuous or quantitative phenotypes, such as in population-based studies, linear regression analysis is appropriate. When phenotypes are binary, such as in case–control studies, logistic regression can be used. Other types of regression are available depending on particular model assumptions [44].

Analysis of variance (ANOVA) is another popular class of methods for association studies. The purpose of ANOVA is to test for significant differences between group means and is equivalent to the Student's t test when only two means are compared. Complex study designs involving repeated measures and nesting can be accommodated under the ANOVA framework, which often is the design used in clinical trials. Multivariate ANOVA (MANOVA) extends the methodology to apply to the analysis of more than one dependent or outcome variable. Additionally within this analysis framework, known clinical or environmental covariates can also be included using analysis of covariance (ANCOVA) and multivariate analysis of covariance (MANCOVA) [45].

Additionally, survival analysis methods play an important role in PGX studies. Survival analysis models time-to-event data, for outcomes such as time to relapse, survival time, and time until an adverse event [46]. By comparing survival time between/among genotype categories, proportional hazards analyses directly compare the hazards ratios/rates for potential associated loci. A hazard rate at a given time is the probability of the given event occurring in that time period, given survival through all prior time intervals. A *hazard ratio*, also called the *hazard function*, is the estimate of the ratio of the hazard rate in one group (often the genotype category) to the hazard rate in another group [46].

It is important to note that these statistical methods have both parametric and nonparametric versions. In parametric methods, both genetic and statistical model assumptions are made and parameters are estimated on the basis of these assumptions. Nonparametric methods are assumption-free approaches, but often come with a loss in power. For example, if the statistical assumptions of ANOVA are not met, both the Kolmogorov–Smirnov two-sample test and the Kruskal–Wallis analysis of ranks are available. A more complete discussion of parametric versus nonparametric methods can be found in an article by moore [47].

There are several advantages to traditional statistical approaches that must not be overlooked. First, they are easily computed, and most methods are readily available in common statistical software packages. Additionally, the results are easily interpreted since the mathematical implications of most parameters have been extensively evaluated, and there is a long history of model interpretation. Finally, these models are readily accepted in both the biological and statistical communities [40,47].

However, there are several disadvantages to traditional methods that must be considered. First, the curse of dimensionality [48] limits the power of traditional methods to detect interactive effects. In regression analysis, for example, this can result in increased type 1 errors, and parameter estimates with very large standard errors simulation studies have demonstrated that 10 outcome events per independent variable are required for each parameter estimate [5]. As the scale of association studies become more common, this is an unrealistic sample size requirement [49].

Variable selection is another concern with the use of traditional methods [40,50]. Most classical statistical tests were designed to test a specific, a priori hypothesis: the association between a prespecified variable(s) and an outcome of interest. They were not designed to identify which variables are the most important in predicting that outcome. Variable selection approaches, such as stepwise selection and best subset selection, are often applied as "wrappers" around traditional methods to try to address this challenge. These wrappers have been most often applied in a regression framework (discussed below), where well-known criteria such as Mallows' C_p, the Akaike information criterion (AIC) and the Bayesian information criterion (BIC) are often used to penalize the number of nonzero parameters. Shrinkage estimation approaches have also been employed to achieve better prediction and reduce the variances of estimators, such as ridge regression [51].

While these procedures can be extremely useful in certain situations, they may not be appropriate for the detection of gene–gene and gene–environment interactions. Stepwise regression, for example, is a well-known and widely used form of variable selection within a regression framework [51]. There are several important limitations with such an approach. Especially in the case of small sample sizes, this approach can yield biased r^2 values, confidence intervals for effects and predicted values that are falsely narrow, p values that do not have proper meaning, and biased regression coefficients that reguire shrinkage [52]. Further, it is based on methods (i.e) F tests for nested models) that were intended to test prespecified hypotheses [11,52]. Additionally, most of these methods rely on some criteria for hierarchical model

TABLE 15.1 Traditional Statistical Analytical Methods

Method	Study Designs	Outcome Variables	Input Variables	Parametric	Genetic	Statistical
Contingency table methods	Pearson's chi-square	Case-control	Discrete	Discrete	Yes	Yes
	Fisher's exact test	Case-control	Discrete	Discrete	Yes	No
	Armitage Cochran	Case-control	Binary	Discrete	Yes	No
	McNemar's chi-square	Case-control	Binary	Discrete	Yes	No
	TDT	Trios	Binary	Discrete	No	Yes
	Sib-TDT	Discordant sibling pairs	Binary	Discrete	No	Yes
	1-TDT	Proband + One parent	Binary	Discrete	No	Yes
	PDT	Extended pedigress	Binary	Discrete	No	Yes
	FBAT	Extended pedigrees	Binary	Discrete	No	Yes
	GTDT	Trios	Binary	Discrete	No	Yes
	Tmhet	Trios	Binary	Discrete	No	Yes
	ccTDT	Mixed designs (Case-control and Family-based)	Binary	Discrete	No	Yes
Generalized linear models	Linear regression	Population-based, Cohort, Family-based	Continuous	Discrete or continuous	Depends on encoding	Yes
	Logistic regression	Case-control	Binary	Discrete or continuous	Depends on encoding	Yes
	Cox proportional hazards regression	Cohort	Binary	Discrete or continuous	Depends on encoding	Yes
	Poisson regression	Cohort	Binary	Discrete or continuous	Depends on encoding	Yes
	Restricted cubic splines regression	Case-control, Cohort, Family-based	Depends on types	Discrete or continuous	Depends on encoding	No
	Kernel regression	Population-based, Cohort, Family-based	Continuous	Discrete or continuous	Depends on encoding	No

	GLM	Population-based; Family-based	Multiple variables; discrete or continuous	Discrete or continuous	No	No
Analysis of variance (ANOVA)	Student's t test	Population-based; Family-based	Continuous	Discrete	Yes	Yes
	MANOVA/MANCOVA	Population-based; Family-based	Continuous	Discrete	No	Yes
	Wald–Wolfowitz runs test	Population-based	Continuous	Discrete	No	No
	Mann–Whitney U test	Population-based	Continuous	Discrete	No	No
	Kolmogorov–Smirnov two-sample test	Population-based	Continuous	Discrete	No	No
	Kruskal–Wallis analysis of ranks	Population-based	Continuous	Discrete	No	No
	Median test	Population-based	Continuous	Discrete	No	No
	Sign test	Population-based; Family-based	Continuous	Discrete	No	No
	Wilcoxon's matched pairs test	Population-based; Family-based	Continuous	Discrete	No	No
	Friedman's two-way ANOVA	Population-based; Family-based	Continuous	Discrete	No	No
	Cochran's Q	Population-based; Family-based	Continuous	Discrete	No	No
	QTDT	Trios	Continuous	Discrete	No	Yes
Survival analysis	Cox proportional hazards	Population-based	Survival	Discrete	Depends on encoding	Semi

building. In a genetic context, this means that they would be dependent on marginal main effects to even begin to build interactive models [11].

Another important consideration with high-dimensional studies is the risk of false discovery due to multiple testing, especially if traditional methods are used to individually test loci or multilocus combinations [49]. As the number of loci increases, so does the number of statistical tests typically performed. This problem may become overwhelming as the field embraces genomewide studies. For example, χ^2 testing of a whole-genome association dataset of 1,000,000 SNPs may yield 50,000 chance associations at $p < 0.05$, and 100 at $p < 0.0001$. Traditional approaches such as the Bonferroni correction adjust for type I error, but are extremely conservative and thus may reject true associations [49]. For genomic studies, these correction procedures may demand unrealistically small significance levels, and often ignore issues of between-test (intertest) dependence due to linkage between markers [53]. It may be more appropriate to correct for multiple testing with the false discovery rate method, which considers the expected number of false rejections divided by the total number of rejections [53]. The false discovery rate method is less conservative than the Bonferroni correction [53], but still may be too conservative for very large numbers of variables. Permutation testing is also used to decrease the impact of multiple comparisons through empirical estimates of significance. Permutation testing is a commonly used nonparametric statistical procedure. Rather than make specific distributional assumptions, a permutation test randomly permutes the data many times to actually construct the distribution of the test statistic under the null hypothesis. If the value of the test statistic based on the original samples is extreme relative to this distribution (i.e.) if it falls far into the tail of the distribution), then the null hypothesis is rejected [54]. The validity of a permutation test relies only on the data maintaining the property of exchangeability under the null hypothesis—so permutation testing makes no statistical or genetic assumptions and produces an unbiased p value [54,55]. Permutation testing can partially control for multiple comparison by significance testing of only the best / or final model as opposed to all individual tests. The chief drawback of this method is that it is computationally expensive, and for extremely large datasets, this limitation may make this type of significance testing prohibitive.

15.6 NOVEL METHODOLOGY FOR COMPLEX PREDICTIVE MODELS

In order to overcome the limitations of traditional methods, a number of novel approaches have been developed. These methods can be described as data mining methods, in contrast to the traditional hypothesis-based approaches, with a main goal of prediction. They are designed to explore large amounts of data (such as in large-scale genetic studies) in search of consistent patterns between variables; applying the detected patterns to new subsets of data then validates the findings. As with traditional methods, these novel methods have been developed for both linkage and association studies. In the current section, we briefly outline some of the basic tools and strategies used by these methods that take a data mining approach to detecting and characterizing epistasis. We discuss the goals and strategies used in a data mining framework, and outline and discuss the most commonly used types of data mining methods. Table 15.2 lists many of the methods used in genetic epidemiology to detect interactive models, and outlines key aspects of the study designs that are appropriate. While the methods covered here do not represent a comprehensive list, many of the most commonly used methods are covered. Again, these tables are meant to serve as a starting point in designing an analysis strategy. A more extensive discussion of these methods can be found in Motsinger et al. [40].

Data mining is an analytical process designed to explore large amounts of data (such as large-scale genetic studies) in search of consistent patterns and/or systematic relationships between variables, and then to validate the findings by applying the detected patterns to new subsets of data. Data mining is often considered "a blend of statistics, AI [artificial intelligence], and database research" [56]. Data mining has sometimes received a tepid reception from traditionalists, even considered by some "a dirty word in statistics" [56]. However, as the practical importance and success of this approach is increasingly recognized, and the scale of genetic studies exponentially expands, this sort of approach is gaining acceptance.

The ultimate goal of any data mining approach is usually prediction—in the case of PGX this prediction is in the form of loci that predict drug response [40]. As opposed to traditional hypothesis testing designed to verify a priori hypotheses about relations between variables, data mining typically falls under an exploratory data analysis framework. It is used to identify relations between variables when there are no, or incomplete, a priori expectations as to the nature of those relations.

There are three general stages to any data mining application [57]:

1. *Data Exploration.* In genetic epidemiology, this may include simply the preliminary analysis discussed above, or a filter step in the analysis, where a certain number of independent variables are selected according to a criterion of choice.
2. *Model Building and Internal Validation.* It is this step that differs greatly from method to method.
3. *Deployment.* This step involves using the model selected as best in the previous stage and applying it to new data to estimate its predictive ability.

Many data mining approaches combine steps 2 and 3 by using a data resampling technique, such as bagging, boosting, cross-validation, jackknifing, or bootstrapping to simultaneously build and test a model. An excellent discussion of resampling and internal model validation techniques can be found in Hastie et al. [58].

There are two general, broad categories of data mining methods: pattern recognition and data reduction. The pattern recognition family of methods considers the full dimensionality of the data, and aims to classify according to information extracted from the patterns [57]. Tree-based methods, neural networks (NN), and clustering algorithms are all included in this family of methods. The term *data reduction* in the context of data mining is usually applied to projects where the goal is

TABLE 15.2 Novel Approaches to Detect Epistasis

Method	Study Design	Outcome	Input	Parametric	Genetically	Statistically
Tree-based	Classification and Regression Trees (CART)	Case-control	Binary	Discrete or continuous	No	No
	Random Forests (RF)	Population-based; Case-control	Discrete, continuous, survival	Discrete or continuous	No	No
	Mutivariate Adaptive Regression Splines (MARS)	Population-based; Case-control	Discrete or continuous; multiple outcome variables	Discrete or continuous	No	No
Combinatorial	Combinatorial Partitioning Method (CPM)	Population-based	Continuous	Discrete	No	No
	Restricted Partition Method (RPM)	Population-based	Continuous	Discrete	No	No
	Multifactor Dimensionality Reduction (MDR)	Case-control	Binary	Discrete	No	No
	MDR-PDT	Family-based	Binary	Discrete	No	No
	Generalized MDR	Case-control; Population-based	Discrete or continuous	Discrete or continuous	No	No
	Patterning and Recursive Partitioning (PRP)	Case-control	Discrete or continuous	Discrete or continuous	No	No
	Detection of Informative Combined Effect (DICE)	Case-control	Discrete or continuous	Discrete or continuous	Yes	No
Neural networks	Parameter Decreasing Method (PDM)	Case-control	Binary	Discrete or continuous	No	No
	Genetic Programming NN (GPNN)	Case-control	Binary	Discrete or continuous	No	No
	Grammatical Evolution NN (GENN)	Case-control	Binary	Discrete or continuous	No	No

Clustering algorithms	CLADHC	Case-control; Family-based	Binary	Discrete	No	Yes or no
	HapMiner	Case-control; Family-based	Discrete or continuous	Discrete	No	Yes
	k-means clustering	Population-based; Family-based	Continuous	Discrete or continuous	No	No
	EM clustering	Population-based; Family-based	Continuous	Discrete or continuous	No	No
Two-step	Set association	Case-control	Binary	Discrete	No	No
	Focused interaction testing framework (FITF)	Case-control	Binary	Discrete	No	No
	Principle components analysis (PCA)	Population-based; Family-based	Continuous	Discrete or continuous	No	No

to aggregate or amalgamate the information contained in large datasets into manageable (smaller) information nuggets. Data reduction methods can include simple tabulation, aggregation (computing descriptive statistics), or more sophisticated techniques such as principal-components analysis. The combinatorial and two-stage approaches discussed below fall into this category.

15.6.1 Pattern Recognition Methods

Pattern recognition methods seek to classify information from patterns extracted from the full data [57,59]. These include neural network approaches, clustering algorithms, and tree-based methods. Clustering algorithms sort objects into groups by maximizing the degree of association of objects in the same group and minimizing the degree of association of objects in different groups. The degree of association is often determined through measures of distance. When applied to genetic data, clusters of individuals are detected whose phenotypic variation is explained by different genetic models.

Arguably the simplest group of data mining approaches used in genetic epidemiology is tree building algorithms [60]. Also referred to as *recursive partitioning methods*, this group of tools determines a set of if–then logical (split) conditions that permit accurate prediction or classification of cases. There are several important advantages to tree-based algorithms that make them particularly useful in the context of genetic epidemiologym [60,61]. First, they can handle a large number of input variables, which is important as the scale of genetic studies increases. Also, learning is fast and computation time is modest even for very large datasets. Additionally, tree methods are suited to dealing with certain types of genetic heterogeneity (roughly, where different variants can lead to the same disease), since splits near the root node define separate model subsets in the data. Also, tree-based algorithms produce an easily interpretable final model that is essentially a set of if–then rules (an example of a "white box" solution representation). Finally, these algorithms can uncover interactions among factors that do not exhibit strong marginal effects, without demanding a prespecified model [61]. One important limitation of these methods to consider when looking for interactions is that they are dependent on slight marginal effects to model epistasis. If marginal main effects are not present, these methods will likely fail to characterize the interaction. Classification and regression trees (CART) [62] and random forests (RF) [48] are two extremely popular variations of tree-based models, and are applicable to a wide range of study designs, including survival outcomes [48].

Neural networks (NN) are machine learning techniques modeled after the cognitive system and neurological processing of the brain [63]. The network "learns" from the existing data and seeks to generate an output pattern (phenotype) that is used to classify the input pattern (genotype) [64]. Two types of neural networks, *genetic programming NN* (GPNN) [65] and *grammatical evolution NN* (GENN) [66], imitate the genetic processes of natural selection in order to construct the network model [67]. Using these ideas, the researcher will select the network with the best predictive capability (i.e., highest fitness). These methods can evaluate both main effect and purely interactive models, and can computationally scale to handle very large-scale data. A more complete review of NN application in genetic epidemiology can be found in a 2008 article [68].

Clustering algorithms are a subgroup of the pattern recognition family [59] that aims to sort different objects into groups such that the degree of association between two objects is maximal if they belong to the same group and minimal otherwise. Clustering approaches have been applied in medicine for clustering diseases, cures for diseases, or symptoms of diseases to generate useful taxonomies. Their application to the identification of genes that predict a phenotype of interest is more novel, and is often used in concert with more traditional measures of association. This class of methods also considers the full dimensionality of the data, so they are also able to cluster according to interactive models. These methods are particularly appealing for cases of genetic heterogeneity, as they can detect "clusters" of individuals whose phenotype variation is explained by different genetic models [9]. Clustering methods have also been used in concert with other computational methodologies to better define phenotypes for analysis or pick-apart genetic heterogeneity [9]. There are several broad classes of clustering techniques available to an epidemiologist: joining (tree clustering), two-way joining, *k*-means, and expectation maximization (EM) clustering [57]. A more complete discussion of the advantages and disadvantages of each of these clustering methods can be found in Motsinger et al. [40].

15.6.2 Data Reduction Methods

In contrast to pattern recognition techniques, data reduction methods seek to reduce the dimensionality of the data, or aggregate the available information. Data reduction methods include combinatorial methods, two-step and multistage approaches, and principal-components analysis.

Combinatorial approaches use an exhaustive search of all possible variable combinations to determine the combination that best predicts the outcome of interest [2]. In our case, combinations of genes are used to predict phenotype. This exhaustive search approach is ideal for detecting interactions, including high-order interactions, since no marginal main effects are needed for variable selection during the training–model building stage. While this is an important theoretical advantage for these methods, the computation time required grows exponentially with the number of markers evaluated. Certainly for genomewide association studies, and even for some large-scale candidate gene studies, computational time may limit the ability to explore high-order interactions with these methods. Three highly successful and closely related methods that fall under this category are the combinatorial partitioning method (CPM) [69], restricted partition method (RPM) [70] and multifactor dimensionality reduction (MDR) [71]. CPM and RPM are designed to detect interactions in quantitative phenotypes of interest, while MDR was originally designed for a binary outcome (although it has more recently been extended) [72]. Cross-validation is then used to assess the model's predictive capability for each of these methods [2]. These methods typically rely on a form of permutation testing to ascribe statistical significance to a final model. Permutation testing has the advantages of being an assumption-free approach to significance testing but is a heavy computational burden, especially for these already computation-heavy methods. MDR particularly has been highly successful in identifying predictive models in PGX for a wide range of drug response outcomes, including response to efavirenz [73]. A more detailed review of the application of MDR to pharmacogenomic data can be found in a 2006 paper [74].

Several novel methods have taken a two-stage approach to detecting genetic associations by first determining a small number of potentially interesting markers, and then modeling interactions between those potential predictors [40]. Focusing on gene–gene and gene–environment interactions, it is crucial that the first step of these approaches consider not only single markers but also sets of markers that could potentially interact. If only markers with strong main effects are considered in the first step, strictly epistatic models will be missed. This multistep approach is not unique to these methods, but is a defining feature. Set association [75] and focused interaction testing framework (FITF) [76] are two popular methods designed specifically to detect interactions with this framework. These methods can be considered data reduction methods because they address the dimensionality problem by reducing the number of variables examined, and try to estimate global levels of significance [40].

Principal-components analysis (PCA) reduces the data dimensionality by examining the correlation between variables and transforming the correlated variables into a smaller number of latent factors [77]. These new underlying factors may be meaningful interactive predictors. PCA has been widely used for microarray analysis and population stratification analysis, and is appropriate for data mining applications in genetics studies with continuous outcome variables.

15.6.3 Network Analysis in Pharmacogenomics

One additional approach to data mining modeling of PGX outcomes capitalizes on the very complex and rich nature of the phenotype data available in the field, and involves complex systems-level modeling utilizing pathway information from the wealth of data available of the known reactions occurring between components in drug metabolism processes. There are a large number of pathway resources publicly available for genetics and genomics generally, and PharmGKB (mentioned above) specifically provides hand-curated and well-documented resources on known drug metabolism pathways. An excellent review on the pathway resources available in PGX can be found in an article by Thorn et al. [78].

15.7 DEVELOPING AN ANALYSIS PLAN

When developing an analysis plan for PGX data, an investigator has broad options. Particularly for large-scale or genomewide studies, investigators may consider using a combination of several of the tools discussed above. For example, the first stage of analysis could involve a filter method, the second stage could involve a novel tool that performs both variable selection and modeling (such as MDR), and as a final step a traditional method such as logistic regression could be used to put the model in a more interpretable or familiar framework. Another option could involve a nonexhaustive combinatorial search to perform variable selection over the entire dataset followed by knowledge-based interpretation of the results. The combinations of choices are effectively infinite, and Tables 15.1 and 15.2 are presented as a launching point for identifying appropriate methods.

The choice comes down to the details of the particular study, and the investigator should carefully consider these details. Are there well-characterized mechanisms or candidate genes in the literature? Is the etiology likely to involve accumulation of minor epistatic effects or one large main effect with modifiers? What is the scale of the study in the number of variables and sample size? Is a validation cohort available?

Continued methods development will help an investigator make these choices, and will hopefully encourage the search for interactions in even more studies. Better curation of a web of knowledge about certain diseases, navigability of knowledge databases, and standards for high-throughput data (genomewide studies, etc.) will all aid in this pursuit.

15.8 CONCLUSIONS

Ultimately, the proof that particular genetic variant impacts a phenotype requires the analysis and investigation of that variation in ways that go well beyond statistical mapping. While statistical analysis can provide evidence of association and, hopefully, predictive value, ultimately the causative nature of these associations can only be confirmed experimentally.

REFERENCES

1. Weiss ST et al. Creating and evaluating genetic tests predictive of drug response. *Nat. Rev. Drug Discov.* 2008;**7** (7):568–574.
2. Wilke RA, Reif DM, Moore JH. Combinatorial pharmacogenetics. *Nat. Rev. Drug Discov.* 2005;**4** (11):911–918.
3. Lanfear DE, McLeod HL. Pharmacogenetics: Using DNA to optimize drug therapy. *Am. Fam. Physician* 2007;**76** (8):1179–1182.
4. Altshuler D, Daly MJ, and Lander ES. Genetic mapping in human disease. *Science* 2008;**322** (5903):881–888.
5. Moore JH. The ubiquitous nature of epistasis in determining susceptibility to common human diseases. *Hum. Hered.* 2003;**56** (1–3):73–82.
6. Moore JH. A global view of epistasis. *Nat. Genet.* 2005;**37** (1):13–14.
7. Moore JH, Williams SM. Traversing the conceptual divide between biological and statistical epistasis: Systems biology and a more modern synthesis. *Bioessays* 2005;**27** (6):637–646.
8. Culverhouse R. et al. A perspective on epistasis: Limits of models displaying no main effect. *Am. J. Hum. Genet.* 2002;**70** (2):461–471.

9. Thornton-Wells TA, Moore JH, Haines JL. Genetics, statistics and human disease: analytical retooling for complexity. *Trends Genet*. 2004;**20** (12):640–647.
10. Wade MJ. Epistasis, complex traits, and mapping genes. *Genetica* 2001;**112–113**:59–69.
11. Moore JH Williams SM. New strategies for identifying gene-gene interactions in hypertension. *Ann. Med.* 2002;**34** (2):88–95.
12. Motsinger Reif AA, Reif DM. Embracing Epistasis: Searching for Gene-Gene and Gene-Environment Interactions in Genetic Epidemiology. In Thangadurai D., Tang W., Pullaiah T. (eds.), *Frontiers in Genome Research*. Regency Publications, New Delhi. *In Press*.
13. Rosand J. Epistasis is coming: Are we ready? *Stroke* 2005;**36** (9):1879–1880.
14. Broeckel U, and Schork, NJ. Identifying genes and genetic variation underlying human diseases and complex phenotypes via recombination mapping. *J. Physiol.* 2004;**554** (Pt. 1):40–45.
15. Giacomini KM et al. When good drugs go bad. *Nature* 2007;**446** (7139):975–977.
16. Wilke R A et al., Identifying genetic risk factors for serious adverse drug reactions: current progress and challenges. *Nat. Rev. Drug Discov.* 2007;**6** (11):904–916.
17. Freimer N Sabatti C. The human phenome project. *Nat. Genet.* 2003;**34** (1):15–21.
18. Klein TE et al. Integrating genotype and phenotype information: An overview of the PharmGKB project. Pharmacogenetics research network and knowledge base. *Pharmacogenomics J.* 2001;**1** (3):167–170.
19. Teorell T. Kinetics of distribution of substances administered to the body. *Arch. Int. Pharmacodyn. Thér.* 1937;**57**:35.
20. Reddy M. *Physiologically Based Pharmacokinetic Modeling: Science and Applications*. Hoboken, NJ: Wiley-Interscience., 2005;
21. Derendorf H et al. Pharmacokinetic/pharmacodynamic modeling in drug research and development. *J. Clin. Pharmacol.* 2000;**40** (12 Pt. 2): 1399–1418.
22. Sheiner LB, Steimer JL. Pharmacokinetic/pharmacodynamic modeling in drug development. *Annu. Rev. Pharmacol. Toxicol.* 2000;**40**:67–95.
23. Korczak JF, Goldstein AM. Sib-pair linkage analyses of nuclear family data: Quantitative versus dichotomous disease classification. *Genet. Epidemiol.* 1997;**14** (6):827–832.
24. Stoll M et al. A genomic-systems biology map for cardiovascular function. *Science* 2001;**294** (5547):1723–1726.
25. Kruglyak L. Prospects for whole-genome linkage disequilibrium mapping of common disease genes. *Nat. Genet.* 1999;**22** (2):139–144.
26. Khoury MJ, Yang Q. The future of genetic studies of complex human diseases: An epidemiologic perspective. *Epidemiology* 1998;**9** (3):350–354.
27. Garrod AE. *Inborn Errors of Metabolism*. Oxford, UK: Oxford Univ. Press, 1909;
28. Malécot G. *Les Mathématiques de l'Hérédité*. Paris: Masson 1948;
29. Kempthorne O. *An Introduction to Genetic Statistics*. New york: Wiley, 1957;
30. Jorde LB, Watkins WS, Bamshad MJ. Population genomics: A bridge from evolutionary history to genetic medicine. *Hum. Mol. Genet.* 2001;**10** (20):2199–2207.
31. Guo SW. Inflation of sibling recurrence-risk ratio, due to ascertainment bias and/or overreporting. *Am. J. Hum. Genet.* 1998;**63** (1):252–258.
32. Watters J.W et al. Genome-wide discovery of loci influencing chemotherapy cytotoxicity. *Proc. Natl. Acad. Sci. USA* 2004;**101** (32):11809–11814.

33. Dolan ME et al. Heritability and linkage analysis of sensitivity to cisplatin-induced cytotoxicity. *Cancer Res.* 2004;**64** (12):4353–4356.
34. Schork NJ et al. Genomic association/linkage of sodium lithium countertransport in CEPH pedigrees. *Hypertension* 2002;**40** (5):619–628.
35. Cheung VG et al. Natural variation in human gene expression assessed in lymphoblastoid cells. *Nat. Genet.* 2003;**33** (3):422–425.
36. Walgren RA, Meucci MA, McLeod HL. Pharmacogenomic discovery approaches: Will the real genes please stand up? *J. Clin. Oncol.* 2005;**23** (29):7342–7349.
37. Guessous I et al. Trends in pharmacogenomic epidemiology: 2001–2007. *Public Health Genomics* 2009;**12** (3):142–148.
38. Risch N. Searching for genes in complex diseases: Lessons from systemic lupus erythematosus. *J. Clin. Invest.* 2000;**105** (11):1503–1506.
39. Daly AK, Day CP. Candidate gene case-control association studies: Advantages and potential pitfalls. *Br. J. Clin. Pharmacol.* 2001;**52** (5):489–499.
40. Motsinger. AA, Ritchie MD, Reif DM. Novel methods for detecting epistasis in pharmacogenomics studies. *Pharmacogenomics* 2007;**8** (9):1229–1241.
41. Motsinger AA, Ritchie MD, Reif DM. Novel Methods for Detecting Epistasis In Pharmacogenomic Studies. *Pharmacogenomics*. 2007 Sep;**8** (9):1229-1241.
42. Spielman RS, McGinnis RE, Ewens WJ. Transmission test for linkage disequilibrium: The insulin gene region and insulin-dependent diabetes mellitus (IDDM). *Am. J. Hum. Genet.* 1993;**52** (3):506–516.
43. Terwilliger JD, Ding Y, Ott J. On the relative importance of marker heterozygosity and intermarker distance in gene mapping. *Genomics* 1992;**13** (4):951–956.
44. Hastie TJ, Tibshirani RJ. *Generalized Additive Models*. New york: Chapman & Hall, 1990;
45. Lindman HR. *Analysis of Variance in Complex Experimental Designs*. San Franscisco: W. H. Freeman, 1974;
46. Collett D. *Modelling Survival Data in Medical Research*, 2nd ed. Boca Raton FL: Chapman & Hall/CRC.
47. Moore JH, Thornton TA, Ritchie MD. Basic statistics. *Curr. Protoc. Hum. Genet.* 2003; Appendix 3M.
48. Bellman R. *Adaptive Control Processes*. Princeton NJ: Princeton Univ. Press, 1961;
49. Moore JH, Ritchie MD. *STUDENTJAMA*. The challenges of whole-genome approaches to common diseases. *JAMA* 2004;**291** (13):1642–1643.
50. Motsinger-Reif AA, Reif DM, Fanelli TJ, Ritchie MD. A Comparison of computational approaches for genetic association studies. *Genetic Epidemiology.* 2008 Dec;**32** (8): 767–78.
51. Draper N, Smith HB. *Applied Regression Analysis*, 2nd ed. New York: Wiley, 1981;
52. Whittingham MJ et al. Why do we still use stepwise modelling in ecology and behaviour? *J. Anim. Ecol.* 2006;**75** (5):1182–1189.
53. Benjamini Y et al. Controlling the false discovery rate in behavior genetics research. Behav. *Brain Res.* 2001;**125** (1–2):279–284.
54. Good P. Extensions of the concept of exchangeability and their applications. *J. Modern Appl. Statist. Methods* 2002;**1**:4.
55. Motsinger-Reif AA. The effect of alternative permutation testing strategies on the performance of multifactor dimensionality reduction. *BMC Res Notes* 2008;**1**:139.

56. Pregibon D. Data mining. *Stat Comput. Graphics.* 1997;**7**
57. Witten I, Frank E. *Data Mining: Practical Machine Learning Tools and Techniques.* New York: Morgan Kaufman, 2000;
58. Hastie TJ, Tibshirani RJ, Friedman JH. *The Elements of Statistical Learning*, Springer Series in Statistics. Basel: Springer-Verlag, 2001;
59. Devijver PA, Kittler J. *Pattern Recognition: A Statistical Approach.* London: Prentice-Hall, 1982;
60. McKinney BA et al. Machine learning for detecting gene-gene interactions: A review. *Appl. Bioinform.* 2006;**5** (2):77–88.
61. Reif DM et al. Integrated analysis of genetic and proteomic data identifies biomarkers associated with adverse events following smallpox vaccination. *Genes Immun.* 2009;**10** (2):112–119.
62. Brieman L et al. *Classification and Regression Trees.* Pacific Grove, CA: Wadsworth and Brooks/Cole Advanced Books and Software, 1984;
63. Beale R Jackson T. In Hilger A, ed: *Neural Computing, an Introduction.* Bristol, UK: IOP Publishing, 1990;
64. Freeman JA Skapura DM. *Neural Networks: Algorithms, Applications, and Programming Techniques.* Boston: Addison-Wesley, 1991;
65. Ritchie MD et al. Optimization of neural network architecture using genetic programming improves detection and modeling of gene-gene interactions in studies of human diseases. *BMC Bioinform.* 2003;**4**:28.
66. Motsinger-Reif AA, Dudek SM, Hahn LW, and Ritchie MD. Comparison of approaches for machine-learning optimization of neural networks for detecting gene-gene interactions in genetic epidemiology. *Genetic Epidemiology.* 2008 May;**32** (4):325–40.
67. Koza J Rice JP. Genetic generation of both the weights and architecture for a neural network. *IEEE Trans.* 1991; **2**.
68. Motsinger-Reif AA Ritchie MD. Neural networks for genetic epidemiology: Past, present, and future. *BioData Mining.* 2008;**1** (1):3.
69. Nelson MR et al. A combinatorial partitioning method to identify multilocus genotypic partitions that predict quantitative trait variation. *Genome Res.* 2001;**11** (3): 458–470.
70. Culverhouse R Klein T, Shannon W. Detecting epistatic interactions contributing to quantitative traits. *Genet. Epidemiol.* 2004;**27** (2):141–152.
71. Ritchie MD et al. Multifactor-dimensionality reduction reveals high-order interactions among estrogen-metabolism genes in sporadic breast cancer. *Am. J. Hum. Genet.* 2001;**69** (1):138–147.
72. Lou XY et al. A generalized combinatorial approach for detecting gene-by-gene and gene-by-environment interactions with application to nicotine dependence. *Am. J. Hum. Genet.* 2007;**80** (6):1125–1137.
73. Motsinger AA et al. Multilocus genetic interactions and response to efavirenz-containing regimens: An adult AIDS clinical trials group study. *Pharmacogenet. Genomics* 2006;**16** (11):837–845.
74. Motsinger AA and Ritchie MD. Multifactor dimensionality reduction: An analysis strategy for modelling and detecting gene-gene interactions in human genetics and pharmacogenomics studies. *Hum. Genomics.* 2006;**2** (5):318–328.

75. Hoh J Wille A, Ott J. Trimming, weighting, and grouping SNPs in human case-control association studies. *Genome Res.* 2001;**11** (12):2115–2119.

76. Millstein J et al. A testing framework for identifying susceptibility genes in the presence of epistasis. *Am. J. Hum. Genet.* 2006;**78** (1):15–27.

77. Pearson K. On lines and planes of closest fit to systems of points in space. *Philos. Mag.* 1901;**2** (6):13.

78. Thorn C.F. et al. Pathway-based approaches to pharmacogenomics. *Curr. Pharmacogenomics.* 2007;**5**:7.

PART V

PHARMACOGENETICS: INDUSTRY AND REGULATORY AFFAIRS

CHAPTER 16

Applications of Pharmacogenetics in Pharmaceutical Research and Development

DANIEL K. BURNS
Duke University, Durham, North Carolina, USA

SCOTT S. SUNDSETH
Cabernet Pharmaceuticals, Durham, North Carolina, USA

16.1 INTRODUCTION

> If it were not for the great variability among individuals, medicine might as well be a science and not an art.
>
> —Sir William Osler (1849–1919)

There continues to be much evidence that the observation by Sir William remains true today. Not every patient responds the same way to a given therapeutic regime [1]. Some derive a beneficial effect, others receive no benefit, and a few experience an adverse event. It is this inherent, individual natural variation, coupled with an inability to predict a clinical outcome that contributes to the practice of trial-and-error medicine. Although conceptually recognized for decades, pharmacogenetics research did not make much progress for a number of years as the tools to study individual human genomes were simply not available. The first draft of the human genome sequence was published in February 2001 [2,3]. This stimulated rapid development of the genomic tools needed to assess DNA variation and, coupled with advances in informatics analyses, has fostered a dynamic field of scientific inquiry. This is reflected in both the growing number of papers appearing in the scientific literature, the appearance of journals dedicated to the field, and, more importantly, by the increasing use of genomic information on drug labels [4].

Pharmacogenetics and Individualized Therapy, First Edition.
Edited by Anke-Hilse Maitland-van der Zee and Ann K. Daly.

Pharmaceutical companies benefit from the general investment into and advancement of science and technologies. As the pace and breadth of scientific discovery has expanded in the last several decades, pharmaceutical companies have actively invested in these new technologies, including genetics. The rationale for bringing new technological solutions to pharmaceutical research and development (R&D) is to increase productivity. The discovery, development, and registration of safe and effective medicines remain a risky venture. The high failure rate of pharmaceutical R&D continues to negatively impact the productivity and therapeutic treatment options for patients. Despite increasing industry expenditures on R&D and increasing financial support for medical research by the US National Institutes of Health (NIH), the productivity of healthcare research, as measured by registration of new chemical entities, is declining [5]. One of the most significant contributors to this decreasing productivity is attrition throughout the pipeline development process. Because of the inherent uncertainties and complexities within pharmaceutical R&D, it is burdened with high levels of failure across all segments of the R&D pipeline [6] (Fig. 16.1). One aspect of this attrition is the inability to predict a clinical outcome (therapeutic benefit, identification of responsive subgroups, or safety events) at each step. This uncertainty does not end once a medicine is approved for general use. A number of medicines have been removed from the marketplace for unexpected serious adverse events [7,8]. These withdrawals are a burden borne by all sectors of healthcare: the drug sponsor, regulators, healthcare providers, and patients. Application of genetics has provided the opportunity to bring more certainty to the discovery, development, and use of therapeutics. By increasing confidence at key decision points in the pharmaceutical pipeline, genetics can maximize the opportunity for each molecule under consideration [9,10]. Used to predict an individual's chance for deriving benefits and/or reducing the risk of an adverse event, widespread adoption of pharmacogenetics will enhance both the benefit/risk ratio and efficient utilization of increasingly limited healthcare resources.

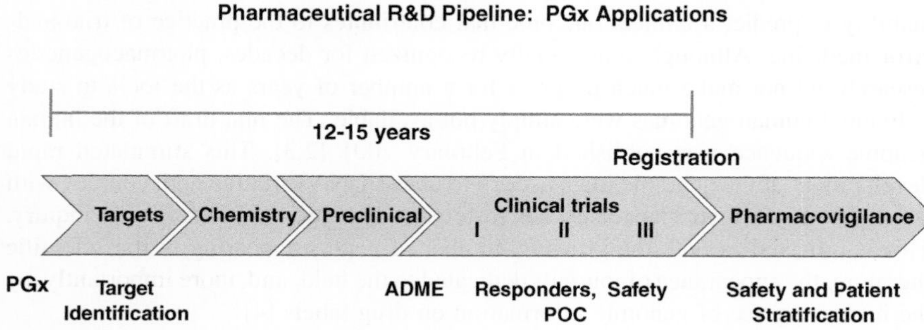

FIGURE 16.1 Pharmaceutical research and development pipeline / pharmacogenetic applications. Integration of PGx activities can occur at several phases along the pipeline from the earliest point (target ID) to postapproval pharmacovigilance and market refinement.

16.2 ENABLING GENETIC DEVELOPMENTS

It has long been known that genes play a fundamental role in physiology and contribute to disease risk. It has been just over a century since Sir Archibald Garrod first made the link between inherited factors and biochemical function [11]. What have been lacking are the experimental tools to enable scientists to probe and investigate the mechanisms by which the information coded in the full complement of the genome results in one's physical characteristics. The ability to manipulate DNA sequences to elucidate gene function began in earnest with the advent of recombinant DNA techniques in the late 1970s [12]. Increasing sophistication of the molecular biology techniques led to the development of methodologies to elucidate the primary nucleotide sequence of DNA strands [13]. With concurrent advances in the fields of automation, robotics, and bioinformatics, the scientific community quickly realized that the capability was now at hand to decipher the human genome, the blueprint for life. This would provide scientists with the basic building blocks that constitute the physical makeup and provide insight into the inherited causes for disease. The rationale was that once genetic factors for disease were identified, new therapeutic approaches could be driven by the knowledge of the molecular basis of disease. The multinational Human Genome Project (HGP) was established in 1990 with the goal of sequencing the entire 3 billion basepairs of the human genome by 2005. Through a combination of publicly funded and private initiatives, this goal was achieved ahead of schedule. In February 2001, the first draft of the human genome sequenced was published and the "finished" sequence was made available to researchers in 2003 [14]. The human genome had become known and bounded. No longer did investigators have to question the existence of a gene; the full complement of gene sequences was now described. Experiments could now focus on gene function and its role in health, pathophysiology, and response to therapeutics. This landmark achievement had created a baseline characterization of a representative human genome. What was needed next was the capability to identify and measure variations from this baseline sequence on a genome wide scale in many individuals. Traditional techniques enabled investigators to examine DNA sequence information at a specific location. A number of genetic technology companies quickly developed and offered standardized platforms that would examine variation at the genome scale. Since the 1990s the number of markers constituting a whole-genome association scan has moved from 10,000 to >1 million single-nucleotide polymorphisms (SNPs). Because DNA is an ordered molecule with defined structure, information is encoded linearly. It is essential to know the precise location of all this variability. With the availability of the baseline human sequence, both private (The SNP Consortium) and publicly supported (HapMap) projects were initiated to map the location of this sequence variation. By 2005 these efforts resulted in the identification and mapping of over 1 million SNPs and placed this information in the public domain [15]. By 2007, further research had mapped over 3.1 million SNPs and made these publicly available [16]. Any investigator, regardless of geographic location or affiliation (public, private, academic, institutional, or government), has the knowledge and tools to elucidate the genetic contribution to the condition under study. This recent and rapid development of the fundamental tools and their widespread availability are fueling the burgeoning field of pharmacogenetics research to the point where it is now viewed as a standard tool in the development of new therapeutics [9,10]. The vast amount of genetic data now in the public domain is creating new developments in systems biology, biochemical, and physiological pathways, statistical analysis methods, and bioinformatics techniques. The coming years will see unparalleled advances in our molecular understanding of human physiology, which will no doubt lead to improved opportunities for the detection, prediction, treatment, and prevention of disease. The challenge for pharmaceutical companies will be to harness this vast genetic information storehouse and develop therapeutics with these new disease insights.

The primary DNA sequence is only one aspect of variation encapsulated in the human genome. New insights into structural types of inherited variation, insertions, deletions, copy number variations, polynucleotide repeats, and other parameters, are increasingly being identified and their role in physiology elucidated. There can be little doubt that new technologies and insight into how the human genome encodes the individual, and knowledge of pathophysiology, will continue to increase. The human genome sequence was not a finish line, but rather the beginning of the journey toward understanding the genome and applying this knowledge to improving human health.

In the late 1990s as the human genome sequencing project was progressing, it was recognized that the identification of genes associated with disease could be the starting point for a drug development program. Earlier genetic linkage or family-based studies had identified genes involved in a number of monogenic Mendelian disorders and also genes involved in a few complex diseases such as Alzheimer's and type 2 diabetes [17–19]. In addition to the genetic tools used to measure DNA variation, this work required the assembly of large collections of families afflicted with the disease being investigated. The identification and recruitment of family members to these types of studies is time-consuming and costly. There was a growing realization that detailed knowledge of genome variation coupled with the tools to measure this variation would permit disease–gene association studies. This approach uses large numbers of unrelated individuals to identify regions of DNA involved in disease. Prior to completion of the human genome sequence or high-throughput and cost-effective methods to measure DNA variation on a large scale, GlaxoSmithKline assembled a disease association collection in a pioneering academic–industrial partnership. The high-throughput disease-specific program (HiTDIP) [20] created a collection of 1000 cases and 1000 matched controls for 14 separate diseases, each subject with systematically collected extensive clinical information with appropriate informed consent. The availability of this collection has been used by both industry scientists and the academic investigators who assembled the collection to perform both candidate genes studies with pharmaceutically tractable or druggable genes and genomewide associations [21–23]. In 2006 a public–private partnership, including the NIH and the Foundation for NIH along with academia and private companies, established the genetic association information network (GAIN) [24,25]. The partnership collected and genetically examined 18,000 samples from six disease collections (ADHD, bipolar disorder, diabetic nephropathy, major depressive disorder, and schizophrenia). Genomewide screens of varying density have been performed and the data deposited in the National Center for Biotechnology Information (NCBI) database of genotypes and phenotypes (dbGaP [26]). In 2007, the Wellcome Trust Case Control Consortium (WTCC) published a landmark paper describing genome wide association studies on seven common diseases (bipolar disorder, coronary artery disease, Crohn's disease, hypertension, rheumatoid arthritis, type 1 and type 2 diabetes) [27]. The investigators typed 500,000 SNPs on each disease collection ($\geq$2000 cases each) and compared these to a common set of 3000 controls. First-pass analysis of the datasets identified positive associations in all the diseases studied except hypertension. These disease gene mapping efforts relied on the HapMap work, which catalogued common variation—present at about 5%. In 2008, Kaiser stated that over the next 3 years using next-generation DNA sequencing technologies, the 1000 genomes projects would seek to identify variation at the 1% level [28]. It is now hoped that rapid technology development and increasing resolution of genetic variation at both SNP and structural levels will increase the ability to understand the role of the human genome in healthcare.

The assembly of large, well-characterized disease collections (including appropriate informed consent) with both phenotypes and DNA samples on hand ensures that with the increasing development of technologies to measure DNA variation, state-of-the-art genetic studies could be rapidly completed without the time-consuming and costly requirement to assemble new patient collections. The ready availability of these genotype/phenotype databases obviates the need for individual investigators to secure the resources to assemble patient collections and genotype the large number of genetic markers, which can be both financially and technologically challenging for laboratories not proficient in these methodologies. In addition, the general availability of these large databases is driving new analytical and bioinformatics methods that explore the genotype–phenotype relationship. There can be little doubt that this vast reservoir of genetic information will lead to an increasing knowledge of the molecular basis of disease and fuel new therapeutic opportunities. In addition, identification of genetic risk factors for disease can support drug discovery for new therapeutic agents and can serve as a means to stratify patients for therapeutic response [10].

Just as subject collections are needed to identify the genetic underpinnings of disease, pharmacogenetics requires the collection of DNA and measures of the efficacy, safety, or dose of a specific therapeutic agent. For several years a number of pharmaceutical companies have been collecting a properly approved DNA sample from subjects enrolled in clinical trials [29]. The objective of this chapter is to highlight how these materials have been put to use to reduce attrition in the pipeline and improve the therapeutic benefit/risk profile for individual patients.

16.3 PHARMACOGENETICS AND THE PHARMACEUTICAL R&D PIPELINE

Figure 16.1 depicts the major elements of the generalized pharmaceutical R&D enterprise. This depiction greatly simplifies the complexity and the continual interplay of biology, chemistry, physiology, pharmacology, and medicine necessary to create new therapeutics. It is important to recognize that the typical time necessary to progress across this continuum is 12–15 years. This time is allocated between the discovery (target, chemistry, preclinical) and development (clinical testing in humans) phases. Furthermore, because of the inherent complexities and uncertainties of developing new therapeutics, the attrition rate across the pipeline is very high. It has been estimated that of 100 compounds that enter clinical testing, only 11 will reach the registration milestone [6], and this does not include attrition of compounds in the pipeline prior to entering human trials. Despite massive investments by both pharmaceutical companies in research and development and basic biomedical research by the NIH [5], neither the attrition rate nor the time it takes to bring a new drug to market have been substantially reduced. This situation has contributed to the increasing cost to bring a new medicine to market, now estimated to be >1 billion US dollars [30], and much has been written about the nonsustainability of this model [31,32]. Recognition of this challenge by the US Food and Drug Administration (FDA) in 2004 led to the creation of the *critical path initiative* [33]. The creation of a new medicine routinely begins with the selection of a molecular target. This selection is based on evidence and optimism that modulating the activity of this target with a therapeutic molecule will prove to be of benefit to a patient. These targets are generally the protein product of genes, such as receptors, enzymes, channels, and signaling molecules. Generally, once selected, a target is then screened against large chemical libraries of small molecules to identify those that interact with the target. The screening "hits" are then developed into "leads" and candidate drug molecules, and the process of refining and optimizing the chemical structure can take several years. Selected compounds continue to be refined for potency, specificity, and selectivity and are evaluated through a variety of preclinical (animal and cellular) models of drug safety. After many years of intense biology and medicinal chemistry effort, selected compounds enter preclinical testing. The route to therapeutic antibodies takes a different course, involving screening of a number of antibodies for the desired attributes prior to testing in humans.

Recognition that genetic variation plays a role in variable therapeutic response has led to significant investments in genetic and pharmacogenetic research by academic institutions and pharmaceutical companies [10,34].

16.3.1 Preclinical Pharmacogenetics Research

Preclinical activities evaluate the pharmacokinetic (PK), pharmacodynamic (PD), and safety profiles of the drug in appropriate animal models to help guide safe dosing decisions in early phase I, or healthy human volunteer, trials. The preclinical data, including *in vitro* drug metabolism and *in vivo* absorption, distribution, metabolism, and excretion (ADME) can be combined with existing knowledge on genetic variation in the drug target, biological pathway, and disease to create genetics-based hypotheses for potential stratification of drug exposure, exposure outliers, and the incorporation of pharmacodynamic biomarkers in phase I study planning. For example, *in vitro* metabolism by CYP2D6 in preclinical studies implies a potential risk for drug overexposure in subjects who have a poor metabolizer phenotype because of their inherent CYP2D6 genotype. Clinical development teams can anticipate this issue and explore its implications for future clinical trial planning in phase 1 studies before proceeding to proof-of-concept studies [35,36].

It is important to recognize that pharmacogenetics research is more than simply assessing genetic risk factors for disease. It is intrinsically a gene-by-environment analysis, the trait of interest only manifests in the presence of the drug. A patient may have a pharmacogenetics research genetic marker with no evident phenotype unless exposed to the drug. Several biological mechanisms (i.e., drug transport, metabolism, degradation, excretion, and modulation of biological response pathways) can impact the efficacy, toxicity, or side effects of a therapeutic, and variations in the corresponding genes have been shown to contribute to drug–response effects.

16.3.2 Pharmacogenetics in Clinical Trials

16.3.2.1 Phase I Pharmacogenetics Research

Phase I studies, which are used to establish the general safety and tolerability of the compound, are usually small ($\sim$10 subjects) and are usually carried out in healthy volunteers. A complete phase I program can consist of a number of separate, distinct studies, each shedding light on the various aspects of the pharmacokinetic parameters of the drug and its tolerability in humans. Because of the poor predictability of animal models of disease and of the animal models used to investigate toxicity characteristics, attrition rates are typically quite high at this stage of development [37].

As compounds transition from the discovery phase to human testing, the focus turns to the drug disposition pathways to gain insight into clearance pathways and pharmacokinetics. Much of the preclinical drug disposition work is done with *in vitro* systems, cell lines, and cell homogenates, and in animal models. Variation in the genes involved in the ADME of xenobiotics provided some of the earliest evidence that pharmacogenetics was clinically relevant. Genetic heterogeneity in the cytochrome P450 oxidative enzyme family has been correlated with functional effects giving rise to extensive and poor metabolizers. These, in turn, can have dramatic consequences on the pharmacokinetic properties of the drug in individuals. Knowledge of an individual's relevant cytochrome P450 makeup can assist in determining the appropriate therapeutic dose for that individual. It is important to remember that the drug has not changed; it is the genetic makeup of the individual patient that leads to a differential outcome. These genes have been studied for a number of years, common variations have been catalogued, and the frequency of these variations has been established in different ethnic groups [38]. Some functional variants can be relatively rare in one ethnic group and more common in another. As medicines are used globally and pharmaceutical companies are increasingly relying on global clinical trials [39], these are important polymorphisms to keep in mind in designing and interpreting global study results. In 2008 a PhRMA sponsored white paper was published that surveyed ADME genetic activities among the study participants [29]. A number of pharmaceutical companies are collecting DNA samples from early clinical studies where rich pharmacokinetic data are collected to permit genetic analysis should there be evidence of variation. This is an important area to investigate as variable PK can contribute to variable PD and therapeutic outcome as well as contribute to adverse events. Another area of attention is the metabolic conversion of a prodrug to the active drug substance. Variants in the enzyme involved in the conversion can have dramatic effects on therapeutic benefit (e.g., codeine, tamoxifen, clopidogrel; discussed below). In addition, commercial technology suppliers are now focusing attention on providing robust genotyping platforms that can reliably measure variation in these pharmacologically important genes, and the FDA has approved a test for measuring cytochrome P450 DNA sequence variations [40].

As phase I studies usually have few subjects, they are best suited for testing a straightforward, single gene/marker hypothesis (e.g., CYP2D6, discussed above). However, multiple phase I studies can be designed with common clinical measurements, thus permitting the study data to be combined and generate sufficient samples for more extensive multigene analyses. If pharmacogenetics research results are critical to development decisionmaking (e.g. PK properties or a safety issue), study subjects can be directly enrolled on the basis of specific genotypes and the phenotype–genotype correlations rapidly tested. One of the greatest values of adopting a cross-pipeline pharmacogenetics research strategy comes from using early-phase pharmacogenetics research results to plan phase II proof-of-concept studies [41]. If pharmacogenetics experiments demonstrate concise data addressing the genotype dependence of observed phenotypic variability, scientists can use the information to design specific next-phase studies. Evidence for genetically defined subpopulations of patients can be leveraged for both smaller, focused trials and early consideration of companion diagnostics as part of the clinical development plan [42]. Finally, pharmacogenetic data addressing PK variability from phase I trials can be incorporated into bridging studies in geographic areas where specific ADME genotypes may be more common, again reducing trial size and costs [43].

16.3.2.2 Phase II

Compounds that are found to be well tolerated, with predictable pharmacokinetic properties, can be advanced to phase II or proof-of-concept studies. These are critical for establishing the therapeutic benefit and provide guidance on the proper dosing regimen. These studies typically can include several hundred patients, subjects with the disease or condition under investigation, and employ either a placebo or standard of care comparison. This is the first glimpse of the drug's potential therapeutic benefit and a full phase II program can involve several distinct studies. Efficacy pharmacogenetics has three components: (1) polymorphisms in ADME genes that determine exposure; (2) polymorphisms in the drug target or its pathway that can influence the PD and, potentially, efficacy; and (3) the underlying genetics components of the disease itself that could influence efficacy.

How genetics is utilized at this stage depends on factors such as novelty of the target, liabilities associated with other members of the drug class, and the clinical and commercial differentiation strategy for the product. Patient stratification may provide another opportunity to pursue pharmacogenetics research during phase II if a drug appears to be, at a population level, less efficacious than a competitor molecule or if the response appears to be variable, which may lead to the need to profile the true or best responders [44]. This research should be incorporated into protocols as secondary or exploratory endpoints if variants with known or suspected function are implicated in the drug response pathway or in stratifying disease pathology.

Phase II studies are relatively small in size, typically consisting of only a few hundred patients, but may be conducted in genetically diverse populations, which increases the possibility of observing variable drug exposure and response. Small subject numbers generally limit pharmacogenetics experiments to testing existing hypotheses on genetic variability associated with pharmacodynamic (PD) endpoints and or clinical efficacy. Exploratory pharmacogenetics studies of either efficacy or PK variability may be in order if genetic effect size appears to be large, or in situations where multiple studies can be combined to increase subject numbers. However, even in these cases, any analysis would be limited to a relatively restricted number, or panel, of common polymorphisms in candidate genes. Review of clinical data from early phase II studies can determine the need for delivering genotype data for inclusion in subsequent studies. Ideally, for pharmacogenetics data to be included as a covariate or to impact development decisions, genotyping must to occur in the same measurement timeframe as other biomarkers during a clinical trial and not following completion of the study.

If efficacy can be stratified according to variation in genotype, there is the potential to use a genetic marker for phase III enrichment with responders. The result could be fewer, smaller, and shorter studies. Similarly, if adverse safety events are associated with a specific genotype, then a subset of patients could be excluded, or more closely monitored during a study to increase the understanding of a drug's safety profile [45,46]. Overall, knowing the potential for genotype-dependent variation in efficacy, dose/response, or safety events can be crucial for proof-of-concept decisions, financial commitment to phase III studies, and commercial planning activities [47].

16.3.2.3 Phase III

Phase III involves testing in many hundred to thousands of patients and provides increased evidence in the therapeutic benefit and provides confidence around the safety profile and informs the benefit/risk equation. Registration is the benchmark for success at this stage. However, it should be noted that only 50% of drugs that enter phase III testing are successfully registered, and many that are do not reach their full potential [6]. Often phase IV or pharmacovigilance studies are requested by regulatory authorities to further establish the safety profile of the therapeutic.

Ideally for late-phase development, genetic markers that were linked to relevant drug response phenotypes in earlier development studies can be confirmed, and the clinical and commercial impact of utilizing genetic stratification can be more thoroughly examined. This is critical if the drug label will depend on patient genotype or if the genetic markers are being developed as a companion diagnostic. In phase III there is an opportunity to power clinical studies with sufficient number of subjects to thoroughly examine genotype by treatment effect(s), particularly in prospective study designs. This is a very efficient strategy to validate a pharmacogenetics research hypothesis in phase III that has emerged from earlier phase I and phase II studies. For example, a retrospective analysis of a phase II study of rosiglitazone-treated Alzheimer's disease patients revealed a very strong genotype by treatment effect. Patients with ApoE4, either homozygous or heterozygous, received no benefit from rosiglitazone, whereas those who were non-ApoE4 did respond positively to treatment [48]. This information was utilized to design the phase III clinical study strategy powered to test the genotype by treatment effect.

In addition, the large number of subjects in phase III studies allows hypothesis-free pharmacogenetics studies that assay very large panels of genetic variants or even use genomewide approaches. These hypothesis-free approaches can be particularly important for identifying genetic contributions to continuous phenotypic variation rather than investigation of distinct outliers or bimodal phenotype distributions [49]. Although pharmacogenetics is an emerging science, there are examples of its contributions at every stage of the pharmaceutical R&D pipeline even benefiting drugs after regulatory approval (see below).

As above, discussed there is a great deal of research activity identifying genes involved in disease. Many of the implicated genes have already entered the pharmaceutical pipeline. Because of the long timelines needed to identify and refine a small molecule to interact with any gene product, it will likely be a decade or more before we realize the benefit of these discoveries in new therapeutics. In addition, one needs to recognize that genetic contributors to disease risk are also being used to stratify patients for efficacy in clinical testing programs. The example of ApoE, a marker associated with age of disease onset for Alzheimer's disease (cited above) is one such example. A number of clinical development programs for new AD treatments have reported efficacy stratification based on patients ApoE4 carriage [50]. Other newly identified disease risk factors are also being evaluated as markers for patient stratification of efficacy [51].

16.3.2.4 Postapproval

Because the application of pharmacogenetics research across the drug discovery–development pipeline is a relatively new practice, there are a number of examples where it has been applied to therapeutics after registration resulting in drug label updates. As pharmacogenetics research becomes integrated into all phases of clinical development there will be an increasing number of examples of new therapeutics launched with genomic information on the labels. Indeed, the US FDA is developing guidelines for drug sponsors on the codevelopment of a therapeutic and an associated test [4]. However, there are a number of considerations that support incorporating a pharmacogenetics research strategy in postapproval drug trials. Postregistration trials can be undertaken to support conditional approval by regulatory authorities, further evaluate efficacy and safety as the number of dosed patients increases, or potentially to investigate expansion to larger patient populations and/or extension to novel indications. There is increasing focus on the risk associated with novel, as well as established, therapeutics [52,53]. In addition, rare, idiosyncratic, adverse drug reactions are only seen when many thousands of patients are treated and the drug is prescribed to more geographically diverse populations.

Some more recent examples of postregistration pharmacogenetics studies that resulted in label changes include:

1. *Warfarin.* Warfarin is an anticoagulant that has been in widespread use for many decades. Several factors must be considered in selecting the appropriate dose for an individual patient (age, gender, weight, etc.). Not achieving the effective dose puts patients at risk by deriving no benefit and increasing the risk for an adverse event, and necessitates multiple physician visits. Variation in a cytochrome P450 (CYP2C9) and the vitamin K epoxide reductase (VKOR1) were found to contribute to the variation in effective dose seen in patients [54,55]. The FDA updated the label for warfarin to reflect these genetic findings in 2007 [56]. More recently, the International Warfarin Pharmacogenetics Consortium reported that use of a pharmacogenetic dosing algorithm was more effective than the clinical algorithm in dosing patients at the lower and higher dose ranges of warfarin to achieve the therapeutic benefit [57]. A number of ongoing prospective studies are underway to assess the clinical utility and pharmacoeconomic benefit of adopting the pharmacogenetics test.
2. *Abacavir.* Abacavir is a nucleoside reverse transcriptase inhibitor (NRTI) used successfully for the treatment of HIV. However, a small percentage of patients have a hypersensitivity reaction with repeated treatment, and this adverse event resulted in a blackbox warning and the institution of a postmarketing pharmacovigilance program. A series of well-designed pharmacogenetic analyses conducted by both the drug manufacturer and academic groups identified a pharmacogenetic marker (*HLA-B**5701*) that demonstrates—via both observational and a prospective, genotype-guided, double-blind, randomized clinical trial—highly specific and sensitive clinical utility, as well as generalizability across racially diverse populations [58,59]. This body of evidence led the FDA to issue a package insert change in July 2008 to include a statement that

    > Prior to initiating therapy with abacavir, screening for the *HLA-B**5701* allele is recommended; this approach has been found to decrease the risk of hypersensitivity reaction. Screening is also recommended prior to re-initiation of abacavir in patients of unknown *HLA-B**5701* status who have previously tolerated abacavir".

    The European Union (EU) product labels were updated earlier in January 2008 with the indication statement that "before initiating treatment with abacavir, screening for carriage of the *HLA-B**5701* allele should be performed in any HIV-infected patient, irrespective of racial origin." The use of the diagnostic test for *HLA-B**5701* increased 9-fold in the first 6 months postannouncement of the results [60], and this increased utilization of the diagnostic test transpired prior to abacavir label changes by the FDA. Clinicians attribute the increased use of the drug to increased confidence in its safety using the diagnostic [61].

3. *Clopidogrel.* Clopidogrel is a prodrug used for antiplatelet therapy, and is one of the most frequently prescribed drugs in the world. The active metabolite is an inhibitor of the platelet cell surface receptor $P2Y_{12}$. There is significant interindividual variation in the PD of clopidogrel, which can lead to increased risk of adverse cardiovascular events and variable efficacy [62]. Some of this variability in PD can be explained by genetic variation in the enzyme (CYP2C19) that converts clopidogrel from a prodrug to the active form [63–66]. In 2009 the FDA updated the drug label to reflect these genetic findings [67]. Ongoing characterization of the clinical utility of these markers may provide physicians with treatment guidelines for antiplatelet therapy, especially as new drugs in the same class that are not as sensitive to PD fluctuations due to genetic variation in ADME genes become available [68]. The pharmacogenetics effect with clopidogrel is a good example of the genetics impacting the PK, the PD, and the clinical outcome of drug therapy with a clear functional underpinning.
4. *Panitumumab and Cetuximab.* These are monoclonal antibodies directed at the extracellular domain of the epidermal growth factor receptor (EGFR) indicated for treatment of colon cancer. Cetuximab was approved by the FDA in 2004, and panitumumab was approved in 2007. After approval, retrospective analysis indicated that patients with tumors carrying a wild-type form of KRAS (the gene product functions in the EGFR signaling cascade) demonstrated improved efficacy response while those with a mutant form of KRAS responded less favorably to therapy with panitumumab or cetuximab [69]. Interestingly, the EMEA approved panitumumab in 2007 for use in patients with a wild-type KRAS. In mid-2009 the FDA updated the US labels to include information reflecting these findings on KRAS status. The use of retrospective data analysis to effect label changes for panitumumab and cetuximab sparked considerable debate in the scientific, pharmaceutical, and regulatory communities regarding about retrospective analysis of clinical data [70].
5. *PegIFNα2a or PegIFNα2b with Ribavarin.* This is the recommended course for treatment of chronic hepatitis C infection. Investigators have published the results of a study of the comparative effectiveness of treatment with one of the two interferons given in combination with ribavarin [71,72]. The investigators went on to study the potential genetic contribution to treatment response. Subjects were genotyped with a high-density array ($>$600,000 markers), and a single SNP was found to be strongly associated with treatment response. The associated SNP is in the vicinity of the IFN3 structural gene. This SNP accounted for a significant portion of the variable treatment response seen in individuals and between ethnic groups. The report is noteworthy in that it used a hypothesis-free, genomewide association scan approach to identify genetic factors for treatment efficacy and identified a host factor that influenced treatment efficacy for an infectious agent. It demonstrates that genomewide

association scan [73] approaches can be used to identify genetic factors contributing to both the efficacy and safety of therapeutics.

These examples are illustrative of the breadth and rapid pace of developments and are not intended as a complete listing. The reader is referred to the FDA website for the table on validated genomic biomarkers included on drug labels [73]. It is important to be recognize that pharmacogenetics effects are being seen for a broad range of widely used drugs, not just for niche products.

Because of the limited number of patients enrolled in clinical trials, and the limited time of drug exposure, the postapproval setting is the only option for investigating drug-associated rare adverse events. It has been recognized for some time that genetics contributes to drug-associated serious adverse events [74]. The Serious Adverse Event Consortium (SAEC) [75] is a public–private partnership combining the expertise of the pharmaceutical industry, the Wellcome Trust, the FDA, and academic experts to investigate the genetic contribution to these events. Using high-density (>1 million SNPs) genomewide association techniques, the SAEC has reported identification of genetic risk markers for drug-associated hepatotoxicity [76]. Drug-associated liver injury is the primary cause of failure for toxicity in development and has been the reason for withdrawal of a number of marketed medicines [77,78]. Identification of genetic markers for risk of rare, serious adverse events may contribute to a reduction of their incidence in clinical practice. The preceding examples highlight the importance of collecting a DNA/biological sample during the course of clinical development. The outcome of clinical trials can be difficult to predict, and having the genetic resources collected and available to address emergent issues is a prudent strategy.

One could speculate on the course of clinical development and use in the practice of healthcare had these genetic tests been pursued as companion diagnostics. Genetically stratified clinical trials may have been performed faster, at less expense, and with less exposure and risk to patients with a more favorable therapeutic outcome. The examples also highlight that once a therapeutic is available on the market; academic and institutional investigators can, and will, explore the genetic effects. Increasingly groups that have access to large patient populations and the associated healthcare/treatment data (e.g., healthcare providers and pharmacy benefits managers) are investigating the role of genetics in therapeutic outcomes [79]. Knowledge of pharmacology does not stop at registration, and regulatory agencies worldwide evaluate and include new findings in drug labels. Making DNA collection a routine component of clinical trials is a prudent step to facilitate new findings and reduce the inherent uncertainty associated with new therapeutics, particularly as they transition to increased patient exposure.

It is important to recognize the unique role of the pharmaceutical industry in the application of pharmacogenetics research. The clinical development process is tightly controlled (with strict inclusion criteria) and focuses on novel therapeutics. These clinical studies offer the opportunity to apply pharmacogenetics research to therapeutics with the highest degree of uncertainty, those transitioning into widespread use following registration. The drug sponsor also has access to a wealth of clinical information that can help to elucidate any potential genetic involvement in drug exposure to patients.

16.4 NONPHARMACEUTICAL INDUSTRY DRIVERS OF PHARMACOGENETICS

Although evidence of pharmacogenetics research effects is well established [34], its routine application to R&D and in providing healthcare to patients is an example of a disruptive technology [80]. As with other disruptive technologies, the existing dominant market entities are generally slow adopters. Market forces that create a pull for the disruptive technology play a significant role in broad uptake of the new technology and this is beginning to be seen for pharmacogenetics research as well. The pharmaceutical and healthcare sectors are undergoing rapid and dramatic change with increasing focus on therapeutic value and a drive for comparative effectiveness studies [81]. Strategies that enable personalized medicine (i.e., pharmacogenetics research), with the goal of increasing the precision and effectiveness of medical treatments for the individual patient are increasingly in demand [81]. A number of academic institutions and medical centers have established personalized medicine programs to enhance medical training and promote research in this field [82]. Increasingly, providers of healthcare services recognize the value in pharmacogenetics strategies and are investing in research and development programs.

As the science of pharmacogenetics moves from bench to bedside, it will require cooperation across a number of constituent groups. Pharmaceutical companies, biotechnology companies, regulatory agencies, diagnostic companies, clinical testing laboratories, physicians, patients, and payers all contribute to assessing the value of a test. Even assessing the economic value of a test or targeted therapeutic will require changes to the way these entities work together and to redefine how value is measured and reimbursed [83]. An important constituency that has only quite recently come under to the discussion is the healthcare payer community. The Drug Information Association (DIA) has sponsored an interactive workshop to bring the payer perspective to the discussions on pharmacogenetics research. The results of that session highlighted payer enthusiasm for this research and the need to demonstrate the clinical utility of the results, understand individual response, and ensure appropriate use of genomic information on drug labels [79]. As the number of examples of predictive genetic tests increases, the data needed to perform pharmacoeconomic modeling to evaluate the cost-effectiveness of using pharmacogenetic tests are becoming sufficient [83,84]. As new pharmacogenetic markers are discovered, research will need to demonstrate the utility and cost-effectiveness of these tests. There will be an increasing need to move from discovering a genetic association to establishing clinical utility for the patient and healthcare providers alike. Collaboration between agencies of the US government (Center for Disease Control and NIH) has established the Genomic Application in Practice and Prevention Network (GAPPNet) to examine the clinical utility of gene discoveries [85].

One fundamental challenge for the pharmaceutical industry is a result of its own success. The decades since 1980 have witnessed an unequaled period of productivity in the discovery and development of new therapeutics. From chronic diseases (e.g., diabetes, heart disease, asthma, hypertension) to acute conditions (antimicrobials, antivirals) to vaccines, today's medicine cabinet contains a large number of treatment options with generally favorable safety profiles. This productivity has benefited all members of the healthcare continuum (patients, physicians, payers, and society) and has enabled the pharmaceutical industry to continue to invest generously in the discovery and development of new therapeutics. With the registration of each of new drug, the acceptance threshold for the subsequent therapeutics is elevated. This is driving an interest in reducing the uncertainty in therapeutic decisionmaking for the individual patient, consistent with the actual practice of medicine.

As the science of pharmacogenetics has matured, global regulatory agencies have increasingly recognized its application in establishing benefit/risk profiles for therapeutics. In particular, the US FDA has advocated use of new science to improve the regulatory process (critical path initiative) and created a mechanism, the voluntary genomic data submission (VGDS), for a drug sponsor to discuss biomarker data with scientists from the agency [86]. The success of the VGDS initiative has led to a broadening of the scope to include exploratory technologies and a rebranding to voluntary exploratory data submission (VXDS). As of this writing, there have been over 50 such discussions, and the format has expanded to joint sessions with scientists from the European and Japanese regulatory agencies. In addition, the FDA has published pharmacogenetic guidance documents for industry (*Pharmacogenetic Tests and Genetic Tests for Heritable Markers*, 2007) and a number of white papers discussing use of pharmacogenetics data in the drug development and review process [87].

The European Medicines Agency (EMEA) has been actively involved in pharmacogenetics research and has incorporated information obtained from this research on approved drug labels. In May 2007, the agency published a reflection paper on the use of pharmacogenetics data in the PK evaluation of medicines [88]. In April 2009, recognizing advances in the field of ADME–pharmacogenetics research, the agency announced its intention to develop guidelines to support integration of this science into the evaluation of medicinal products [89].

In 2008 the International Committee on Harmonization of Technical Requirements for Registration of Pharmaceuticals for Human Use (ICH) provided guidance on pharmacogenetics research to the drug development industry [90]. The E15 *Definitions for Genomic Biomarkers, Pharmacogenomics, Pharmacogenetics, Genomic Data and Sample Coding Categories* provides important standardization of terms for the field—an important step toward incorporating these data in worldwide registration packages. The support for, and utilization of, pharmacogenetics by regulatory agencies indicates that pharmacogenetics research is becoming a routine tool in the approval and use of therapeutics. The ability to sequence an individual's entire genome is becoming increasingly cost-effective [91]. The long-term impact on healthcare of the escalating trend toward personal genomics (individuals obtaining their own genetic/genomic profile [92]) is unknown at this time.

16.5 CONCLUSION

It is now evident to all the stakeholders within the healthcare continuum (patients, physicians, regulators, payers) that the tools, technologies, and strategies to used elucidate the genetic contributions to pathophysiology and therapeutic response have proved successful. A number of trends are aligning to foster change in the discovery, development, and use of new therapeutics, and all healthcare stakeholders acknowledge that the status quo in pharmaceutical R&D is nonsustainable. The high attrition rates and reduced productivity cannot be continued indefinitely. Patients will continue to display variable responses to therapeutics, in part because of the inherent variation in their underlying genetic makeup. Regulatory agencies, healthcare providers, and healthcare payers will require evidence of positive benefit/risk ratios on the individual level. There is wide recognition that harnessing the information in the genome will be a significant contributor to individualized patient care and will significantly inform the value proposition for individual patients.

More recent progress in understanding the science of the genome, technological developments, and bioinformatic/analytical approaches demonstrates that we can identify genetic markers that contribute to the safe and efficacious use of therapeutics. The rapidly evolving regulatory and business climate is putting a premium on increasing specificity and certainty around therapeutic choice. The pharmaceutical industry has recognized the opportunity for improved precision and decreased attrition during the drug development cycle and has invested in pharmacogenetic capabilities. Routine application of pharmacogenetics will benefit patients, healthcare providers, payers, and the pharmaceutical industry.

REFERENCES

1. Spear BB, Heath-Chiozzi M, Huff J. Clinical application of pharmacogenetics. *Trends Mol. Med.* 2001; **7**(5):201–204.
2. Lander ES, Linton LM, Birren B, Nusbaum C, Zody MC, Baldwin J, Devon K, Dewar K, Doyle M, FitzHugh W, Funke R, Gage D, Harris K, Heaford A, Howland J, et al. Initial sequencing and analysis of the human genome. *Nature* 2001; **409**(6822):860–921.
3. Venter JC, Adams MD, Myers EW, Li PW, Mural RJ, Sutton GG, Smith HO, Yandell M, Evans CA, Holt RA, Gocayne JD, Amanatides P, Ballew RM, Huson DH, et al. The sequence of the human genome. *Science* 2001; **291**(5507):1304–1351.
4. US Food and Drug Administration (FDA) Genomics Website. (`http://www.fda.gov/Drugs/ScienceResearch/ResearchAreas/Pharmacogenetics/default.htm`).
5. US FDA. *Innovation or Stagnation: Challenge and Opportunity on the Critical Path to New Medical Products*. available at `http://www.fda.gov/downloads/ScienceResearch/SpecialTopics/CriticalPathInitiative/CriticalPathOpportunitiesReports/ucm113411.pdf`; accessed 3/04).
6. Kola I, Landis J. Can the pharmaceutical industry reduce attrition rates? *Nat. Rev. Drug. Discov.* 2004; **3**(8):711–715.

7. Shah RR. Can pharmacogenetics help rescue drugs withdrawn from the market? *Pharmacogenomics* 2006; **7**(6):889–908.
8. US FDA. List of drug products that have been withdrawn or removed from the market for reasons of safety or effectiveness. Food and Drug Administration, HHS. Final rule. *Fed Regist*, 1999; **64**(44):10944–10947.
9. Roses AD. Pharmacogenetics and the practice of medicine. *Nature* 2000; **405** (6788):857–865.
10. Roses AD. Pharmacogenetics in drug discovery and development: A translational perspective. *Nat. Rev. Drug Discov.* 2008; **7**(10):807–817.
11. Garrod AE. *Inborn errors of metabolism*, 2nd ed. London: H. Frowde and Hodder & Stoughton, 1923.
12. Morrow JF. Recombinant DNA techniques. *Methods Enzymol.* 1979; **68**:3–24.
13. Sanger F, Nicklen S, Coulson AR. DNA sequencing with chain-terminating inhibitors. *Proc. Natl. Acad. Sci. USA*, 1977; **74**(12):5463–5467.
14. Anonymous. Finishing the euchromatic sequence of the human genome. *Nature* 2004; **431** (7011):931–945.
15. Sachidanandam R, Weissman D, Schmidt SC, Kakol JM, Stein LD, Marth G, Sherry S, Mullikin JC, Mortimore BJ, Willey DL, Hunt SE, Cole CG, Coggill PC, et al. A map of human genome sequence variation containing 1.42 million single nucleotide polymorphisms. *Nature* 2001; **409**(6822):928–933.
16. Frazer KA, Ballinger DG, Cox DR, Hinds DA, Stuve LL, Gibbs RA, Belmont JW, Boudreau A, Hardenbol P, Leal SM, Pasternak S, Wheeler DA, Willis TD, et al. A second generation human haplotype map of over 3.1 million SNPs. *Nature*, 2007; **449** (7164):851–861.
17. Koenig M, Hoffman EP, Bertelson CJ, Monaco AP, Feener C, Kunkel LM. Complete cloning of the Duchenne muscular dystrophy (DMD) cDNA and preliminary genomic organization of the DMD gene in normal and affected individuals. *Cell* 1987; **50** (3):509–517.
18. Roses AD, Saunders AM. APOE is a major susceptibility gene for Alzheimer's disease. *Curr. Opin. Biotechnol.* 1994; **5**(6):663–667.
19. Florez JC, Hirschhorn J, Altshuler D. The inherited basis of diabetes mellitus: Implications for the genetic analysis of complex traits. *Annu. Rev. Genomics Hum. Genet* 2003; **4**:257–291.
20. Roses AD, Burns DK, Chissoe S, Middleton L, St. Jean P. Disease-specific target selection: A critical first step down the right road. *Drug Discov. Today* 2005; **10**(3):177–189.
21. Kraus VB, Jordan JM, Doherty M, Wilson AG, Moskowitz R, Hochberg M, Loeser R, Hooper M, Renner JB, Crane MM, Hastie P, Sundseth S, Atif U. The genetics of generalized osteoarthritis (GOGO) study: Study design and evaluation of osteoarthritis phenotypes. *Osteoarthritis Cartila.* 2007; **15**(2):120–127.
22. Stirnadel H, Lin X, Ling H, Song K, Barter P, Kesaniemi YA, Mahley R, McPherson R, Waeber G, Bersot T, Cohen J, Grundy S, Mitchell B, Mooser V, Waterworth D. Genetic and phenotypic architecture of metabolic syndrome-associated components in dyslipidemic and normolipidemic subjects: The GEMS study. *Atherosclerosis* 2008; **197** (2):868–876.
23. Pillai SG, Ge D, Zhu G, Kong X, Shianna KV, Need AC, Feng S, Hersh CP, Bakke P, Gulsvik A, Ruppert A, Lodrup Carlsen KC, Roses A, Anderson W, Rennard SI, et al. A

genome-wide association study in chronic obstructive pulmonary disease (COPD): Identification of two major susceptibility loci. *PLoS Genet.* 2009; **5**(3):e1000421.

24. Manolio TA, Rodriguez LL, Brooks L, Abecasis G, Ballinger D, Daly M, Donnelly P, Faraone SV, Frazer K, Gabriel S, Gejman P, Guttmacher A, Harris EL., et al. New models of collaboration in genome-wide association studies: The Genetic Association Information Network. *Nat. Genet.* 2007; **39**(9):1045–1051.
25. The Genetic Assocation Information Network (GAIN) (available at `http://www.genome.gov/19518664`.)
26. NCBI. The Database of Genotypes and Phenotypes (dbGaP) (available `http://www.ncbi.nlm.nih.gov/sites/entrez?db=gap`).
27. Anonymous. Genome-wide association study of 14,000 cases of seven common diseases and 3,000 shared controls. *Nature* 2007; **447**(7145):661–678.
28. Kaiser J. DNA sequencing. A plan to capture human diversity in 1000 genomes. *Science* 2008; **319**(5862):395.
29. Williams JA. Andersson T, Andersson TB, Blanchard R, Behm MO, Cohen N, Edeki T, Franc M, Hillgren KM, Johnson KJ, Katz DA, Milton MN, Murray BP, et al. PhRMA white paper on ADME pharmacogenomics. *J. Clin. Pharmacol.* 2008; **48**(7):849–889.
30. DiMasi JA, Hansen RW, Grabowski HG. The price of innovation: New estimates of drug development costs. *J. Health Econ.* 2003; **22**(2):151–185.
31. Garnier JP. Rebuilding the R&D engine in big pharma. *Harv. Business. Rev.* 2008; **86** (5):68–70, 72–76 128.
32. Cuatrecasas P. Drug discovery in jeopardy. *J. Clin. Invest.* 2006; **116**(11):2837–2842.
33. Woodcock J, Woosley R. The FDA critical path initiative and its influence on new drug development. *Annu. Rev. Med.* 2008; **59**:1–12.
34. Roden DM, George AL, Jr. The genetic basis of variability in drug responses. *Nat. Rev. Drug. Discov.* 2002; **1**(1):37–44.
35. Dickinson GL, Rezaee S, Proctor NJ, Lennard MS, Tucker GT, Rostami-Hodjegan, A. Incorporating in vitro information on drug metabolism into clinical trial simulations to assess the effect of CYP2D6 polymorphism on pharmacokinetics and pharmacodynamics: dextromethorphan as a model application. *J. Clin. Pharmacol.* 2007; **47** (2):175–186.
36. Gibbs JP, Hyland R, Youdim K. Minimizing polymorphic metabolism in drug discovery: Evaluation of the utility of in vitro methods for predicting pharmacokinetic consequences associated with CYP2D6 metabolism. *Drug Metab. Dispos.* 2006; **34**(9):1516–1522.
37. Hou T, Wang J, Zhang W, Wang W, Xu X. Recent advances in computational prediction of drug absorption and permeability in drug discovery. *Curr. Med. Chem.* 2006; **13** (22):2653–2667.
38. Pharm GKB.The pharmacogenomics knowledge base (PharmGKB), (available at `http://www.pharmgkb.org/`).
39. Glickman, SW, McHutchison JG, Peterson ED, Cairns CB, Harrington RA, Califf RM, Schulman KA. Ethical and scientific implications of the globalization of clinical research. *New Engl. J. Med.* 2009; **360**(8):816–823.
40. FDA. Roche AmpliChip Cytochrome P450 Genotyping test and Affymetrix GeneChip Microarray Instrumentation System—K042259, 2004 (information available at `http://www.fda.gov/MedicalDevices/ProductsandMedicalProcedures/`

DeviceApprovalsandClearances/Recently-ApprovedDevices/ucm078879.htm).

41. Katz DA, Murray B, Bhathena A, Sahelijo L. Defining drug disposition determinants: A pharmacogenetic-pharmacokinetic strategy. *Nat. Rev. Drug. Discov.* 2008; **7**(4):293–305.
42. Hinman L, Spear B, Tsuchihashi Z, Kelly J, Bross P, Goodsaid F, Kalush F. Drug-diagnostic codevelopment strategies: FDA and industry dialog at the 4th FDA/DIA/PhRMA/PWG/BIO Pharmacogenomics Workshop. *Pharmacogenomics* 2009; **10**(1):127–136.
43. Myrand SP, Sekiguchi K, Man MZ, Lin X, Tzeng RY, Teng CH, Hee B, Garrett M, Kikkawa H, Lin CY, Eddy SM, Dostalik J, Mount J, Azuma J, Fujio Y, et al. Pharmacokinetics/genotype associations for major cytochrome P450 enzymes in native and first- and third-generation Japanese populations: Comparison with Korean, Chinese, and Caucasian populations. *Clin. Pharmacol. Ther.* 2008; **84**(3):347–361.
44. Klotsman M, York TP, Pillai SG, Vargas-Irwin C, Sharma SS, van den Oord EJ, Anderson WH. Pharmacogenetics of the 5-lipoxygenase biosynthetic pathway and variable clinical response to montelukast. *Pharmacogenet. Genomics.* 2007; **17**(3):189–196.
45. Ingelman-Sundberg M. Pharmacogenomic biomarkers for prediction of severe adverse drug reactions. *New Engl. J. Med.* 2008; **358**(6):637–639.
46. Woodcock J, Lesko LJ, Pharmacogenetics—tailoring treatment for the outliers. *New Engl. J. Med.* 2009; **360**(8):811–813.
47. Roses AD. The medical and economic roles of pipeline pharmacogenetics: Alzheimer's disease as a model of efficacy and HLA-B(*)5701 as a model of safety. *Neuropsychopharmacology* 2009; **34**(1):6–17.
48. Risner ME, Saunders AM, Altman JF, Ormandy GC, Craft S, Foley IM, Zvartau-Hind ME, Hosford DA, Roses AD. Efficacy of rosiglitazone in a genetically defined population with mild-to-moderate Alzheimer's disease. *Pharmacogenomics J.* 2006; **6**(4):246–254.
49. Nelson MR, Bacanu SA, Mosteller M, Li L, Bowman CE, Roses AD, Lai EH, Ehm MG. Genome-wide approaches to identify pharmacogenetic contributions to adverse drug reactions. *Pharmacogenomics J.* 2009; **9**(1):23–33.
50. Roses AD, Saunders AM, Huang Y, Strum J, Weisgraber KH, Mahley RW. Complex disease-associated pharmacogenetics: Drug efficacy, drug safety, and confirmation of a pathogenetic hypothesis (Alzheimer's disease). *Pharmacogenomics J.* 2007; **7**(1):10–28.
51. Cowey CL, Rathmell WK. VHL gene mutations in renal cell carcinoma: Role as a biomarker of disease outcome and drug efficacy. *Curr. Oncol. Rep.* 2009; **11**(2):94–101.
52. US FDA. *The Sentinel Initiative: National Strategy for Monitoring Medical Product Safety* (available at http://www.fda.gov/downloads/Safety/FDAsSentinelInitiative/UCM124701.pdf; accessed 5/08).
53. US FDA. FDA Sentinel Initiative Homepage.
54. Cavallari, LH, Limdi NA. Warfarin pharmacogenomics. *Curr. Opin. Mol. Ther.* 2009; **11**(3):243–251.
55. Kim MJ, Huang SM, Meyer UA, Rahman A, Lesko LJ. A regulatory science perspective on warfarin therapy: A pharmacogenetic opportunity. *J. Clin. Pharmacol.* 2009. **49**(2):138–146.
56. Press release, FDA approves updated warfarin (coumadin) prescribing information New genetic information may help providers improve initial dosing estimates of the anticoagulant for individual patients (available at http://www.fda.gov/NewsEvents/Newsroom/PressAnnouncements/2007/ucm108967.htm; accessed 8/07).

57. Klein TE, Altman RB, Eriksson N, Gage BF, Kimmel SE, Lee MT, Limdi NA, Page D, Roden DM, Wagner MJ, Caldwell MD, Johnson JA. Estimation of the warfarin dose with clinical and pharmacogenetic data. *New Engl. J. Med.* 2009; **360**(8):753–764.

58. Saag M, Balu R, Phillips E, Brachman P, Martorell C, Burman W, Stancil B, Mosteller M, Brothers C, Wannamaker P, Hughes A, Sutherland-Phillips D, Mallal S, Shaefer M. High sensitivity of human leukocyte antigen-b*5701 as a marker for immunologically confirmed abacavir hypersensitivity in white and black patients. *Clin. Infect. Dis.* 2008; **46** (7):1111–1118.

59. Mallal S, Phillips E, Carosi G, Molina JM, Workman C, Tomazic J, Jagel-Guedes E, Rugina S, Kozyrev O, Cid JF, Hay P, Nolan D, Hughes S, Hughes A, Ryan S, et al. HLA-B*5701 screening for hypersensitivity to abacavir. *New Engl. J. Med.* 2008; **358** (6):568–579.

60. Lai-Goldman M, Faruki H. Abacavir hypersensitivity: A model system for pharmacogenetic test adoption. *Genet. Med.* 2008; **10**(12):874–878.

61. Rockstroh, JK, Hay PE, Leather DA. Personal expereinces of HLA-B*5701 genetic screening in routine clinical practice. *Touch Briefings: European Infectious Disease–HIV and AIDS*, 2007; Issue II (available at `http://www.touchbriefings.com/cdps/cditem.cfm?cid=5&nid=3024`).

62. Arguello Viudez L. Do antiplatelet agents (aspirin and other antiplatelets such as clopidogrel) increase the risk of hemorrhagic complications after endoscopic polypectomy or endoscopic sphincterotomy and should these drugs therefore be withdrawn 7-10 days before these procedures are performed?. *Gastroenterol. Hepatol.* 2009; **32**(4):318–320.

63. Collet JP, Hulot JS, Pena A, Villard E, Esteve JB, Silvain J, Payot L, Brugier D, Cayla G, Beygui F, Bensimon G, Funck-Brentano C, Montalescot G. Cytochrome P450 2C19 polymorphism in young patients treated with clopidogrel after myocardial infarction: A cohort study. *Lancet* 2009; **373**(9660):309–317.

64. Freedman JE, Hylek EM. Clopidogrel, genetics, and drug responsiveness. *New Engl. J. Med.* 2009; **360**(4):411–413.

65. Mega JL, Close SL, Wiviott SD, Shen L, Hockett RD, Brandt JT, Walker JR, Antman EM, Macias W, Braunwald E, Sabatine MS. Cytochrome p-450 polymorphisms and response to clopidogrel. *New Engl. J. Med.* 2009; **360**(4):354–362.

66. Simon T, Verstuyft C, Mary-Krause M, Quteineh L, Drouet E, Meneveau N, Steg PG, Ferrieres J, Danchin N, Becquemont L. Genetic determinants of response to clopidogrel and cardiovascular events. *New Engl. J. Med.* 2009; **360**(4):363–375.

67. Press release, Plavix (clopidogrel bisulfate) 75 mg tablets: Safety labeling changes approved by FDA Center for Drug Evaluation and Research (CDER) (available at `http://www.fda.gov/Safety/MedWatch/SafetyInformation/ucm165166.htm`; accessed 5/09).

68. Montalescot G, Wiviott SD, Braunwald E, Murphy SA, Gibson CM, McCabe CH, Antman EM. Prasugrel compared with clopidogrel in patients undergoing percutaneous coronary intervention for ST-elevation myocardial infarction (TRITON-TIMI 38): Double-blind, randomised controlled trial. *Lancet* 2009; **373**(9665):723–731.

69. Benvenuti S, Sartore-Bianchi A, Di Nicolantonio F, Zanon C, Moroni M, Veronese S, Siena S, Bardelli A. Oncogenic activation of the RAS/RAF signaling pathway impairs the response of metastatic colorectal cancers to anti-epidermal growth factor receptor antibody therapies. *Cancer Res.* 2007; **67**(6):2643–2648.

70. Mack GS. FDA holds court on post hoc data linking KRAS status to drug response. *Nat. Biotechnol.* 2009; **27**(2):110–112.

71. Ge D, Fellay J, Thompson AJ, Simon JS, Shianna KV, Urban TJ, Heinzen EL, Qiu P, Bertelsen AH, Muir AJ, Sulkowski M, McHutchison JG, Goldstein DB. Genetic variation in IL28B predicts hepatitis C treatment-induced viral clearance. *Nature* 2009; **46** (7262):399–401.

72. McHutchison JG, Lawitz EJ, Shiffman ML, Muir AJ, Galler GW, McCone J, Nyberg LM, Lee WM, Ghalib RH, Schiff ER, Galati JS, Bacon BR, Davis MN, et al. Peginterferon alfa-2b or alfa-2a with ribavirin for treatment of hepatitis C infection. *New Engl. J. Med.* 2009; **361**(6):580–593.

73. *Table of Valid Genomic Biomarkers in the Context of Approved Drug Labels*, 2008 (available at `http://www.fda.gov/Drugs/ScienceResearch/ResearchAreas/Pharmacogenetics/ucm083378.htm`).

74. Wilke RA, Lin DW, Roden DM, Watkins PB, Flockhart D, Zineh I, Giacomini KM, Krauss RM. Identifying genetic risk factors for serious adverse drug reactions: Current progress and challenges. *Nat. Rev. Drug Discov.* 2007; **6**(11):904–916.

75. Holden AL. The innovative use of a large-scale industry biomedical consortium to research the genetic basis of drug induced serious adverse events. *Drug Discov. Today Technol.* 2007; **4**(2):75–87.

76. Daly AK, Donaldson PT, Bhatnagar P, Shen Y, Pe'er I, Floratos A, Daly MJ, Goldstein DB, John S, Nelson MR, Graham J, Park BK, Dillon JF, Bernal W, et al. HLA-B*5701 genotype is a major determinant of drug-induced liver injury due to flucloxacillin. *Nat. Genet.* 2009; **41**(7):816–819.

77. Kaplowitz N. Idiosyncratic drug hepatotoxicity. *Nat. Rev. Drug Discov.* 2005; **4** (6):489–499.

78. Navarro VJ, Senior JR. Drug-related hepatotoxicity. *N Engl. J. Med.* 2006; **354**(7):731–739.

79. Epstein RS, Frueh FW, Geren D, Hummer D, McKibbin S, O'Connor S, Randhawa G, Zelman B. Payer perspectives on pharmacogenomics testing and drug development. *Pharmacogenomics* 2009; **10**(1):149–151.

80. Christensen CM, Bohmer R, Kenagy J. Will disruptive innovations cure health care? *Harv. Bus. Rev.* 2000; **78**(5):102–112, 199.

81. Priorities for Personalized Medicine, Report of the President's Council for Economic Advisors on Science and Tehcnology (available at `http://www.ostp.gov/galleries/PCAST/pcast_report_v2.pdf`; accessed 9/08).

82. Personalized Medicine Coalition. *The Case for Personalized Medicine* (available at `http://www.personalizedmedicinecoalition.org/about/about-personalized-medicine/the-case-for-personalized-medicine`; accessed 5/09).

83. Davis JC, Furstenthal L, Desai AA, Norris T, Sutaria S, Fleming E, Ma P. The microeconomics of personalized medicine: today's challenge and tomorrow's promise. *Nat. Rev. Drug Discov.* 2009; **8**(4):279–286.

84. Dervieux T, Bala MV. Overview of the pharmacoeconomics of pharmacogenetics. *Pharmacogenomics*, 2006; **7**(8):1175–1184.

85. Khoury MJ, Feero WG, Reyes M, Citrin T, Freedman A, Leonard D, Burke W, Coates R, Croyle RT, Edwards K, Kardia S, McBride C, Manolio T, Randhawa G. et al. The

genomic applications in practice and prevention network. *Genet. Med.* 2009; **11** (7):488–494.

86. US FDA. Genomic data submissions (available at http://www.fda.gov/Drugs/ScienceResearch/ResearchAreas/Pharmacogenetics/ucm083641.htm).
87. US FDA. Genomics at FDA—guidances, concept papers, and MaPPs (available at http://www.fda.gov/Drugs/ScienceResearch/ResearchAreas/Pharmacogenetics/ucm083673.htm).
88. EMEA. Reflection Paper on the use of pharmacogenetics in the pharmacokinetic evaluation of medicinal products (available at http://www.emea.europa.eu/pdfs/human/pharmacogenetics/12851706enfin.pdf; accessed 5/07).
89. EMEA. Concept paper on the development of a guideline on the use of pharmacogenomic methodologies in the pharmacokinetic evaluation of medicinal products (available at http://www.emea.europa.eu/pdfs/human/pharmacogenetics/6327009en.pdf; accessed 4/09).
90. US FDA. *Guidance for Industry: E15 Definitions for Genomic Biomarkers, Pharmacogenomics, Pharmacogenetics, Genomic Data and Sample Coding Categories* (available at http://www.fda.gov/downloads/Drugs/GuidanceComplianceRegulatoryInformation/Guidances/ucm073162.pdf; accessed 4/08).
91. Tucker T, Marra M, Friedman JM. Massively parallel sequencing: The next big thing in genetic medicine. *Am. J. Hum. Genet.* 2009; **85**(2):142–154.
92. McGuire AL, Cho MK, McGuire SE, Caulfield T. Medicine. The future of personal genomics. Science 2007; **317**(5845):1687.

CHAPTER 17

Role of Pharmacogenetics in Registration Processes

MYONG-JIN KIM, ISSAM ZINEH, SHIEW-MEI HUANG, and LAWRENCE J. LESKO
Food and Drug Administration, Silver Spring, Maryland, USA

17.1 INTRODUCTION

One of the major challenges in drug development and clinical practice is interindividual drug response variability. Genetic predisposition may be a significant contributor to individual drug response variation in clinical studies across all phases of a drug development program, and in clinical practice for already approved drugs. Understanding of the genetic variations in drug response opens the door to individualized therapy by identifying patients who are more (1) prone to experience adverse events from a drug and (2) likely to benefit from a particular therapy. Pharmacogenomics–pharmacogenetics research (the two terms will be used interchangeably here and abbreviated PGX, referring to either term) is positioned to be an important scientific tool in drug development and regulatory decisionmaking to improve the efficacy of drugs, personalize drug dosing, and minimize adverse drug reactions.

17.1.1 FDA Role in Pharmacogenomics/Pharmacogenetics and Personalized Medicine

The US Food and Drug Administration (FDA) recognizes the importance of pharmacogenomics and biomarkers and encourages the integration of their use in drug development and their appropriate use in clinical practice [1–3]. To facilitate this integration, the agency understands that an adequate framework for pharmacogenomic data assessment needs to be provided in a regulatory context. For example, the agency engages industry and other stakeholders in continuous dialog

Pharmacogenetics and Individualized Therapy, First Edition.
Edited by Anke-Hilse Maitland-van der Zee and Ann K. Daly.

by developing workshops dedicated to pharmacogenomics [4–10], developing infrastructure to address voluntary genomic data submissions [11], issuing guidances as the science matures [12–15], and assessing the impact of pharmacogenomics on public health [2]. The FDA works to advance its capabilities to analyze and interpret genomic data that come into the agency, and to communicate the relevant information in an understandable way in drug labels. Also, the agency is working to coordinate the efficient and timely review between centers in the agency as drugs are developed through the use of genetic and other biomarkers. These initiatives are discussed in detail below.

17.1.2 FDA Initiatives and Pharmacogenomics

In 2002, the Center for Drug Evaluation and Research (CDER) of the FDA articulated its commitment to pharmacogenetics in drug development and regulatory science [16]. In the subsequent 5 years, CDER took a leadership role through a series of workshops, guidances, and harmonization efforts dedicated to pharmacogenomic data submissions (Fig. 17.1) [17]. Other related activities that have become flagships of FDA genomics activities since 2002 include establishment of voluntary genomic submission [12] and biomarker qualification programs [18,19], formation of the Interdisciplinary Pharmacogenomics Review Group (IPRG) for review of voluntary pharmacogenomic data submissions, formation of a genomics group within the Office of Clinical Pharmacology to review pharmacogenomics data in regulatory submissions, development of data analysis tools for use in regulatory review and drug development [20], organization of the public–private–academia–government Micro-Array Quality Control (MAQC) consortium [21], development of online educational

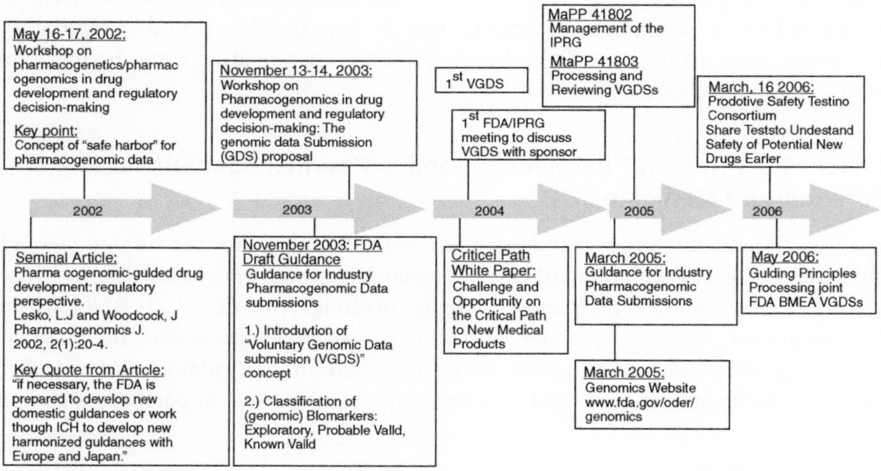

FIGURE 17.1 Role of the FDA Center for Drug Evaluation and Research (CDER) in regulation of pharmacogenomic data submissions.

tools, and updating drug labels to ensure the integration of pharmacogenomic information [3,11,22,23].

In May 2002, a workshop was held to discuss aspects surrounding genomic data submission to the FDA and to evaluate the regulatory impact of genomic data in current drug development. In this workshop on pharmacogenetics/pharmacogenomics (PGX) in drug development and regulatory decisionmaking, the concept of a safe harbor for the submission of pharmacogenomic data was first introduced [4,16]. Shortly thereafter, a draft guidance on pharmacogenomic data submissions was developed. In the following year, a second workshop on pharmacogenomics in drug development and regulatory decisionmaking, specifically, the genomic data submission (GDS) proposal, was held to gather public feedback on the FDA *Draft Guidance for Industry: Pharmacogenomic Data Submissions*. This guidance also introduced the concept of voluntary genomic data submissions (VGDSs) (Fig. 17.1) [5,17].

In 2004, FDA launched the *critical path initiative* [1], a national effort to stimulate and facilitate the modernization of the sciences through which regulated products are developed, evaluated, and manufactured. In March 2005, the FDA released a guidance on the agency's current thinking about pharmacogenomics and on data submission [12] and created a "genomics at FDA" web portal [2] that provides regulatory and background information on genomics. The program itself has recently been renamed VXDS, where the X stands simply for *exploratory*. The intent of this change was to reflect the diverse nature of exploratory biomarker data being received by the agency.

17.2 CRITICAL PATH INITIATIVES

Advances in preclinical and biomedical research have heightened expectations that more effective and safe medical products would quickly enter the marketplace. However, this anticipated surge in drug development is likely to take time, and has not yet occurred, as illustrated by the decreased number of new drug and biologic applications submitted to FDA more recently [1]. The number of new drug approvals have has decreased and remains low (Fig. 17.2). In 2008, only 17 new molecular entity drugs were approved [24]—a reflection of the decreased number of regulatory submissions over time.

Recognizing the slowdown in innovative medical therapies reaching patients, the FDA issued a report entitled Innovation or Stagnation: Challenge and Opportunity on the Critical Path to New Medical Products in 2004 [1]. The critical path initiative is aimed at facilitating development of innovative tools, such as predictive genetic tests, valid biomarkers, and information technology, to enable the efficient development and evaluation of safe and more effective drugs [1,25]. This document details why the agency believes drug development to be stagnant and highlights concerns regarding the rising cost of drug development coupled with the decline in new drug and biologic submissions to the FDA. It also emphasizes the urgent need to modernize the medical product development process to keep pace with scientific innovation, and proposes a series of opportunities to increase productivity. In March 2006, the FDA published

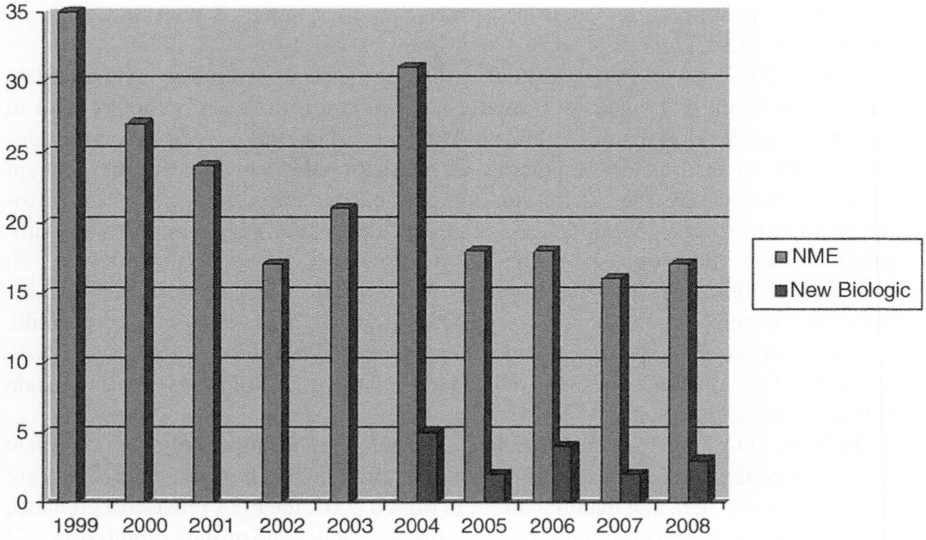

FIGURE 17.2 The number of new drug applications has decreased.

the second of two reports on the critical path to medical product development, the *Critical Path Opportunities Report and List* [26,27]. These documents recognize 76 specific scientific activities identified through outreach to patient groups, pharmaceutical industry, academia, other federal agencies, and other health-related organizations that are anticipated to bring promising new products to patients.

A key prospect described in the *Critical Path* document, and illustrated with a series of concrete proposals in the list of opportunities [26,27], is the use of pharmacogenomics and biomarkers in drug development. The emerging techniques of pharmacogenomics show great promise for contributing biomarkers to target responders, monitoring clinical response, identifying patients at risk for an adverse event, and serving as biomarkers of drug effectiveness. Therefore, integration of pharmacogenomics and biomarkers can serve as a bridge between discovery and the product development process. As a scientific opportunity to streamline the critical path, the use of pharmacogenomics can improve lead compound selection, better characterize disease, identify prognostic and predictive biomarkers, inform dose selection in later-phase clinical studies, and elucidate heterogeneity in drug exposure or response.

17.3 GUIDANCE FOR INDUSTRY

The FDA, as a regulatory agency, has a responsibility to provide a consistent policy and framework for pharmacogenomic data collection, submission, and assessment. To provide guidance about their use and clarify regulatory consequences of using these genomic markers, several guidance documents were developed that provide information on the agency's current thinking and the use of pharmacogenomics for regulatory decision making.

17.3.1 Guidances on Pharmacogenomic Data Submissions and Harmonization of Terms

In March 2005, the agency issued the *Guidance for Industry: Pharmacogenomic Data Submissions* [12]. This guidance explains when and how to submit pharmacogenomic data to the FDA, and introduces a novel, voluntary submission path for early, exploratory research data. This guidance also addresses related labeling. The main purpose of this guidance is to promote the use of pharmacogenomics in drug development and to encourage open and public sharing of data and information on pharmacogenomic test results. In general, the guidance addresses the following: (1) when to submit pharmacogenomic data to the agency, (2) what format and content to provide for submissions, and (3) how and when the genomic data would be used in regulatory decisionmaking. More specifically, this guidance lays out the cases when the regulations required pharmacogenomic data to be submitted and when the submission of such data would be on a voluntary basis. Depending on the cases, complete reports of pharmacogenomic studies, an abbreviated report, or synopsis would be submitted. In addition, the guidance addresses when the pharmacogenomic data would be considered sufficiently reliable to serve as the basis for regulatory decisionmaking, when these data would be considered only supportive to a decision, and when the data would not be used in regulatory decisionmaking.

The guidance defines categories of biomarkers as exploratory, probably valid, and known valid biomarkers. Although most pharmacogenomic measurements are considered exploratory biomarkers, many of those related to drug metabolism have well-established mechanistic and clinical significance and are currently being integrated into drug development and clinical practice. The guidance gives three decision trees based on the categories of biomarkers and the stage of drug development. These decision trees can be used to determine when genomic data can be submitted voluntarily, and when submissions of the data are required by FDA regulations. In addition, the guidance describes the format for submitting such data.

In addition to the abovementioned guidance, the FDA is a participating member of the International Conference on Harmonization of Technical Requirements for Registration of Pharmaceuticals for Human Use (ICH). ICH is a consortium of regulatory agencies from the United States, Europe, and Japan, and pharmaceutical industry representatives in the three regions with the goal of discussing scientific and technical issues around product registration. ICH issues guidelines related to a variety drug development topics, including pharmacogenomics. One such guidance is the E15 *Definitions for Genomic Biomarkers, Pharmacogenomics, Pharmacogenetics, Genomic Data and Sample Coding Categories* [13]. In the effort to develop harmonized approaches to drug regulation and ensure that consistent definitions of terminology are being applied to avoid the potential for either conflicting use of terms in regulatory documentation and guidelines or inconsistent interpretation, this guidance contains definitions of genomic biomarkers, pharmacogenomics, pharmacogenetics, and genomic data and sample coding categories.

17.3.2 Pharmacogenetic Tests and Genetic Tests for Heritable Markers

The *Guidance for Industry and FDA Staff—Pharmacogenetic Tests and Genetic Tests for Heritable Markers* was issued in draft in February 2006, and the final version was issued in June 2007 [14]. This guidance provides recommendations in preparing and reviewing premarket approval applications (PMA) and premarket notification [510(k)] submissions for pharmacogenetic and other human genetic tests. For an application for premarket approval or clearance of a device, a statement of the intended use of the device needs to be included. In addition, the intended use of the device for which approval or clearance is sought should specify the marker that the device is intended to measure, the clinical purpose of measuring the marker, and the populations to which the device is targeted. The following additional aspects are also covered in the guidance: analytical studies, software and instrumentation, comparison studies using clinical specimens, clinical evaluation studies comparing device performance to accepted diagnostic procedure(s), effectiveness of the device, and labeling.

17.4 VOLUNTARY EXPLORATORY DATA SUBMISSION (VXDS)

The US *FDA Guidance for Industry*: *Pharmacogenomic Data Submissions* first introduced the new concept of *voluntary genomic data submissions* (VGDSs). The purpose of this type of submission path is to create an environment in which regulators and sponsors can interact without making a regulatory decision. Specifically, this mechanism is recognized as a scientific, nonregulatory, nonbinding exchange regarding data on exploratory biomarkers not yet ready for use in regulatory decisionmaking. In addition, the program has created a novel way to interact with industry on a more informal level, with a focus on the scientific rather than regulatory interpretation of the results presented. This approach has greatly facilitated an early interaction between the two parties and allowed several biomarker-driven drug development programs to move forward effectively. Since its first introduction in 2003, the voluntary submission program has expanded so that all other -omic (or exploratory) data can be submitted under the new *voluntary exploratory data submission* (VXDS) program.

Pharmacogenomic data that are required to be submitted follow the existing regulations when such data are used for regulatory decisionmaking, provide supportive information, and are derived from known valid or probable valid pharmacogenomic biomarkers. However, exploratory or research data or reports are not required to be submitted under an investigational new drug (IND), new drug application (NDA), or biologics license application (BLA) under the VXDS. Voluntary submissions can benefit both the industry and the FDA in a general way by providing a means for sponsors to ensure that regulatory scientists are familiar with, and prepared to appropriately evaluate, future genomic submissions [11].

To facilitate VXDSs, FDA has established a cross-center IPRG to ensure high-quality review of these voluntary submissions, to work on policy development, and, on request, to advise review divisions on interpretation and evaluation of pharmacogenomic data. The IPRG is responsible for establishing a scientific and regulatory framework for reviewing genomic data. The process for voluntarily submitting genomic data to the agency is further detailed in the document on processing and reviewing voluntary genomic data submissions (VGDSs) [28].

Finally, joint VXDS meetings with the European Medicines Agency (EMA) have helped generate consensus on opportunities and limitations of genomic data in drug development and regulatory review. The two agencies issued in 2006 the *Guiding Principles for Processing Joint FDA/EMEA VGDSs*, which describe how bilateral VXDSs are being processed and reviewed [15].

17.5 BIOMARKER QUALIFICATION PROCESS

Pharmacogenomics and the characterization of genomic biomarkers have become a part of research and development for new therapeutics since the 1990s. However, if these biomarkers are to be used as definitive evidence suitable for supporting registration, they must be validated. The analytical and clinical validity of biomarkers must be demonstrated using relevant clinical samples to assure performance in drug development and clinical practice [3].

A *valid biomarker* is defined as "a biomarker that is measured in an analytical test system with well-established performance characteristics and for which there is an established scientific framework or body of evidence that elucidates the physiologic, toxicologic, pharmacologic, or clinical significance of the test results" [12]. An example of biomarker validity is implicit in the definition of biomarker use in approved drug labels [19]. A table of valid genomic biomarkers in the context of approved drug labels can be found on the FDA website [29]. It provides a list of valid genomic biomarkers, links to pharmacogenomic data that support their validity, and recommendations for the clinical use of some of these biomarkers.

Biomarkers can be classified as exploratory, probably valid, or known valid [12]. In order to facilitate the use of biomarkers in drug development and regulatory review, qualification of biomarkers is an important activity. *Biomarker qualification* can be defined as the conclusion that within the stated context of use, the results of biomarker measurements can be relied on to have a stated interpretation and value. The regulatory implication of biomarker qualification is substantial. Namely, the pharmaceutical and biologics industry can rely on using the biomarker in the approved manner in regulatory submissions, and CDER regulatory reviews in all offices and disciplines will accept the biomarker as valid.

To help qualify biomarkers for a specific (often narrow) context of use, the FDA has developed a biomarker qualification process (BQP) [11,18,19] and corresponding interdisciplinary *biomarker qualification review team* (BQRT). The BQP is generally divided into two phases: the evaluation phase and the review phase. During evaluation, the BQRT examines information from the sponsor/consortium such as summary analyses of data on the biomarker to be qualified. During review, the BQRT receives and reviews detailed data from biomarker studies. Ultimately, the BQRT makes a recommendation for or against qualification of a given biomarker in a proposed context for use. The first biomarkers to be qualified under this mechanism are the preclinical renal toxicity markers of the Predictive Safety Testing Consortium, KIM1, albumin, total protein, B2-microglobulin, cystatin C, clusterin, and trefoil factor-3.

17.6 LABELING AND PHARMACOGENOMICS

Information about the impact of genetic variations on drug therapy can provide an additional and more precise set of tools for clinicians to use for diagnosis and treatment. The FDA plays a role in making this information available to clinicians through the inclusion of pharmacogenomic biomarker information in drug labels and the clearance of devices for genetic testing. The labeling of drugs is performed in the context of the available knowledge and applicable standards at the time when the labeling process takes place, and it is updated as new information becomes available. Pharmacogenomic biomarkers have been identified for drugs in many treatment areas, and information regarding their use has been provided to clinicians through drug labels [22,30,31].

17.6.1 Pharmacogenomics/Pharmacogenetics (PGX) in IND/NDA Submissions to the FDA

In order to gain insight into how sponsors were utilizing PGX in drug development, the agency evaluated a subset of INDs and NDAs submitted since mid-2000 [30]. A total of 70 INDs and or NDAs were reviewed. Overall, genes encoding CYP2D6 activity were the most frequently examined and accounted for 73% of all tests, followed by CYP2C19, CYP3A4, transferases, CYP1A2, certain receptors, CYP2C9, and *p*-glycoprotein. In many occasions, multiple genetic variations were tested, and both phenotyping and genotyping methods were used in the same submission. This informal survey indicated increased integration of pharmacogenomics and pharmacogenetics in the drug development process.

In another survey, nearly one-fourth of all outpatients received one or more drugs that have pharmacogenomic information in the label for that drug [22]. Of 1200 drug labels reviewed for the years 1945–2005, 121 drug labels were found to include pharmacogenomic biomarker information. Of these 121 labels, 69 referred to human genomic biomarkers, or information related to the genetics of normal or cancerous tissue. An additional 52 labels referred to microbial genomic biomarkers, or information based on the genetics of infectious agents and used in microbial typing. A summary of these human genomic biomarkers, the drug label context of use, and the associated drugs is available on the FDA website [29]. Of the labels referring to human biomarkers, 43 (62%) pertained to polymorphisms in CYP enzyme metabolism, with CYP2D6 as most common. Biomarkers related to CYP enzymes were cited in 43 (62%) of the 69 identified labels. The CYP enzymes identified most frequently were CYP2D6 (24 labels, 35%), CYP2C19 (12 labels, 17%), and CYP2C9 (7 labels, 10%). When the labels containing pharmacogenomic information were sorted by therapeutic class (after removal of antimicrobial drugs), oncology drug products showed the highest percentage of labels with pharmacogenomic content (22 labels, 32%), followed by cardiology drugs (18 labels, 26%), neurology and psychiatry drugs (12 labels, 17%), and drugs for other therapeutic areas (17 labels, 25%).

17.6.2 Postmarketing Label Updates

There are several examples of drugs with labels that contain pharmacogenomic information (Table 17.1) [23,29]. In most cases, the identified drug labels provide pharmacogenomic information without recommending a specific action. However, a

TABLE 17.1 Examples of More Recent FDA Drug Product Labeling that Included Genetic Information

Therapeutic Area	Drug	Genetic Information
Transplant	Azathioprine	Dose adjustments for TPMT variants
Oncology	Trastuzumab	Indicated for HER2 overexpression
	Irinotecan	Dose reduction for UGT1A1*28
	6-Mercaptopurine	Dose adjustments for TPMT variants
Antiviral	Maraviroc	Indicated for CCR5-positive patients
	Abacavir	Boxed warning for HLA-B*5701 allele
Pain	Codeine	Warnings for nursing mothers that CYP2D6 UM-metabolized codeine to morphine more rapidly and completely[a]
Hematology	Warfarin	Genotype-guided dosing recommendation based on patient's CYP2C9 and VKORC1 information
Psychopharmacological	Thioridazine	Contraindication for CYP2D6 PM
	Atomoxetine	Dosage adjustments for CYP2D6 PM; no drug interactions with strong CYP2D6 inhibitors expected for PM
Neuropharmacological	Carbamazepine	Boxed warning for Asians with variant alleles of HLA-B*1502

Notation: TPMT—thiopurine methyltransferase; HER2—human epidermal growth factor receptor 2; UGT—uridine diphosphate glucuronosyltransferase; CCR5—chemokine (C–C motif) receptor 5; HLA—human leukocyte antigen; UM—ultra-rapid metabolizer; VKORC1—vitamin K reductase complex 1; PM—poor metabolizer.

[a]Based on information from `http://www.fda.gov/Drugs/DrugSafety/PostmarketDrugSafetyInformationforPatientsandProviders/ucm124889.htm`.

Source: Data from `http://www.accessdata.fda.gov/scripts/cder/drugsatfda/index.cfm`.

few labels recommend or require biomarker testing as a basis for reaching a therapeutic decision. For example, testing for *HER2/neu* and epidermal growth factor receptor (EGFR) overexpression is required before starting therapy with trastuzumab [32]; the drug should be prescribed only if the test results are positive for a potential patient. Testing is recommended for common polymorphisms in the human uridine diphosphate glucuronosyltransferase 1A (UGT1A1) gene locus (which is associated with irinotecan toxicity) [33], deficient thiopurine methyltransferase (TPMT) activity before treatment with azathioprine [34] or 6-mercaptopurine [35], and protein C deficiency in patients who will receive warfarin therapy [36].

Labels that have been updated with pharmacogenetic information include the HIV drug abacavir [37] and antiepileptic carbamazepine [38], in which associations between genetic markers in the HLA family and severe cutaneous reactions are described. The label of atomoxetine [39], a selective norepinephrine reuptake inhibitor indicated for the treatment of attention deficit–hyperactivity disorder (ADHD), states that dosage adjustments of atomoxetine may be necessary when administered to CYP2D6 poor metabolizers (PMs). The labels for the antineoplastic drugs irinotecan [33] and 6-mercaptopurine [35] are updated to inform of severe toxicities associated with deficiencies in UGT1A1 and TPMT, respectively. Another example is warfarin, an anticoagulant indicated for the treatment and/or prevention of chronic conditions such as atrial fibrillation and deep-vein thrombosis. The label was updated to include genotype-guided dosing recommendation based on patient's CYP2C9 and vitamin K epoxide reductase complex 1 (VKORC1) information [36].

17.7 LEVEL OF EVIDENCE IN PHARMACOGENOMICS AND PHARMACOGENETICS

There is considerable debate about the quality, quantity, and type of evidence needed to change clinical practice by introducing genetic testing for drugs [23,40–43]. The evidence base for genetic testing should be informed by the pharmacologic characteristics of the drug and the characteristics of the outliers [43]. Critical factors that add strength to observed genotype–phenotype associations include (but are not limited to) strength of the association, replication across multiple independent populations, and mechanistic or experimental corroboration. A prospective, randomized clinical trial may not be a feasible or appropriate pharmacogenetic design in some cases (e.g., rare adverse events). In large observational studies of serious conditions, if lack of drug benefit is robustly demonstrated in a given genetic subgroup, the risks to individuals in that subgroup may be inferred without a randomized clinical trial [43]. Using principles of bioequivalence and quantitative pharmacology, pharmacogenetics-based dosing may be recommended without the need for additional prospective studies. On the other hand, prospectively designed studies to support dosage modifications may be critical when the mechanistic consequences of genetic differences are less clear. The exact evidence needed to determine the significance of a pharmacogenetic association will likely vary on a casespecific basis, and will likely be impacted by the severity of the clinical event, the

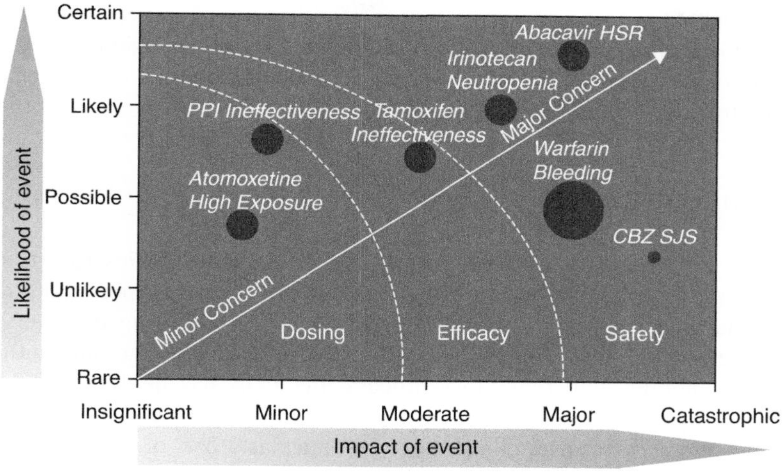

FIGURE 17.3 Factors involved in determining the significance of a pharmacogenetic association.

size of the population likely to be affected, and the penetrance of the genetic variant as it relates to the drug response phenotype (Fig. 17.3).

17.8 GENETICS AND GENOMIC TESTS

Numerous metabolism biomarker tests are available on the market as FDA-approved or laboratory-developed tests. For example, the FDA cleared the AmpliChip Cytochrome P450 Genotyping Test® (Roche Diagnostics) in December 2004 [44]. AmpliChip analyzes a patient's DNA for the presence of genetic variations in two drugmetabolizing enzymes, CYP2C19 and CYP2D6. This type of genotyping knowledge may assist the treating clinician in selecting the appropriate dose for a given patient to achieve target systemic drug exposure.

Another example is the utility of UGT1A1 genotype information in the therapeutic application of irinotecan. In August 2005, the FDA cleared the *invader UGT1A1 molecular assay*, which detects variations in a gene that affects the patient's ability to break down the major active metabolite of irinotecan [45].

In addition to genetic (i.e., genetic variation) tests, new genomic (i.e., gene expression) tests are becoming rapidly available. MammaPrint®, a test that relies on microarray analysis to predict whether existing cancer will metastasize, was approved in February 2007 [46]. This is the first cleared *in vitro* diagnostic multivariate index assay device that relies on the geneexpression profiles of 70 genes, the results of which are converted to scores using an algorithm that is used to determine whether the patients are at low or high risk for metastasis.

In the area of antiretroviral treatment, HIV genomes are constantly and rapidly evolving. An FDA-approved kit, the TRUGENE HIV-1 genotyping kit, detects HIV genomic mutations that confer resistance to specific types of antiretroviral drugs, as an aid in monitoring and treating HIV infection [47]. These two regions are targets of anti-retroviral treatments. If drug resistance is found to be present, the physician can alter the treatment regimen accordingly.

17.9 EDUCATION AND TRAINING

The FDA has created a training program in pharmacogenomics for all stakeholders and engages in several applied research projects to support and promote the translation of pharmacogenomics from basic science, drug discovery, and drug development into clinical practice [3]. To facilitate the integration of pharmacogenomics into regulatory process, the FDA has held several lecture series and reviewer training courses to educate the FDA scientists on the latest developments and research in pharmacogenomics as a part of ongoing training. In addition to offering an introduction to the basic principles of pharmacogenomics, the courses were designed to promote and create regulatory consensus based on appropriate scientific and regulatory interpretation of genomic data [48]. The agency offers weekly scientific seminars or round table discussions, on various topics, including pharmacogenomics, and invites speakers from diagnostic and pharmaceutical industries, academia, and institutions such as the National Institutes of Health, to provide different aspects of pharmacogenomics from their own perspectives. It is valuable experience for the FDA reviewers to participate in these educational programs. These training opportunities can help the FDA reviewers to implement the use of pharmacogenomics into their review process in a positive manner.

17.10 CONCLUSION

The FDA CDER has a dual role (i.e., mission) of (1) protecting public health by ensuring the safety and efficacy of drugs and biological products and (2) promoting efficient, informative, and innovative ways to improve the benefit/risk ratio of drugs in all subsets of patients. As part of the critical path initiative, the FDA has undertaken several initiatives in the field of pharmacogenomics that are intended to achieve the goals of this mission. The FDA has been proactive in encouraging the use of genomics across the spectrum of drug development through guidance, public meetings, and meetings with industry, and in translating genomics from data to knowledge by way of the product label. It has encouraged the identification of patient subsets using genomic tests to improve the dosing of widely used drugs. As the field of genomics continues to expand, and as the critical mass of advocates for individualization in drug development and clinical practice continues to grow, we expect that genomics will gradually change the focus of benefit and risk from populations to individuals. This shift in focus will improve the medical meaningfulness of genetic tests and pharmacotherapy.

REFERENCES

1. *US FDA Critical Path Initiative* (available at http://www.fda.gov/ScienceResearch/SpecialTopics/CriticalPathInitiative/defaulthtm).
2. *US FDA Genomics at FDA* (available at http://www.fda.gov/drugs/scienceresearch/researchareas/pharmacogenetics/default.htm).
3. Amur S, Frueh F, Lesko L, Huang SM. Integration and use of biomarkers in drug development, regulation and clinical practice: A US regulatory perspective. *Biomarkers Med.* 2008;**2**:305–311.
4. *FDA/PhRMA/DruSafe/PWG* 2002 Workshop on Pharmacogenetics/Pharmacogenomics in Drug Development and Regulatory Decision-Making, Rockville, MD, May 16–17, 2002.
5. FDA/DIA/PhRMA/PWG/Bio 2003 Workshop on Pharmacogenomics in Drug Development and Regulatory Decision-Making: The Genomic Data Submission (GDS) Proposals, Washington, DC, Nov. 13–14, 2003.
6. Lesko LJ, Salerno RA, Spear BB, et al. Pharmacogenetics and pharmacogenomics in drug development and regulatory decision making: Report of the first FDA-PWG-PhRMA-DruSafe Workshop. *J. Clin. Pharmacol.* 2003;**43**:342–358.
7. FDA/DIA 2004 Pharmacogenomics Workshop: Co-Development of Drug, Biological, and Device Products, Arlington, VA, July 29, 2004.
8. FDA/IA/PWG/PhRMA/BIO 2005 Pharmacogenomics in Drug Development and Regulatory Decision Making—Workshop 3: Three Years of Promise, Proposals, and Progress on Optimizing the Benefit/Risk of Medicines, Bethesda, MD, April 11–13, 2005.
9. FDA/DIA 2007 Workshop on Pharmacogenomics in Drug Development and Regulatory Decision Making, Bethesda, MD, Dec. 10–12, 2007.
10. Frueh FW, Salerno RA, Lesko LJ, Hockett RD. 4th US FDA-Drug Information Association pharmacogenomics Workshop, held 10–12 December, 2007. *Pharmacogenomics* 2009;**10**:111–115.
11. Goodsaid F, Frueh FW. Implementing the U. S. FDA guidance on pharmacogenomic data submissions. *Environ. Mol. Mutagen.* 2007;**48**:354–358.
12. *US FDA Guidance for Industry: Pharmacogenomic Data Submissions* (available at http://www.fda.gov/downloads/RegulatoryInformation/Guidances/ucm126957.pdf; accessed 3/05).
13. *US FDA Guidance for Industry: E15 Definitions for Genomic Biomarkers, Pharmacogenomics, Pharmacogenetics, Genomic Data and Sample Coding Categories* (available at http://www.fda.gov/downloads/Drugs/GuidanceComplianceRegulatoryInformation/Guidances/ucm073162.pdf; accessed 4/08).
14. *US FDA Guidance for Industry and FDA Staff: Pharmacogenetic Tests and Genetic Tests for Heritable Markers* (available at http://www.fda.gov/downloads/MedicalDevices/DeviceRegulationandGuidance/GuidanceDocuments/ucm071075.pdf; accessed 6/07).
15. *US FDA. Guiding Principles for Processing Joint FDA/EMEA Voluntary Genomic Data Submissions (VGDSs) within the Framework of the Confidentiality Arrangement* (available at http://www.fda.gov/downloads/Drugs/ScienceResearch/ResearchAreas/Pharmacogenetics/ucm085378.pdf).
16. Lesko LJ, Woodcock J. Pharmacogenomic-guided drug development: Regulatory perspective. *Pharmacogenomics J.* 2002;**2**:20–24.

17. Orr MS, Goodsaid F, Amur S, Rudman A, Frueh FW. The experience with voluntary genomic data submissions at the FDA and a vision for the future of the voluntary data submission program. *Clin. Pharmacol. Ther.* 2007; **81**:294–297.

18. Goodsaid F, Frueh F. Process map proposal for the validation of genomic biomarkers. *Pharmacogenomics* 2006;**7**:773–782.

19. Goodsaid F, Frueh F. Biomarker qualification pilot process at the US Food and Drug Administration. *Am. Assoc. Pharm. Sci. J.* 2007;**9**:E105–E108.

20. Tong W, Cao X, Harris S, et al. ArrayTrack-supporting toxicogenomic research at the U. S. Food and Drug Administration National Center for Toxicological Research. *Environ. Health Perspect.* 2003;**111**:1819–1826.

21. Canales RD, Luo Y, Willey JC, et al. Evaluation of DNA microarray results with quantitative gene expression platforms. *Nat. Biotechnol.* 2006;**24**:1115–1122.

22. Frueh FW, Amur S, Mummaneni P, Epstein RS, Aubert RE, DeLuca TM, Verbrugge RR, Burckart GJ, Lesko LJ. *Pharmacogenomic biomarker information in drug labels approved by the United States Food and Drug Administration: Prevalence of related drug use. Pharmacotherapy* 2008;**28**:992–998.

23. Huang SM, Temple R. Is this the drug or dose for you? Impact and consideration of ethnic factors in global drug development, regulatory review, and clinical practice. *Clin. Pharmacol. Ther.* 2008;**84**:287–294.

24. US FDA. *CDER Drug and Biologic Approval Reports* (available at `http://www.fda.gov/Drugs/DevelopmentApprovalProcess/HowDrugsareDevelopedandApproved/DrugandBiologicApprovalReports/default.htm`).

25. Buckman S, Huang SM, Murphy S. Medical product development and regulatory science for the 21st century: The critical path vision and its impact on health care. *Clin. Pharmacol. Ther.* 2007;**81**:141–144.

26. US FDA. *Innovation or Stagnation? Critical Path Opportunities Report* (available at `http://www.fda.gov/ScienceResearch/SpecialTopics/CriticalPathInitiative/CriticalPathOpportunitiesReports/ucm077262.htm`).

27. US FDA. *Innovation or Stagnation? Critical Path Opportunities List* (available at `http://www.fda.gov/downloads/ScienceResearch/SpecialTopics/CriticalPathInitiative/CriticalPathOpportunitiesReports/UCM077258.pdf`).

28. US FDA. *Manual of Policies and Procedures, Processing and Reviewing Voluntary Genomic Data Submissions (VGDSs)* (available at `http://www.fda.gov/downloads/AboutFDA/CentersOffices/CDER/ManualofPoliciesProcedures/ucm073575.pdf`).

29. US FDA. *Table of Valid Genomic Biomarkers in the Context of Approved Drug Labels* (available at `http://www.fda.gov/Drugs/ScienceResearch/ResearchAreas/Pharmacogenetics/ucm083378.htm`).

30. Chou W, Huang S, Sahajwalla CG, Lesko LJ.An informal survey of pharmacogenetics/pharmacogenomics (PGtx) in a sample of IND's and NDA's. *Proc. 9th Annual FDA Science Forum*, board number P-03, Washington, DC, April 24–25, 2003.

31. Zineh I, Gerhard T, Aquilante CL, Beitelshees AL, Beasley BN, Hartzema AG. Availability of pharmacogenomics-based prescribing information in drug package inserts for currently approved drugs. *Pharmacogenomics J.* 2004;**4**:354–358.

32. US FDA. Herceptin (trastuzumab) product label (information available at http://www.accessdata.fda.gov/drugsatfda_docs/label/2010/103792s5250lbl.pdf).

33. US FDA. Camptosar (irinotecan hydrochloride) product label (information available at http://www.accessdata.fda.gov/drugsatfda_docs/label/2010/020571s031s032s033s036s037lbl.pdf).

34. US FDA. Imuran (azathioprine) product label (information available at http://www.accessdata.fda.gov/drugsatfda_docs/label/2008/016324s031,017391s014lbl.pdf).

35. US FDA. Purinethol (mercaptopurine) product label (information available at http://www.accessdata.fda.gov/drugsatfda_docs/label/2004/09053s024lbl.pdf).

36. US FDA. Coumadin (warfarin sodium) product label (information available at http://www.accessdata.fda.gov/drugsatfda_docs/label/2010/009218s108lbl.pdf).

37. US FDA. Ziagen (abacavir sulfate) product label (information available at http://www.accessdata.fda.gov/drugsatfda_docs/label/2008/020977s019,020978s022lbl.pdf).

38. US FDA. Tegretol (carbamazepine) product label (information available at http://www.accessdata.fda.gov/drugsatfda_docs/label/2009/016608s101,018281s048lbl.pdf).

39. US FDA. Strattera (atomoxetine hydrochloride) product label (information available at http://www.accessdata.fda.gov/drugsatfda_docs/label/2010/021411s032lbl.pdf).

40. Woodcock J. The prospects for "personalized medicine" in drug development and drug therapy. *Clin. Pharmacol. Ther.* 2007;**81**:164–169.

41. Lesko LJ. Personalized medicine: Elusive dream or imminent reality? *Clin. Pharmacol. Ther.* 2007;**81**:807–816.

42. Roses A. Personalized medicine: elusive dream or imminent reality? A commentary. *Clin. Pharmacol. Ther.* 2007;**81**:801–805.

43. Woodcock J, Lesko LJ. Pharmacogenetics—tailoring treatment for the outliers. *New Engl. J. Med.* 2009;**360**:811–813.

44. US FDA. *Roche AmpliChip CYP450 test* (information available at http://www.fda.gov/MedicalDevices/ProductsandMedicalProcedures/DeviceApprovalsandClearances/Recently-ApprovedDevices/ucm078879.htm).

45. US FDA. *Invader UGT1A1 molecular assay* (information available at http://www.fda.gov/NewsEvents/Newsroom/PressAnnouncements/2005/ucm108475.htm).

46. US FDA. *MammaPrint* (information available at http://www.fda.gov/NewsEvents/Newsroom/PressAnnouncements/2007/ucm108836.htm).

47. US FDA. *TRUGENE HIV-1 test* (information available at http://www.fda.gov/NewsEvents/Newsroom/PressAnnouncements/2005/ucm108475.htm).

48. Frueh FW, Goodsaid F, Rudman A, Huang SM, Lesko LJ. The need for education in pharmacogenomics: A regulatory perspective. *Pharmacogenomics J.* 2005;**5**:218–220.

PART VI

CONCLUSIONS

CHAPTER 18

Pharmacogenetics: Possibilities and Pitfalls

ANKE-HILSE MAITLAND-VAN DER ZEE
Utrecht University, Utrecht, The Netherlands

ANN K. DALY
Newcastle University, Newcastle upon Tyne, UK

18.1 INTRODUCTION

In Chapters 3–6 we described the basic pharmacokinetic and pharmacodynamic principles that play a role in pharmacogenetics. Then in Chapters 7–14 we described the state-of-the-art information on pharmacogenetics in many disease areas. In Chapters 16 and 17 new techniques in genotyping and in data analyses are described. In Chapter 15 different angles on how pharmacogenetics might play a role in clinical practice were discussed. In this final discussion and concluding chapter we would like to discuss the current role of pharmacogenetics in clinical practice, and describe hurdles and challenges that are leading to the low implementation grade that we are seeing today.

We will also discuss the impact of the genomewide association studies (GWASs) on pharmacogenetics as well as the impact of GWAS disease studies on the development of new drugs. Finally, we will consider the future of studies in pharmacogenetics. Proteomics, transcriptomics, metabolomics, and other "-omics" fields may enlighten biological mechanisms and support findings from pharmacogenetics. Furthermore, sequencing is becoming cheaper, with technologies enabling analysis of whole-genome and whole-exome sequences now available. It seems likely that sequencing will provide important new insights in the (pharmaco)genetics field in the near future.

Pharmacogenetics and Individualized Therapy, First Edition.
Edited by Anke-Hilse Maitland-van der Zee and Ann K. Daly.

18.2 PHARMACOGENETICS IN CLINICAL PRACTICE

Even though many studies have been performed and several pharmacogenetic interactions have been well established, only a handful of interactions have been implemented in general practice. As described in Chapter 1, the field with the best implementation of pharmacogenetics is the cancer field. Both tumor and host genetics are considered in the choice of therapy. In other areas implementation is very slow. Pharmacogenetic knowledge on the cytochromes P450 (CYP450) is implemented in daily care only in rare cases. For example, some psychiatric hospitals use information on CYP2D6 for prescribing antipsychotics and antidepressants. However, knowledge of P450 genotypes is also relevant to the prescription of a wider group of drugs. Guidelines for interpreting information from genotyping tests and for translating this into interventions in clinical practice, and easy access to genotyping facilities/genotype data, are pivotal for the chance of success for implementation. In The Netherlands a module has been introduced in the medical information system in pharmacies that provides the opportunity to monitor drug–gene interactions [1]. However, patient genotypes are seldom available, and therefore the module is still scarcely used.

A good example of an association that is now successfully implemented in clinical practice is relates to abacavir (also see Chapter 10) [2]. Genotyping HLA-B*5701 before beginning therapy with abacavir is standard in many hospitals. Physicians now appear more likely to use abacavir after implementation of the test because it is possible to predict who is prone to develop the severe side effects. However, this genotyping was implemented only after a clinical trial was performed (despite the massive amount of evidence from previous observational research) [2].

Coumarins are a group of anticoagulation agents that play a role in the prevention of blood clots in, for example, patients with atrial fibrillation or deep-vein thrombosis. Coumarins have a very narrow therapeutic window, and there is wide inter- and intraindividual variation in the dose that is needed to reach treatment goal. Genetic differences in the CYP450 2C9 and VKORC1 genes have been shown to predict the stable dose needed by a patient [3,4]. More about this relationship can be found in Chapter 7. The FDA has added a warning to the drug leaflet that states that a patient's genotype should be taken into account when dosing coumarins. However, there are no guidelines on how to adjust the dose if one or more of the genetic changes are present. Furthermore, physicians still seem to be reluctant to start genetic testing before the utility has been shown in a randomized controlled trial. In both the United States and Europe trials to study the efficacy of genotyping before start of coumarin therapy have been established [5]. Therefore, at present, only pharmacogenetic effects that have been proved in prospective trials seem to be implemented in routine care. It is questionable whether this is favorable for the future, although it seems possible that if genotyping before starting drug therapy becomes more common, it will be easier to implement new pharmacogenetic tests in clinical practice.

18.3 SAFETY

Drug safety continues to be an enduring problem for both the pharmaceutical industry and all healthcare systems in the EU. This has been illustrated by the withdrawals of several drugs from the market, such as the COX2 inhibitor rofecoxib, because of the occurrence of cardiovascular events [6]. The *prevention* of adverse reactions for drugs that are on the market would be highly beneficial for patients, governments, and pharmaceutical industries. Moreover, safety issues play an important role in drug development, as knowing which genes or which drug characteristics play a role in, for example, drug-induced liver injury or cardiotoxicity will be of utmost importance in compound selection in the drug development process. Studying the pharmacogenetic background of adverse drug reactions would require a biobank including large number of samples. These numbers of patients will never be found in one country because of the rarity of most adverse reactions, and therefore it is important that several international initiatives [such as the Serious Adverse Events Consortium (SAEC)] have been established to collect the numbers of samples necessary to find and validate novel pharmacogenetic relationships. Importantly for drug-induced liver injury (DILI), it has already been shown that pharmacogenetic tests can predict those at risk of developing DILI when using flucloxacillin and lumiracoxib [7,8]. We expect that pharmacogenetic tests will play an important role in the prevention of adverse reactions in the future. For example, drugs that are associated with severe side effects in a small group of patients might remain available for patients who do not experience these side effects if genetic tests can predict who is prone to experience the severe side effects.

18.4 GWAS

The first genuine genomewide association study was published in 2005 [9]. Now (as of 2011), 718 studies have been published and 3593 SNPs were found associated [10]. Because large numbers are usually necessary to find the relationships and because replication of results is an important issue, the value of collaborative efforts across studies is increasingly recognized. The unraveling of the genetics of common diseases might provide the pharmaceutical industry with new leads for the development of drugs.

In pharmacogenetics increasing numbers of GWAS studies have been published [11]. One of the first GWAS studies in pharmacogenetics analyzed the relationship between statin use and myopathy. In only a small set of patients the researchers showed a significant effect from a mutation in the SLCO1B1 transporter gene (see also Chapter 6) [12]. This study showed the possibility of finding a significant relation within only 85 cases and 90 controls. Furthermore, it underlined the importance of transporter genes in the occurrence of side effects.

18.5 NEW DEVELOPMENTS

The field of pharmacogenetics has developed very rapidly since 2009, and it is expected that many things will happen in the coming years. The use of GWAS studies in many pharmacogenetic datasets will lead to the discovery of SNPs that were not associated before. Furthermore, sequencing studies will help pinpoint which SNPs play a functional role, especially where rare variants are involved. Proteomics, transcriptomics, and other -omics research areas will also help to provide biological mechanisms for pharmacogenetic interactions. Large consortia will be able to cross-validate and replicate associations that are found.

18.6 CONCLUSION

Because of these developments, clinical implementation of pharmacogenetics will become much more accepted and therefore much easier. Variability in response and in adverse reactions to therapy has many causes (e.g., age of patient, severity of disease, quality of prescribing and dispensing, compliance of the patient), but genetic differences definitely play a role. Pharmacogenetics will become increasingly important in individualizing patient treatments in the near future, especially as simple tests that can be performed in a clinic or pharmacy become available.

REFERENCES

1. Swen JJ, Nijenhuis M, de Boer A, Grandia L, Maitland-van der Zee AH, Mulder H, et al. Pharmacogenetics: from bench to byte–an update of guidelines. *Clin Pharmacol Ther.* 2011;**89**:662–73.
2. Mallal S, Phillips E, Carosi G, Molina JM, Workman C, Tomazic J, et al. HLA-B*5701 screening for hypersensitivity to abacavir. *New Engl. J. Med.* 2008;**358**(6):568–579.
3. Sconce EA, Khan TI, Wynne HA, Avery P, Monkhouse L, King BP, et al. The impact of CYP2C9 and VKORC1 genetic polymorphism and patient characteristics upon warfarin dose requirements: Proposal for a new dosing regimen. *Blood* 2005;**106**(7): 2329–2333.
4. Schalekamp T, Brasse BP, Roijers JF, Chahid Y, van Geest-Daalderop JH, de Vries-Goldschmeding H, et al. VKORC1 and CYP2C9 genotypes and acenocoumarol anticoagulation status: Interaction between both genotypes affects overanticoagulation. *Clin. Pharmacol. Ther.* 2006;**80**(1):13–22.
5. van Schie RM, Wadelius MI, Kamali F, Daly AK, Manolopoulos VG, de Boer A, et al. Genotype-guided dosing of coumarin derivatives: The European pharmacogenetics of anticoagulant therapy (EU-PACT) trial design. *Pharmacogenomics* 2009;**10**(10): 1687–1695.
6. Gislason GH, Rasmussen JN, Abildstrom SZ, Schramm TK, Hansen ML, Fosbol EL, et al. Increased mortality and cardiovascular morbidity associated with use of nonsteroidal anti-inflammatory drugs in chronic heart failure. *Arch. Intern. Med.* 2009;**169**(2):141–1419.

7. Daly AK, Donaldson PT, Bhatnagar P, Shen Y, Pe'er I, Floratos A, et al. HLA-B*5701 genotype is a major determinant of drug-induced liver injury due to flucloxacillin. *Nat. Genet.* 2009;**41**(7):816–819.
8. Singer JB, Lewitzky S, Leroy E, Yang F, Zhao X, Klickstein L, Wright TM, Meyer J, Paulding CA. A genome-wide study identifies HLA alleles associated with lumiracoxib-related liver injury. *Nat. Genet.* 2010;**42**(8):711–714.
9. Klein RJ, Zeiss C, Chew EY, Tsai JY, Sackler RS, Haynes C, et al. Complement factor H polymorphism in age-related macular degeneration. *Science* 2005;**308**(5720):385–389.
10. http://www.genome.gov/GWAstudies/; accessed 12/08/10).
11. Daly AK. Genome-wide association studies in pharmacogenomics. *Nat. Rev. Genet.* 2010;**11**:241–246.
12. Link E, Parish S, Armitage J, Bowman L, Heath S, Matsuda F, et al. SLCO1B1 variants and statin-induced myopathy—a genomewide study. *New. Engl. J. Med.* 2008;**359**(8): 789–799.

INDEX

Sections giving detailed accounts of specific topics are shown in bold

Pharmacogenetics and Individualized Therapy, First Edition.
Edited by Anke-Hilse Maitland-van der Zee and Ann K. Daly.

Printed and bound by CPI Group (UK) Ltd, Croydon, CR0 4YY

16/04/2025

14658518-0004